Advances in
Assisted Reproductive Technology

Advances in Assisted Reproductive Technology

Editor

Nayana H Patel MD (Obs & Gyn)
Managing Director and Medical Director
Akanksha Hospital and Research Institute
Anand, Gujarat, India

Co-Editor

Sandro C Esteves MD PhD
Medical and Scientific Director
ANDROFERT—Andrology and Human Reproduction Clinic
Center for Male Reproduction
Campinas, Brazil

Forewords

Liselotte Mettler
Sadhana Desai
Kamini A Rao

JAYPEE

JAYPEE BROTHERS MEDICAL PUBLISHERS
The Health Sciences Publisher
New Delhi | London

Jaypee Brothers Medical Publishers (P) Ltd

Headquarters

Jaypee Brothers Medical Publishers (P) Ltd
4838/24, Ansari Road, Daryaganj
New Delhi 110 002, India
Phone: +91-11-43574357
Fax: +91-11-43574314
E-mail: jaypee@jaypeebrothers.com

Overseas Office

J P Medical Ltd
83 Victoria Street, London
SW1H 0HW (UK)
Phone: +44 20 3170 8910
Fax: +44 (0)20 3008 6180
E-mail: info@jpmedpub.com

Website: www.jaypeebrothers.com
Website: www.jaypeedigital.com

Advances in Assisted Reproductive Technology

First Edition: **2020**

ISBN: 978-93-88958-99-8

Printed at: Samrat Offset Pvt. Ltd.

Dedicated to

All my surrogate mothers of yesterday, today and tomorrow.
You have the womb of the "Universe" and the heart of gold.
You continue to inspire us always....
Salute to you all... Stay blessed!

Contributors

Abha Majumdar MS FICS
Director and Head
Centre of IVF and Human Reproduction
Sir Ganga Ram Hospital
New Delhi, India

Aditi Nadkarni MBBS DGO
Embryologist
21st Century Hospital and IVF Centre
Surat, Gujarat, India

Akanksha Allahbadia Gupta MBBS
Observer Fellow
Rotunda—The Center for Human Reproduction
Mumbai, Maharashtra, India

Alpesh Doshi MSc Dip RC Path
Consultant Clinical Embryologist and Co-founder
London Fertility Institute
London, UK

Anuradha Rathi MBBS DGO
Fellow in Assisted Reproductive Technology
Nadkarni Hospital and Test Tube Baby Center
Surat, Gujarat, India

Arpita Patel MSc
Junior Embryologist
Akanksha Hospital and Research Institute
Anand, Gujarat, India

Arunima Halder MS DNB (Obs & Gyn) FNB (Reproductive Medicine)
Consultant (Reproductive Medicine)
Milann—The Fertility Center
Bengaluru, Karnataka, India

Asha Baxi MBBS MS (Obs & Gyn) Fellow of FRCOG (London) Fellow of FICOG
Director and Chief (Obstetrics and Gynecology)
Disha Fertility and Surgical Centre
Indore, Madhya Pradesh, India

Asha Rao MBBS, DNB (Obs & Gyn)
Infertility Specialist
Obstetrician and Gynecologist
Rao Hospital
Coimbatore, Tamil Nadu, India

Atsushi Tanaka MD (Obs & Gyn)
Founder and Current Director
Saint Mother Hospital
Kitakyushu, Fukuoka, Japan

Bhavana Singla MD
Consultant Doctor
Advance Fertility and Gynecology Centre
New Delhi, India

C Rathi Lavanya MBBS MD (Obs & Gyn)
Consultant—Obstetrician and Gynecologist and Infertility
Rao Hospital
Coimbatore, Tamil Nadu, India

Christophe Blockeel PhD
Medical Director
Centre of Reproductive Medicine
University Hospitals
Brussels, Belgium

Devika Gunasheela MBBS MRCOG (UK) Fellowship in Reproductive Medicine
Director
Gunasheela Surgical and Maternity Hospital
Gunasheela Assisted Reproduction Center Pvt Ltd
Bengaluru and Mysuru
Karnataka, India

Dhaval Baxi MS (Obs & Gyn)
Consultant
Disha Fertility and Surgical Centre
Indore, Madhya Pradesh, India

Diksha Goswami MBBS MD MRCOG (UK) Fellowship in Reproductive Medicine
Infertility Specialist and Obstetrician
Global Rainbow Hospitals
Agra, Uttar Pradesh, India

Divyesh V Shukla MD (Obs & Gyn)
Director
Isha Hospital
Vadodara, Gujarat, India

Duru Shah MD FRCOG FCPS FICS FICOG FICMCH DGO DFP
Scientific Director and Fertility Expert
Gynaecworld Fertility Center, Kemps Corner
Mumbai, Maharashtra, India

Faram E Irani MD FCPS DGO DFP
Director
Southern Cross Fertility Center
Mumbai, Maharashtra, India

Firuza R Parikh MBBS MD (Obs & Gyn) Dip (Obs & Gyn)
Director
Assisted Reproduction and Genetics
Jaslok Hospital and Research Centre
Mumbai, Maharashtra, India

Gautam Nand Allahbadia MD DNB FNAMS FCPS DGO DFP FICOG FICMU
Medical Director
Millennium Medical Center MMC IVF
Villa 1089, Al Thanyah
Al Wasl Road, Dubai, UAE

Goral Gandhi MSc
Clinical Director
Indo Nippon IVF Director
Department of IVF Laboratory
Lead Faculty, ISRME
Mumbai, Maharashtra, India

Harsha Bhadarka MSc (Microbiology) PhD Pursuing
Chief Embryologist and IVF Lab Director
Akanksha Hospital and Research Institute
Anand, Gujarat, India

Hrishikesh Pai MD FCPS FICOG MSc (USA)
Gynecologist and Head of IVF Unit
Lilavati Hospital and Research Centre
Scientific Director, Bloom IVF
Mumbai, Maharashtra, India

Jaideep Malhotra MD FICMCH FICOG FICS FMAS FIAJAGO
Managing Director
Rainbow IVF
Agra, Uttar Pradesh, India

Jatin P Shah MD DGO
ART Specialist and Director
Mumbai Fertility Clinic and IVF Centre
Mumbai, Maharashtra, India

Kaberi Banerjee MD (AIIMS) MRCOG MNAMS
Medical Director
Infertility and IVF Specialist
Advanced Fertility and Gynecology Center
New Delhi, India

Kamini A Rao MBBS DGO MCh FRCOG FNAMS FICOG PGDMLE (Law)
Medical Director
Milann—The Fertility Center
Bengaluru, Karnataka, India

Kanthi Bansal MD DGO FICOG
Director
Safal Fertility Foundation
Director
Brij Basant Hospital Pvt Ltd
Ahmedabad, Gujarat, India

Keiji Kuroda MD (Obs & Gyn)
Medical Doctor and Researcher
Department of Obstetrics and Gynecology
Juntendo University Hospital
Juntendo University
Tokyo 113-0033, Japan

Keshav Malhotra MBBS MCE
Embryologist
Rainbow IVF, Agra
Director
Global Rainbow Healthcare, Agra
Director of Training
Rainbow IVF
Agra, Uttar Pradesh, India

Kruti Patel MSc
Senior/Assistant Embryologist
Akanksha Hospital and Research Institute
Anand, Gujarat, India

Mackens Shari MD
Resident Obstetrics-Gynecology-Fertility
Centre for Reproductive Medicine
Universitair Ziekenhuis Brussel (UZ Brussel)
Laarbeeklaan 101, 1090 Brussels
Belgium

Maham AS MBBS
Unit Head and Clinical Director
Millennium Medical Center (MMC) IVF
Dubai, UAE

Mala Arora FRCOG FICOG D'Obst (UK)
Director
Noble IVF Center
Noble Hospital
Faridabad, Haryana, India
Past Chairperson, ICOG

Manchi Bharucha PhD (Reproductive Endocrinology/Infertility Residency Program)
Medical Director (Consultant)
Neuosaante Pharmaceuticals Pvt Ltd
Mumbai, Maharashtra, India

Manish Pandya MD FICOG FICMCH Endoscopy (CICE France)
Professor and Head
Scientific Research Institute
Mahavir Hospital
Surendranagar, Gujarat, India
ART (EART—Mumabi, CRM—Cleveland, Ohio, USA)

Markus Eckart Nitzschke MD
Scientific Director
Medical Director
Specialist in Obstetrics and Gynecology
Superspecialist in Reproductive Medicine
Canary Institute of Infertility
Las Palmas de Gran Canaria
Canary Islands, Spain

Masahiko Ito MD (Obs & Gyn)
Associate Doctor
Saint Mother Obstetrics and Gynecology Clinic
Institute for ART
Kitakyushu, Fukuoka, Japan

Matheus Roque MBBS PhD
Scientific Director
ORIGEN—Center for Reproductive Medicine, Brazil

Meenal Khandeparkar MBBS MS (Obs & Gyn)
Clinical Fellow
Jaslok Hospital and Research Centre
Mumbai, Maharashtra, India

Molina Patel MBBS MD (Obs & Gyn)
Gynecologist and Infertility Specialist
Akanksha Hospital and Research Institute
Anand, Gujarat, India

Nalini Mahajan MD MMed Sci (ART) (UK) FICOG
Director
Mother and Child Hospital
New Delhi, India

Narendra Malhotra MBBS (Obs & Gyn) MD FICMCH FIAJAGO FICOG FICMU FRSH
Managing Director
Rainbow Hospital
Agra, Uttar Pradesh, India

Nayana H Patel MD (Obs & Gyn)
Managing Director and Medical Director
Akanksha Hospital and Research Institute
Anand, Gujarat, India

Neharika Malhotra MBBS MD (Obs & Gyn)
Infertility Specialist and Obstetrician
Global Rainbow Hospital
Agra, Uttar Pradesh, India

Niket Patel MBBS MD (Obs & Gyn)
Director and Gynecologist
Akanksha Hospital and Research Institute
Anand, Gujarat, India

Nisha Bhatnagar MBBS MD (Obs & Gyn)
Infertility Specialist, Gynecologist and Obstetrician
EyeFem and Aveya IVF and Fertility Centre
New Delhi, India

Padmashri MBBS PGDip USG
Sonologist
Rao Hospital
Coimbatore, Tamil Nadu, India

Pankaj Talwar MBBS MD
Head (ART)
Department of Obstetrics and Gynecology
Army Hospital (R&R)
New Delhi, India

Partha Guha Roy MD DGO
Senior Clinical Associate
Fertility Clinic and IVF Center
Mumbai, Maharashtra, India

Payal Bajaj MBBS DGO Diploma in Sonography Diploma in Reproductive Medicine and Embryology
Infertility Specialist and Gynecologist
Aveya IVF and Fertility Centre
New Delhi, India

Piyush Chudasama MSc PhD (Pursuing)
Research Scientist (R & D Unit)
Sat Kaival Hospital Pvt Ltd
Anand, Gujarat, India

Pooja Awasthi MSc (Applied Biochemistry)
Head and Clinical Embryologist
Origin IVF and Fertility Centre
Ghaziabad, Uttar Pradesh, India
Head and Consultant
Reproductive Medicine and Embryology
Manipal Hospital
Dwarka, New Delhi, India

Pratap Kumar MD DGO FICS FICOG
Professor
Kasturba Medical College
Manipal, Karnataka, India

Priya Kannan MBBS MMed MCE
Embryologist
Garbba Rakshambigai Fertility Center
Chennai, Tamil Nadu, India

Purnima Nadkarni MD DGO
Director
21st Century Hospital and IVF Centre
Surat, Gujarat, India

Racca Annalisa MD
Clinical Fellow
Centre for Reproductive Medicine
Universitair Ziekenhuis Brussel
Brussels, Belgium

Rahul Gajbhiye MBBS PhD
Scientist D
Department of Clinical Research
National Institute for Research in Reproductive Health
Indian Council of Medical Research
Mumbai, Maharashtra, India

Rajam Murali MBBS MD Fellowship in Reproductive Medicine
Consultant Gynecologist
Gunasheela Surgical and Maternity Hospital
Bengaluru, Karnataka, India

Rajvi H Mehta PhD (Human IVF)
Director
Trivector Embryology Support Academy
Mumbai, Maharashtra, India

Rishabh Bora MBBS MD (Radiology)
Consultant Radiologist
Global Rainbow Hospital
Agra, Uttar Pradesh, India

Roshi Satija MBBS MS FNB
IVF Consultant
Dr Sunder Lal Memorial Hospital
New Delhi, India

Rupin Shah MBBS MS (Surgery) MCh (Urology)
Consultant Andrologist and Micro Surgeon
Department of Andrology
Lilavati Hospital and Research Centre
Mumbai, Maharashtra, India

Sabahat Rasool MD MRCOG DNB MNAMS FMAS
Infertility Consultant and Reproductive Medicine Specialist
Gynaecworld Fertility Center
Kemps Corner
Mumbai, Maharashtra, India

Sadhana Desai MD FRCOG
Founder Director
Fertility Clinic and IVF Centre
Mumbai, Maharashtra, India

Sambit Nanda MS (Obs & Gyn)
FMAS Dip Advanced Gyne-endoscopy (Kiel Germany) Dip Gyneoncology (Giessen Germany)
Consultant Gyne-Laparoscopic Surgeon
Pattnaik Hospital
Guru Nanak Hospital
Mumbai, Maharashtra, India

Sangeeta Deshmukh MD (Obs & Gyn)
Consulting Doctor IVF
Jaslok Hospital and Research Centre
Mumbai, Maharashtra, India

Sanjay Patel MD (Obs & Gyn)
Gynec–Endoscopic Surgeon
Infertility and IVF Specialist
Director
Mayflower Women's Hospital
Ahmedabad, Gujarat, India

Santos-Ribeiro Samuel MD PhD
Scientific Coordinator and Senior Gynecologist in Reproductive Medicine
Instituto Valenciano de Infertilidad
Lisbon, Portugal

Shailesh Puntambekar MS (General Surgery)
Professor, Onco Surgeon and Consultant
Medical Director
Galaxy Care Laparoscopy Institute
Pune, Maharashtra, India

Shally Gupta MBBS DGO DNB
Infertility Specialist and Obstetrician
Global Rainbow Hospital
Agra, Uttar Pradesh, India

Shilpi Shukla MD (Obs & Gyn)
Consultant Obstetrician, Gynecologist and Infertility Specialist
Isha Hospital
Vadodara, Gujarat, India

Sonal Panchal MD
Consultant Ultrasound Specialist
Dr Nagori's Institute of Infertility and IVF
Ahmedabad, Gujarat, India

Sugandha Goel MS
Gynecologist, Infertility Specialist
Safal Fertility Foundation
Ahmedabad
Director
Brij Basant Hospital Pvt Ltd
Ahmedabad, Gujarat, India

Takashi Yamaguchi MD PhD
Associate Doctor
Saint Mother Obstetrics and Gynecology Clinic
Institute for ART
Kitakyushu, Fukuoka, Japan

Trupti Mehta MBBS DGO DNB
Consulting Doctor IVF
Jaslok Hospital and Research Centre
Mumbai, Maharashtra, India

Unnati Mamtora MD (Obs & Gyn)
Obstetrician and Gynecologist
Mumbai, Maharashtra, India

Urmila Sunda MBBS MS (Gyn) FMAS
Fellow in Obstetrics and Gynecology
Nadkarni Hospital and Test Tube Baby Center
Surat, Gujarat, India

van de Vijver Arne MD PhD
ART Specialist
Centre for Reproductive Medicine
Universitair Ziekenhuis Brussel
Brussels, Belgium

Vedapriya MBBS MD (Radiation Oncology)
Consultant Radiation Oncologist
Mazumdar Shaw Cancer Centre
Bengaluru, Karnataka, India

Vijay Mangoli MSc PhD
Laboratory Director
Fertility Clinic and IVF Center
Mumbai, Maharashtra, India

Yuvraj Jadeja MBBS MD (Obs & Gyn) FRM DRM
Gynecologist and Infertility Specialist
Akanksha Hospital and Research Institute
Anand, Gujarat, India

Foreword

Assisted reproductive technologies have evolved rapidly over the past few decades. Given that this mode of infertility treatment is rapidly becoming the standard of care, the relevance of this textbook is greater than ever. We live in an era where the term "Assisted Reproductive Technologies" are becoming redundant and we have to thank the pioneers in the field for getting us there. One of those pioneers is Dr Nayana H Patel. She has seen the incredible evolution of this field since the first test tube baby, Louise Brown, first hand and actively contributed to this evolution. I therefore cannot think of a better author for a textbook in the field.

I first met Dr Nayana H Patel really only 2 years back in one of our common ART teaching courses in Akanksha Hospital and Research Institute, Anand, Gujarat, India, and am highly impressed by her activities.

The collaboration between so many eminent authors in our field has created an outstanding textbook that offers practical and comprehensive information for the novice and advanced ART specialists alike. Every chapter is written by authorities in the field and the chapters cover old and new features in our field of ART. This book is therefore an outstanding resource and will serve the reader well. I would like to congratulate the authors and editors for a job well done.

Advances in Assisted Reproductive Technology covers almost all the recent developments in this specialty. It is a complete book with contributions from Indian and international authors.

Professor Dr med Dr hc mult Liselotte Mettler
PhD MD
Patroness
Kiel School of Gynaecological Endoscopy
Emeritus Professor
Department of Obstetrics and Gynecology
University Hospitals Schleswig-Holstein
Kiel, Germany
Executive Director
International Academy of Human Reproduction (IAHR)

Foreword

It is a pleasure to pen the foreword to a book of great clinical utility titled *"Advances in Assisted Reproductive Technology"* edited by eminent Infertility and ART Specialist of India, Dr Nayana H Patel from Gujarat.

In an age, when conventional diagnostic and therapeutic treatments are being challenged and replaced by newer innovations, the infertility specialists must know all recent advances and their advantages and pitfalls while managing women undergoing assisted reproduction.

Today, the field of ART is rapidly expanding with new tests, new treatments and researches particularly in the field of embryo implantation, molecular genetics, and improving the quality of gametes and even forming new gametes *in vitro*.

Dr Nayana H Patel has taken a lot of efforts in compiling various aspects of current developments in the field of ART. The various chapters of her book are written by nationally and internationally renowned IVF experts.

This book will be useful to both upcoming ART specialists as well as postgraduates interested in field of infertility. I congratulate Dr Nayana H Patel for compiling this ready-reckoner.

Sadhana Desai
MD FRCOG
Founder Director
Fertility Clinic and IVF Centre
Mumbai, Maharashtra, India

Foreword

Over the last few decades, there have been dramatic advances in the field of reproductive medicine. In 1978, the world witnessed the birth of the first "test tube baby" and ever since with the ever-expanding horizons of science and technology, infertility treatment has taken a quantum leap, making available a great many treatment options that will help eliminate most of the barriers to conception. The advent of advanced imaging techniques, state-of-the-art laboratory equipment and the emergence of related technologies, such as embryonic genetic testing and oocyte preservation have very dramatically developed into a revolution of new ways of seeing and doing things. These developments now occur at such a rapid pace that unless we keep up with the developing technology, we will inevitably and inexorably fall behind. Concurrent with the advancements in IVF are the development of newer technologies, such as ovarian tissue freezing, preimplantation genetic diagnosis, genetic screening of embryos, uterus transplant, stem cell biology, etc. All of which, potentially have broad applications for fertility. ART is directly challenging society to re-evaluate the way in which the origins of human life are viewed. As these relevant applications of ART become increasingly utilized, society has a responsibility to ensure that the advances achieved through ART are implemented in a morally responsible manner.

Advances in Assisted Reproductive Technology by Dr Nayana H Patel is a laudable effort to help the reproductive medicine fraternity keep abreast with the latest developments in the field. The book has 42 chapters covering almost all the recent developments in the field of ART. With contributions from eminent national and international authors, the book is a comprehensive learning manual providing important information for both scientists and clinicians. Every chapter is focused on a specific topic and uses international scientific standards of evidence-based medicine. This timely publication brings the latest advances in IVF within reach of practicing specialists and will be a useful learning tool in their day-to-day practice.

Kamini A Rao
MBBS DGO MCh FRCOG FNAMS FICOG PGDMLE (Law)
Medical Director
Milann—The Fertility Center
Bengaluru, Karnataka, India

Preface

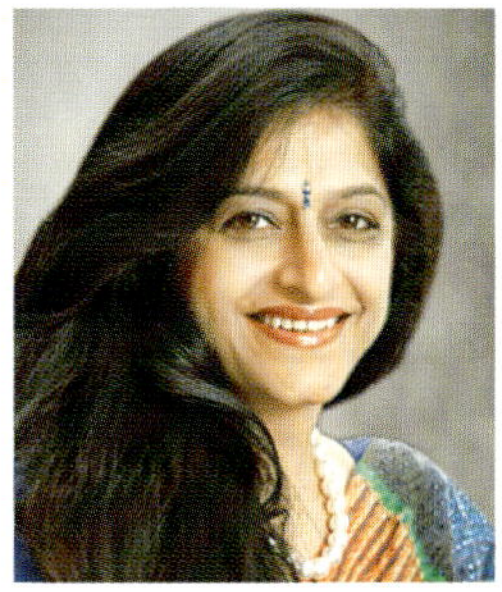

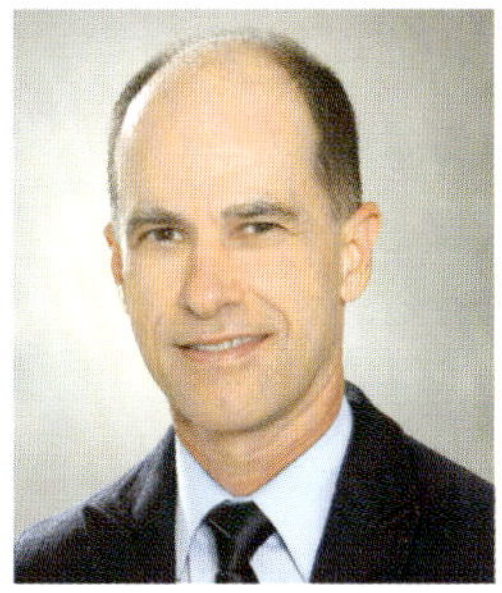

World over, Assisted Reproductive Technology is seen in the light of a super-specialized and advanced treatment modality. Since the inception, the spectrum of treatment options available are vast and mind boggling. An accurate profile and understanding of the various aspects of infertility, trends of the various conditions and recent advances for management are essential for practical approaches for the practicing clinicians.

This book aims to highlight the most recent advances in assisted conception and highlights ongoing and potential future of this field.

Each of the contributing authors have summarized their respective chapters into few crisp take home messages that are indicative of the gist of the topic.

With a compilation of the most recent advances of infertility, the book also stimulates its reader for future scientific research.

The contributors involved are acknowledged pioneer in their respective fields, this book in-turn provides confidence and harness authenticity to the experience-based treatment protocols suggested by them. Hence, this book holds promise for all practicing infertility experts, clinicians, embryologists and postdoctoral fellows, etc.

This book endeavors to provide an in-depth insight into every aspect of reprodcutive technology.

It is our hope and expectation that it justifies its objectives and all the readers enjoy this textbook as much as we have enjoyed compiling it!

Nayana H Patel
Sandro C Esteves

Acknowledgments

After 30 years of my practice in the field of ART, I have experienced and witnessed a drastic evolution of our understanding and knowledge in the field of Infertility. This inspired me to put on a platter all the information in the form of a book.

I would like to express my sincere thanks to all the contributors for their time, effort and commitment for sharing their knowledge.

My deep gratitude to Drs Manchi Bharucha and Faram E Irani, under whose guidance, I started with IVF in 1995–1996. I extend my heartfelt gratitude for Dr Harsha Bhadarka, my embryologist. Her hardwork and support is an eminent part of my success till date. Dr Yuvraj Jadeja, who gave me the idea of the book and drafted the rough contents. Drs Niket Patel and Molina Patel, who have been my backbone throughout. Also, grateful to Ms Dipali Patel, Ms Harmi Thakkar, Ms Nilofar Sodagar, and Mr Piyush Chudasama, for their relentless support and inputs in compiling this book.

I would also take this opportunity to thank all my patients, hospital staff, my family and my husband, Dr Hitesh Patel, for being constant source of support.

Last but not the least, I thank Almighty for making this happen.

I am especially thankful to Shri Jitendar P Vij (Group Chairman), Mr Ankit Vij (Managing Director), Mr MS Mani (Group President), Ms Chetna Malhotra Vohra (Associate Director—Content Strategy), Ms Pooja Bhandari (Production Head) and Ms Kritika Dua (Development Editor) of M/s Jaypee Brothers Medical Publishers (P) Ltd, New Delhi, India, for giving a go-ahead at the very beginning and helping us in every way possible to bring out this book.

Nayana H Patel

Contents

1

CHAPTER

Controlled Ovarian Hyperstimulation for IVF Embryo Transfer and its Influence on Outcomes

Manchi Bharucha, Faram E Irani

INTRODUCTION

Several million oocytes are residing in each ovary at mid-gestation. Let us look at the journey of primordial follicles from conception to birth and until menopause and thereafter. The resting primordial follicles are initiated in the fetus and some 100–2,000 primordial germ cells enter the massive proliferation process that results in about 70 million potential oocytes at mid-gestation and about 85% of these oocytes are lost before birth. The decline in number of follicles continues throughout the woman's reproductive life and reaching negligible level at menopause, resulting in impaired quality of life, thereafter. The life expectancy of 48.3 years in 1900 has now increased to 80 years or beyond in 2000 due to various advancements in improved healthcare, both in diagnosis and treatment areas. In this chapter, we shall deal with some of these developments in the area of reproduction. In our view, the two major areas are: (1) Young women suffering from cancer being able to produce their own genetic children after treatment and (2) Women being able to postpone menopause by 5–10 years and lead better quality of life through ovarian tissue freezing and reimplantation at convenience.

RECENT ADVANCEMENTS

During the last decade or so, highly significant advances aimed at optimizing results, both on clinical and laboratory sides, with the approach of individualizing diagnosis and treatment rather than adopting "one size fits all" approach, have taken place. This patient-centric approach, aided by advancements in imaging techniques, has satisfied increasing patient requirements and challenging scenario to the clinician and embryologist alike resulting in enhanced patient satisfaction, perhaps with reduced cost in some. Notable advancements have been made in the areas of determining ovarian reserve prior to treatment cycle, reducing length of treatment cycle with enhanced safety and neither under nor over response, greater dependence on laparoscopic intervention for treatment of common ailments associated with infertility like uterine leiomyomas, pelvic and ovarian endometriosis, increasing demand for preimplantation genetic screening, especially beneficial to women of advanced age, women with history of recurrent implantation failure with *in vitro* fertilization (IVF), women experiencing repeated early pregnancy loss and last but not the least, cryofreezing techniques resulting in higher pregnancy and live birth rates (LBRs) and found beneficial to young women suffering from pelvic cancer desiring future pregnancies with their own genetic children.

In this chapter, we shall deal with selected few developments, viz. determination of ovarian reserve prior to treatment cycle for IVF, refinements in stimulation for optimal mature oocyte recovery, adoption of single embryo transfer (SET) to avoid multiple pregnancy and consequent perinatal morbidity, adoption of freeze all strategy and policy for attaining higher pregnancy rates without complications like ovarian hyperstimulation syndrome (OHSS).

Determination of Ovarian Reserve

The ovarian reserve is typically referred to as population of primordial follicles. The model devised by Wallace and Kelsey in 2010 allows estimation of primordial follicles at any age of a woman. In practice, we find three types of response in women undergoing treatment for IVF-ET. They are normal response, poor response, and hyper response. Anticipation of the right response helps devising the most appropriate strategy in terms of the gonadotropin selection and its dosage for maximizing mature oocyte recovery (MII oocytes) with safety from complications and avoidance of suboptimal or poor response. It should be noted that maximum mature oocyte recovery has direct relationship with prospect of pregnancy. Earlier, determination of ovarian reserve used to be on determination of basal follicle stimulating hormone (FSH). However, it was soon realized after multiple studies that the sensitivity and positive predictive value of FSH was far from satisfactory and least reliable for prediction of right type of response. A potential, highly sensitive, and far more reliable is the anti-Müllerian hormone (AMH) or Müllerian inhibitory substance (MIS) test.

Estimation of AMH

Anti-Müllerian hormone is a dimeric glycoprotein belonging to the family of transforming growth factor-beta (TGF-β). AMH is involved in regression of Müllerian ducts during male fetal development and is expressed in Sertoli cells from testicular differentiation up to puberty. In females, it is exclusively produced in granulosa cells from birth to menopause. AMH production starts once the primordial follicles have differentiated to primary stage and it continues until the follicles have reached the antral stage corresponding to diameter of 2–6 mm. The number of small antral follicles is related to the size of the primordial follicle pool and with decrease in number of antral follicles with age, AMH production appears to get diminished and it invariably becomes undetectable at and after menopause. There is increasing accumulated evidence demonstrating usefulness of AMH as a cycle-independent biomarker of ovarian reserve which is in contrast to FSH, serum estradiol (E2), and inhibin B. In women, serum AMH expression can first be observed in granulosa cells of primary follicles and the expression is strongest in preantral and small antral follicles. Expression of AMH disappears in follicles of increasing size and is almost lost in follicles of >8 mm. Another advantage is AMH can be measured at any stage of the menstrual cycle, though recent evidence suggests that AMH attains its peak on Day 7 corresponding to 4–5 days before ovulation of idealized cycle of 28 days. Another observation made is the predictive power of AMH for poor response to controlled ovarian hyperstimulation (COH) and is comparable to that of AFC, another useful biomarker to be dealt with later. AFC is cycle specific and it can concomitantly predict high and low or poor responders. In one study, a strong association was found between mid-luteal, early follicular, and pre-ovulatory AMH levels and number of oocytes retrieved. It was concluded by the authors that mid-luteal and early follicular AMH levels could offer good prognostic value for prediction of clinical pregnancy. The cutoff value observed for prediction of pregnancy in this study was 2.7 ng/mL.

A number of other studies have advocated the level of AMH at below 1 ng/mL for prediction of poor response and even lower chances of pregnancy. Further, as per one study, AMH levels have been shown to be independently associated with occurrence of miscarriage. Higher AMH levels (5.61–35.00 ng/mL) have also been shown to be associated with lowest miscarriage rates and lowest AMH levels (0.08–1.60 ng/mL) with lowest response to COH and negligible chance of pregnancy, regardless of age of women. Overall, it appears from this study and other studies that AMH is not only a useful biomarker quantitatively but also qualitatively, including oocyte/embryo competence. In fact, diminished ovarian reserve has been found to be a cause of recurrent miscarriage defined as 3–4 failed clinical pregnancies of <20 weeks of gestational or fetal weight of <500 g.

Polycystic ovarian syndrome (PCOS) is known to be associated with raised levels of AMH at >4 ng/mL and high AFC.

Estimation of Antral Follicle Count

Ovarian reserve can also be estimated by transvaginal ultrasound by counting number of antral follicles in both the ovaries. AFC consists of counting antral follicles of 2–8 mm. Both AMH and AFC reflect the age-dependent decline in ovarian function. The difference between the two is, whereas AMH indicates ovarian reserve in general, AFC is more cycle specific as it could differ in each cycle. To elaborate further, AMH can be the same in the age range of 10 years in different women, but AFC can be different amongst them and that too different in each cycle in each woman. Hence AFC is more dependable for response in a particular treatment cycle. It should be noted that AFC must be measured in the treatment cycle only on any day from Day 2 to Day 4 and not in the cycle of evaluation or downregulated cycle. AMH has been shown to be a weak marker of pregnancy, but AMH and AFC combined together may indicate higher chance of pregnancy. AMH of <1 ng/mL and/or AFC of <8 has been shown to indicate low response to stimulation suggesting aggressive approach to stimulation in terms of higher doses of gonadotropins and perhaps longer duration of stimulation in some. There is consistent biological evidence suggesting detrimental effect of endometrioma and even stripping during surgery, on ovarian reserve resulting from reduced AFC. In cases where the endometriotic or any other functional cyst, unilateral or bilateral, AMH reading becomes debatable, in which case AFC would be the only dependable marker of ovarian reserve. There is high evidence in the literature validating the use of AFC as a surrogate marker of ovarian reserve. However, based on currently accepted recommendations, AFC assessment in women with ovarian endometriosis or in women having undergone previously ovarian surgery has been questioned. Hence, ovarian responsiveness to COH is actually considered the best noninvasive surrogate marker of ovarian reserve in these women.

Conclusively, it can be said and believed that the predictive power of AMH for live birth is higher than that of AFC with the predictive error of 1% to <5% with AMH, both being regarded independent of age. Further, it has been suggested that antral follicles of 5–8 mm size make greatest contribution to AMH levels compared to follicles of 2–6 mm size, providing the most accurate estimate of ovarian response.

Controlled Ovarian Hyperstimulation

Since the birth of Louise Brown 39 years before, IVF centers worldwide have been utilizing COH to enhance oocyte recovery to maximize development of good quality viable embryos for transfer to optimize chances of pregnancy. Care is taken in devising the protocol that no woman is excessively stimulated to avoid OHSS and at the same time she is not understimulated to avoid low or poor response. This dual objective calls for individualized patient tailored strategy in devising stimulation. The physician, today, is required to consider a number of parameters, partly based on findings of determination of ovarian reserve, and others like age, BMI, cause and duration of infertility, other existing comorbid illnesses, menstrual irregularity, etc. Care should be taken to see that duration of stimulation is not too long as too long a stimulation could compromise the result. Equal care needs to be taken for choosing single or combination of gonadotropins considering age, BMI, and ovarian reserve. Dyssynchronous growth of follicles is a known phenomenon and this is avoidable by the use of FSH and luteinizing hormone (LH) together right from the start and so also chance of poor response. Minimum possible dosage is used, avoiding chance of over response. Before starting stimulation, uterine status must be evaluated by transvaginal ultrasonography, 3D or 4D, and if necessary, by hysteroscopy. History and findings of sonography should be carefully weighed to rule out need for surgical intervention prior to IVF in case of common illness like uterine leiomyoma, pelvic endometriosis, etc.

Controlled ovarian hyperstimulation is considered to be a key factor for success of IVF, enabling recruitment of multiple dominant follicles to realize maximum mature oocyte recovery. The current standard of care is to use combination of FSH and LH as either human menopausal gonadotropin (hMG) or combination of rFSH and rLH in suitable dosages and to avoid single gonadotropin like FSH alone for reasons to be cited later.

ENDOCRINE REGULATION OF OVARIAN FUNCTION AND FOLLICULOGENESIS

Folliculogenesis is the result of complex and closely integrated series of events which start soon after conception and end about five decades later with menopause. The ovulatory menstrual cycle is the final result of these processes and it relies upon a complex series of physiological mechanisms that link the hypothalamus, the pituitary gland, and the ovary. Although gonadotropins are the key drivers of the menstrual cycle, other compounds such as ovarian steroids and inhibins critically affect and modulate hypothalamic and pituitary hormone selection as well as local gonadal function. Further, folliculogenesis and oocyte maturation depend upon an integration of cellular and endocrine mechanisms which are only in part under gonadotropin control. Much of the germ cell maturation occurs during intrauterine life (Adashi, 1996). These germ cells undergo mitosis and achieve their peak number (6–7 million) by mid-gestation; thereafter, due to initiation of meiosis and follicular atresia, the number of female germ cells drastically declines, so that about 300,000 oocytes are present at puberty.

Gonadotropin levels are low in the prepubertal period, but during fetal life, gonadotropin stimulation may be relevant even in these early stages of development (Gulyas et al., 1977). After attaining antral stage, FSH plays only permissive role in follicular development and ovarian follicles grow slowly. At the recruitable stage which begins in the luteal phase of the cycle, preceding ovulation, follicles can be stimulated by FSH to grow rapidly and enlarge beyond 2 mm diameter. The selective rise of FSH that occurs during luteal-follicular transition is a potent stimulus for follicle recruitment and several early antral follicles respond by beginning to enlarge. Endogenous and exogenous gonadotropins can now exert their full traditional stimulating effects and follicular growth becomes rapid.

Luteinizing hormone is also critically involved in the physiological events that lead to development of reproductively competent preovulatory follicle. LH is capable of stimulating androgen substrate from theca cells in fetal life, as attested by the elevated steroid levels found in female neonates (Winter et al., 1995). This modular action of gonadotropins has been named "two-cell two-gonadotropin model" (Dorrington and Armstrong, 1979). Estrogens in turn play fundamental role through improving follicle and oocyte maturity, in priming the hypothalamus-pituitary unit in preparation for the preovulatory gonadotropin surge as well as inducing the morphological uterine and endometrial changes needed for embryo implantation. Finally, LH-follicle intersections disrupt theca cell contacts in the cumulus and induce oocyte meiotic maturation to cause follicular rupture (Espey, 1974; Lawrence et al., 1980) and induce granulosa cell luteinization (Brailly et al., 1981).

In the course of follicular phase, FSH stimulates granulosa cells to express LH receptors and this action is facilitated by estrogens (Rani et al., 1981). Thus, in the late stages of follicular development, once antral follicle diameter increases beyond 10 mm, LH receptors are expressed by granulosa cells which become receptive to LH stimulation. LH then is capable of exerting its actions on both granulosa and theca cells (Hillier, 1994). At this stage, LH can exert virtually all physiological actions of FSH on granulosa cells, including stimulation of aromatase system (Zeleznik and Hillier, 1984). Serum FSH levels are reduced during most of the luteal phase, beginning to increase only a few days before menses, and are elevated throughout luteal–follicular transition. FSH thus progressively declines across the follicular phase until the mid-cycle surge is triggered by rising estrogen and progesterone concentrations.

Thus, it is evident that physiological follicular growth and maturation is dependent upon the dynamic interplay between FSH and LH, key physiological events such as follicular recruitment and dominant follicle selection rely upon both the prevalence of FSH and LH activity.

Selective LH activity in Controlled Ovarian Hyperstimulation

Selective LH activity administration in the mid and late stages of ovulation induction, both in COH and anovulatory patients has been demonstrated. Low dose of 75 IU/day of rLH administration, after at least one 14 mm follicle development, has impact on oocyte yield and pregnancy rates in assisted reproductive technology (ART) (Ben-AMOL, 2000). Available data suggests that LH activity can be used to improve and optimize FSH stimulation for COH. LH activity during ovulation induction also causes noticeable and significant modifications in ovarian response. The addition of LH to the FSH therapy during COH consistently and significantly shortens the duration of treatment and reduces the amount of FSH required for final oocyte maturation [Filicori et al., (1999b, 2001)], especially toward the end. Gonadotropin releasing hormone (GnRH) analog type, formulation, and route of administration can undoubtedly contribute to results, when both FSH and LH preparations, individually or in combined form as hMG, are used. GnRH antagonist when started from Day 6 of stimulation or when lead follicle attains 12–14 mm size is known to synergize with exogenous FSH and provide adequate follicle stimulation. In the short flare-up protocol of GnRH agonists (GnRHa), supported by hMG, endogenous FSH and LH are elevated for the first 3 days of administration and thereafter endogenous LH secretion is maintained till the day of trigger. Intranasal administration of GnRHa is associated with low absorption (about 3%) rate and less profound suppression of FSH and LH (Filicori, 1994). In the long mid-luteal suppression protocol, where GnRHa is administered from mid-luteal phase of the previous cycle, downregulation is achieved in about 10–20 days of administration and then switched over to stimulation by hMG or rFSH + rLH till the day of trigger. It is also recognized that during highly purified hMG (HP hMG) administration, estradiol level rise is brisk as compared to slow rise in case of HP FSH.

Effect on Progesterone

Serum levels of progesterone usually remain low during natural cycle or during COH. GnRHa or GnRH antagonist prevents untimely LH surge leading to premature ovulation (Filicori, 1996). Moderate rise of P, around 1.3 ng/mL, is occasionally observed during COH and is equated with premature follicle luteinization (Silverberg et al., 1991; Fanchin et al., 1993). This phenomenon, however, does not affect oocyte or embryo quality (Hofmann et al., 1993a; Legro et al., 1993) but may reduce IVF success through secretory endometrial transformation and impair chance of embryo implantation. Progesterone rise can take place with any preparation like hMG or FSH or rFSH + rLH and in spite of using GnRHa or GnRH antagonist. However, in practice, P rise is observed more often with increased dosage of FSH at the end of stimulation. Hence, it is considered prudent to reduce the dose of FSH and proportionately increase the dose of LH. It is further observed from some studies that if P level on the day of trigger is above 2.5 ng/mL, it is better to avoid fresh transfer and consider frozen embryo transfer (FET) in subsequent natural or modified natural cycle.

The phenomenon of dyssynchronous follicular growth between both ovaries is well known during the beginning of COH. This is largely due to use of FSH alone, which stimulates unselectively or due to differential uptake of FSH by multitude of follicles. Hence, it is better to start with FSH + LH or hMG, which could provide a means to selectively achieve both large follicles and curtailment of small follicular development (Marco Filicori et al., 2002). In addition to supporting the growth of larger follicles, LH activity appears to exert other important actions on the dynamics of folliculogenesis. In 2001, (Filicori et al., 2001) it was shown that hMG administration leads to progressive decline in number of small follicles (<10 mm) and this was significantly more marked than with HP FSH. This finding was confirmed by significant inverse relationship between the amount of LH administered and the number of small follicles in a study on 120 patients (Filicori et al., 2002a).

Conclusively, therefore administration of rFSH + rLH or hMG promotes synchronized growth of follicles which in turn could help realizing greater yield of mature oocytes. In case of hyper responders, care has to be taken especially in case of younger women. In case of women of advanced age (≥ 35 years) and/or women with high BMI (>29 kg/m^2), this procedure may be found equally useful. In women with PCOS, both GnRHa long protocol and fixed protocol of GnRH antagonist can be used. In the case of young lean women with PCOS (BMI < 28 kg/m^2 and basal LH >5 mIU/mL), GnRH antagonist in the dose of 0.25 mg/day and FSH 150 or 225 IU from Day 1 of cycle may be preferred, the antagonist continued till the day of trigger. In these patients in whom antagonist is started on Day 1 of cycle, more rapid follicular development and earlier rise in E2 levels can be expected; another advantage being, LH can be suppressed within a matter of hours of starting the antagonist, whereas in case of GnRHa long protocol, suppression takes nearly 2 weeks, not to speak of higher gonadotropin requirement.

Oral contraceptive pill (OCP) pretreatment is used by some physicians for suppression in women with normal basal levels of FSH and LH for not more than 15 days. Women with OCP intake of >15 days are known to consume more gonadotropins and have longer duration of treatment. The antagonist usage is known for much lesser or negligible prevalence of OHSS compared to usage of long GnRHa protocol, both in normal and hyper responders.

UNEXPECTED LOW OR POOR RESPONSE IN WOMEN WITH NORMAL BASELINE HORMONAL LEVELS

Adequate follicular development in response to gonadotropic treatment is a prerequisite to successful IVF program. However, many women respond poorly or not at all to the standard COH protocols. Such patients account for 10–25% of IVF population. Some of these patients have age-related decline in their reproductive performance. Also, a low response is one of the most problematic issues in reproductive medicine.

It has been reported that the follicular fluid (FF) secretes multiple autocrine and paracrine factors that affect follicular development (Weng et al., 2006; Choi YS et al., 2006). There is evidence suggesting that ovarian insulin-like growth factor (IGF-II), insulin-like growth factor binding protein 4 (IGFBP4), and pregnancy-associated plasma protein-A (PAPP-A) system plays a major role in follicular development (Keay SD et al., 2003; Choi YS et al., 2006). Thus, FF levels are significantly lower in poor responders. A correlation is also reported between AMH levels in FF and the responsiveness to stimulation (Fallet ME et al., 1997). In addition, other follicular markers like soluble Fas and vascular endothelial growth factors (VEGFs) could be altered in ovarian response to stimulation (Hasyakor D, 2004; Neulan J et al., 2001). Soluble Fas is anti-apoptotic molecule reported to be positively correlated with oocyte maturation (Malamutsi-Puckner A et al., 2004). A negative correlation has also been suggested between VEGF in FF and the number of follicles (Tokuyama O et al., 2002). In one study (Young AG; Koo et al., 2009), multiple follicular development was found associated with higher levels of VEGF expression in FF and the same was observed in unexpected low responders and normal responder patients. Several other studies have also reported that regulation of follicular angiogenesis is important for normal development of follicles (Fauser BCJM, 1997; Schimizu T et al., 2003; Taylor PD et al., 2004).

EXPLORING UNCHARTED TERRITORIES IN CONTROLLED OVARIAN HYPERSTIMULATION

There are several situations we come across in practice during COH, considered uncommon, but of practical importance and without knowledge of which, they could become hazardous and/or not cost-effective to implement, though they are evidence-based. Let us deal with them individually.

- *Pretreatment with OCP*: OCP is being used by some in antagonist cycle for the dual purpose of suppression and planning the cycle, both for convenience of patient and the physician. A systematic review and meta-analysis conducted revealed no difference in pregnancy rates between patients who used OCP and those who did not. But gonadotropin consumption and duration of treatment cycle were increased significantly after OCP pretreatment (Georg Griesinger et al., 2008).

- *Importance of LH supplementation*: Utilizing beneficial effect of LH activity routinely helps realizing greater yield of mature oocytes and preventing P rise on the day of trigger, thus protecting favorable implantation prospect in fresh ET cycle, as P rise is known to impair implantation by disturbing the window of implantation.

During mid and late follicular phase of natural menstrual cycle, preovulatory follicular development proceeds despite progressive fall in serum FSH level. Studies conducted in women of reproductive age, using rFSH and rLH after downregulation of pituitary in the long protocol with leuprolide acetate (LA) demonstrated that LH sustains follicular E2 production in presence of falling FSH and E2 levels, which were used as index of follicular development (Michael Sullivan et al., 1999). The E2 levels of women receiving LH toward the final stage of stimulation increase throughout despite declining FSH level. It was also observed that thecal androgen production was exquisitely sensitive to LH.

The hypothesis is LH protects the maturing follicles from declining FSH levels. In this study, the FSH treatment was arbitrarily discontinued, when lead follicles reached 14 mm or more in diameter and LH treatment introduced till the end of the cycle. In practical terms it can be stated that when lead follicles reached 14 mm size or so, rFSH dose could be reduced by 75 IU or more depending on size of follicles lagging behind and rLH in the proportionate dose of 75 IU or more introduced and continued till the end of the cycle.

- *Inadequate response to FSH in the beginning of COH is a frequent occurrence*: After 5 days of stimulation with FSH alone. This phenomenon is observed in about 12–14% of young normogonadotropic women treated with long mid-luteal GnRHa protocol. In such an event, rLH can be introduced from Day 6 of stimulation in the dose of 75 IU or more, depending upon size of growing follicles on Day 6, which are usually <11 mm in diameter. With this strategy, good response can be expected on Day 8 or Day 9 in terms of increased size of follicles coupled with rising level of E2 and this combination continued till the day of trigger. In one study with this strategy, it was found that LH supplementation was more effective than increasing the dose of FSH in terms of mature oocyte outcome (G De Placido et al., 2005).

There are a number of situations where gonadotropin-deficient women do not respond to FSH alone adequately in the initial stage, and the E2 level on Day 6 of stimulation is lower than expected (<250 pg/mL), the follicles stimulated with FSH alone do not consistently rupture after hCG administration and they luteinize poorly and their oocytes may have lower fertilization rates. In this population of women, addition of rLH from Day 6 of stimulation in the dose of 75 IU/day or 150 IU/day has been shown to be effective to achieve adequate follicular development and steroidogenesis (European rLH study group, 1998).

- After pituitary downregulation with GnRHa in the long protocol, suppression of endogenous LH is more profound than of FSH. These are young normogonadotropic women in whom, if FSH is used alone, the oocyte yield is not seen to be adequate and their developmental competence is compromised. They develop poorly as zygotes and their embryos show lower implantation rates compared to those in whom rLH was administered along with rFSH during COH. A number of studies have shown higher implantation and pregnancy rates with combined administration of rFSH and rLH for COH (Jan Tesarik and Carman Mendoza, 2002; Westrgard LG et al., 1996).
- The phenomenon of premature LH surge is known to occur in many women, regardless of age, during COH, it is known to occur even in natural cycle resulting in premature ovulation. This is more commonly encountered in women of advanced age (>35 years). In such women, when GnRHa or GnRH antagonist is used, suppression of LH is seen to be more profound and if FSH is used alone for stimulation, the cycle outcome in terms of oocyte yield becomes suboptimal and consequently number of viable embryos may be less for transfer. Several studies performed to investigate whether the cycle outcome improves if rLH is added to rFSH during initial stage of stimulation. One such study has demonstrated that addition of rLH is essential for oocyte maturation (Mochtiar, 2011). Even in natural cycle, LH is shown to be essential for oocyte maturation (Hillier, 2001). Low LH levels in IVF cycles have been found to be associated with availability of fewer embryos for cryopreservation and transfer (Fleming et al., 1998; Marrs et al., 2004). Bosch et al., 2011, in their study in GnRH antagonist cycles further confirmed this finding and found higher clinical and ongoing pregnancy rates in women of 36–39 years.
- Faultless completion of meiosis I and II is crucial to chromosomal integrity of oocyte and hence oocyte diploidy (Verlinsky and Kuliev, 1996). If meiosis, a process extremely sensitive to disruption, was to be influenced by the presence or lack of appropriate LH level, LH supplementation in the course of fertility treatment could indeed influence diploidy rates in cleavage stage embryos. It has also been observed that diploid embryos are more likely to implant (Santiago Munne et al., 2005) and hence higher percentage

of diploid embryos would ultimately lead to higher pregnancy chances. These data have also been confirmed by studies by Lisi et al., 2005, and Anderson et al., 2006, who reported higher pregnancy rates in women receiving LH supplemented stimulation rather than stimulation with FSH alone.

Younger women, especially those with normal ovarian reserve or function, are more likely to have low basal LH level and are therefore at higher risk of profound LH suppression during pituitary downregulation (Flamming et al., 1998). The data on beneficial influence LH supplemented embryo diploidy are particularly evident in women who lack adequate endogenous LH level. This interpretation has been supported by Van Waly et al., 2003a, who reported in younger women, significantly higher clinical pregnancy rates after long agonist protocol for COH, using hMG in comparison to using FSH alone. The likely beneficial effect of hMG stimulation in poor responders has also been supported by Cochrane working group (Van Waly et al., 2003b).

In conclusion, the data presented provides overwhelming evidence that in selected patient population, LH supplemented ovarian stimulation protocols could beneficially affect diploidy rates in preimplantation embryos.

- *Beneficial effect of androgens in COH*: In some cases of poor response to FSH alone or rFSH + rLH or hMG, androgenic agents like hCG and testosterone (T) do impart beneficial effect to folliculogenesis in patients who fail to show adequate response to conventional therapy. Even these agents can be straight away incorporated in stimulation protocol in patients with documented or clinical poor response. This alternative can be deployed in all types of cases except in women with PCOS. In this alternative, downregulation is carried out with long mid-luteal GnRHa protocol. Once downregulation is confirmed by clinical and laboratory criteria, testosterone in the form of intradermal patch in the dose of 1.2 mg/day for 5 days is administered followed by hMG or rFSH + rLH in the appropriate doses is given till lead follicles of minimum 17 mm are seen (Lossi et al., 2006). If T patch is not available, hCG in a small dose of 1,250 IU/day could be used at least for 8 days in the same manner.
- *Does growth hormone (GH) has a place in poor responders?*: The incidence of poor ovarian response to COH varies from 9% to 24% (Surrey ES et al., 2000).

How do we define poor response?

A consensus study organized by European Society of Human Reproduction and Embryology (ESHRE) 2011 defined poor ovarian response (POR) to include any two of the following three features. They are also referred to as Bologna criteria.

1. Maternal age (≥ 40 years) or any other risk factor for POR.
2. Clinical evidence of POR [Three or fewer oocytes with ovulation induction in earlier cycle(s)].
3. Documented POR by ovarian reserve testing. AMH <0.5–1.1 ng/mL and/or AFC of <8 between both ovaries.

Deficiency of GH causes delay in onset of puberty in addition to growth retardation during childhood. Treatment of these patients with human GH induces sexual maturation (Zachman et al., 2003). These findings suggest that GH influences gonadal function. GH is reported to enhance responsiveness of follicles to gonadotropins leading to stimulation of folliculogenesis in infertile women who fail to respond to exogenous gonadotropins (Burger HG et al., 1991). The action of GH is partly mediated by IGF-1 production from the liver (Homburg R et al., 1996). Both GH and IGF-1 are detected in FF and their receptors are also expressed in the ovary (Givdice LC, 1992; Johnson MC et al., 1996). The role of GH and IGF-1 in follicular development has been examined in humans (Givdice LC, 1992; AdashI EY, 1985).

Growth hormone is also known to influence luteal function, directly or indirectly, to affect P production by luteal cells *in vitro* (Bergh C et al., 1991).

One of the options to improve the situation of poor response is addition of GH as an adjuvant to other ovulation inducing agents like FSH, LH, etc. (Kucvk T et al., 2008). The efficacy of GH in improving cycle outcome has been controversial till today. A recent, parallel, open-label, randomized study conducted from 2014 to 2016 (Yasmin Ahmed Bassionny, 2016) incorporated GH in antagonist cycles of proven poor responders. The protocol in the study group consisted of hMG 300–450 IU/day from Day 1 or Day 2 of the cycle depending on age and ovarian reserve markers like FSH, AMH, and AFC. GnRH antagonist added when lead follicles were 12–14 mm and GH added from Day 6 of stimulation in the dose of 2.5 mg/day SC, until the day of trigger. Norditropin (Novo Nordisk) 2.5 mg is equivalent to 7.5–8.0 IU/day or 0.1 IU/kg/day. The control group consisted of hMG + antagonist given in the same manner as in the study group patients. The total number of patients was 140 and the results were as below:

- Duration of treatment in both groups, study group and control group, was 10.77 days and 12.02 days, respectively.
- Total dose of GT was 3,900 IU and 4,906 IU.
- E2 on day of trigger was 1,862 and 1,854.
- Number of MII oocytes was 4.53 and 2.53.

Reproductive outcomes were as below:

- Implantation rates were 11.98% and 9.88%.
- Clinical pregnancy rate/cycle was 22.1% and 15%.
- Live birth rate was 17.5% and 13.6%.

Several studies to improve results in poor responders have reported increase in number of retrieved and MII oocytes (Kucuk T et al., 2008; Effthekar M et al., 2013; Bergh C et al., 1994). One meta-analysis suggested that GH administration is associated with increased proportion of patients who reach ET stage and are thus exposed to chance of pregnancy (Kolibianaskis EM et al., 2009). This finding, in our view, appears illusory. In another systematic review and meta-analysis, different interventions to improve outcome in poor responders were investigated and two interventions with a favorable impact and increased pregnancy rates were the use of GH and Day 2 transfer (Kyton D et al., 2009). The data provided above shows that GH cotreatment with antagonist results in improved parameters assessed, including LBR, and the differences between study group patients and control group patients did not reach statistical significance. Although these data are encouraging, the use of GH as an adjunct treatment in poor responders should be implemented cautiously till further larger and conclusive systematic studies, reviews, and meta-analysis are available.

Additional useful information on poor responders: In view of increasing prevalence of poor or low response to COH, more and more studies are forthcoming leading to availability of beneficial information on the subject, which are as below:

- Poor ovarian response is observed more in younger women of <35 years than in women of advance age.
- Poor ovarian response can be anticipated through determination of ovarian reserve; AMH of <1 ng/mL and/or AFC of <8 is indicative.
- Ultrashort protocol of GnRHa for first 3 days with added hMG from Day 1 till the day of trigger works well in some women.
- GnRH antagonist is known not to act in many of these cases in whom AMH is <1 ng/mL and AFC <8. Hence, use of progestogens like medroxyprogesterone acetate (MPA), Utrogestan, and Duphaston have been tried and found successful. In this protocol, Utrogestan 100 mg/day or MPA 10 mg/day or Duphaston 10 mg/day along with hMG 375–450 IU/day are started from Day 1 or Day 2 or Day 3 till the day of trigger.
- The protocol of double stimulation can be attempted in some. In this protocol, start stimulation with any of aforesaid formulations from Day 1 or Day 2 till follicles of 17–18 mm are seen and proceed with oocyte pickup (OPU) after the trigger. Freeze the embryos and after 3–5 days, assess E2 and P levels and E2, if found at 35 pg/mL or less, and P of up to 2.5 ng/mL, resume stimulation again as earlier, at once and proceed with 2nd OPU, and freeze the additional embryos for transfer of good quality selected embryos in natural or modified natural cycle.

NEWER DEVELOPMENTS IN GONADOTROPIN RESEARCH FOR CONTROLLED OVARIAN HYPERSTIMULATION

There are two new drugs in the category of rFSH under clinical trials for stimulation during COH for IVF patients. They are follitropin delta and corifollitropin. Both appear to be promising. Corifollitropin is long acting rFSH with single dose administration from Day 1 having duration of 7 days, after which current rFSH with one dose/day in the aqueous form is to be administered till the day of trigger. Follitropin delta is rFSH, uniquely expressed in fetal retinal cell line, which owing to differences in glycosylation profile, has a lower clearance and induces higher ovarian response than the existing rFSH preparations, when administered in equal doses of biological activity (IU).

Additional useful information on prevention of premature LH surge: The phenomenon of premature LH surge has been known for a number of years, not only in COH but even in natural cycle. It can take place anywhere from early follicular phase to the point where the follicles of 12–14 mm, inducing ovulation before trigger, thus impairing oocyte recovery and culminating into empty follicle syndrome in some cases. It is also known that P inhibits E2-induced positive feedback by reduced GnRH pulse frequency. It has also been seen that GnRH antagonist does not work in some cases where AMH is <1 ng/mL in which case, as per early preliminary studies, both MPA and Utrogestan can be used as they have been validated as effective oral alternatives to GnRH antagonist for prevention of this phenomenon. Didrogestral (Duphaston), a synthetic P, differing from Utrogestan in its molecular structure and pharmacological effects, has also been found useful for this purpose but not to have androgenic effects, even at high doses. Utrogestan, a natural micronized P, is fit for both oral and vaginal administration. Duphaston 20 mg has been found to be equivalent to Utrogestan 200 mg. Both have been found to be effective in preventing premature LH surge in a randomized controlled trial (RCT). In the same study, it was also observed that high doses of progestins could swiftly decrease circulating LH levels and low doses could achieve the same effect by prolonged duration. Such a “dose–time” effect has been elucidated in large scale investigations for endometrial transformation or ovulatory inhibition. In another similar study, Utrogestan 100 mg/day was found to be as effective as Utrogestan 200 mg/day in preventing premature LH surge.

Further, it is suggested that for optimal effect of preventing premature LH surge, both Utrogestan and Duphaston must be given simultaneously with hMG or rFSH + rLH from Day 1 of stimulation till the day of trigger. MPA in 10 mg/day dosage is also effective in preventing premature LH surge.

Conclusively, it can be said that for poor responder women in whom GnRH antagonist may not work for the purpose of preventing premature LH surge, we have a choice of three progestins. Besides, oral progestins may be more cost-effective than the antagonist.

Application of GnRHa as a Trigger during Controlled Ovarian Hyperstimulation

In the history of IVF over nearly four decades, extraordinary advances have been made by physicians and scientists alike to increase its efficiency and safety. Equally important are the techniques introduced. One such technique is the use of GnRHa as a trigger instead of hCG in the antagonist based protocol to reduce or to avoid the likelihood of OHSS. Initial concerns over altered luteal phase E2 levels in the antagonist cycles with GnRHa as trigger were largely alleviated by administering aggressive luteal support. However, despite its demonstrated efficacy and safety, some clinicians hesitate to use it widely because a small subset of women do not respond with adequate LH rise, which is the obligatory finding or signal for final oocyte maturation. The following information would adequately explain what is the optimal LH rise level desirable for attaining oocyte maturity and what are the factors or reasons why some patients do not adequately respond to GnRHa trigger for oocyte maturity. The contribution made on this subject by Weill Cornell Medical Center, New York and George Washington University, Washington DC has been more than significant. Their study involving 500 fresh IVF cycles over a period of 6 years has suggested the optimal LH level, post-trigger with GnRHa on the day of trigger, required for adequate response and the risk factors present in women not responding adequately to post-GnRHa trigger for oocyte maturity. A number of outcome variables were assessed in this study, viz. suboptimal response to GnRHa trigger in the morning after the trigger, optimal response in the morning after the trigger, age, BMI, trigger type, i.e. single versus double trigger, history of irregular menses or amenorrhea, insignificant basal FSH and LH levels, and OCP pretreatment. The cycle evaluated showed that those patients who had single GnRHa trigger and who exhibited LH level of ≥15–30 mIU/mL had at least eight mature oocytes retrieved with an oocyte maturity rate of 68–100% and had a LBR of 57%. But those who had post-trigger LH of <15 mIU/mL in the morning after trigger, had either three or fewer mature oocytes or had OPU cancelled. Statistical analysis further revealed that suboptimal responders had post-trigger LH of <15 mIU/mL and normal responders, some of them having been given dual GnRHa trigger, had ≥15 mIU. The GnRHa used was LA 2 mg or 4 mg or triptorelin 0.2 mg (decapeptyl). The dual trigger consisted of GnRHa + hCG 1,500 IU immediately after post-trigger LH level was available.

The authors suggested that certain demographic parameters like irregular menses, BMI of < 29 kg/m^2, FSH level of <0.1 IU/mL, LH level of <4 mIU/mL on the day of trigger, and OCP intake of >2 weeks, should be regarded as risk factors for optimal response. The authors contend that suboptimal group of patients almost always occurs and advance identification of this group should be guided by the risk factors present, so that precautionary measure like use of double trigger can be taken to avoid cancellation of the cycle. The GnRHa trigger has an added advantage of inducing mid-cycle FSH surge which also contributes to oocyte maturity. It is noteworthy to consider that though LH surge induced by GnRHa trigger effectively secures oocyte maturity, low circulating level of endogenous LH level during early luteal phase could result in corpus luteum demise and poor reproductive outcome, unless the standard luteal phase support is modified and made more aggressive.

Luteal Phase Support by GnRH Agonist as a Sole Support in Antagonist Cycles

Luteal phase deficiency is being observed as an unfavorable sequela to OPU in all IVF-intracytoplasmic sperm injection (ICSI) cycles. Therefore luteal support is being offered routinely in all IVF cycles in the form of P or P + E. Administration of a single or multiple boluses of luteal GnRHa has been gaining popularity in recent years as it has been observed to improve pregnancy rates and LBR. The beginning was made in 2004–2005 by Pirard et al., who investigated use of GnRHa as a substitute to P for luteal support. The same authors conducted a feasibility study followed by pilot study in 2006 and in 2015. All the above studies demonstrated efficiency of GnRHa as a sole luteal support in non-downregulated cycles. Subsequently, a large randomized control study on 2,529 antagonist cycles on 1,479 women, aged 25–41 years by Itai Bar Hava et al., conducted over a period of 6 years from 2009–2015, showed a higher LBR in the entire GnRHa group as compared with the P group. GnRHa administration was by intranasal route and P by vaginal route. In the GnRHa group, significantly higher levels of mid-luteal E2 and P were observed. Clinical pregnancy rates were also higher in GnRHa group (27.9% vs. 19.8%). In our opinion, luteal support with intranasal GnRHa spray has several advantages over P by vaginal or P by IM or SC route. It is much more convenient without any irritation and not at all painful unlike P by IM or SC.

The above large study also illustrates that GnRHa as luteal support not only rescues corpus luteum function but is also sufficient to support embryo implantation and further development without any other luteal phase support. The luteal support needs to be given only implantation and on embryonic β-human chorionic for 2 weeks after ET. The observed effects of GnRHa on implantation and on embryonic β-human chorionic gonadotropin (β-hCG) secretion are attributed to direct effect on embryo and on endometrium mediated by LH, in accordance with the previous observations on the effects of LH activity on endometrial receptivity, independent of ovarian function. Further studies have also shown similar beneficial effects of GnRHa administration on implantation. At present, many centers worldwide have been using GnRHa as an effective luteal support. As per our knowledge, GnRHa for luteal support is likely to replace currently used P administration, given higher pregnancy rates and LBRs.

FROZEN VERSUS FRESH EMBRYO TRANSFER

In vitro fertilization with FET has become increasingly common with IVF centers the world over. The number of FETs increased by 80% in the US from 2006–2012, which far outpaced the rate of increase of fresh ETs over the same period. Advances in cryopreservation of embryos have contributed immensely to this trend, as newer vitrification techniques have improved embryo survival rates as compared with slow freezing. In addition, there is increasing evidence of FET leading to more favorable perinatal and live birth outcomes including a lower risk of preterm birth (PTB), low birth weight (LBW), placenta previa, and placenta abruption. One large multicenter matched cohort study on over 2,900 cycles found significantly higher implantation rates and ongoing pregnancy rates with FET cycles compared with fresh transfers. The ongoing PRs with FET cycles were 52% and with fresh cycles it was 45.3%. This effect was most pronounced with P >1 ng/mL on the day of trigger and also in women of advanced age. There are a number of RCTs reporting higher PRs in normal and high responders.

Frozen embryo transfer protocols are thought to have several potential advantages over fresh transfer protocols. Multiple mechanisms have been suggested for the negative impact of COH on implantation and on pregnancy. Hormone regulation plays a large role in endometrial receptivity and high E2 and P levels from COH may affect hundreds of genes involved in implantation. High E2 levels during COH have also been hypothesized to interfere with endometrial perfusion. On the other hand, endometrium in an unstimulated cycle is more receptive to early placentation and embryogenesis than endometrium during COH.

It is believed by most centers that FET is most likely to yield higher implantation and clinical pregnancy rates than fresh transfers, regardless of age, infertility cause, duration of infertility, etc. In fact, many have adopted FET as policy in their centers. In our center, we have adopted FET as a policy for all patients since a year and we have observed more than double the PRs with FET than what it was with fresh transfers.

There are two major considerations for FET as a policy: (1) Premature rise in P is known to occur in most cases, making difficult the determination of opening and closing of the window of implantation (WOI), affecting adversely the chance of fresh embryo implantation. (2) It is much easier for the clinician to determine WOI in natural or modified natural cycle to facilitate FET and to maximize the pregnancy rates.

CORRELATION BETWEEN EMBRYO DEVELOPMENTAL STAGE AND ENDOMETRIAL STATUS

Asynchrony between embryo developmental stage and endometrium can result from COH leading to advanced histology and downregulation of P receptors. Prior to this event, COH may lead to premature rise in P, which is more due to FSH than to LH. Hence higher dependence on LH than on FSH toward the end of stimulation may prevent rise in P on the day of trigger, which can induce premature decidualization disrupting or advancing WOI, which is known to last for about 48 hours. It has also been hypothesized that the freeze-thaw process in freeze-only cycles serves as filter for embryos of poor quality, which may not survive the thaw process, FET procedure can also reduce the risk of OHSS.

Failure of implantation is the biggest challenge to IVF today. Uterine contribution to implantation success should never be underestimated. Uterine receptivity, which facilitates implantation besides embryo quality, is controlled by hormonal milieu during COH and the appropriate timing of embryo transfer, which in turn depends upon whether the WOI is open. The WOI opens with the appearance of P (including endogenous P) in serum, which is difficult to determine in stimulated cycles but not in unstimulated ones.

Another important factor for effective implantation is the endometrial thickness (EnT) on the day of ET influenced by rising E2 level. However, contribution of EnT to implantation is considered controversial. EnT of 6–7 mm or >10–14 mm has been reported to affect implantation adversely. Other studies have shown no association between EnT and implantation process. In view of this controversy, some studies have advocated using endometrial pattern on the day of ET for implantation. The reduced implantation rate in patients with a particular type of endo pattern suggests that premature luteinization leading to uterine-embryo asynchrony is a significant contributor to implantation failure.

MAXIMIZING LIVE BIRTH WITH SINGLE EMBRYO TRANSFER

Today, every couple desires birth of one healthy child at a time. However, in India, a woman willingly and gracefully accepts twins or triplets under compelling circumstances. So is the gentle nature of an Indian woman. The increase in multiple births observed in the last 25 years or so is largely attributed to ART. Many consider multiple births as an adverse outcome because of the associated maternal and neonatal morbidity as well as adverse economic impact. The risks with multiple pregnancies include prematurity, intrauterine growth restriction, LBW, cerebral palsy, learning disabilities, and developmental delays. Strategies to curb multiple births, to improve implantation by transfer of single blastocyst transfer, preferably FET, are being increasingly adopted all over the world, including India, today. In the US, the practice of SET increased from 2% in 2002 to 12% in 2011. However, it appears underutilized compared to European countries, particularly Sweden, which was 73.3%. The number of SETs performed in the US increased by 82.5% from 2006 to 2012. It is well established and acknowledged now that SET reduces multiple births and improves neonatal end points, while providing acceptable LBRs.

In Japan, in early 2000s, conflict developed between ART specialists and obstetricians. The neonatal intensive care units (NICUs) throughout the country were occupied by babies born after infertility treatment. ART specialists were accused of producing multiple pregnancies by their ignorance. Since then, the need for SET has been seriously contemplated. The study by Takeshima et al. highlights the success of SET policy for improvement of perinatal outcome and mortality rate. SET policy was adopted by the entire country. It is noteworthy that Japanese medical practices for ART are self-regulated by the rules of the society and not by legislation. The policy, thereafter, produced SET rate of 82.6% in 2012.

The important pre-requisite for the success of SET policy is the "normal euploid embryo". There are several methods to ensure euploid embryo morphology, the latest being preimplantation genetic screening (PGS). The study by Kazumi Takeshima et al., reviewed retrospectively the total of 140,718 live births and 510 stillbirths (after 22 weeks of gestation) conceived by ART between 2007 and 2012. The following were the findings, based on analysis of Japanese registry data:

- The practice of SET increased from 52.2% in 2007 to 82.6% in 2012.
- The multiple pregnancy prevalence decreased from 10.7% to 4.1% during the same period.
- The prevalence of PTB, LBW, and small for gestational age (SGA) decreased significantly while that of large for gestational age (LGA) increased.
- Perinatal morbidity decreased from 0.7% to 0.4% in fresh cycles, while that of FET cycles did not change.

The scenario in South Asian countries, as indicated by one British study, showed higher cancellation rates and lower LBRs. Another collaborative study by two centers based in the US demonstrated lower implantation rates in south Asian women versus Caucasian women (28% vs 39%) and lower LBRs among South Asian women versus Caucasians (24% vs 41%).

Summarily, there is enough data to support transfer of single frozen blastocyst, providing excellent LBRs, greatly reduced multiple and preterm births. In our view all patients should be encouraged to opt for frozen thawed blastocyst transfer with autologous oocytes and sperm.

Why euploid blastocysts do not always implant?

Early on, higher number of oocytes harvested could produce higher number of embryos to enable transfer of multiple embryos because of enhanced efficacy of ovarian stimulation to establish implantation and possibly pregnancy.

Today, this practice has changed. Improvements in IVF technology have rendered multiple embryo transfer unacceptable to both, clinicians and patients. The obligation to foster SET for reducing multiple pregnancy has underscored the need for ideal endometrial receptivity conditions prior to transfer. To achieve the ideal eutopic endometrial status, the clinician may be required to look at number of abnormalities, both in the woman's pelvis and the uterus itself. There could be several abnormal conditions, such as inflammation of the endometrium arising from primary infection, other conditions distorting the pelvic anatomy such as endometriosis, and/or adenomyosis, asymptomatic endometriosis producing P resistance or P block, leiomyomatosis requiring surgical intervention prior to IVF treatment, numerous endometrial gene expressions known to occur after COH rendering endometrium simply abnormal, etc. In fact, when office hysteroscopy is performed in women undergoing first IVF attempt and in women with history of repeat implantation failures or early pregnancy failures, uterine abnormalities are detected in as much as 11–22% and 26–45%, respectively. Myometrial pathologies like leiomyoma or fibroids, submucosal or intramural myomas are known to encroach uterine cavity with associated reduced implantation and increased miscarriage rates. Adenomyosis, which is steroid dependent and which is identified in 27–79% of infertile women and up to 90% of women with endometriosis, has been shown to significantly reduce pregnancy rates as per recent meta-analysis.

In view of the above conditions, impairing endometrial receptivity, euploid blastocyst, certified by PGS, cannot be expected to implant or to produce pregnancy.

CONCLUSION

Quite often, question is raised, especially in non-medical society, are we moving forward with assisted reproductive technology? Some say Yes and some No.

We shall attempt to answer. Let us look at the journey that began about 30 years back. The process was termed inefficient, full of failures like multiple births, intolerable prevalence of implantation failures and early pregnancy loss, no cost-effectiveness, to name the few. The positive side of the scenario has been contributed by advancements like extended culture of cleavage stage embryos, cryopreservation techniques, especially, the vitrification process, time lapse morphokinetics, preimplantation genetic screening, oocyte and embryo freezing techniques, ovarian tissue freezing and reimplantation, uterine transposition and transplant, preservation of fertility in young women suffering from pelvic and uterine cancers, etc. The future, in our view, appears full of promise. Already, young cancer survivors are having better quality of life and expecting their own genetic children. Shortly, women will be able to postpone menopause by at least 5–10 years, possibly because of depleted ovarian reserve, to have better quality of living, with no possibility of early menopause, reduction in the incidence of aneuploidy in embryos of women of advance age, and so on.

Taking stock of all these and other positive developments and future possibilities, we can confidently say that we have progressed well through the journey and the future is highly promising.

Lastly, we wish all readers a happy reading and hope that they would add to their skills and efficiency. Thank you all.

EDITORS' COMMENTS

1. Demographic characteristics, genetic predisposition, and diverse pathologies should also be considered and extensively studied while performing COS and while assessing its response.
2. Individualized COS (iCOS) optimizes outcomes and safety issues by adapting patient specific characteristics. With endocrine, paracrine, and genetic biomarkers iCOS can be refined further.
3. Natural and modified natural cycle protocols may be discussed to complete knowledge on COS.
4. Assisted reproductive technology is such an ever expanding field, that to summarize it in a few words is next to impossible. From discovering the importance of sex hormones, studying impact of age, hormones on eggs, understanding ovum and embryo genetics, to newer advances in ART technology like Embryoscope, Poloscope, etc., the infertility specialist is exposed to wide option to maximise the success.

SUGGESTED READING

1. Alcoba DD, Pimentel AM, Brum IS, et al. Developmental potential of in vitro or in vivo mature oocytes. Zygote. 2015;23(1):93-8.
2. Atasever M, Soyman Z, Demirel E, et al. Diminished ovarian reserve: is it a neglected cause in the assessment of recurrent miscarriage? A cohort study. Fertil Steril. 2016;105(5): 1236-40.
3. Balaban B, Urman B, Ata B, et al. A randomized controlled study of human Day 3 embryo cryopreservation by slow freezing or vitrification: vitrification is associated with higher survival, metabolism and blastocyst formation. Hum Reprod. 2008;23:1976-82.
4. Bar Hava I, Blueshtein M, Ganer Herman H, et al. Gonadotropin-releasing hormone analogue as sole luteal support in antagonist-based assisted reproductive technology cycles. Fertil Steril. 2017;107(1):130-5.e1.

5. Behringer RR, Finegold MJ, Cate RL. Müllerian inhibiting substance function during mammalian sexual development. Cell. 1994;79:415-25.
6. Benaglia L, Candotti G, Busnelli A, et al. Antral follicle count as a predictor of ovarian responsiveness in women with endometriomas or with a history of surgery for endometriomas. Fertil Steril. 2015;103(6):1544-50.
7. Bodri D, Colodron M, Vidal R, et al. Prognostic factors in oocyte donation: an analysis through egg-sharing recipient pairs showing a discordant outcome. Fertil Steril. 2007; 88(6):1548-53.
8. Broekmans FJ, de Ziegler D, Howles CM, et al. The antral follicle count: practical recommendations for better standardization. Fertil Steril. 2010;94(3):1044-51.
9. Broekmans FJ, Kwee J, Hendriks DJ, et al. A systematic review of tests predicting ovarian reserve and in vitro fertilization outcomes. Hum Reprod Update. 2006;12(6):685-718.
10. Chabbert-Buffeta N, Skinner DC, Caraty A. Neuroendocrine effects progesterone. Steroids. 2001;65(10-11):613-20.
11. Chen ZJ, Shi Y, Sun Y, et al. Fresh versus frozen embryos for infertility in the polycystic ovary syndrome. N Engl J Med. 2016;375(6):523-35.
12. Chian RC, Buckett WM, Abdul Jalil AK, et al. Natural-cycle in vitro fertilization combined with in vitro maturation of immature oocytes is a potential approach in infertility treatment. Fertil Steril. 2004;82(6):1675-8.
13. Chian RC, Uzelac PS, Nargund G. In vitro maturation of human immature oocytes for fertility preservation. Fertil Steril. 2013; 99(5):1173-81.
14. Choavaratana R, Thanaboonyawat I, Laokirkkiat P, et al. Outcomes of FSH priming and nonpriming in in vitro maturation of oocytes in infertile women with polycystic ovarian syndrome: a single blinded randomized study. Gynec Obstet Invest. 2015;79(3):153-9.
15. Csokmay JM, Hill MJ, Chason RJ, et al. Experience with patient-friendly, mandatory single blastocyst transfer policy: the power of one. Fertil Steril. 2011;96(3):580-4.
16. Dain L, Bider D, Levron J, et al. Thin endometrium in donor oocyte recipients: enigma or obstacle for implantation? Fertil Steril. 2013;100(5):1289-95.
17. de Ziegler D, Pirtea P, Galliano D, et al. Optimal uterine anatomy and physiology necessary for normal implantation and placentation. Fertil Steril. 2016;105(4):844-54.
18. Durlinger AL, Kramer P, Karels B, et al. Control of primordial follicle recruitment by anti-Müllerian hormone in the mouse ovary. Endocrinology. 1999;140:5789- 96.
19. Durlinger AL, Vissar JA, Themmen AP. Regulation of ovarian function: the role of anti-Müllerian hormone. Reproduction. 2002;124(5):601-9.
20. Elgindy EA, El-Haieg DO, El-Sebaey A. Anti-Müllerian hormone: correlation of early follicular, ovulatory and midluteal levels with ovarian response and cycle outcome in intracytoplasmic sperm injection patients. Fertil Steril. 2008;89(6):1670-6.
21. Engmann L, Benadiva C. Agonist trigger: what is the best approach? Agonist trigger with aggressive luteal support. Fertil Steril. 2012;97(3):531-3.
22. Fitzpatrick LA, Good A. Micronized progesterone: clinical indications and comparison with current treatments. Fertil Steril. 1999;72(3):389-97.
23. Grande M, Borobio V, Bennasar M, et al. Role of ovarian reserve markers, antimüllerian hormone and antral follicle count, as aneuploidy markers in ongoing pregnancies and miscarriages. Fertil Steril. 2015;103(5):1221-7.
24. Grunfeld L, Walker B, Bergh PA, et al. High resolution endovaginal ultrasonography of the endometrium: a non-invasive test for endometrial adequacy. Obstet Gynecol. 1991;78(2):200-4.
25. Harris TG, Dye S, Robinson JE, et al. Progesterone can block transmission of the estradiol-induced signal for luteinizing hormone surge generation during a specific period of time immediately after activation of the gonadotropin-releasing hormone surge-generating system. Endocrinology. 1999;140(2):827-34.
26. Hehenkamp WJ, Looman CW, Themmen AP, et al. Anti-Müllerian hormone levels in the spontaneous menstrual cycle do not show substantial fluctuation. J Clin Endocrinol Metab. 2006;91(10):4057-63.
27. Homburg R, Ray A, Bhide P, et al. The relationship of serum anti-Müllerian hormone with polycystic ovarian morphology and polycystic ovary syndrome: a prospective cohort study. Hum Reprod. 2013;28(4):1077-83.
28. Horcajadas JA, Riesewijk A, Polman J, et al. Effect of controlled ovarian stimulation in IVF on endometrial gene expression profiles. Mol Hum Reprod. 2005;11(3):195-200.
29. Huang R, Fang C, Xu S, et al. Premature progesterone rise negatively correlated with live birth rate in IVF cycles with GnRH agonist: an analysis of 2,566 cycles. Fertil Steril. 2012;98(3):664-70.
30. Humaidan P, Kol S, Papanikolaou EG; Copenhagen GnRH Agonist Triggering Workshop Group. GnRH agonist for triggering of final oocyte maturation: time for a change of practice? Hum Reprod Update. 2011;17(4):510-24.
31. Jayaprakasan K, Deb S, Batcha M, et al. The cohort of antral follicles measuring 2-6 mm reflects the quantitative status of ovarian reserve as assessed by serum levels of anti-Müllerian hormone and response to controlled ovarian stimulation. Fertil Steril. 2010;94(5):1775-81.
32. Kansal Kalra S, Ratcliffe SJ, Milman L, et al. Perinatal morbidity after IVF is lower with frozen embryo transfer. Fertil Steril. 2011;95(2):548-53.
33. Kasius A, Smit JG, Torrance HL, et al. Endometrial thickness and pregnancy rates after IVF: a systematic review and meta-analysis. Hum Reprod Update. 2014;20:530-41.
34. Kiliçdag EB, Haydardedeoglu B, Cok T, et al. Premature progesterone elevation impairs implantation and live birth rates in GnRH-agonist IVF/ICSI cycles. Arch Gynecol Obstet. 2010;281(4):747-52.
35. Kitajima M, Defrère S, Dolmans MM, et al. Endometriomas as a possible cause of reduced ovarian reserve in women with endometriosis. Fertil Steril. 2011;96(3):685-91.
36. Kitajima M, Dolmans MM, Donnez O, et al. Enhanced follicular recruitment and atresia in cortex derived from ovaries with endometriomas. Fertil Steril. 2014;101(4):1031-7.

37. Kuang Y, Chen Q, Fu Y, et al. Medroxyprogesterone acetate is an effective oral alternative to preventing premature LH surge in women undergoing controlled ovarian hyperstimulation for in vitro fertilization. Fertil Steril. 2015;104(1):62-70.
38. Kunz G, Beil D, Huppert P, et al. Adenomyosis in endometriosis—prevalence and impact on fertility. Evidence from MRI. Hum Reprod. 2005;20(8):2309-16.
39. Kwee J, Schats R, McDonnell J, et al. Evaluation of anti-Müllerian hormone as a test for the prediction of ovarian reserve. Fertil Steril. 2008;90;3737-43.
40. La Marca A, Stabile G, Artenisio AC, et al. Serum anti-Müllerian hormone throughout the human menstrual cycle. Hum Reprod. 2006;21(12):3103-7.
41. La Marca A, Sunkara SK. Individualization of controlled ovarian stimulation in IVF using ovarian reserve markers: from theory to practice. Hum Reprod Update. 2014;20(1):124-40.
42. Lambert-Messerlian G, Plante B, Eklund EE, et al. Levels of anti-müllerian hormone in serum during the normal menstrual cycle. Fertil Steril. 2016;105(1):208-13.
43. Lashen H, Afnan M, Sharif K, et al. A controlled comparison of ovarian response to controlled stimulation in first generation Asian women compared with white Caucasians undergoing in vitro fertilisation. Br J Obstet Gynaecol. 1999;106(5):407-9.
44. Lopata A, Johnston IW, Hoult IJ, et al. Pregnancy following intrauterine implantation of embryo obtained by in vitro fertilization of a preovulatory egg. Fertil Steril. 1980;33(2):117-20.
45. Maheshwari A, Bhattacharya S. Elective frozen replacement cycles for all: ready for prime time? Hum Reprod. 2013;28(1):6-9.
46. Maheshwari A, Pandey S, Shetty A, et al. Obstetric and perinatal outcomes in singleton pregnancies resulting from the transfer of frozen thawed versus fresh embryos generated through in vitro fertilization treatment: a systematic review and meta-analysis. Fertil Steril. 2012;98(2):368-77.e1-9.
47. Mahmud G, López Bernal A, Yudkin P, et al. A controlled assessment of the in vitro fertilization performance of British women of Indian origin compared with white women. Fertil Steril. 1995;64(1):103-6.
48. Marinov B, Petkova S, Dukovski A, et al. Utrogestan and high risk pregnancy. Akush Ginekol (Sofiia). 2004;43(5):22-4.
49. Meyer L, Murphy LA, Gumer A, et al. Risk factors for a suboptimal response to gonadotropin-releasing hormone agonist trigger during in vitro fertilization cycles. Fertil Steril. 2015;104(3):637-42.
50. Nelson SM. Biomarkers of ovarian response: current and future applications. Fertil Steril. 2013;99(4):963-9.
51. Nelson SM, Fleming R, Gaudoin M, et al. Anti-müllerian hormone levels and antral follicle count as prognostic indicators in a personalized prediction model of live birth. Fertil Steril. 2015;104(2):325-32.
52. Pigny P, Jonard S, Robert Y, et al. Serum anti-Müllerian hormone as a surrogate for antral follicle count for definition of the polycystic ovary syndrome. J Clin Endocrinol Metab. 2006;91(3):941-5.
53. Pirard C, Donnez J, Loumaye E. GnRH agonist as luteal phase support in assisted reproduction technique cycles: results of a pilot study. Hum Reprod. 2006;21(7):1894-900.
54. Pirard C, Donnez J, Loumaye E. GnRH agonist as novel luteal support: results of a randomized, parallel group, feasibility study using intranasal administration of buserelin. Hum Reprod. 2005;20(7):1798-804.
55. Pirard C, Loumaye E, Laurent P, et al. Contribution to more patient-friendly ART treatment: efficacy of continuous low-dose GnRH agonist as the only luteal support-results of a prospective, randomized, comparative study. Int J Endocrinol. 2015;2015:727569.
56. Practice Committees of the American Society for Reproductive Medicine and the Society for Assisted Reproductive Technology. In vitro maturation: a committee opinion. Fertil Steril. 2013;99(3):663-6.
57. Raffi F, Metwally M, Amer S. The impact of excision of ovarian endometrioma on ovarian reserve: a systematic review and meta-analysis. J Clin Endocrinol Metab. 2012;97(9):3146-54.
58. Reh A, Fino E, Krey L, et al. Optimizing embryo selection with day 5 transfer. Fertil Steril. 2010;93(2):609-15.
59. Rodin DA, Bano G, Bland JM, et al. Polycystic ovaries and associated metabolic abnormalities in Indian subcontinent Asian women. Clin Endocrinol. 1998;49(1):91-9.
60. Roque M, Valle M, Guimarães F, et al. Freeze-all policy: fresh vs. frozen-thawed embryo transfer. Fertil Steril. 2015;103(5):1190-3.
61. Schindler AE, Campagnoli C, Druckmann R, et al. Classification and pharmacology of progestins. Maturitas. 2003; 46:S7-16.
62. Shah MS, Caballes M, Lathi RB, et al. In vitro fertilization outcomes after fresh and frozen blastocyst transfer in South Asian compared with Caucasian women. Fertil Steril. 2016;105(6):1484-7.
63. Shahine LK, Lamb JD, Lathi RB, et al. Poor prognosis with in vitro fertilization in Indian women compared to Caucasian women despite similar embryo quality. PloS One. 2009; 4(10):e7599.
64. Shapiro BS, Daneshmand ST, Garner FC, et al. Clinical rationale for cryopreservation of entire embryo cohorts in lieu of fresh transfer. Fertil Steril. 2014;102(1):3-9.
65. Shapiro BS, Daneshmand ST, Garner FC, et al. Freeze all can be a superior therapy to another fresh cycle in patients with prior fresh blastocyst implantation failure. Reprod Biomed Online. 2014;29(3):286-90.
66. Shih W, Rushford DD, Bourne H, et al. Factors affecting low birth weight after assisted reproductive technology: difference between transfer of fresh and frozen embryo transfer suggests an adverse effect of oocyte collection. Hum Reprod. 2008;23(7):1644-53.
67. Smith LC, Olivera-Angel M, Groome NP, et al. Oocyte quality in small antral follicles in the presence or absence of a large dominant follicle in cattle. J Reprod Fertil. 1996;106(2):193-9.
68. Somigliana E, Berlanda N, Benaglia L, et al. Surgical excision of endometriomas and ovarian reserve: a systematic review on serum anti-müllerian level modifications. Fertil Steril. 2012;98:1531-8.

69. Somigliana E, Vercellini P, Daguati R, et al. Fibroids and female reproduction: a critical analysis of the evidence. Hum Reprod Update. 2007;13(5):465-76.
70. Stillman RJ, Richter KS, Banks NK, et al. Elective single embryo transfer: a 6-year progressive implementation of 784 single blastocyst transfers and the influence of payment method on patient choice. Fertil Steril. 2009;92(6):1895-906.
71. Takeshima K, Jwa SC, Saito H, et al. Impact of single embryo transfer policy in fresh and frozen cycles—analysis of the Japanese Assisted Reproduction Technology registry in Japan between 2007 and 2012. Fertil Steril. 2016;105(2):337-46.
72. Tarasconi B, Tadros T, Ayoubi JM, et al. Serum antimüllerian hormone levels are independently related to miscarriage rates after in vitro fertilization-embryo transfer. Fertil Steril. 2017;108;3:518-24.
73. Tesarik J, Hazout A, Mendoza C. Enhancement of embryo developmental potential by a single administration of GnRH agonist at the time of implantation. Hum Reprod. 2004;19(5):1176-80.
74. Trounson A, Wood C, Kausche A. In vitro maturation and fertilization and developmental competence of oocytes recovered from untreated polycystic ovary syndrome patients. Fertil Steril. 1994;62:353-62.
75. van Rooij IA, Broekmans FJ, Scheffer GJ, et al. Serum anti-müllerian hormone levels best reflect the reproductive decline with age in normal women with proven fertility: a longitudinal study. Fertil Steril. 2005;83(4):979-87.
76. van Rooij IA, Tonkelaar Id, Broekmans FJ, et al. Anti-müllerian hormone is a promising predictor for the occurrence of the menopausal transition. Menopause. 2004;11:601-6.
77. Vercellini P, Consonni D, Dridi D, et al. Uterine adenomyosis and IVF outcome: a systematic review and meta-analysis. Hum Reprod. 2014; 29(5):964-77.
78. Vigier B, Tran D, Legeai L, et al. Origin of anti-Müllerian hormone in bovine freemartin fetuses. J Reprod Fertil. 1984;70:473-9.
79. Wang A, Santistevan A, Hunter Cohn K, et al. Freeze-only versus fresh embryo transfer in a multicenter matched cohort study: contribution of progesterone and maternal age to success rates. Fertil Steril. 2017;108(2):254-61.e4.
80. Weissman A, Gotlieb L, Casper RF. The detrimental effect of increased endometrial thickness on implantation and pregnancy rates and outcome in IVF program. Fertil Steril. 1999;71(1):147-9.
81. Yding Andersen C, Leonardsen L, Ulloa-Aguirre A, et al. FSH-induced resumption of meiosis in mouse oocytes: effect of different isoforms. Mol Hum Reprod. 1999;5(8):726-31.
82. Zhao J, Zhang Q, Wang Y, et al. Endometrial pattern, thickness and growth in predicting pregnancy outcome following 3319 IVF cycle. Reprod Biomed Online. 2014;29(3):291-8.
83. Zhu X, Ye H, Fu Y, et al. Use of Utrogestan during controlled ovarian hyperstimulation in normally ovulating women undergoing in vitro fertilization or intracytoplasmic sperm injection treatments in combination with a "freeze all" strategy: a randomized controlled dose-finding study of 100 mg versus 200 mg. Fertil Steril. 2017;197(2):379-86.
84. Zhu X, Ye H, Fu Y. The Utrogestan and hMG protocol in patients with polycystic ovarian syndrome undergoing controlled ovarian hyperstimulation during IVF/ICSI treatments. 2016;95(28):e4193.

2

CHAPTER

Individualized Controlled Ovarian Stimulation

Abha Majumdar, Roshi Satija

DEFINITION

The assessment of ovarian reserve and subsequently its response to any previous stimulation, in terms of poor, normal or over responder, enables us to choose the ideal treatment protocol as well as gonadotropin dose for subsequent treatment cycles. These individualized treatment protocols called as "individualized controlled ovarian stimulation" (ICOS) not only aim at achieving the best possible response in terms of follicular recruitment and oocyte recovery but also minimize complications in terms of ovarian hyperstimulation as well as the frequency of cycle cancellation.

With regards to refusal of *in vitro* fertilization (IVF) treatment for women who have been predicted as poor responders, it is commonly agreed not to exclude anyone from their first IVF attempt only on the basis of the ovarian reserve test, as the accuracy of these tests can be poor for the prediction of pregnancy. Antral follicle count (AFC) and anti-Müllerian hormone (AMH) appear to be amongst the best predictive markers of ovarian reserve, but neither are completely reliable, with a false positive rate of 10–20%.

PATIENT PROFILE

Prediction of ovarian response can be done by taking into account various clinical as well as investigative parameters of a woman. Table 1 tends to profile patients so as to identify them regarding their expected normal, hyper, and poor response.

The success of assisted reproductive technology (ART) is the ability to have a single healthy child per initiated cycle while minimizing the associated risks. This can only be achieved if we could offer every woman treatment based on assessment of her previous ovarian response and unique characteristics defining her ovarian reserve, associated pathology or hormonal imbalances. This ICOS should not only enable us at having the best results in terms of single live birth per started cycle, but also minimize iatrogenic complications and associated costs, so as to also prevent couples from dropping out of ART treatment.

Pre-requisites to optimize ICOS with the right protocol and right gonadotropin for women undergoing IVF (Box 1).

TABLE 1 Identification of hyper, normal, and poor responders.

Hyper-responder	*Normal responder*	*Poor responder*
Oligo/amenorrhea PCOS	Regular cycles	Regular or short cycles
Thin built	Normal built	Obese
Age <30 years	Age <37 years	Age >37 years
FSH <8 mIU/mL	FSH <12 mIU/mL	FSH >12 mIU/mL
AMH >25 pmol/L (>3.5 ng/mL)	AMH 10–25 pmo/L (1.5–3.4 ng/mL)	AMH <3–9 pmol/L (0.5–1.4 ng/mL)
AFC >12 each ovary	AFC 7–11	AFC <7
Previous hyper-response to stimulation	Previous normal response to stimulation	Previous poor response to stimulation

(AFC: antral follicle count; AMH: anti-Müllerian hormone; FSH: follicle-stimulating hormone; PCOS: polycystic ovarian syndrome)

BOX 1 Right protocol and right gonadotropin for women undergoing IVF.

- Prospective identification of the ovarian response
- Determine coexisting hormonal imbalances affecting COS
- Determining underlying pathology which could change the need for protocol as well as dosing of the drugs used for optimal ICOS
- Ensure complete safety for oocyte donors undergoing COS without compromising oocyte quality
- Adopt protocols to fit the need of an individual patient as per the time available to her for an ART cycle
- Respect a woman's desire of minimal stimulation and adopt suitable protocols accordingly
- Gonadotropin protocols for patients with oncologic issues in urgent need of oocyte or embryo preservation
- Developing protocols suitable for women with prothrombotic conditions or estrogen-dependent cancers at risk with high estrogen levels during COS
- Optimization of the total reproductive potential of a couple by use of embryo cryopreservation technology.

(COS: controlled ovarian stimulation; ICOS: individualized controlled ovarian stimulation; ART: assisted reproductive technology)

The first step toward personalized medicine for a women undergoing IVF, appears to be ICOS. Apart from all parameters which help pick up the most optimal appearing protocol as well as gonadotropin dose for a set of patients with identical profile, there still could be instances of paradoxically different response within the group. This is probably where gene polymorphism of follicle-stimulating hormone (FSH) and luteinizing hormone (LH) receptors may have a role to play. The knowledge of this helps us to correlate between gene expression or single-nucleotide polymorphisms and the efficacy or toxicity of a drug which is also known as pharmacogenomics. Analysis of patient's genotype may therefore, ensure better optimization of drug therapy, to ensure maximum efficacy with minimal adverse effects.

Proposed treatment protocols for personalized or individualized COS:

Protocols after Prospective Identification of the Ovarian Response

Normal responder: Long agonist as well as antagonist protocol, both work well with this group of women. However, there could be a wide range of response in terms of ovarian stimulation in this group of women, depending on the pool of gonadotropin sensitive follicles they have. Researchers have been on the lookout for determining means to tailor the need of gonadotropins for these patients according to their response looking at doses which would uniformly create an average of 12–16 oocytes which could serve for a fresh as well as frozen embryo transfer, in addition to preventing the occurrence of a hypo as well as hyper-response. As per recently published several studies AMH and AFC are nowadays considered two markers with similar diagnostic performance and are actually measuring the same thing: the pool of recruitable follicles. Although tailored therapy based on markers of ovarian reserve appears to be an agreed upon approach by most, studies suggesting how to determine individualized therapy are not too many. On the use and efficacy of the single value of AMH in tailored treatment, two studies had been published. In both studies the FSH starting dose decreased with increasing basal serum AMH and both studies indicated that the treatment strategy based on AMH may lead to a reduction of both excessive responses as well as canceled cycles. Another more complete and easy to use nomogram has been elaborated in order to calculate the most appropriate FSH starting dose in IVF cycles. The nomogram is based on patient's age, serum Day 3 FSH and AMH and may be the basis for the individualization of the FSH dose for all patients in IVF cycles (Fig. 1).

Hyper-responder: The term "hyper-response" refers to the retrieval of 15–20 or more oocytes following a conventional COS protocol. It is of great importance to accurately predict women who are likely to have a high response to COS as it is the main risk factor for ovarian hyperstimulation syndrome (OHSS) the most dreaded complication of COS.

Prediction of high response is currently based on clinical criteria and patient characteristics, such as young age, delayed menstrual cycles, evidence of symptoms of Polycystic ovarian syndrome (PCOS) and hyper-response in a previous cycle.

Use of gonadotropin-releasing hormone (GnRH) antagonist protocol with lower doses of gonadotropins (100–150 unit recombinant FSH) for hyper-responder with GnRH agonist trigger for ovulation is the most preferred protocol. This leads to a smaller cohort of growing follicles when compared with the standard long GnRH agonist protocol. Studies have shown that antagonist protocol requires fewer days of stimulation than the GnRH agonist protocol (9 days vs 13 days) and is associated with reduced hospitalization for OHSS (13.9% in the agonist group vs 0.0% in the antagonist group).

Other protocols which can be used for hyper-responders are milder stimulation regimes or use of anti-estrogens such as clomiphene citrate (CC) with lower dose of gonadotropins and antagonist.

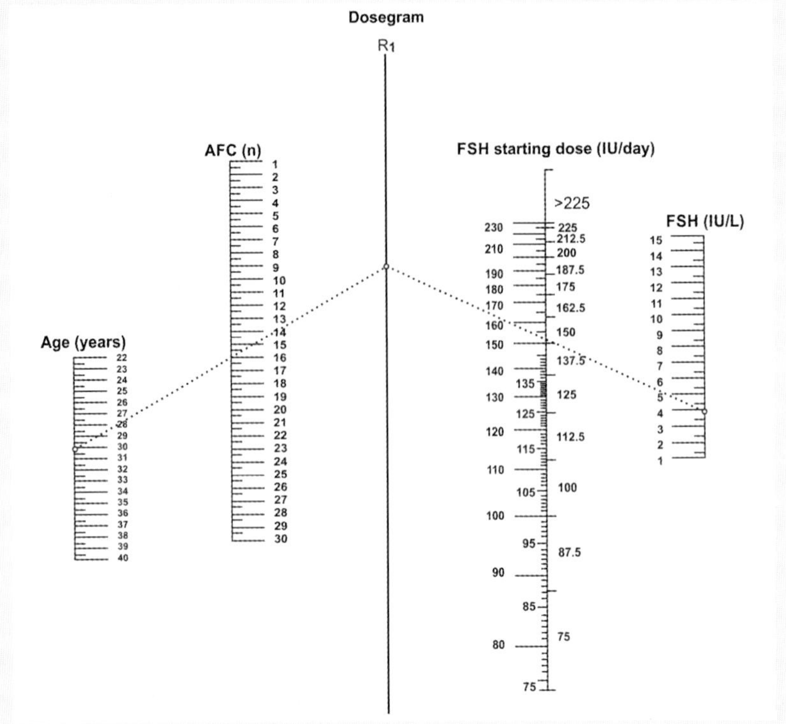

Fig. 1: The nomogram for the calculation of the FSH starting dose based on age, AFC, and serum Day 3 FSH. In the example, for a 30-year-old woman with AFC = 16 and Day 3 FSH = 4 IU/L, the FSH starting dose is 152 IU/day. Since the new FSH delivery system will have the dosage dial based on doses of FSH of 12.5 IU, on the right side of the FSH starting dose column, the FSH dose as selected for the delivery system is reported (150 IU/day for the example).
(AFC: antral follicle count; FSH: follicle-stimulating hormone)

Poor responder: The protocol favored for poor responders is mostly antagonist protocol. However, this protocol requires the addition of adjuvants in the late luteal phase of the previous cycle to maximize the cohort of recruitable follicles before starting gonadotropins. For this, one of the four options can be used; addition of oral contraceptive pills (OCPs) from Day 2 of a menstrual cycle for 14–21 days, medroxyprogesterone acetate (MPA) 10 mg twice a day for 5 days from Day 21 of the cycle, estradiol valerate orally in doses of 2–4 mg daily from Day 21 of cycle or antagonist 0.25 mg injection from Day 25 in the previous cycle till the day of menstruation followed by gonadotropin stimulation. These protocols generally use higher doses of gonadotropins such as 225–450 IU daily. Addition of recombinant luteinizing hormone from Day 1 of stimulation is sometimes associated with better response especially in the poseidon group 1 and 2 of poor responders. However, even the addition of human menopausal gonadotropin (hMG) may enhance the ovarian response in poor responders.

Microdose flare is another method of ovarian stimulation for this group of patients where GnRh agonist is given from Day 1 of menses for 2–3 days in doses of 20–25 µg twice a day followed by gonadotropins and antagonist as flexible regime.

Long protocol still enjoys a reasonable choice in the ovarian stimulation for this group also and this is probably because it makes the best cohort despite the need for higher doses of gonadotropins for longer period of time.

Mild ovarian stimulation has also been proposed by International Society for Mild Approaches in Assisted Reproduction (ISMAAR) for women with poor ovarian reserve. This is based on the fact that these women have a very modest pool of recruitable follicles. No significant improvements in oocyte and embryo yield or pregnancy rates have been observed following an upward adjustment of FSH with starting dose of 150 IU/day. There appears no benefit to use doses above 300 IU of FSH to increase the pregnancy rate in poor responders. However, individualized FSH-dosing algorithms targeting poor responders are not yet available.

Duo-stimulation protocols "Duplex protocol" (DPX): The emergence of these protocols occurred with data coming from researchers which fuelled the concept that ovarian stimulation can be dissociated from the follicular phase and its hormonal environment, as long as no fresh embryo transfer takes place. Oocyte yields of the "random-start" protocols were found to equal those of ovarian stimulation started in the early follicular phase. These data indicate that ovarian stimulation can be totally disconnected from the cycling phases of endogenous gonadotropins without any detrimental consequences, on the resultant embryo which can be transferred later in a natural or hormonal replacement cycle.

The duo-stimulation protocol is best suited for women with low ovarian reserve (AMH <1.5 ng/mL, AFC 6 follicles), or have shown a poor response in the previous COS for cycle with less than 5 oocytes retrieved especially for patients who need to have preimplantation genetic testing (PGT), so that more embryos could be accumulated before sending them for genetic testing.

Protocol

- *Follicular phase*: High-dose gonadotropins such as recombinant FSH 300 IU along with recombinant LH 75 IU with follicular monitoring, till one or more 18 mm dominant follicles are seen after which GnRH agonist trigger is given followed by oocyte retrieval 35 hours later with "freeze all embryos" strategy.
- *Luteal phase*: After the first stimulation and OCR, gonadotropins can be started again within 5 days of oocyte retrieval to promote growth of the second wave of follicular growth. Antagonist needs to be given once the progesterone declines and the lead follicle is 14 mm in size, trigger is given again.

Protocols for Coexisting Hormonal Imbalances affecting Controlled Ovarian Syndrome

Polycystic ovarian syndrome: 30% to 40% of PCOS hypersecrete LH with concerns regarding its ill effects on oocyte quality and endometrium. There are various views regarding the best protocol which can be used to optimize ovarian stimulation and pregnancy rates in this group of women.

- Ignore basal high LH levels and start with fixed antagonist protocol as routine practice in normal responders.
- Suppress basal high levels of LH with antagonist for 2–3 days before starting stimulation with gonadotropins. One can reevaluate LH levels to ensure suppression after which conventional antagonist protocol can be followed.
- Pretreatment with oral contraceptives for 2–3 months or ovarian drilling may also reduce LH hypersecretion in considerable number of cases.
- Use of long *GnRH agonist* protocol suppresses serum LH levels fully before starting stimulation with gonadotropins. The drawback of this protocol is the high risk of OHSS in these patients.

Hypogonadotropic hypogonadism: Women with this hormonal imbalance are unique in respect to complete absence of LH surge even after ovulatory follicular size is achieved. Therefore, there appears no need to control pituitary LH by either agonist or antagonist as their pituitary is unable to synthesize FSH or LH. These women are best treated by combination of FSH and LH, i.e. by hMG or recombinant FSH and LH combined. There is evidence to support that LH is required in small amounts only, hence it may be mandatory to step up the dose of FSH every 5–7 days but LH can be kept constant at 75 units in most cases. The trigger before oocyte retrieval is always hCG and not GnRH agonist. Luteal support is preferable with hCG along with vaginal progesterone till pregnancy is confirmed and then till 8 weeks gestation. It is recommended to give pretreatment with estrogen and progesterone cyclically for 6–9 months till the mid cycle endometrium appears ideal for implantation unless the patient is already on cyclical hormone replacement therapy.

Development of Protocols for Underlying Pathology which Perform Poorly with Conventional Controlled Ovarian Syndrome

Severe endometriosis: Use of the traditional agonist long or antagonist short protocol, has been used in women with endometriosis and compromised ovarian reserve with variable results. However, it has been seen that ultra long protocol—administration of GnRH agonist for 3–6 months prior to ovarian stimulation for especially in women with good ovarian reserve increases clinical pregnancy rate fourfold and live birth rate 9 times. The Cochrane database systematic review 2010 also concluded the same.

Controlled Ovarian Syndrome to Ensure Complete Safety for Oocyte Donors without Compromising Oocyte Quality

Oocyte donor: A qualitative follow-up study of experiences with oocyte donors was done by Kalfoglou who concluded that matching agencies and IVF clinics may improve donor satisfaction by minimizing the donor's trips to the clinic, using protocols that limit their number of intramuscular injections and reduce their risk of hyperstimulation syndrome. Improved donor satisfaction is likely to improve donor recruitment and retention.

Antagonist protocol with agonist trigger appears the safest method of stimulating donors for oocyte retrieval. This protocol not only minimizes the risk of hyperstimulation to the lowest possible but also maintains the number and quality of mature oocytes comparable to hCG trigger.

Attempts are being made to develop even simpler protocols for oocyte donors which would not only eliminate use of GnRH analogs in controlled ovarian hyperstimulation (COH) cycles but also reduce monitoring too. These involve use of progestational agents from the start of stimulation to hCG trigger. Starting of gonadotropin stimulation in the luteal phase or use of a progestin or progesterone along with COH in the follicular phase suppresses the LH surge. These protocols on the one hand eliminate restrictions imposed by the dates of the menstrual cycle and on the other hand limit the ovarian stimulation agents to gonadotropin and trigger injections only.

Medroxyprogesterone acetate 10 mg orally daily once from the start of stimulation to the day of trigger is seen to block LH surge effectively. Alternatively, MPA could be replaced with 100 mg twice daily of oral micronized progesterone, which could also effectively block LH surge.

It appears pragmatic to extrapolate a role for these new protocols in oocyte donors, especially with the emerging use of long-acting FSH which is effective for approximately 7 days, given once only on Day 2 or 3 of the cycle. Situations involving normal responders not in need of fresh transfer are the preferred target and hence at the forefront of these situations are oocyte donors and woman requiring preservation. Nevertheless, it remains to be investigated whether the total dose and the duration of stimulation are increased, as seems to have been shown by the Asian retrospective studies.

Alternatively use of CC from Day 2 of cycle and addition of gonadotropin a few days later may not only reduce the total dose and cost of gonadotropin, but continuation of CC till trigger can effectively control LH surge too by blocking the hypothalamic-pituitary gonadotropin receptors.

Miscellaneous Group Desiring Milder Stimulation or have Time Constraints for *in vitro* Fertilization

Women desiring milder stimulation: The ISMAAR has advocated regimes for ovarian stimulation for IVF which aim at retrieval of seven or less oocytes in women with normal ovarian reserve. Under these regimes low doses of gonadotropins are used or they are coupled with oral ovulation inducing agents with flexible antagonist protocol. This protocol not only optimizes retrieval of oocytes but also results in a more favorable endometrium for implantation compared to that seen after conventional IVF. Natural cycle IVF or modified natural cycle aims at retrieval of a single oocyte only, with minimal disturbance of endometrium. However, these cycles do not culminate in a reasonable pregnancy rate with laboratories having suboptimal performance.

Women with time constraints: For women who are traveling and have time constraints can go through IVF using modified natural cycle. For women who are ovulating, cycle stimulation can be started any day in the follicular phase later than Day 5 after counseling for single oocyte retrieval. Lastly, women with PCOS who have prolonged periods of amenorrhea and normal endometrium can be started with stimulation on any day, provided their base line hormones are in the normal range.

Gonadotropin Protocols for Patients with Oncologic Issues in Urgent Need of Oocyte or Embryo Preservation

For young cancer patients awaiting chemotherapy, a random start of ovarian stimulation on any day of the follicular phase or in the luteal phase post ovulation is most appropriate considering the time constraint they have. Even two back-to-back COS in one cycle by starting again in the luteal phase after 5 days of OCR, has been used to maximize the number of oocytes retrieved without wasting their time to chemotherapy. In stimulation protocols starting in the luteal phase GnRH-antagonist could be added in case progesterone levels drop and menstruation ensues in the same manner as in conventional COS, to prevent a premature LH surge, and is continued till hCG or GnRH agonist trigger.

Waves of folliculogenesis have been proposed during the menstrual cycle contrary to the traditional theory that a single cohort of antral follicles grows only at the beginning of the follicular phase. Ultrasound monitoring of follicles have shown, that 68% of women have two waves of follicular growth, and 32% have three waves during a single menstrual cycle. The first follicular wave that emerges at start of menstrual cycle is ovulatory while the wave or waves emerging in the luteal phase are anovulatory. It is important to recognize that folliculogenesis is independent from the rhythm of the menstrual cycle.

Women Requiring Low Estrogen Levels During COS Owing to Prothrombotic Conditions or Estrogen-Dependent Cancers

For the group of women with prothrombotic conditions or estrogen-dependent breast or endometrial cancers, where high serum estrogen levels are undesirable, different ovarian stimulation regimes have been developed. These regimes are being used clinically and involve the use of gonadotropin along with letrozole, an aromatase inhibitor which reduces the estrogen production to bare minimum during ovarian stimulation. Letrozole is used in doses of 2.5 mg/day to as much as 10 mg/day during the whole stimulation cycle, till hCG trigger is given to keep follicular estrogen levels to less than 500 pg/mL yet optimize the number of oocytes retrieved.

CONCLUSION

Conventional stimulation protocols for women undergoing IVF were developed initially to optimize its outcome. However, the associated complications in terms of OHSS and multiple gestations, and the financial burden along with physical and emotional stress seemed to be counterproductive. To combat these side effects came in use of milder stimulation regimes, which lead to development of fewer embryos, with possibly more synchronized endometrium and hence better implantation rates. However, even this did not work too well in terms of live birth rate per cycle thus hence forth ICOS with selection of the right protocol with the right gonadotropin is being developed for personalized care of women undergoing IVF which aims at not only optimizing its outcome but also minimizing complications.

EDITORS' COMMENTS

In this chapter, Prof. Majumdar provides readers a well-written and practical review about individualized controlled ovarian stimulation (iCOS). The author begins by highlighting the importance of ovarian biomarkers, in particular, anti-Müllerian hormone and antral follicle count, for helping to identify women with predictive normal, hyper, and poor response to ovarian stimulation. Then, Dr Majumdar expands on other clinical scenarios in which the iCOS approach is also sound, including endometriosis, PCOS, oocyte donation, as well as taking into account the patient's preferences.

Ovarian stimulation (OS) is an essential process of assisted reproductive technology (ART) as it allows multifollicular development and maturation of multiple oocytes. A critical aspect to keep in mind when planning iCOS is oocyte number. The number of oocytes retrieved is associated with the size of the resulting embryo cohort. Therefore, the higher the oocyte number, the higher the likelihood of cumulative pregnancy success.

Another critical issue is the patient-centered COS. Indeed, many patients drop out from treatment after one or more failed cycles. Patients refer that the burden associated with multiple injections and procedures, a lack of adequate medical and psychological support, as well as a poor organization of Fertility Centers are the leading factors for treatment dropout. In the modern ART era, it is therefore desirable to implement patient-oriented treatment strategies focusing on improving the quality of care. While effectiveness is a critical issue in that regard, other equally important aspects include safety, timeliness, efficiency, equity, and patient-centeredness. Most of these requirements can be applied to OS. This means that OS should be aimed not only to maximize effectiveness regarding oocyte number but also to improve patient satisfaction as well as to minimize its adverse effects.

Over the last years, quality management systems (QMS) have been implemented in an increasing number of Fertility Centers worldwide as a means to improve the quality of care delivered to patients. Ideally, OS should be planned accordingly to allow a balanced distribution of oocyte retrievals over the weekdays, thus securing an organized workflow that ultimately results in increased effectiveness, safety, as well as patient and staff satisfaction. QMS models applied to ART give the opportunity to achieve a well-organized workflow while securing optimal service provision.

In a recent study, we described a protocol for IVF cycle programming consistent with the concept of a patient-centered iCOS approach.[1] The method was designed to be broadly applied to OS in the context of IVF but is of particular interest to Fertility Centers running QMS models.

SC Esteves, Campinas, Brazil

REFERENCE

1. Fischer R, Nakano FY, Roque M, et al. A quality management approach to controlled ovarian stimulation in assisted reproductive technology: the "Fischer protocol". Panminerva Med. 2019;61(1):11-23.

SUGGESTED READING

1. Azim A, Oktay K. Letrozole for ovulation induction and fertility preservation by embryo cryopreservation in young women with endometrial carcinoma. Fertil Steril. 2007;88:657-64.

2. Baerwald AR, Adams GP, Pierson RA. Characterization of ovarian follicular wave dynamics in women. Biol Reprod. 2003;69:1023-31.
3. Berkkanoglu M, Ozgur K. What is the optimum maximal gonadotropin dosage used in microdose flare-up cycles in poor responders? Fertil Steril. 2010;94:662-5.
4. Bodri D, Sunkara SK, Coomarasamy A. Gonadotropin-releasing hormone agonists versus antagonists for controlled ovarian hyperstimulation in oocyte donors: a systematic review and meta-analysis. Fertil Steril. 2011;95:164-9.
5. Broer SL, Dólleman M, Opmeer BC, et al. AMH and AFC as predictors of excessive response in controlled ovarian hyperstimulation: a meta-analysis. Hum Reprod Update. 2011;17:46-54.
6. Cakmak H, Katz A, Cedars MI, et al. Effective method for emergency fertility preservation: random-start controlled ovarian stimulation. Fertil. Steril. 2013;100;1673-80.
7. Carone D, Caropreso C, Vitti A, et al. Efficacy of different gonadotropin combinations to support ovulation induction in WHO type I anovulation infertility: clinical evidences of human recombinant FSH/human recombinant LH in a 2:1 ratio and highly purified human menopausal gonadotropin stimulation protocols. J Endocrinol Invest. 2012;35:996-1002.
8. Chen Q, Wang Y, Sun L, et al. Controlled ovulation of the dominant follicle using progestin in minimal stimulation in poor responders. Reprod Biol Endocrinol. 2017;15(1):71.
9. Damario MA, Moomjy M, Tortoriello D, et al. Delay of gonadotropin stimulation in patients receiving gonadotropin-releasing hormone agonist (GnRH-a) therapy permits increased clinic efficiency and may enhance in vitro fertilization (IVF) pregnancy rates. Fertil Steril. 1997;68:1004-10.
10. Fanchin R, Salomon L, Castelo-Branco A, et al. Luteal estradiol pre-treatment coordinates follicular growth during controlled ovarian hyperstimulation with GnRH antagonists. Hum Reprod. 2003;18:2698-703.
11. Galindo A, Bodri D, Guillén JJ, et al. Triggering with HCG or GnRH agonist in GnRH antagonist treated oocyte donation cycles: a randomised clinical trial. Gynecol Endocrinol. 2009;25:60-6.
12. Gardner DK, Weissman A, Howles CM, et al. (Eds). Textbook of Assisted Reproductive Techniques, 4th edition; 2012.
13. Geng X, Ou X, Liao Y, et al. Effect of basal serum luteinizing hormone and luteinizing hormone/follicle-stimulating hormone ratio on outcomes of in vitro fertilization-embryo transfer in patients with polycystic ovarian syndrome. Nan Fang Yi Ke Da Xue Xue Bao. 2013;33:857-60.
14. Griesinger G, Diedrich K, Devroey P, et al. GnRH agonist for triggering final oocyte maturation in the GnRH antagonist ovarian hyperstimulation protocol: a systematic review and meta-analysis. Hum Reprod Update. 2006;12:159-68.
15. Gupta S, Satwik R, Majumdar A, et al. Clomiphene based ovarian stimulation in a commercial donor program. J Hum Reprod Sci. 2015;8:142-5.
16. Huirne JA, Homburg R, Lambalk CB. Are GnRH antagonists comparable to agonists for use in IVF? Hum Reprod. 2007;22:2805-13.
17. Humaidan P, Ejdrup Bredkjaer H, Westergaard LG, et al. 1,500 IU human chorionic gonadotropin administered at oocyte retrieval rescues the luteal phase when gonadotropin-releasing hormone agonist is used for ovulation induction: a prospective, randomized, controlled study. Fertil Steril. 2010;93:847-54.
18. Humaidan P, Quartarolo J, Papanikolaou EG. Preventing ovarian hyperstimulation syndrome: guidance for the clinician. Fertil Steril. 2010;94:389-400.
19. Kalfoglou AL, Gittelsohn J. A qualitative follow-up study of women's experiences with oocyte donation. Hum Reprod. 2000;15:798-805.
20. Kuang Y, Chen Q, Fu Y, et al. Medroxyprogesterone acetate is an effective oral alternative for preventing premature luteinizing hormone surges in women undergoing controlled ovarian hyperstimulation for in vitro fertilization. Fertil Steril. 2015;104:62-70.e3.
21. Kuang Y, Chen Q, Hong Q, et al. Double stimulations during the follicular and luteal phases of poor responders in IVF/ICSI programmes (Shanghai protocol). Reprod Biomed Online. 2014;29:684-91.
22. La Marca A, Papaleo E, Grisendi V, et al. Development of a nomogram based on markers of ovarian reserve for the individualisation of the follicle-stimulating hormone starting dose in in vitro fertilisation cycles. BJOG. 2012;119:1171-9.
23. La Marca A, Sighinolfi G, Radi D, et al. Anti-Müllerian hormone (AMH) as a predictive marker in assisted reproductive technology (ART). Hum Reprod Update. 2010;16:113-30.
24. La Marca A, Spada E, Sighinolfi G, et al. Age-specific nomogram for the decline in antral follicle count throughout the reproductive period. Fertil Steril. 2011;95:684-8.
25. La Marca A, Sunkara SK. Individualization of controlled ovarian stimulation in IVF using ovarian reserve markers: from theory to practice. Hum Reprod Update. 2014;20:124-40.
26. Lie Fong S, Baart EB, Martini E, et al. Anti-Müllerian hormone: a marker for oocyte quantity, oocyte quality and embryo quality? Reprod Biomed Online. 2008;16:664-70.
27. Loutradis D, Patsoula E, Minas V, et al. FSH receptor gene polymorphisms have a role for different ovarian response to stimulation in patients entering IVF/ICSI-ET programs. J Assist Reprod Genet. 2006;23:177-84.
28. Malmusi S, La Marca A, Giulini S, et al. Comparison of a gonadotropin-releasing hormone (GnRH) antagonist and GnRH agonist flare-up regimen in poor responders undergoing ovarian stimulation Fertil Steril. 2005;84:402-6.
29. Massin N. New stimulation regimens: endogenous and exogenous progesterone use to block the LH surge during ovarian stimulation for IVF. Hum Reprod Update. 2017;23: 211-20.
30. Melo M, Busso CE, Bellver J, et al. GnRH agonist versus recombinant HCG in an oocyte donation programme: a randomized, prospective, controlled, assessor-blind study. Reprod Biomed Online. 2009;19:486-92.
31. Mohiyiddeen L, Nardo LG. Single-nucleotide polymorphisms in the FSH receptor gene and ovarian performance: future role in IVF. Human Fertil (Camb). 2010;13:72-8.
32. Moon KY, Kim H, Lee JY, et al. Nomogram to predict the number of oocytes retrieved in controlled ovarian stimulation. Clin Exp Reprod Med. 2016;43:112-8.

33. Nargund G, Fauser BC, Macklon NS, et al. The ISMAAR proposal on terminology for ovarian stimulation for IVF. Hum Reprod. 2007;22:2801-4.
34. Nathalie Massin. New stimulation regimens: endogenous and exogenous progesterone use to block the LH surge during ovarian stimulation for IVF. Hum Reprod Update. 2017;23:211-20.
35. Nazari A, Dietterich et al. Comparison of androgen levels in conception vs. non-conception cycles following controlled ovarian stimulation using luteal phase gonadotropin-releasing hormone agonist protocol. Gynecol Endocrinol. 1995;9:209-14.
36. Nelson SM, Yates RW, Fleming R. Serum anti-Müllerian hormone and FSH: prediction of live birth and extremes of response in stimulated cycles—implications for individualization of therapy. Hum Reprod. 2007;22:2414-21.
37. Nelson SM, Yates RW, Lyall H, et al. Anti-Müllerian hormone-based approach to controlled ovarian stimulation for assisted conception. Hum Reprod. 2009;24:867-75.
38. Orvieto R, Meltcer S, Homburg R, et al. What is the preferred GnRH analogue for polycystic ovary syndrome patients undergoing controlled ovarian hyperstimulation for in vitro fertilization? Fertil Steril. 2009;91:1466-8.
39. Papaleo E, Vanni VS, Viganò P, et al. Recombinant LH administration in subsequent cycle after "unexpected" poor response to recombinant FSH monotherapy. Gynecol Endocrinol. 2014;30:813-6.
40. Poseidon Group (Patient-Oriented Strategies Encompassing IndividualizeD Oocyte Number), Alviggi C, Andersen CY, et al. A new more detailed stratification of low responders to ovarian stimulation: from a poor ovarian response to a low prognosis concept. Fertil Steril. 2016;105:1452-3.
41. Rashidi B, Nasiri R, Rahmanpour H, et al. Luteal phase estradiol versus luteal phase GnRH antagonist administration: their effects on antral follicular size coordination and basal hormonal levels. Iran J Reprod Med. 2011;9:315-31.
42. Requena A, Cruz M, Collado D, et al. Evaluation of the degree of satisfaction in oocyte donors using sustained-release FSH corifollitropin α. Reprod Biomed Online. 2013;26:253-9.
43. Sallam HN, Garcia-Velasco JA, Dias S, et al. Long-term pituitary down-regulation before in vitro fertilization (IVF) for women with endometriosis. Cochrane Database Syst Rev. 2006;(1):CD004635.
44. Shrestha D, La X, Feng HL. Comparison of different stimulation protocols used in in vitro fertilization: a review. Ann Transl Med. 2015;3:137.
45. Sismanoglu A, Tekin HI, Erden HF, et al. Ovulation triggering with GnRH agonist vs. hCG in the same egg donor population undergoing donor oocyte cycles with GnRH antagonist: a prospective randomized cross-over trial. J Assist Reprod Genet. 2009;26:251-6.
46. Smeenk JM, Sweep FC, Zielhuis GA, et al. Antimüllerian hormone predicts ovarian responsiveness, but not embryo quality or pregnancy, after in vitro fertilization or intracyoplasmic sperm injection. Fertil Steril. 2007;87:223-6.
47. Sönmezer M, Türkçüoğlu I, Coşkun U, et al. Random-start controlled ovarian hyperstimulation for emergency fertility preservation in letrozole cycles. Fertil Steril. 2011;95:2125.e9-11.
48. Thessaloniki ESHRE/ASRM-Sponsored PCOS Consensus Workshop Group. Consensus on infertility treatment related to polycystic ovary syndrome. Hum Reprod. 2008;23:462-77.
49. Ubaldi FM, Capalbo A, Vaiarelli A, et al. Follicular versus luteal phase ovarian stimulation during the same menstrual cycle (DuoStim) in a reduced ovarian reserve population results in a similar euploid blastocyst formation rate: new insight in ovarian reserve exploitation. Fertil Steril. 2016;105:1488-95.
50. Verberg MF, Macklon NS, Nargund G, et al. Mild ovarian stimulation for IVF. Hum Reprod Update. 2009;15:13-29.
51. von Wolff M, Thaler CJ, Frambach T, et al. Ovarian stimulation to cryopreserve fertilized oocytes in cancer patients can be started in the luteal phase. Fertil Steril. 2009;92:1360-5.
52. Wennerholm UB, Bergh C. What is the most relevant standard of success in assisted reproduction? Singleton live births should also include preterm births. Hum Reprod. 2004;19:1943-5.
53. Yates AP, Rustamov O, Roberts SA, et al. Anti-Müllerian hormone-tailored stimulation protocols improve outcomes whilst reducing adverse effects and costs of IVF. Hum Reprod. 2011;26:2353-62.
54. Youssef MA, Van der Veen F, Al-Inany HG, et al. Gonadotropin-releasing hormone agonist versus HCG for oocyte triggering in antagonist-assisted reproductive technology. Cochrane Database Syst Rev. 2014;(10):CD008046.
55. Zarek SM, Muasher SJ. Mild/minimal stimulation for in vitro fertilization: an old idea that needs to be revisited. Fertil Steril. 2011;95:2449-55.
56. Zhu X, Zhang X, Fu Y. Utrogestan as an effective oral alternative for preventing premature luteinizing hormone surges in women undergoing controlled ovarian hyperstimulation for in vitro fertilization. Medicine (Baltimore). 2015;94:e909.

3

CHAPTER

Treatment for Poor Responders: Recent Consensus

Trupti Mehta, Sangeeta Deshmukh, Meenal Khandeparkar, Firuza R Parikh

INTRODUCTION

One of the greatest challenges facing the reproductive endocrinologist is managing the infertile woman who has a poor ovarian response (POR) to standard methods of ovulation induction. The poor response to ovarian stimulation results in poor quality and quantity of oocytes which in-turn results in reduced implantation and pregnancy rates.

There is no well-understood definition of poor ovarian responders because this clinical condition has been described in several different ways using different modalities. The lack of universal terminology makes it challenging to study this group of women. This may be accounted for by the fact that women with a poor ovarian response may fulfill some but not all criteria to define them. The three main parameters used to describe this condition are: advanced age of the woman, abnormal ovarian reserve testing and previous poor response to ovarian stimulation. The clinical setting in which a woman fits into this condition varies and the terms diminished ovarian reserve (DOR) or primary ovarian insufficiency (POI) are sometimes used interchangeably.

The first description of a woman who had a poor ovarian response was given by Garcia et al. 35 years ago.

In fact there are 38 different definitions to describe this condition.

In view of there being no uniform definition, the European Society of Human Reproduction and Embryology organized a workshop in 2011 and published the "Bologna Criteria (BC) to define Poor Responders". A consensus was reached that at least two of the following three features should be present to define POR.

1. Advanced maternal age (≥40 years) or any other risk factor for POR.
2. A previous POR (≤3 oocytes with a conventional stimulation protocol)
3. An abnormal ovarian reserve test (ORT) [antral follicle count (AFC) less than 5–7 follicles or anti-Müllerian hormone (AMH) <0.5–1.1 ng/mL].

Two episodes of POR after maximum stimulation are sufficient to define a patient as a poor responder in absence of advanced maternal age or abnormal ORT. Since the Bologna criteria were designed to identify PORs for research purposes only, most clinicians are reluctant to use them.

There are a few drawbacks of the Bologna criteria:

- An abnormal reserve testing of AMH <0.5–1.1 ng/mL would be in the normal range for women more than 40 years.
- The Bologna criteria are not representative of a homogeneous group of women.
- Regardless of age, the Bologna criteria use the same threshold of 3 or less than 3 oocytes retrieved.
- The cut-off age is arbitrarily fixed at 40 years.
- Other factors such as oocyte quality, smoking, medical and genetic disorders are also considered.

THE POSEIDON STRATIFICATION FOR WOMEN WITH POOR OVARIAN RESPONSE

The POSEIDON (Patient Oriented Strategies Encompassing IndividualizeD Oocyte Number) group showed a new stratification for women with a decreased ovarian reserve or an unsuitable response to exogenous gonadotropins.

The group has suggested four subgroups based on quantitative and qualitative parameters.

- Age and the expected aneuploidy rate.
- Ovarian biomarkers such as AFC and AMH.
- Ovarian response—provided a previous stimulation cycle was performed.

The POSEIDON criteria: are they an answer to the Bologna criteria?

The POSEIDON group introduced a new measure which is more practical—the ability to retrieve the number of oocytes needed for a specific patient to obtain at least one euploid embryo for transfer.

This classification would overcome the problem of wider heterogeneity in this population and also guide the clinician in a pragmatic manner.

The four stratifications are as follows:

Group 1:

Young patient <35 years with adequate ovarian reserve; parameters (AFC >5; AMH >1.2 ng/mL) and with an unexpected poor or suboptimal ovarian response.

Subgroup 1a: < 4 oocytes

Subgroup 1b: 4–9 oocytes retrieved.*

Group 2:

Older patient ≥35 years with adequate ovarian reserve; parameters (AFC > 5; AMH > 1.2 ng/mL) with an unexpected poor or suboptimal ovarian response.

Subgroup 2a: <4 oocytes

Subgroup 2b: 4–9 oocytes retrieved.*

Group 3:

Young patient (<35 years) with poor ovarian reserve; prestimulation parameters (AFC < 5; AMH < 1.2 ng/mL).

Group 4:

Older patient (>35 years) with poor ovarian reserve; prestimulation parameters (AFC < 5; AMH < 1.2 ng/mL).

ETIOPATHOLOGY OF POOR OVARIAN RESPONSE

There are many factors contributing to poor ovarian response.

Advancing Age of the Woman

Women are born with a finite number of oocytes. Attrition of these oocytes occurs throughout the reproductive span. Follicular atresia accelerates after the age of 38 years. A DOR can affect younger women too as they may have an accelerated decline in the follicular pool. Some of these women may have a larger nongrowing follicular (NGF) pool and this may cause a lowered response to changes in hormone levels associated with the woman's age.

Age-related changes in the quality of the granulosa cells surrounding the oocyte can impact on the quality of oocytes. Advancing age impacts on the transcriptome profile of the cumulus cells which is linked to oocyte quality. In women over the age of 37 years it has been shown that the angiogenic genes ANGPTLA, LEPR, and TOTFBR3 are significantly overexpressed compared to younger patients and in contrast, genes implicated in the TGF-B signaling pathway—AMH, TGFB1, inhibin and activin receptors are underexpressed. This in turn has an impact on the quality of the oocytes.

A study done at Yale identified the molecular pathways involved in the aging of human eggs. The authors found that degeneration of oocyte quality with advancing age was linked to oxygen deprivation in the cumulus cells. This triggers a cascade of biochemical changes which may ultimately affect the chromosomal integrity of aging oocytes.

Another study showed that in older women's granulosa cells, follicle-stimulating hormone (FSH) receptor expression was downregulated and progesterone receptor (PGR) expression was upregulated. These changes cause premature luteinization and therefore impact on egg quality.

Al-Edani et al. analyzed the transcriptomes of cumulus cells (CCs) from women in different age categories. In this elegant study, they showed that transcriptome profiles of cumulus cells showed a substantial difference between older and younger women's cumulus cells. They identified 2,186 transcripts that significantly distinguished the CCs in the three groups of women, CC younger (age <30 years), CC median (age 31–34 years), and CC older (age >37 years).

In the CC younger group, overexpression of inflammatory response genes such as CIS, FNI, and OSMR was observed. In the CC median group, overexpression of genes involved in insulin signaling pathways such as IGFBP3 and IGFBP5 was seen. The CC older group was enriched by genes involved in angiogenesis such as VEGFC and FGF2. Many genes involved in cumulus-oocyte dialog were downregulated

*After standard ovarian stimulation

in CC older. In CC older, there was upregulation of genes involved with angiogenesis. This may be as a result of hypoxia due to insufficiency of oxygen. This stimulation appears to be a compensation mechanism to modulate the deleterious effects of hypoxia.

Their study has shown that the use of human CC gene expression can be a powerful noninvasive tool to predict oocyte quality and developmental potential.

Endometriosis

The presence of ovarian endometriosis and ovarian endometrioma can contribute to POR due to a decline in vascularity and alteration of the cortical stroma of the ovary. Also the endometriosis can harm the follicular and endocrine environment and thus contribute to POR. Endometriomas cause chronic pelvic inflammation thus affecting the oocyte environment. Ovarian endometrioma can also activate ovarian connective tissue resulting in production of excess testosterone which affects egg quality. Endometriosis triggers natural killer cell activation, which over time can cause deterioration of ovarian function.

Ovarian Surgery

Ovarian cystectomy for endometrioma can also diminish the ovarian reserve. Removal of one ovary can cause POR. Prior ovarian surgery which involves ablation of the ovarian cortex can also contribute to POR. One of the iatrogenic causes of POR is the vigorous electrocauterization of follicles in women with polycystic ovarian syndrome (PCOS).

Surgical treatment for ovarian endometrioma can cause a quantitative and qualitative impairment of ovarian reserve.

Genital Tuberculosis, Pelvic Infection and Pelvic Adhesions

These are major contributors to POR. In fact, it is a well-known observation that women with genital TB require a higher dose for ovarian stimulation and yield less number of oocytes.

Genital TB is associated with ovarian adhesions. Healing in genital TB is associated with fibrosis. The fibrosis and adhesions can impair blood supply to the ovary and thereby compromise ovarian reserve. A study by Hans PS et al. showed that the ovarian volume was significantly larger in TB negative women as compared to TB positive women. The authors also demonstrated higher baseline FSH levels and less number of follicles in women who had genital TB.

A study by Keay et al. showed that pelvic infection decreases the ovarian response to ovarian stimulation.

Obesity and Increased BMI

These also contribute to POR. In an interesting study on the effect of obesity on serum AMH levels in women with different racial backgrounds, Moy et al. studied the medical records of 350 women of different races. They showed that BMI had a negative correlation with AMH in Caucasian women but not in African-American, Hispanic or Asian women.

Other studies have shown that older obese women have a mean AMH level that is 65% lower than AMH levels in nonobese women.

The mechanism by which obesity affects AMH levels and the ovarian reserve is by its potential disruption of the ovarian follicular environment and increasing both oxidative stress and inflammatory responses in the follicular fluid of obese women.

Loh and her group showed that non-PCOS women undergoing OI with high basal FSH showed a poor response to ovarian stimulation. Obese patients showed a varying response to ovulation induction resulting in more cancellation of cycles.

Older women in spite of being normogonadotropic and with normal BMI required higher amounts of gonadotropins for ovulation induction.

Smoking

One of the dangers of smoking is the poor response to ovulation induction. This may be due to advanced follicular atresia. In a paper presenting original data, Firns and her group showed that female smoking had an adverse effect on ovarian reserve. Cigarette smoke contain cotinine and benzo(a)pyrene which are mutagenic and carcinogenic. Female active and passive smoking carried a risk of increased miscarriage. It also had an impact on the age of onset of menopause. They showed that basal FSH increased in tandem with the years of smoking. Fertilization rates with *in vitro* fertilization (IVF) decreased as female years of smoking increased. Interestingly, the clomiphene citrate challenge test (CCCT) which is one of the markers for ovarian reserve testing was looked at by Sharara and group. They showed that the incidence of DOR was increased in women who smoked as compared to age-matched controls who did not smoke.

Uterine Artery Embolization for Attenuation of Fibroids

This can compromise the blood flow to the ovaries and cause POR. There are several theories as to how uterine artery embolization as conservative treatment of fibroids can cause DOR. The embolic material may reach the ovarian circulation causing damage to the ovaries. The incidence of ovarian failure after uterine artery embolization (UAE) is about 7%. The authors have also described a fall in AMH in women who have undergone UAE.

Chemotherapy and Radiotherapy

Since these modalities affect actively dividing cells with high metabolic activity, these cause an attrition and sometimes a complete destruction of the follicles resulting in POR. Iwase et al. conducted a computer based search to look at various studies evaluating ovarian reserve after toxic ovarian interventions such as chemotherapy and radiotherapy. Most of the studies looked at basal FSH and AMH and reported rise in basal FSH and decreased AMH following such treatment.

Lower Gonadotropin Surge Attenuating Factor

It has been observed that women with poor response to IVF have lowered circulating gonadotropin surge-attenuating factor (GnSAF) bioactivity during spontaneous and stimulated cycles.

Ethnicity

Ethnicity has a strong association with POR. An Indian study has shown that Indian ethnicity may contribute to poor ovarian reserve and that Indian Women shared an ovarian response similar to Spanish women 6.3 years older than them. Another study of ethnicity and ovarian reserve showed that Chinese, Latino, and African women had a lower ovarian reserve compared to Caucasian women of similar age.

Genetic Association with Diminished Ovarian Reserve

Multiple genes play a role in folliculogenesis. Diminished ovarian reserve, resulting in POR could be because of decreased production of oocytes embryologically, abnormal follicular development, increased follicular atresia or defects in the communication between oocytes and granulosa cells. The article by Greene et al. carried out a review of 21 articles to identify gene mutations, polymorphisms and epigenetics associated with DOR, which helped to isolate eight such genes.

FMR1 Gene

A premutation in the fragile X mental retardation 1 *(FMR1)* gene of 55–200 CGG repeats can contribute to premature ovarian failure (POF) in female carriers. A positive correlation between rising FSH levels, falling AMH levels and CGG repeats above 32 has been reported.

Gene Polymorphisms and Diminished Ovarian Reserve

The promoter region of genes contains polymorphisms which contain a huge amount of genetic variation.

- Polymorphism of growth differentiation factor 9 (GDF9) has been associated with DOR, poor ovarian response during IVF, and poor quality of oocytes.
- Polymorphism of FSH receptor (FSHR) which is located on granulosa cells also contributes to DOR.
- Polymorphism of estrogen alpha receptor (ESR1). This receptor is expressed more in the theca cells of the follicle. The homozygous CC (cytosine–cytosine) allele of the PvuII polymorphic variant of the *ESR1* gene is associated with POI and these women show higher baseline FSH.

Gene Expression Profiling

Many genes are differentially expressed in women with DOR. These include forkhead-like 13 transcription factor, Pumilio 2, Notch 3, and STAT-induced STAT inhibitor 3.

The DOR patients have cells of the membrana granulosa type which showed a differential gene expression in which the gene for AMH is also present and there was a higher gene expression of LHCGR and a lower expression of the gene for AMH in the DOR group.

Gremlin 1 *(GREM1)* is a downstream effector of the *GDF9* gene. In women with DOR, there is decreased expression of this gene.

Greenseid et al. studied granulosa cell expression for insulin-like growth factor 1 (IGF-1), IGF-2 and their receptors IGF1R and IGF2R and results depicted downregulation in women with DOR.

Diminished Ovarian Reserve and Genes in Mice

Generally identification of genes is first established in animal models and then similar models are used to detect genes in human beings.

Six candidate genes have been associated in mice with DOR that elaborate the phenotype of the mice. Similar genes have been found in humans.

These are:

- Forkhead transcription factor Forkhead L2 (FOXL2) protein
- Growth differentiation factor 9
- Bone morphogenetic protein 15 (BMP15)
- Autoimmune regulator (AIRE)
- Wingless-type MMTV integration site family, member 4 (WNT4).
- G protein-coupled receptor 3 (GPR3).

Translocations in chromosomes are seen when there is interchanging and rearrangements in the parts of the nonhomologous chromosomes. DOR has been observed in women with translocations particularly involving chromosome 21 as premature menopause is seen in these patients which may be related to disruption in chromosome 21.

Epigenetic Carriers of Diminished Ovarian Reserve

Epigenetics describes hereditary changes in gene formation without a change in the DNA sequence. Many environmental toxins and endocrine disruptors can cause a diminishing follicular pool over three generations. Many of these endocrine disruptors cause differential DNA methylation patterns suggesting epigenetic effects.

Ovarian Antibodies and Diminished Ovarian Reserve

One-third of patients with premature ovarian insufficiency (POR) or DOR have antiovarian (AOA) and antithyroid antibodies in their serum. About 2–10% of POI cases are known to be associated with adrenal autoimmunity. The presence of these pathogenic factors may accelerate the process of apoptosis and atresia of ovarian follicles. Abnormalities of cellular immunity of T lymphocytes, macrophages, and dendritic cells play an important role in these autoimmune events. This study showed decreased peripheral regulatory T-lymphocytes (CD25+ high) and increased peripheral blood B cells (CD19+). CD25+ peripheral regulatory lymphocytes could contribute to the formation of an autoimmune response in association with the presence of AOA and antithyroid antibodies.

In our study on anti-ovarian antibodies (AOA), 20/70 (28.56%) women who were AOA positive were poor responders. We also showed that post-corticosteroid administration for 3 months reversed their positive AOA status to negative AOA status in 70/138 women.

To summarize, many factors contribute to POR. Research in these factors will help the clinician to counsel women showing a poor ovarian response as to their choices for treatment.

The importance of testing and interpreting measures of ovarian reserve in order to understand the concept of diminished ovarian reserve.

The Committee Opinion of the American Society of Reproductive Medicine (ASRM) is very helpful as it uses biological markers to define this condition.

DEFINING OVARIAN RESERVE

Only a tiny fraction of the millions of primordial follicles initially present at birth will survive to maturity. This remaining pool of ovarian follicles defines a woman's ovarian reserve.

The definition of DOR is vague and generally signifies varied outcomes of oocyte quantity, quality, and the fertility of the patient according to the ASRM Committee.

Diminished ovarian reserve describes women of reproductive age whose response to ovarian stimulation or fecundity is reduced as compared to women of comparable age.

Need to Measure Ovarian Reserve

Although oocyte number and quality decline with age, fertility varies significantly among women of similar age.

Ovarian reserve testing is done with the aim of predicting reproductive potential and when menopause is to be expected. It is done with the idea of adding prognostic information to counseling, planning, and treatment options. Evidence of DOR does not necessarily mean an inability to conceive.

OVARIAN RESERVE TESTS

Ovarian reserve tests include biochemical, biological, histological, and biophysical tests of the ovaries which may predict the response and reproductive outcome. ORTs are an indirect estimate of a woman's remaining follicular pool. An ideal ovarian reserve test should be able to differentiate between a normal and a poor ovarian response. To determine the ovarian reserve certain tests such FSH, estradiol (E2), inhibin B, and AMH, and others such as the CCCT are available. The availability of multiple ovarian tests suggests that none of them are ideal. They have a role in identifying women with OHSS as well as DOR. These tests predict response to ovarian stimulation and do not predict pregnancy or its outcome.

How are ovarian reserve tests used?

Diminished ovarian reserve has been defined in different ways, including reduced fecundability and poor ovarian response to gonadotropin stimulation, measures of ovarian response such as the number of follicles, the number of oocytes retrieved, the number of embryos formed, and the cancellation rate of the cycle are surrogates for clinically important outcomes, viz. pregnancy and live birth. These surrogate outcomes are clinically important but are not synonymous with the outcome of POR. Heterogeneity in study populations and varied exposures and outcomes have resulted in a wide range of test characteristics for measures of ovarian reserve as reported in literature. Therefore, the reported "effectiveness" of ORTs varies. Accordingly, it is important to consider study designs carefully when applying the results of these screening studies to individual patients.

BIOLOGICAL MARKERS

Age as a Biological Marker

Since ovarian reserve reduces with age, fecundity in both natural and stimulated cycles declines with age. Secondary to decline in the ovarian follicle pool, the ovarian response to FSH decreases with advancing maternal age showing that there is a linear relationship of age and poor response.

Basal Follicle-stimulating Hormone

Serum FSH is the primary stimulus for final follicle maturation. FSH is under the negative feedback of estradiol (E2) and inhibin B. Basal serum concentrations (Day 2, 3 of the menstrual cycle) increase with advancing reproductive age. Inhibin B depends on the number of follicles in the ovary. As the number of follicles decline, inhibin B levels reduce and FSH levels rise. The measurement of FSH is easy and inexpensive.

There are a lot of diurnal, intercycle, and intracycle variations in the FSH levels. But repeating FSH in order to wait for a good cycle has not been shown to improve reproductive outcome. There is no universally accepted cut-off value for poor response.

Assays standardized against the WHO second international standard demonstrate high specificity (83–100% range) for predicting poor response to stimulation (usually defined as < 2–3 follicles or <4 retrieved oocytes) using multiple cut-off points above 10 IU/L of FSH (10–20 IU/L).

Ovarian aging begins several years before any elevation in FSH levels. Combined with other markers it can be used to counsel patients regarding a poor ovarian response.

Estradiol

Basal Estradiol Levels

Smotrich et al. evaluated the prognostic value of Day 3 E2 levels independent of Day 3 FSH levels, in response to ovulation induction and subsequent pregnancy rates in IVF-ET patients. They showed that women with elevated E2 level (E2 ≥ 80 pg/mL) on cycle Day 3 achieved a lower pregnancy rate and had a higher cancellation rate as compared to women with E2 levels < 80 pg/mL. Even after eliminating patients with elevated basal FSH levels of ≥ 15 mIU/mL those with higher basal E2 levels had a lower pregnancy rate and higher cancellation rate. They showed that when Day 3 E2 levels were ≥100 pg/mL, no pregnancies were achieved. A Day 3 E2 level in addition to a Day 3 FSH level helped the authors to counsel women undergoing IVF regarding their pregnancy outcome.

Clomiphene Citrate Challenge Test

It is a dynamic test for ovarian function. The CCCT involves measurements of serum FSH before CC treatment (cycle Day 3) and after CC treatment (cycle Day 10) (100 mg daily, cycle Days 5–9). An elevated FSH concentration after clomiphene stimulation suggests DOR. Studies of CCCT results have shown a lot of inter-cycle variability in FSH levels, basal and stimulated estradiol and inhibin B concentrations. Hence it is not a very reliable test. In addition, like any other dynamic test it is time consuming, more invasive, expensive, and may have some side effects.

ANTI-MÜLLERIAN HORMONE

Anti-Müllerian hormone is a dimeric glycoprotein exclusively produced by the granulosa cells of the preantral and small antral follicles.

When applying AMH cut-off points in clinical practice, care has to be exercised that the assay used to measure AMH is the same in the study group as used in the original assay.

Anti-Müllerian hormone can be measured on any day of the menstrual cycle and does not show inter-cycle variability and can predict hyperresponse also.

Serum AMH is the best indicator of ovarian reserve with high sensitivity and specificity. Levels of serum AMH can predict the number of oocytes with positive predictive value of 96%. Measurement of AMH is a promising screening test and is more likely to be useful in women at a high risk for DOR than in women at low risk for DOR. Low AMH cut-off points are fairly specific for poor ovarian response, but not for pregnancy.

Antral Follicle Count

Antral follicle count is the sum of the antral follicles in both ovaries, as observed by transvaginal ultrasonography during the early follicular phase. Most studies have defined antral follicles as those measuring 2–10 mm in mean diameter in the greatest two-dimensional (2D) plane; a count of 8–10 is considered as a predictor of normal response. An AFC of four or fewer is associated with a significant increase in cycle cancellation and decrease in pregnancy success in patients without canceled cycles. Repeated measurements have shown that there is limited inter-cycle variability. More than 14 antral follicles are considered to be predictive of ovarian hyperstimulation.

Low AFC is highly specific for predicting POR but has got low sensitivity.

Inhibin B

Inhibin B is a heterodimeric glycoprotein released by the granulosa cells of follicles. Inhibin B is lower in poor responders than in women with normal ovarian response to stimulation. Women with a low Day 3 inhibin B concentration (<45 pg/mL) have a poor response to superovulation during IVF and are less likely to conceive.

Large-scale studies have demonstrated that inhibin B does not discriminate between being able to or not able to conceive.

Ovarian Volume

The ovarian volume is measured by transvaginal ultrasonography applying the formula for an ellipsoid (D1 × D2 × D3 × 0.52) = ovarian volume. The volume of each ovary is calculated by measuring the ovary in three perpendicular directions and arriving at the mean average volume of both ovaries in the same individual.

Ovarian volume has limited value for detection of DOR. A decline in ovarian volume is a late event noticed in women greater than 40 years.

Ovarian Response

The ORT indicates ovarian reserve at a point in time whereas ovarian response represents the effect following ovarian stimulation. Two episodes of poor ovarian response after maximal stimulation are sufficient to define a patient as a poor responder in the absence of advanced maternal age or an abnormal ORT.

Table 1 outlines the various screening tests of ovarian reserve as outlined by the Practice Committee, Ovarian Reserve Testing, Fertil Steril. 2015.

DISCUSSION

Women in their late 30s and early 40s form a large part of the infertile population. Many of them require assisted reproductive technology (ART) treatment. The ORT gives important information regarding the ovarian reserve and hence helps the infertility specialist deciding treatment. The ideal test to measure ovarian reserve should be measurable, minimally invasive, not expensive, and have a good predictive value.

Ovarian reserve tests can identify poor responders as well as hyper-responders. This also helps in deciding the ovarian stimulation dose. Basal FSH levels rise late in case of POF and have intra-cycle and inter-cycle variability. Basal estradiol and inhibin B levels are not better predictors than FSH. CCCT is less sensitive for detection of DOR than basal FSH. AMH and AFC are found to be better predictors of DOR and hyper-response, are more sensitive and specific and show less inter-cycle and intra-cycle variation.

Ovarian reserve tests have a moderate ability to predict DOR and hyperresponse. The present evidence shows that AFC and AMH are the best markers of ovarian reserve in addition to chronological age.

Since AMH can detect DOR before it reaches a critical level, it can help women make an informed decision regarding their reproductive choices.

TABLE 1 Summary of the value of screening tests of ovarian reserve.

		Poor response		*Nonpregnancy*				
Test	*Cutpoint*	*Sensitivity (%)*	*Specificity (%)*	*Sensitivity (%)*	*Specificity (%)*	*Reliability*	*Advantages*	*Limitations*
FSH	10–20 IU/L	10–80	83–100	7–58	43–100	Limited	Widespread use	• Reliability • Low sensitivity
AMH	0.2–0.7 ng/mL	40–97	78–92	a	a	Good	Reliability	• Limit of detectability • Does not predict nonpregnancy
AFC	3–10	9–73	73–100	8–33	64–100	Good	Reliability	Low sensitivity
Inhibin B	40–45 pg/mL	40–80	64–90	a		Limited	Widespread use	• Reliability • Does not predict nonpregnancy
CCCT (Day-10 FSH)	10–22 IU/L	35–98	68–98	23–61	67–100	Limited	Higher sensitivity than basal FSH	• Reliability • Limited additional value to basal FSH • Requires drug administration

Note: Laboratories ELISA.

[a]Insufficient evidence.

(FSH: follicle-stimulating hormone; AMH: anti-Müllerian hormone; AFC: antral follicle count; CCCT: clomiphene citrate challenge test)

Source: Practice Committee. Ovarian reserve testing. Fertil Steril; 2015.

MANAGEMENT OF POOR OVARIAN RESPONDERS

Various controlled ovarian hyperstimulation (COH) protocols and strategies have been used to improve reproductive outcome in poor ovarian responders (PORs).

Several systematic reviews have evaluated the existing protocols for PORs. These include evidence generated from randomized clinical trials (RCTs). The majority of strategies aim to recruit a higher number of follicles either by increasing the dosage of gonadotropins, decreasing the dose of gonadotropin-releasing hormone (GnRH) analogs, suppressing an early rise in FSH with "estrogen priming," or optimizing the endogenous FSH flare effect.

A comprehensive review of available literature to analyze the efficacy of various protocols is reviewed here.

PRETREATMENT AND ADJUNCTIVE THERAPY

Dehydroepiandrosterone

Dehydroepiandrosterone (DHEA) supplementation in a dose of 25 mg thrice a day for 4 months is helpful in increasing oocyte yield in PORs by the accumulation of androgens in the ovary. This stimulates early stages of follicular growth, augments the expression of FSH receptors in granulosa cells and thus, potentially causes an enhanced responsiveness of the ovaries to FSH. A recent meta-analysis, evaluating the role of androgens or androgen-modulating agents concluded that pretreatment with them increases clinical pregnancy and live birth rates.

It appears to be devoid of major side effects. However, due to lack of data supporting its effectiveness in other studies, it is not used on a wide scale.

Human Growth Hormone

Human growth hormone (HGH), either directly or indirectly via IGF-1, regulates oocyte maturation and increases the sensitivity of the ovaries to gonadotropins and promotes early follicle development. The use of 2–4 IU of HGH from Day 3 of exogenous gonadotropin administration until the day following hCG injection has been studied.

In a recently updated Cochrane review of all RCTs using HGH for ovarian stimulation, no beneficial effects were shown in normal responders, however, a significant improvement in pregnancy and live birth rates was seen in PORs. However, the exact subgroup which would benefit from HGH augmentation needs be identified.

A recent study revealed that in PORs and women with one or more previous IVF treatment failures, the HGH adjuvant therapy significantly improved the number of oocytes and embryos and rates of implantation and pregnancy.

Low-dose Aspirin

Increased intra-ovarian vascularity has been linked to improved delivery of gonadotropic hormones and other growth factors required for folliculogenesis. However, a recent meta-analysis and systematic review concluded that clinical pregnancy rate per embryo transfer was not found to be different between patients who received low-dose aspirin and the control group.

Resveratrol

Resveratrol administration orally, exerts benefits against loss of ovarian follicles and these actions may be mediated at least in part via anti-inflammatory, insulin-sensitizing, and antihyperandrogenism effects.

Coenzyme Q10 Supplementation

Oral supplementation of coenzyme Q10 (CoQ10) holds a lot of promise in the treatment of PORs. Studies on bovine oocytes suggest that CoQ10 could be added to culture media of the embryos for significantly improving mitochondrial function and ATP production. The age-related decline in oocyte quality and quantity could be reversed by the administration of CoQ10.

A strategy of supplementation of mitochondrial nutrients may lead to improvement in oocyte and embryo quality, and subsequently, a healthy pregnancy outcome for older women.

A recently conducted RCT showed that pretreatment with CoQ10 improved ovarian response to stimulation and embryological parameters in young women with poor ovarian reserve in IVF-intracytoplasmic sperm injection (ICSI) cycles.

Precycle Oral Contraceptive Pills

Using a long protocol with genre agonists leads to more pituitary downregulation as compared to oral contraceptive pills (OCPs).

Increased doses of gonadotropins can significantly improve the pregnancy outcome in PORs where OCPs have been given for a short period of time to suppress the pituitary ovarian axis.

Oral contraceptive pill pretreatment in PORs undergoing GnRH antagonist cycles does not influence cancellation rates, oocyte yield, pregnancy or implantation rates as per Min et al.

Luteal Phase Estrogen with Antagonist Suppression

Due to the effect of precycle use of OCPs in ovarian suppression, interest has been generated in giving estrogen in the luteal phase to upregulate the FSH receptors and produce a better response with FSH stimulation thereby promoting oocyte maturation. This has resulted in better stimulation outcomes, has reduced cycle drop out rates and has shown a slight increase in pregnancy rates.

Objectives of Controlled Ovarian Hyperstimulation

From the early 90s, the combination of GnRH agonists administered in the luteal phase of the previous cycle, followed by gonadotropins (long protocol), has been considered the protocol of choice in normally responding women. However, this may lead to increased ovarian suppression which will lead to a decreased or an absent follicular response. For this reason, the strategies used would be to:

- Reduce the duration of suppression by reducing the duration of GnRH agonist use (short and ultrashort, mini- and microdose flare-up regimens)
- Lower or to stop (after pituitary suppression) the dose of GnRH agonists initiated during the luteal phase
- Use GnRH antagonists in combination with gonadotropins to prevent premature luteinizing hormone (LH) rise during the mid-late follicular phase.

Controlled Ovarian Hyperstimulation Protocols in Poor Responders

Gonadotropin-releasing Hormone Agonist Flare Protocol

Gonadotropin-releasing hormone agonists are started shortly before beginning with gonadotropin injections in the follicular phase of a stimulation cycle. GnRH agonist is given in the dose of 100 µg in divided doses starting from Day 1 to Day 3 of menses followed by gonadotropins till day of hCG trigger. Reported clinical pregnancy rates have ranged from 12% to 26.3%. In one of the trials, pretreatment with OCPs had outcomes of around 30%. Most practitioners prefer the GnRH agonist flare protocols over the long GnRH protocols due to their efficacy as this trend has been observed over the last two decades (Fig. 1).

Modified GnRH Agonist Flare Protocol

Suppression by GnRH agonists is significant in a flare protocol. To decrease this effect a very low dose (microdose) GnRH agonist protocol was studied. In this study one dose of 25–50 µg od GnRH was given from the 1st day of menses for 3 days prior to starting gonadotropins and was continued till day of hCG trigger, which showed a rise in both FSH and LH levels. In addition to this pretreatment with OCPs in the cycle prior to stimulation by the above protocol averts a rise in progesterone production.

Using microdose protocols in PORs has resulted in improvement in the number of retrieved oocytes, pregnancy rates and cancellation rates as compared to long GnRH agonist protocols in retrospective studies (Fig. 2).

Agonist versus Antagonist Protocol

Gonadotropin-releasing hormone (GnRH) antagonists arrest a premature LH surge and do not lead to early suppression of follicular development. Their use in IVF protocols for POR is well justified (Fig. 3).

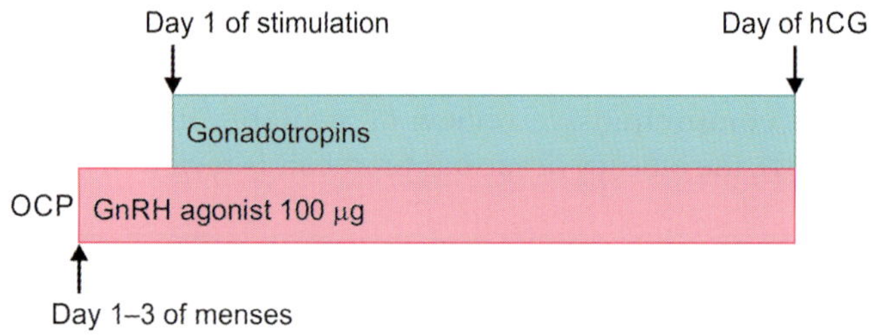

Fig. 1: Gonadotropin-releasing hormone (GnRH) agonist flare protocol.

Source: Modified from Talwar P, Verma S, Nayar KA, et al. Poor Ovarian Responders. E-bulletin ARText: Third Issue, Volume III. Indian Fertility Society; 2017.

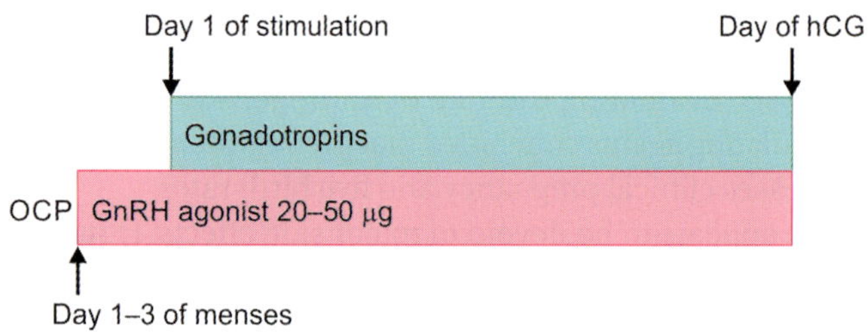

Fig. 2: Gonadotropin-releasing hormone (GnRH) agonist microdose flare protocol.

Source: Modified from Talwar P, Verma S, Nayar KA, et al. Poor Ovarian Responders. E-bulletin ARText: Third Issue, Volume III. Indian Fertility Society; 2017.

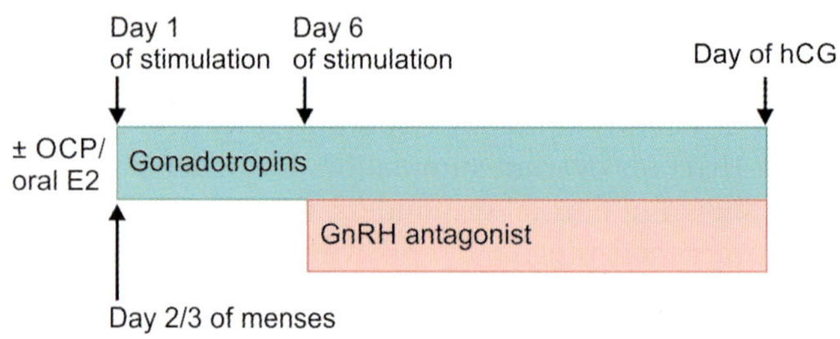

Fig. 3: Gonadotropin-releasing hormone (GnRH) antagonist protocol.

Source: Modified from Talwar P, Verma S, Nayar KA, et al. Poor Ovarian Responders. E-bulletin ARText: Third Issue, Volume III. Indian Fertility Society; 2017.

Pregnancy rates were not considerably different when the agonist versus antagonist protocols were used according to multiple prospective RCTs. However, the antagonist protocol seemed to be more beneficial to PORs. To conclude this more robust clinical trials are required.

To prevent the increase in progesterone and corpus luteum activity OCPs are used prior to the flare protocol as against the antagonist protocol in which pretreatment with OCPs is not given.

Clomiphene Flare Protocol

Early clomiphene citrate (CC) administration in a dose of 100 mg everyday can also lead to a flare of endogenous gonadotropins. In such cases, there is a rise in LH which can be prevented by administration of antagonists and the CC flare resulted in a decrease in cancellation rates, increase the number of oocytes retrieved, leading to higher implantation and pregnancy rates in women with POR versus the long GnRH agonist protocol.

Letrozole Flare Protocol

Letrozole is administered in any given cycle along with gonadotropins and a GnRH antagonist. The requirement of FSH in the long agonist protocol is reduced with the addition of letrozol but it does not seem to have an advantage when antagonists are being used, according to an RCT in 38 PORs. Further RCTs are therefore needed to assess the value of this protocol.

Minimal Stimulation Protocol

In PORs, the oocyte recovery can be significantly low in spite of administering elevated doses of gonadotropin injections. It has been seen that oral medication or even low-dose gonadotropin injections can give a satisfactory oocyte yield in PORs.

A natural cycle with low-dose gonadotropin injections can achieve pregnancy rates equivalent to the high-dose gonadotropins.

However in natural cycles, there is unpredictability and the cycle can get canceled easily. Despite GnRH antagonists used in the follicular phase at a late stage have shown some good results.

Two such comparative studies showed that the oocytes retrieved and the embryos transferred though low in number had similar pregnancy rates.

Most recent evidence on low-dose gonadotropins in POR in a systematic review and meta-analysis of 14 RCTs in 2104 women has shown similar clinical pregnancy rates and live birth rates between women treated with low-dose versus high-dose gonadotropins.

RESULTS OF IVF CYCLES WITH FULL DOSE GONADOTROPINS VERSUS NATURAL CYCLES VERSUS CLOMIPHENE ALONE VERSUS LETROZOLE ALONE

In 1,800 natural IVF cycles in PORs, there were 7.2% ongoing pregnancy rates per cycle and 15.8% ongoing pregnancy rates per transfer. If one compares another study where full dose gonadotropins were administered to patients, then the natural cycle ICSI group had a better implantation rate. The reason for this could be a superior follicular development and better recruitment of this follicle in a natural cycle leading to improved oocyte quality and thicker endometrium.

In various different RCTs comparison between CC stimulation alone IVF and the natural cycle IVF showed to have similar pregnancy rates as compared to full-dose gonadotropins. In fact CC, IVF may have a slight edge over natural cycle IVF in PORs.

Mohsen and El Din, showed no difference in clinical pregnancy rates in PORs when comparing a GnRH agonist microflare protocol to a letrozole antagonist protocol but the days of stimulation and total dose of gonadotropins were significantly lower in the letrozole group. Despite these findings more studies are needed to evaluate minimal stimulation IVF with letrozole alone.

Madani et al. have suggested that the pregnancy outcomes with the long, short, miniflare agonist, and antagonist protocols are similar in PORs. However, Ubaldi et al. have indicated that the antagonist protocol in PORs has advantages over agonist protocols. Avoiding luteal GnRH agonist or protocols using suppression with OCPs in favor of flare and antagonist protocols seem to most used protocols in PORs.

Although short and ultrashort flare protocols are widely used in PORs for more than 20 years, all published studies, prospective nonrandomized trials with or without control or retrospective ones were unable to demonstrate clearly any significant beneficial effect on the clinical outcome in this group.

Gonadotropins: Dose and Types

Dose

In women who have a reduced ovarian reserve, the recruitable follicles are fewer and the gonadotropins, independently of the dosage administered, can only support the cohort of follicles receptive to stimulation without manufacturing follicles *de novo*.

In PORs, it is best to start with at least 300 IU of FSH and one can go up to 450 IU per day. However a maximum dose of 450 IU should be started at the earliest which can be reduced, if the response is satisfactory. Yet more prospective trials are necessary to evaluate the exact dosage in such patients.

Few studies have shown to give a better outcome in PORs with the use of human menopausal gonadotropin (hMG) as against recombinant follicle-stimulating hormone (rFSH) and combination protocols of rFSH and hMG are now being used to give a high FSH dose and some LH but have not yet been proven to be superior. But most randomized prospective trials have shown no difference among various gonadotropins available.

Role of Luteinizing Hormone

Addition of LH to rFSH stimulation in IVF has not been studied at length in PORs. Numerous studies have been done with addition of recombinant luteinizing hormone (rLH) in doses ranging from 37.5 to 225 IU starting from Day 1 to Day 8 of rFSH and continued till the day of hCG trigger.

It was found that giving rLH along with FSH in PORs increases the IVF rates in few select patients and thus no extra benefit was attributed to this. This was also confirmed by a Cochrane data base in 2007. LH always proved to be beneficial during the cycle for PORs and therefore many infertility specialists are using both FSH and LH for stimulation in this group. It has been noticed that in PORs very few oocytes are picked up (<5) and therefore formation of good quality embryos is diminished.

Intracytoplasmic sperm injection in such cases may be useful over IVF but as it stands today due to a small number of studies ICSI and conventional IVF showed no difference in the final pregnancy outcome.

Techniques for Embryo Culture

Co-culture

Following a follicular stimulation treatment that leads to successful oocyte collection, further measures may be taken in the laboratory to improve pregnancy rates for PORs. The traditionally recommended procedure has been co-culture, where fertilized eggs are co-cultured in media with purified cells from the maternal uterine lining. In our program, we use cumulus co-culture in this set of women.

Assisted Hatching

Another postfertilization procedure that improves pregnancy rates in PORs is assisted hatching. A significant increase in pregnancy rates has been demonstrated when this procedure was utilized.

Collection of Oocytes over Multiple Cycles

Another strategy would be to collect embryos over several cycles, cryopreserve them and subsequently perform the embryo transfer after an adequate number of embryos are available.

Preimplantation Genetic Screening

Today with availability of aCGH analysis one can perform biopsies on trophectoderm using the same. The result of this is satisfactory then these euploid embryos can be transferred in POR patients after vitrification. However not many trials have been done with this respect except a few to render any significant conclusions.

In PORs, there is practically no risk of OHSS and therefore, a mild stimulation protocol is not a must. Once women are adequately stimulated and wish to conceive with their own eggs, oocyte retrieval and preimplantation genetic screening (PGS) may be continued even with very low number (<7) of embryos. Routine canceling of PGS cycles because of poor response should be reconsidered, especially for younger women.

When to Transfer?

It is indeed difficult to pinpoint the day of transfer in POR patients. Day 3 postretrieval transfers have shown to have no advantage over Day 2 with regards to clinical outcome. If one prolongs the embryos in *in vitro* culture, then one can select the better quality embryos with a higher chance of successful implantation.

It has been noticed that embryos of PORs are prone to arrest and damage when exposed to *in vitro* conditions.

Anti-Müllerian Hormone and Donor Oocytes

Recently, serum levels of AMH have gained popularity as a measure for ovarian reserve, partly because of its intra-cycle stability, where it appears superior to FSH in predicting oocyte yield and pregnancy potential in women undergoing ART.

It appears that reducing the AMH cut-off level below 1 ng/mL by itself does not improve the predictive capacity of pregnancy occurrence following IVF. Therefore, extremely low cut-off AMH values should not be used to exclude couples from IVF treatment. There have been encouraging studies in patients younger than 42 years of age who present with extremely low AMH levels to continue to pursue treatment after failed IVF procedures. Lehmann et al., advised counseling the patients about poor prognosis when levels were < 0.47 ng/mL (<3.3 pmol/L).

Some authors have reported that live birth rate is highest when AMH levels were > 2 ng/mL (>14.2 pmol/L), significantly lower when the levels reached 1 ng/mL (7.1 pmol/L), and 0% when the levels were -0.1 ng/mL (0.7 pmol/L).

PORs with many failed IVF cycles, or the ones who have a very poor prognosis prior to IVF, should be counseled appropriately and advised for either oocyte donation, adoption or to abandon fertility treatment.

Thus egg donation may be the mainstay of management in these women who have not conceived with various techniques of COH.

FUTURE PROSPECTS

It has become standard practice in assisted reproduction where IVM, cryopreservation of donor oocytes from multiple pick up cycles and donor oocyte freezing allowing for commercial egg banking.

Some of the novel interventions which seem to hold promise for the future are stem cell therapy, plasma rich protein (PRP) injection into ovaries and the techniques of augment, OvaPrime and OvaTure as therapies propagated by a company called OvaScience.

Stem cells have self-renewing and pluripotent functions. They can not only repair tissue cells but also regulate immune function. Thus, the role of the therapeutic potential of autologous mesenchymal bone marrow stem cells (BMSCs) transplantation in women with POF is being studied.

Plasma rich protein is a relatively new and promising regenerative therapeutic application which can offer several benefits without detrimental side effects as it is a direct product of one's own blood sample. PRP is rich in several growth factors that have a significant role in tissue regeneration. According to the latest research by Harvard scientists, PRP application to the ovarian cortex can possibly stimulate the germ cell lines into developing into ovarian oocytes. So far, there is only one published scientific document that has studied the effects of ovarian PRP infusion on eight perimenopausal women. According to the results of this study, following an ovarian PRP infusion, return of ovarian function was observed within 3 months in all women.

Energy-producing mitochondria from a woman's own egg precursor cells which are immature egg cells found in the protective ovarian lining, are added to the patient's mature eggs to supplement the existing mitochondria. Improved egg health may thus offer the potential for enhanced IVF. Commercially marketed as augment treatment, this is specifically designed to improve a woman's egg health.

OvaPrime treatment is a potential fertility treatment that could enable a woman to increase her egg reserve. This treatment is designed to transfer cells extracted from the protective outer lining of the ovary, isolated, and then reimplanted into the main part of the ovary, where they are projected to mature into healthy and viable eggs. Thus the procedure is designed to help women with a very low ovarian reserve.

In another program, called OvaTure, the method hopes eventually to perform IVF without hormones. Hormones are needed to stimulate a woman's ovary to release as many eggs as possible. With OvaTure, the woman would have some of her egg precursor cells removed, and cultured in the laboratory to mature into fully functional eggs, all without hormones. In this way, the side effects of hormone injections would be avoided. The last two techniques, however, are still in research.

CONCLUSION

Despite the two decades of attempts at improving results in PORs, there is still no international consensus for the definition of a poor responder and that the varying treatment strategies used, do not result in high pregnancy rates. Also one should remember that not all women who respond poorly to ovarian simulation have poor pregnancy rates.

Poor ovarian responders will keep challenging reproductive specialists until a scientific breakthrough is achieved that has the capability to restore the continuously depleting ovarian reserve with aging, that being the most common cause of the problem.

ACKNOWLEDGMENT

We would like to thank Mr Arvind Shirodkar for his excellent typing skills in preparing this manuscript.

EDITORS' COMMENTS

In this chapter, Drs Trupti Mehta and colleagues eloquently summarized the current knowledge about poor responders. They described the existing criteria and challenges to identify this prevalent patient population in our daily practice. Subsequently, they pointed out the main reasons explaining decreased ovarian reserve and consequently the POR. The authors also discussed the treatment options for this subset of women undergoing IVF.

Clinical trials using the current standards to define POR failed to show evidence in favor of a particular treatment modality. Also, critical factors for reproductive success, such as the age-dependent embryo aneuploidy rates and the intrinsic ovarian resistance to gonadotropin stimulation are not taken into consideration by the current POR criteria. As a result, the accepted definitions for POR have been criticized for their inadequacy concerning the proper patient characterization and for not providing clinicians a guide for therapeutic management.

The novel system to classify infertility patients with "expected" or "unexpected" inappropriate ovarian response to exogenous gonadotropins—the POSEIDON criteria—was developed to provide a more nuanced picture of POR and to guide physicians in the management of such patients.[1] The new standards are provoking as they challenge the current terminology of POR in favor of the newly defined concept of "low prognosis." Thus, the POSEIDON group proposes a change in the definition of POR, with subgrouping, resulting in more homogeneous populations. Hopefully, this new classification system will prove to be of daily help for clinicians as well as for patients, ultimately facilitating treatment and resulting in a shorter time to pregnancy and live birth.

REFERENCE

1. Esteves SC, Roque M, Bedoschi GM, et al. Defining low prognosis patients undergoing assisted reproductive technology: POSEIDON criteria—The Why. Front Endocrinol (Lausanne). 2018;9:461.

SUGGESTED READING

1. Al-Edani T, Assou S, Ferrieres A, et al. Female aging alters expression of human cumulus cells genes that are essential for oocyte quality. Biomed Res Int. 2014;2014:964614.
2. Al-Fozan H, Al-Khadouri M, Tan SL, et al. A randomized trial of letrozole versus clomiphene citrate in women undergoing superovulation. Fertil Steril. 2004;82:1561-3.
3. Al-Inany HG, Abou-Setta AM, Aboulghar MA, et al. Highly purified hMG achieves better pregnancy rates in IVF cycles but not ICSI cycles compared with recombinant FSH: a meta-analysis. Gynecol Endocrinol. 2009;25:372-8.
4. Alisch A, Roiha K, Finas D, et al. Extreme suppression of LH within 3 hours after GnRH-antagonist administration in COH: results of pulsatility pattern analysis. Hum Reprod. 2004;19:61.
5. Badawy A, Wageah A. Strategies for pituitary down-regulation to optimize IVF/ICSI outcome in Poor Ovarian Responders. J Reprod Infertil. 2012;13:124-30.
6. Bahceci M, Ulug U, Ciray HN, et al. Efficiency of changing the embryo transfer time from Day 3 to Day 2 among women with poor ovarian response: a prospective randomized trial. Fertil Steril. 2006;86:81-5.
7. Barasoain M, Barrenetxea G, Huert I, et al. Study of *FMR1* gene association with ovarian dysfunction in a sample from the Basque country. Gene. 2013;52:145-9.
8. Bassil S, Wyns C, Toussaint-Demylle D, et al. The relationship between ovarian vascularity and the duration of stimulation in in vitro fertilization. Hum Reprod. 1997;12:1240-5.
9. Ben-Meir A, Burstein E, Borrego-Alvarez A, et al. Coenzyme Q10 restores oocyte mitochondrial function and fertility during reproductive aging. Aging Cell. 2015;14:887-95.
10. Bentov Y, Casper RF. The aging oocyte-can mitochondrial function be improved? Fertil Steril. 2013;99:18-22.
11. Bleil ME, Greogorich SE, Adler NE, et al. Race/ethnic disparities in reproductive age: an examination of ovarian reserve estimates across four race/ethnic groups of healthy, regularly cycling women. Fertil Steril. 2014;101:199-207.
12. Blumenfeld Z, Amit T. The role of growth hormone (GH), GH receptor and GH-binding protein in reproduction and ovulation induction. J Pediatr Endocrinol Metabol. 1996;9:145-62.
13. Boots CE, Bernardi LA. Bologna criteria: clinically or academically relevant? Fertil Steril. 2018;109:59-60.
14. Bosdou JK, Venetis CA, Kolibianakis EM, et al. The use of androgens or androgen-modulating agents in poor responders undergoing in vitro fertilization: a systematic review and meta-analysis. Hum Reprod Update. 2012;18:127-45.
15. Brodin T, Hadziosmanovic N, Berglund L, et al. Anti-Müllerian hormone levels are strongly associated with live-birth rates after assisted reproduction. J Clin Endocrinol Metabol. 2013;98:1107-14.
16. Cabello E, Garrido P, Moran J, et al. Effects of resveratrol on ovarian response to controlled ovarian hyperstimulation in ob/ob mice. Fertil Steril. 2015;103:570-9.
17. Carlos M, Amparo R. Intracytoplasmic sperm injection as a routine indication in low responder patients. Hum Reprod. 1998;13:2126-9.
18. Chang EM, Han JE. Effect of estrogen priming through luteal phase and stimulation phase in poor responders in in vitro fertilization. J Assist Reprod Genet. 2012;29:225-30.
19. Chapel S. The Role of Mitochondria from Mature Oocyte to Viable Blastocyst. Obstet Gynecol Int. 2013;2013:18302.
20. Chin KV, Seifer DB, Feng B, et al. DNA microanalysis of the expression profiles of luteinized granulosa cells as a function of ovarian reserve. Fertil Steril. 2002;77:1214-8.
21. Cosgrave MP, Tyrrell J, McCarron M, et al. Age at onset of dementia and age of menopause in women with Down's syndrome. J Intellect Disabil Res. 1999;43:461-5.
22. Czuczwar P, Stepniak A, Wojciech W, et al. The influence of uterine artery embolization on ovarian reserve, fertility and pregnancy outcomes: a review of literature. Prz Menopauzalny. 2016;15:205-9.
23. D'Amato G, Caroppo E, Pasquadibisceglie A, et al. A novel protocol of ovulation induction with delayed gonadotropin-releasing hormone antagonist administration combined with high-dose recombinant follicle-stimulating hormone and clomiphene citrate for poor responders and women over 35 years. Fertil Steril. 2004;81:1572-7.
24. Davar R, Aflatoonian A. Clinical effects of a microdose GnRH agonist flare regimen administered to poor responders

undergoing ART cycles. Acta Medica Iranica. 2009;47: 263-7.
25. Dayal MB, Frankfurter D, Athanasiadis I, et al. Day 2 embryo transfer (ET) and day 3 ET afford similar reproductive outcomes in the poor responder. Fertil Steril. 2011;95:1130-2.
26. Desai SG, Cooper AR, Hagemann AR, et al. Assisted hatching may benefit young women with poor ovarian response. Fertil Steril. 2013;100:S506.
27. Desai SS, Roy BS, Mahale SD. Mutations and polymorphisms in FSH receptor: functional implications in human reproduction. Reproduction. 2013;146:R235-48.
28. Duffy JMN, Ahmad G, Mohiyiddeen L, Nardo LG, Watson A. Growth hormone for in vitro fertilization. Cochrane Database Syst Rev. 2010;(1):CD000099.
29. Edessey M, Hosni H. Stem cells transplantation in premature ovarian failure. World J Med Sci. 2014;10:12-16.
30. Elizur SE, Aslan D, Shulman A, et al. Modified natural cycle using GnRH antagonist can be an optional treatment in poor responders undergoing IVF. J Assist Reprod Genet. 2005; 22:75-9.
31. Faddy MJ, Gosden RG, Gougeon A, et al. Accelerated disappearance of ovarian follicles in mid-life: Implications for forecasting menopause. Hum Reprod. 1992;7:1342-6.
32. Fasouliotis SJ, Laufer N, Sabbagh-Ehrlich S, et al. Gonadotropin-releasing hormone (GnRH)-antagonist versus GnRH-agonist in ovarian stimulation of poor responders undergoing IVF. J Assist Reprod Genet. 2003;20:455-60.
33. Ferraretti AP, La Marca A, Fauser BC, et al. ESHRE consensus on the definition of 'poor response' to ovarian stimulation for in vitro fertilization: the Bologna criteria. Hum Reprod. 2011;26:1616-24.
34. Ficicioglu C, Kutlu T, Baglam E, et al. Early follicular anti-Müllerian hormone as an indicator of ovarian reserve. Fertil Steril. 2006;85:592-6.
35. Firns S, Cruzet VF, Keena KN, et al. The effect of cigarette smoking, alcohol consumption and fruit and vegetable consumption on IVF outcomes: a review and presentation of original data. Reprod Biol Endocrinol. 2015;13:134.
36. Frattarelli JL, Levi AJ, Miller BT, et al. A prospective assessment of the predictive value of basal antral follicles in in vitro fertilization cycles. Fertil Steril. 2003;80:350-5.
37. Freeman E, Gracias C, Sammel MD, et al. Association of anti-Müllerian hormone levels with obesity in late reproductive-age women. Fertil Steril. 2007;87:101-6.
38. Galey-Fontaine J, Cédrin-Durnerin I, Chaïbi R, et al. Age and ovarian reserve are distinct predictive factors of cycle outcome in low responders. Reprod Biomed Online. 2005;10:94-9.
39. Garcia JE, Jones GS, Acosta AA, et al. HMG/hCG follicular maturation for oocytes aspiration: Phase II, 1981. Fertil Steril. 1983;39:174-9.
40. Gelbaya TA, Kyrgiou M, Li TC, et al. Low-dose aspirin for in vitro fertilization: a systematic review and meta-analysis. Hum Reprod Update. 2007;13:357-64.
41. Gleicher N, Weghofer A, Barad DH. A pilot study of premature ovarian senescence: I. Correlation of triple CGG repeats on the *FMR1* gene to ovarian reserve parameters FSH and anti-Müllerian hormone. Fertil Steril. 2009;91:1700-6.
42. Goswami SK, Das T, Chattopadhyay R. A randomized single-blind controlled trial of letrozole as a low-cost IVF protocol in women with poor ovarian response: a preliminary report. Hum Reprod. 2004;19:2031-5.
43. Greene AD, Patounakis G, Segars JH. Genetic associations with diminished ovarian reserve: a systematic review of the literature. J Assist Reprod Genet. 2014;31:935-46.
44. Greenseid K, Jindal S, Hurwitz J, et al. Differential granulosa cell gene expression in young women with diminished ovarian reserve. Reprod Sci. 2011;18:892-9.
45. Hagerman R, Hagerman P. The fragile X permutation: into the phenotypic fold. Curr Opin Genet Dev. 2002;12:278-83.
46. Hans PS, Swarankar ML, Garg S, et al. Effect of tuberculosis on ovarian reserve of patients undergoing in vitro fertilization. Int J Infert Fetal Med. 2015;6:73-83.
47. Hansen KR, Knowlton NS, Thyer AC, et al. A new model of reproductive aging: The decline in non-growing follicular number from birth to menopause. Hum Reprod. 2008;23:699-708.
48. Hendricks DJ, Broekmans FJ, Bancsi LF, et al. Repeated clomiphene citrate challenge testing in the prediction of outcome in IVF: a comparison with basal markers for ovarian reserve. Hum Reprod. 2005;20:163-9.
49. Ho HY, Lee RK, Hwu YM, et al. Poor response of ovaries with endometrioma previously treated with cystectomy to controlled ovarian hyperstimulation. J Assist Reprod Genet. 2002;19:507-11.
50. Ho YK, Lee TH, Lee CI, et al. Effects of growth hormone plus gonadotropins on controlled ovarian stimulation in infertile women of advanced age, poor responders, and previous in vitro fertilization failure patients. Taiwanese J Obstet Gynecol. 2017;56:806-10.
51. Hull MG, Fleming CF, Hughes AO, et al. The age-related decline in female fecundity: a quantitative controlled study of implanting capacity and survival of individual embryos after in vitro fertilization. Fertil Steril. 1996;65:783-90.
52. Iglesias C, Banker M, Mahajan N, et al. Ethnicity as a determinant of ovarian reserve: differences in ovarian aging between Spanish and Indian women. Fertil Steril. 2014; 102(1):244-9.
53. Iwase A, Nakamura T, Nakahara T, et al. Anti-Müllerian hormone and assessment of ovarian reserve after ovarian toxic treatment: A systematic narrative review. Reprod Sci. 2015;22:519-26.
54. Jenkins JM, Davies DW, Devonport H. Comparison of 'poor' responders with 'good' responders using a standard buserelin/human menopausal gonadotropin regime for in vitro fertilization. Hum Reprod. 1991;6:918-21.
55. Jindal S. Greenseid K, Berger D, et al. Impaired gremlin 1 (GREM1) expression in cumulus cells in young women with diminished ovarian reserve (DOR). J Assist Reprod Genet. 2012;29:159-65.

56. Keay SD, Liversedge NH, Jenkins JM. Could ovarian infection impair ovarian response to gonadotropin stimulation? Br J Obstet Gynaecol. 1998;105:252-3.
57. Kedem A, Haas J, Geva LL, et al. Ongoing pregnancy rates in women with low and extremely low AMH levels. A multivariate analysis of 769 cycles. PLoS One. 2013;8:e81629.
58. Keltz M, Gera PS, Skorupski J, et al. Comparison of FSH flare with and without pretreatment with oral contraceptive pills in poor responders undergoing in vitro fertilization. Fertil Steril. 2007;88:350-53.
59. Keltz M, Sauerbrun-Cutler MT, Breborowicz A. Managing poor responders in IVF. Expert Rev Obstet Gynecol. 2013;8:121-34.
60. Kyrou D, Kolibianakis EM, Venetis CA, et al. How to improve the probability of pregnancy in poor responders undergoing in vitro fertilization: a systematic review and meta-analysis. Fertil Steril. 2009;91:749-66.
61. Laverge H, De Sutter P, Van der Elst J, et al. A prospective, randomized study comparing day 2 and day 3 embryo transfer in human IVF. Hum Reprod. 2001;16:476-80.
62. Lehmann P, Velez MP, Saumet J, et al. Anti-Müllerian hormone (AMH): a reliable biomarker of oocyte quality in IVF. J Assisted Reprod Genet. 2014;31:493-8.
63. Lindheim SR, Barad DH, Witt B, et al. Short-term gonadotropin suppression with oral contraceptives benefits poor responders prior to controlled ovarian hyperstimulation. J Assist Reprod Genet. 1996;13:745-7.
64. Loh S, Wang JX, Mathews CD. The influence of body mass index basal FSH and age on the response to gonadotropin stimulation in non-polycystic ovarian syndrome patients. Hum Reprod. 2002;17:1207-11.
65. Loutradis D, Patsoula E, Minas V, et al. FSH receptor gene polymorphisms have a role for different ovarian response to stimulation in patients entering IVF/ICSI-ET programs. J Assist Reprod Genet. 2006;23:177-84.
66. Lukaszuk K, Liss J, Kunicki M, et al. Anti-Müllerian hormone (AMH) is a strong predictor of live birth in women undergoing assisted reproductive technology. Reprod Biol. 2014;14: 176-81.
67. Luterman J, White Yvonne AR. Preclinical data support the safety of egg precursor cell repositioning using a method designed to address poor response to controlled ovarian stimulation. Ovascience Inc. Mid-west Reproductive Symposium International; 2017.
68. M'Rabet N, Moffat R, Helbling S, et al. The CC-allele of the Pvu11 polymorphic variant in intron 1 of the α-estrogen receptor gene is significantly more prevalent among infertile women at risk of premature ovarian aging. Fertil Steril. 2012;98:965-72.
69. Madani T, Ashrafi M, Yeganeh LM. Comparison of different stimulation protocols efficacy in poor responders undergoing IVF: a retrospective study. Gynecol Endocrinol. 2012;28: 102-5.
70. Malhotra N, Sharma V, Bahadur A, et al. The effect of tuberculosis on ovarian reserve among women undergoing IVF in India. Int J Gynaecol Obstet. 2012;117:40-4.
71. Martinez F, Barn PN, Coroleu B, et al. Women with poor response to IVF have lowered circulating gonadotropin surge-attenuating factor bioactivity during spontaneous and stimulated cycles. Hum Reprod. 2002;17:634-40.
72. Min JK, Claman P. Oral Contraceptive (OC) Pre-treatment Does not Influence Oocyte Yield in Poor Responders Undergoing Gonadotropin Releasing Hormone (GnRH) Antagonist Cycles for In Vitro Fertilization (IVF). Oral presentation.O-109. Fertil Steril. 2005;84:S45-6.
73. Mochtar MH, Van der Veen, Ziech M, et al. Recombinant luteinizing hormone (rLH) for controlled ovarian hyperstimulation in assisted reproductive cycles. Cochrane Database Syst Rev. 2007;18:CD005070.
74. Mohsen IA, El Din RE. Minimal stimulation protocol using letrozole versus microdose flare up GnRH agonist protocol in women with poor ovarian response undergoing ICSI. Gynecol Endocrinol. 2013;29:105-8.
75. Molinari E, Bar H, Pyle AM, et al. Transcriptome analysis of human cumulus cells reveals hypoxia as the main determinant of follicular senescence. Mol Hum Reprod. 2016;22:866-76.
76. Morgia F, Sbracia M, Schimberni M. A controlled trial of natural cycle versus microdose gonadotropin-releasing hormone analog flare cycles in poor responders undergoing in vitro fertilization. Fertil Steril. 2004;81:1542-7.
77. Moy V, Jindal S, Lieman H, et al. Obesity adversely affects Serum anti-Müllerian hormone (AMH) levels in Caucasian women. J Assist Reprod Genet. 2015;32:1305-11.
78. Nargund G, Bromhan D. Comparison of endocrinological and clinical profiles and outcomes of IVF cycles in patients with one ovary and two ovaries. J Assist Reprod Genet. 1995;12:458-60.
79. Nelson SM. Biomarkers of ovarian response: current and future applications. Fertil Steril. 2013;99:963-9.
80. Pantos K, Nitsos N, Kokkali G, et al. Ovarian rejuvenation and folliculogenesis reactivation in peri-menopausal women after autologous platelet-rich plasma treatment. Proceedings of the 32nd Annual Meeting of ESHRE: Helsinki, Finland; 2016.
81. Parikh FR, Nadkarni SG, Naik NJ, et al. Cumulus co-culture and cumulus-aided embryo transfer increases pregnancy rates in patients undergoing in vitro fertilization. Fertil Steril. 2006;86:839-47.
82. Pellicer A, Albert C, Mercader A, et al. The follicular and endocrine environment in women with endometriosis: local and systemic cytokine production. Fertil Steril. 1998;70: 425-31.
83. Pires E, Parikh FR, Khole VV. Can anti-ovarian antibody testing be useful in an IVF-ET clinic? J Assist Reprod Genet. 2011;28:55-64.
84. Pogacnik R, Vrtovec H, Ihan A, et al. Possible role of autoimmunity in patients with Premature Ovarian Insufficiency. Int J Fert Steril. 2014;7:281-90.

85. Polyzos NP, Devroey P. A systematic review of randomized trials for the treatment of poor ovarian responders: is there any light at the end of the tunnel? Fertil Steril. 2011;96:1058-61. e7.
86. POSEIDON Group (Patient-Oriented Strategies Encompassing IndividualizeD Oocyte Number), Alviggi C, Andersen CY, et al. A new more detailed stratification of low responders to ovarian stimulation: from a poor ovarian response to a low prognosis concept. Fertil Steril. 2016;105:1452-3.
87. Practice Committee of the American Society for Reproductive Medicine. Testing and interpreting measures of ovarian reserve: a committee opinion. Fertil Steril. 2015;103:e9-17.
88. Practice Committee of the American Society for Reproductive Medicine. Diagnostic Evaluation of the infertile female: a committee opinion. Fertil Steril. 2015;103:e 44-50.
89. Schoolcraft WB, Fragouli E. Clinical application of comprehensive chromosomal screening at the blastocyst stage. Fertil Steril. 2010;94:1700-6.
90. Scott RT, Navot D. Enhancement of ovarian responsiveness with microdoses of gonadotropin-releasing hormone agonist during ovulation induction for in vitro fertilization. Fertil Steril. 1994;61:880-5.
91. Sharara FI, Beatse SN, Leonardi MR, et al. Cigarette smoking accelerates the development of diminished ovarian reserve as evidenced by the clomiphene citrate challenge test. Fertil Steril. 1994;62:257-62.
92. Siristatidis CS, Hamilton MP. What should be the maximum FSH dose in IVF/ICSI in poor responders? J Obstet Gynaecol. 2007;27:401-5.
93. Skiadas CC, Duan S, Correll M, et al. Ovarian reserve status in young women is associated with altered gene expression in membrana granulosa cells. Mol Hum Reprod. 2012;18:362-71.
94. Smotrich DB, Widra EA, Gindoff PR, et al. Prognostic value of day 3 estradiol on in vitro fertilization outcomes. Fertil Steril. 1995;64:1136-40.
95. Talwar P, Verma S, Nayar KA, et al. Poor Ovarian Responders. E Bulletin ARText:3, Volume III. Indian Fertility Society; 2017.
96. Te Velde ER, Pearson PL. The variability of female reproductive ageing. Hum Reprod Update. 2002;8:141-54.
97. Tur-Kaspa I. The management of poor responder for IVF with PGD. Institute for Human Reproduction (IHR) and IVF-PGD Program, 10th International Congress on Preimplantation Genetic Diagnosis C-33. Reproductive Genetics Institute, Chicago, IL: USA; 2010.
98. Ubaldi F, Vaiarelli A, D'Anna R, et al. Management of poor responders in IVF: Is there anything new? Biomed Res Int. 2014;2014: 352098.
99. Urman B, Yakin K. DHEA for poor responders: can treatment be justified in absence of evidence? Reprod Biomed Online. 2012;25:103-7.
100. Wang TT, Wu YT, Dong MY, et al. G546A polymorphism of growth differentiation factor-9 contributes to the poor outcome of ovarian stimulation in women with diminished ovarian reserve. Fertil Steril. 2010;94:2490-2.
101. Weghofer A, Margreiter M, Bassim S, et al. Minimal stimulation using recombinant follicle-stimulating hormone and a gonadotropin-releasing hormone antagonist in women of advanced age. Fertil Steril. 2004;81:1002-6.
102. Wu YG, Barad DH, Kushnin VA, et al. Age-related premature luteinization of granulosa cells is avoided by early oocyte retrieval. J Endocrinol. 2015;226:167-80.
103. Xu Y, Nisenblat V, Lu C, et al. Pretreatment with coenzyme Q10 improves ovarian response and embryo quality in low-prognosis young women with decreased ovarian reserve: a randomized controlled trial. Reprod Biol Endocrinol. 2018;16:29.
104. Yadava BJ, Bhandari HM. Effective treatment protocol for poor ovarian response: a systematic review and meta-analysis. J Hum Reprod Sci. 2016;9:70-81.
105. Youssef Mohamed AF, Wely Madelon V. Low dosing of gonadotropins in in vitro fertilization cycles for women with poor ovarian reserve: systematic review and meta-analysis. Fertil Steril. 2018;109:289-301.
106. Zama AM, Uzumcu M. Epigenetic effects of endocrine-disrupting chemicals on female reproduction: an ovarian perspective. Front Neuroendocrinol. 2010;31:420-39.

4

CHAPTER

IVF Lite: Is this the Future of Assisted Reproductive Technology?

Gautam Nand Allahbadia, Goral Gandhi, Akanksha Allahbadia Gupta, Maham AS

INTRODUCTION

Infertility is one of the major medical problems in the western world caused by genetic or epigenetic factors, or both, which has led to continuous research and advancements in the field of assisted reproductive technology (ART). Many stimulation protocols are available for controlled ovarian hyperstimulation (COH) in *in vitro* fertilization (IVF). An inverse relationship between oocyte efficiency and ovarian response was reported in conventional IVF. The purpose of a new study by Zhang et al. was to report metaphase II (MII) oocyte efficiency according to oocyte yield in minimal/mild-stimulation IVF (mIVF) and to assess whether oocyte yield affects live birth rate (LBR). Infertile women ($n = 264$) aged <39 years old with normal ovarian reserve who had mIVF were recruited. All participants received the same protocol for ovarian stimulation. All the embryos were cultured to the blastocyst stage and vitrified using a freeze-all approach. This was followed by a single blastocyst transferred to each participant in subsequent cycles over a 6-month period. Ovarian response was categorized according to the number of MII oocyte yield (low: 1–2, intermediate: 3–6, and high: ≥7 MII oocytes). MII oocyte utilization rate was calculated as the number of live births divided by the number of MII oocytes produced after only one oocyte retrieval and subsequent transfers of vitrified/warmed blastocysts. The main outcome measure was cumulative LBR over a 6-month period. Among all the participants, 1,173 total retrieved oocytes (4.4 ± 0.2 per patient) resulted in 1,019 (3.9 ± 0.2 per patient) total MII oocytes, a clinical pregnancy rate (PR) of 48.1% and a LBR of 41.2%. Oocyte utilization rate was inversely related to ovarian response where it was 30.3% in the "low" versus 9.3% in the "intermediate" versus 4.3% in the "high" oocyte yield groups ($p < 0.05$). Implantation rate significantly dropped as the number of MII oocytes increased and was highest in the "low" oocyte yield group ($p < 0.0001$). Cumulative LBR was similar in "low", "intermediate", and "high" oocyte yield groups ($p > 0.05$). The number of MII oocytes had poor sensitivity and specificity for predicting a live birth. These data extend the hypothesis of oocyte efficiency reported in conventional IVF protocols to mIVF protocols.

Why more is less and less is more?

It has been proven that the use of high-gonadotropin dose does not necessarily improve the final outcome of IVF. Mild ovarian stimulation is based on the principle of optimal utilization of competent oocytes/embryos and endometrial receptivity. There is growing evidence that the pregnancy or LBRs with mild-stimulation protocols are comparable to those with conventional IVF; the cumulative pregnancy outcome has been shown to be no different, despite having fewer numbers of oocytes or embryos available with milder ovarian stimulation. Although equally effective, mild-stimulation IVF is associated with a greater safety profile, in terms of the incidence of ovarian hyperstimulation syndrome (OHSS) and venous thromboembolism. It is also found to be better tolerated by patients and less expensive. Emerging research evidence may lead to widespread acceptance of mild IVF, by both patients and IVF providers, and make IVF more accessible to women and couples worldwide.

Blumenfeld searched the pertinent English literature (PubMed) addressing mild stimulation for IVF/ART and publications addressing "mild" or "soft" controlled ovarian stimulation (COS) versus conventional COS for IVF, OHSS, natural cycle IVF, and IVF outcome in association with COS. Four possible mechanisms can be put forward to explain the apparent paradox of "less is more". (1) In the natural- or mild-stimulation cycles, the healthiest follicles are selected by the principle of "quality for quantity"; (2) high estradiol (E2) in the late follicular phase significantly correlated with higher rates of small for gestational age (SGA) and low-birth-weight (LBW) neonates; (3) anti-Müllerian hormone (AMH), luteinizing hormone (LH), testosterone, and E2 are significantly higher in natural cycle (NC)-IVF than in stimulated IVF follicles, suggesting an alteration of the follicular metabolism in stimulated cycles; and (4) supraphysiological E2 may increase the growth hormone-binding protein (GHBP) by neutralizing GH and diminishing the resultant insulin-like growth factor (IGF) levels, necessary for optimal synergism with follicle-stimulating hormone (FSH). The author suggested to aim at the retrieval of around eight to ten eggs. Mild stimulation should be the common practice for IVF. In cases where more than ten ova are retrieved or high E2 levels are reached, either intentionally or unintentionally, "freeze-all policy" should be considered and embryo transfer (ET) done in a subsequent natural cycle.

Baker et al. published a retrospective study to evaluate the correlation between total gonadotropin dose and LBR. A total of 658,519 fresh autologous cycles of IVF were reported to the Society for Assisted Reproductive Technology from 2004 to 2012. Logistic regression models were fitted to LBRs with the use of categorized values for total FSH dose and number of oocytes retrieved as the primary predictor variables. To reduce the effect of the most significant confounders that may lead physicians to prescribe higher doses of FSH, additional analyses were performed limited to good-prognosis patients (<35 years of age, body mass index <30 kg/m^2, and no diagnosis of diminished ovarian reserve, endometriosis, or ovulatory disorder) and including duration of gonadotropin treatment. LBR significantly decreased with increasing FSH dose, regardless of the number of oocytes retrieved. The statistically significant decrease in LBR with increasing FSH dose remained in patients with good prognosis, and regardless of female age, except for women aged ≥35 years with 1–5 oocytes retrieved. This analysis suggests that physicians may wish to avoid prescribing a high dose of FSH.

UAE PERSPECTIVE

In the UAE, for the last decade, IVF clinics were allowed to cryopreserve only gametes and not embryos. This law has changed this year and the clinics can now take individual patient permissions to freeze embryos from the Ministry of Health, UAE. Over the past decade in contradiction to the world, IVF laboratories were vitrifying oocytes and accumulating them in cases of poor responders and older women. IVF Lite in the country was done using oocyte accumulation and segmented IVF with or without genetic screening. When the requisite number was collected over multiple egg retrievals, the oocytes were thawed and injected and the generated embryos were either transferred directly or subjected to preimplantation genetic screening (PGS) and then screened euploid embryos transferred. The efficiency of a good vitrification system continued giving the UAE clinics results comparable to embryo vitrification over the last decade. The rate-limiting step was the method used and the training and experience of the laboratory staff. From 2014, we were using published data to counsel our patients about the noninferiority status of oocyte vitrification at the time of recruiting them for IVF Lite.

The aim of a prospective observational study by Herero et al. was to compare multiple embryological and pregnancy outcomes for vitrified oocytes against the same outcomes using vitrified embryos in patients at risk for OHSS. 96 patients were included and allocated to vitrification of oocytes (Group 1) or embryos (Group 2). No statistical differences in baseline characteristics between groups were detected. No differences were observed in outcomes according to vitrification timing. Oocyte vitrification achieved the same LBR as embryo vitrification.

The aim of an American study was to report the oocyte-freezing experience in women aged 40 years and older at a single fertility center. 158 women (mean age 43.9 ± 0.2) who underwent minimal ovarian stimulation IVF were enrolled. IVF protocol included the use of clomiphene citrate (CC) (50 mg/day) or letrozole (2.5 mg/day) with or without low-dose gonadotropins (started at 75 IU/day and increased as needed to 150 IU/day). 584 retrieved oocytes (2.1 ± 0.15 per patient) yielded 532 mature MII oocytes that were frozen. After thawing and fertilization by ICSI, a total of 344 embryos (1.9 ± 0.1 per patient) were formed. A total of 57 relatively good embryos were transferred and yielded three live births (5.3% per embryo transfer), three spontaneous abortions, and one chemical pregnancy. These data are important in counseling older women who desire autologous oocyte freezing.

RATIONALE OF DEFERRED EMBRYO TRANSFER

The rationale of a deferred ET whether following a conventional stimulation of a minimal stimulation is the same. Roque et al. setup a prospective study to compare IVF outcomes between fresh ET and frozen-thawed ET (the "freeze-all" policy), with fresh ET performed only in cases without progesterone (P) elevation. A total of 530 patients submitted to COS with a gonadotropin-releasing hormone (GnRH) antagonist protocol, and cleavage stage, Day 3 ET. A total of 530 cycles were included in the analysis: 351 in the fresh ET group (when P levels were ≤1.5 ng/mL on the trigger day); and 179 cycles in the freeze-all group (ET performed after endometrial priming with estradiol valerate, at 6 mg/day, taken orally). For the fresh ET group versus the freeze-all group, the implantation rate was 19.9% and 26.5%; clinical PR was 35.9% and 46.4%, respectively; and ongoing PR was 31.1% and 39.7%. The IVF outcomes were significantly better in the group using the freeze-all policy, compared with the group using fresh ET. These results suggest that even in a selected group of patients who underwent fresh ET (P levels ≤1.5 ng/mL), endometrial receptivity may have been impaired by COS, and outcomes may be improved by using the freeze-all policy.

MODIFIED NATURAL CYCLE IVF

The first live birth after IVF was achieved in a purely natural cycle. Because early attempts at IVF were associated with low efficiency, ovarian stimulation was added to achieve a greater margin for error in oocyte retrieval, fertilization, and thus, overall pregnancy success. As technology improved, the intuitive appeal of the natural cycle led investigators to once again attempt IVF without antecedent gonadotropin stimulation. Triggering of ovulation with human chorionic gonadotropin (hCG) was added to allow for accurate scheduling of oocyte retrieval and thus increased oocyte yield. When GnRH antagonists became available, premature ovulations could be prevented, albeit at the cost of adding some form of ovarian stimulation to continue follicle development until ovulation triggering. This type of cycle came to be known as the "modified natural cycle" (MNC-IVF). These modified natural IVF cycles are associated with decreased medication costs; they produce acceptable PRs and they may be particularly appropriate for patients at increased risk of OHSS, poor responders, and those wishing to avoid supernumerary embryo production. In MNC-IVF, spontaneous ovulation is prevented with a minimal amount of hormones and spontaneous monofollicular growth is supported. As a result, there is no risk of OHSS, and the risk of a multiple pregnancy is low. There is a 9.1% chance of pregnancy after one MNC-cycle and the cumulative PR after a maximum of six MNC-IVF cycles is 33.4%. The cumulative results of a maximum of six MNC-IVF cycles are comparable to those of the first COS-IVF treatment cycle including transfer of cryopreserved embryos produced as a result of the treatment (33.4% versus 37.7%). The risk of a twin pregnancy following MNC-IVF is 0.1%, and 18.3% following COS-IVF. This means that MNC-IVF is a good alternative for COS-IVF.

A Korean prospective randomized study was performed to investigate the effectiveness of minimal stimulation using recombinant human FSH (rhFSH) and GnRH antagonist compared with GnRH antagonist multiple-dose protocol (MDP) in low responders undergoing IVF/ICSI. The study demonstrated that minimal stimulation in natural cycles provides similar PRs to the GnRH antagonist MDP with fewer dose and days of rhFSH used and thus can be a cost-effective alternative as a last chance before oocyte donation in low responders.

CLOMIPHENE CITRATE OR LETROZOLE

There has been increasing interest in combining the oral agents CC and letrozole with gonadotropins in IVF—for poor responders to reduce the amount of gonadotropins used, and in normal responders to reduce the incidence of OHSS. In normal responders, mild stimulation with the use of CC and gonadotropins was found to decrease the number of oocytes retrieved and result in good PRs, but in most studies, the cumulative PR was lower compared with conventional ovarian stimulation when frozen embryo transfers were considered. Coadministration of letrozole and gonadotropins has mainly been used in patients with breast cancer to prevent the massive elevation of serum E2 concentrations with the use of standard COH. CC and letrozole have both been used with gonadotropins in poor responders and have been shown to reduce the amount of gonadotropin used without reducing the PR. Letrozole use with gonadotropins in IVF cycles may increase endometrial receptivity by increasing integrin expression in the endometrium and by lowering estrogen concentrations to more physiologic levels.

The objective of study by Rose et al. was to compare the use of CC and letrozole in an IVF setting in which the objective was to produce only one or two embryos. Either CC or letrozole was used in conjunction with gonadotropins without the use of GnRH antagonists. Sixty-two patients received either CC or letrozole with low-dose gonadotropins in 128 non-randomized treatment cycles. hCG was given when one follicle was at least 17 mm. Oocyte retrieval was done 34 hours later and fertilization was performed using ICSI. There were no statistically significant differences in the number of large follicles produced, oocytes fertilized, endometrial thickness, clinical PRs, or delivery rates in patients taking letrozole compared to CC. More mature oocytes were retrieved after CC, but a subset analysis of patients undergoing both treatments did not support this difference. The only statistically different finding in both analyses was the peak estradiol levels during treatment, which averaged 516 pg/mL with letrozole and 797 pg/mL with CC ($p = 0.005$). Overall, the cancellation rate due to a premature LH surge was 5%. An average of 2.8 mature oocytes were recovered, 2.1 oocytes were fertilized, and 1.6 embryos were transferred. The overall clinical PR per transfer was 25% [95% confidence interval (CI) 17.7–33.3%] and the overall LBR per transfer was 19.2% (95% CI, 11.6–26.8%). Other than peak estradiol levels, there were no clinically significant differences when letrozole or CC was used for mild ovarian stimulation for IVF. There were only rare cancellations because of premature LH surges.

MILD STIMULATION VERSUS CONVENTIONAL STIMULATION FOR IVF

Lazer et al. examined whether treatment with minimum-dose stimulation (MS) protocol enhances clinical PRs compared to high-dose stimulation (HS) protocol. A retrospective cohort study was performed by comparing IVF and pregnancy outcomes between MS and HS gonadotropin-antagonist protocol for patients with poor ovarian reserve. Inclusion criteria included patients with an AMH ≤8 pmol/L and/or antral follicle count (AFC) ≤5 on Days 2–3 of the cycle. Patients in 2008 exclusively had a HS protocol treatment, while patients in 2010 had treatment with a MS protocol exclusively. The MS protocol involved letrozole at 2.5 mg over 5 days, starting from Day 2, overlapping with gonadotropins, starting from the 3rd day of letrozole at 150 units daily. GnRH antagonist was introduced once one or more follicles reached 14 mm or larger. The HS group received gonadotropins (≥300 IU/day) throughout their antagonist cycle. Clinical PR was significantly higher in the MS protocol compared to the HS protocol ($p = 0.007$). Furthermore, the live birth rate was significantly higher in the MS group compared to the HS group ($p = 0.034$). In conclusion, the MS IVF protocol is less expensive (lower gonadotropin dosage) and resulted in a higher clinical PR and LBR than a HS protocol for poor responders.

Zhang et al. performed a randomized noninferiority controlled trial with a prespecified border of 10% that compared 1 cycle of mini-IVF with single-embryo transfer (SET) with 1 cycle of conventional IVF with double-embryo transfer. Around 564 infertile women (<39 years old) who were undergoing their first IVF cycle were allocated randomly to either mini-IVF or conventional IVF. The primary outcome was cumulative LBR per woman over a 6-month period. Secondary outcomes included OHSS, multiple PRs, and gonadotropin use. The primary outcome was cumulative live birth per randomized woman within a time horizon of 6 months. 564 couples were assigned randomly between February, 2009 and August, 2013 with 285 couples allocated to mini-IVF and 279 couples allocated to conventional IVF. The cumulative LBR was 49% (140/285) for mini-IVF and 63% (176/279) for conventional IVF [relative risk (RR), 0.76; 95% CI, 0.64–0.89]. There were no cases of OHSS after mini-IVF compared with 16 moderate/severe OHSS cases (5.7%) after conventional IVF. The multiple PRs were 6.4% in mini-*IVF* compared with 32% in conventional IVF (RR, 0.25; 95% CI, 0.14–0.46). Gonadotropin consumption was significantly lower with mini-IVF compared with conventional IVF (459 ± 131 vs 2079 ± 389 IU; $p < 0.0001$). Compared with conventional IVF with double-embryo transfer, mini-IVF with SET lowers LBRs, completely eliminates OHSS, reduces multiple PRs, and reduces gonadotropin consumption.

POOR OVARIAN RESERVE

Pilehvari et al. setup a study to compare the pregnancy outcomes achieved by IVF between minimal stimulation and conventional antagonist protocols in poor ovarian responders (PORs). In this randomized controlled trial, 77 PORs undergoing IVF were selected and divided into two groups. First group was the minimal stimulation group ($n = 42$) receiving 100 mg/day CC on Day 2 of the cycle for 5 day that was followed by 150 IU/day human menopausal gonadotropin (hMG) on Day 5 of the cycle. Second group was the conventional group ($n = 35$) receiving at least 300 IU/day gonadotropin on Day 2 of the cycle. GnRH antagonist protocol was applied for both groups according to flexible protocol. Number of retrieved oocytes and chemical PR were the main outcomes. There was no difference in number of retrieved oocyte and PR (2.79 ± 1.96 vs 2.20 ± 1.71 and 5.6% vs 4.1%; $p > 0.05$) between both groups. The gonadotropin dose used in the minimal stimulation group was lower than conventional group (1,046 ± 596 vs 2,806 ± 583). Minimal stimulation protocol with lower gonadotropin used is likely to be considered as a patient-friendly and cost-effective substitute for PORs.

A recent study compared the IVF outcomes of letrozole/antagonist and microdose GnRH agonist flare up protocols in PORs undergoing ICSI. 60 proven POR patients were randomized by computer-generated list to receive either letrozole/antagonist (mild stimulation) $n = 30$ or GnRHa protocol (microdose flare) $n = 30$. Both groups were similar with respect to background and hormonal characteristics (age, duration of infertility, BMI, FSH, LH, and E2). The clinical PR per cycle was similar in both groups (13.3 vs 16.6%; OR = 0.769; 95% CI = 0.185, 3.198). The doses of used gonadotropins and the number of stimulation days were significantly lower in the letrozole/antagonist protocol. The peak E2 level on the day of hCG, the endometrial thickness, the retrieved oocytes, the number of fertilized oocytes, the number of transferred embryos, and the cancellation rate were statistically similar in both groups. The letrozole/antagonist protocol is a cost-effective and patient-friendly protocol that may be used in PORs for IVF/ICSI.

The objective of a French study was to assess the reproductive competence of oocytes obtained by follicular flushing in poor responder patients. This prospective comparative study, at the University of Paris XI, Assistance Publique des Hopitaux de Paris, INSERM Unit 782, was performed on 165 infertile IVF embryo transfer candidates. A total of 271 consecutive minimal stimulation IVF (msIVF) cycles were studied. Oocyte retrieval was performed 34 hours after hCG administration and oocytes were allocated into two groups according to their retrieval method: oocytes obtained in the first follicular aspiration (FA, $n = 127$) and oocytes retrieved in the subsequent follicular flushing (FF, $n = 102$). The principal outcome was to evaluate clinical pregnancy and embryo implantation rates. Thus, patient characteristics, fertilization rate, and clinical PR per oocyte were comparable in both of groups. In contrast, embryo morphology (41% vs 59%, $p < 0.01$) and implantation rates (20.4% vs 34.8%, $p < 0.04$) were better in the FF group. In conclusion, an optimal reproductive competence was observed in oocytes retrieved by follicular flushing in msIVF in poor responder patients.

The use of progestin (P) during ovarian stimulation is effective in blocking the LH surge in women with normal ovarian reserve; however, its effects have not been determined in poor responders. A recent study by Chen et al. aimed to explore the follicular dynamics in P-primed minimal stimulation in poor responders. A total of 204 infertile women with diminished ovarian reserve were allocated into the medroxyprogesterone acetate (MPA) group or the natural cycle control group in an alternating order. MPA (10 mg) was administered daily beginning from the early follicular phase and a low dose of hMG was added in the late follicular phase, if the serum FSH level was lower than 8.0 mIU/mL. When a dominant follicle reached maturity, triptorelin 100 µg and hCG 1,000 IU were used for trigger, and oocytes were retrieved 34–36 hours later. All viable embryos were cryopreserved for subsequent frozen embryo transfer. Natural cycle IVF was used as controls. Compared with the natural cycle group, the MPA group exhibited a larger preovulatory follicle (18.7 ± 1.8 mm vs 17.2 ± 2.2 mm), a longer follicular phase (13.6 ± 3.6 days vs 12.3 ± 3.2 days), and higher peak estradiol values (403.88 ± 167.16 vs 265.26 ± 122.16 pg/mL), while maintaining lower LH values ($p < 0.05$). The incidences of spontaneous LH surge and premature ovulation decreased significantly (1.0% vs 50% and 2% vs 10.8%, respectively; $p < 0.05$). A greater number of oocytes and viable embryos were harvested from the MPA group than from the natural cycle group ($p < 0.05$). Moreover, the clinical PR was slightly higher in the MPA group than in the natural cycle controls, but the difference was not significant (11.8% vs 5.9%, $p > 0.05$). This study supported the hypothesis that P-primed minimal stimulation achieved ovulation control of the dominant follicle and did not adversely affect the quality of oocytes in poor responders. Therefore, P-priming is a promising approach to overcome premature ovulation in minimal stimulation for poor responders.

OLDER WOMEN

There were few reports about infertile women aged 45 years and above undergoing IVF/ICSI. Yan et al. reported the case of a 49-year-old woman who delivered twins after ICSI using autologous oocytes with mild ovarian stimulation. The patient was presented with 26-year primary infertility caused by bilateral fallopian tube obstruction and severe oligoasthenozoospermia in her husband. She was given a mild ovarian stimulation cycle of CC and low-dose FSH with ICSI, and two blastocysts were transferred. Twins were delivered by cesarean section at 37 weeks for moderate pregnancy-induced hypertension.

For women of advanced age with abnormally increased FSH levels, standardized hormonal stimulation often represents a cost-intensive procedure with a low success rate. It is well established now that with mild ovarian stimulation, there is a greater percentage of good-quality eggs (although a smaller number) than with higher-dose conventional stimulation. Mild-stimulation protocols reduce the mean number of days of stimulation, the total amount of gonadotropins used, and the mean number of oocytes retrieved. The proportion of high-quality and euploid embryos seems to be higher compared with conventional stimulation protocols, and the PR per embryo transfer is comparable. Moreover, the reduced costs, the better tolerability for patients, and the less time needed to complete an IVF cycle make mild approaches clinically and cost-effective over a given period of time. The low number of embryos available for transfer poses a great challenge in the management of older women going in for IVF. A potential management of these older women is to create a sufficient pool of embryos by accumulating vitrified good-grade embryos over several minimal stimulation and modified natural cycles. At the end of the accumulation process, these embryos can be subjected to a PGS using next-generation sequencing and then the pool would have only chromosomal normal embryos with maximal chances of implantation. This would potentially make the chances of success for older women similar to normal responders. This management, however, is unthinkable without an outstanding vitrification program. The option of accumulating embryos has become a promising reality with the advent of vitrification technologies.

MINIMAL STIMULATION AND SINGLE-EMBRYO TRANSFER WITH SEGMENTED IVF

In Zhang's series, patients were not denied the treatment based on their Day 3 FSH value or ovarian reserve. Yet, very acceptable PRs were achieved (20% for fresh embryo transfers and 41% for cryopreserved embryo transfers). These results strengthen the argument for a mini-IVF protocol and vitrification as an alternative to standard conventional IVF stimulation protocols.

A retrospective, cohort study was performed in private infertility center to evaluate the embryological and clinical results of a large exclusively SET program according to patient's age (≤29, 30–34, 35–39, 40–44, and ≥45 years). A total of 7,244 infertile patients had undergone 20,244 cycles with a clomiphene-based minimal stimulation or natural cycle IVF protocol during 2008. Following oocyte retrieval, fertilization, and embryo culture, a total of 10,401 fresh or frozen SET procedures were performed involving cleavage-stage embryos or blastocysts. Successful oocyte retrieval rate (78.0%) showed no age-dependent decrease until 45 years. Fertilization (80.3%) and cleavage (91.1%) rates were not significantly different between age groups. Blastocyst formation (70.1–22.8%) and overall LBRs (35.9–2%) showed an age-dependent decrease. Frozen-thawed blastocyst transfer cycles gave the highest chance of live birth per embryo transfer (41.3–6.1%). High-fertilization and cleavage rates were obtained regardless of age, whereas blastocyst formation and LBRs showed an age-dependent decrease. An elective SET program based on a minimal ovarian stimulation protocol yields acceptable LBRs per embryo transfer in infertile patients up until their mid-40s. However, in very advanced age patients (≥ 45 years old), success rates fall below 1%.

A 3-year, retrospective, single-center cohort study was conducted in a private infertility center to determine cumulative LBRs per scheduled oocyte retrieval following minimal ovarian stimulation/natural cycle IVF in unselected infertile patients. A total of 727 consecutive infertile patients were analyzed who underwent 2,876 (median 4) cycles with scheduled oocyte retrieval from November, 2008 to December, 2011. Natural cycle IVF or clomiphene-based minimal ovarian stimulation was coupled with SET and increased use of delayed vitrified-warmed blastocyst transfer. Main outcome measures were crude and expected age-specific cumulative LBR per scheduled oocyte retrieval. Crude cumulative LBRs were 65%, 60%, 39%, 15%, and 5% in patients aged 26–34, 35–37, 38–40, 41–42, and 43–44 years, respectively. No live births occurred in patients aged ≥ 45 years. Dropout rates per cycle were 13–25%. Success rates gradually reached a plateau, with few additional live births after six cycles. Most of the expected success rate was reached within 6 months with almost maximal rates within 15 months of the first oocyte retrieval. Acceptable cumulative LBR are reached with an exclusive minimal ovarian stimulation/SET policy, especially in patients aged <38 years but also in intermediate aged patients (38–40 years).

MILD STIMULATION USING CORIFOLLITROPIN ALFA

Mild COH, combined with oocyte retrieval (OR) under local anesthesia (LA), may provide low-impact IVF. Since a single injection of corifollitropin alfa (CFA) provides 7 days of COH, the authors hypothesized that CC followed by CFA may provide adequate COH response from one single FSH injection. Their aim was to assess IVF outcomes after a novel CC/CFA protocol, compared to women undergoing standard rFSH COH protocols (good prognosis comparative cohort: GPCC) in a 1:2 matched design. In this pilot study of 25 patients, they examined the effectiveness of oral clomiphene (100 mg; days 2–6) followed by CFA in a GnRH antagonist protocol producing a single injection COH stimulation regime. All ORs were conducted under LA preovarian block. Cycle outcomes were compared to a matched GPCC undergoing standard rFSH COH. Mild stimulation was achieved with less oocytes being collected compared to the GPCC (6.4 ± 0.7 vs 10.7 ± 0.9, $p < 0.001$), resulting in a reduced number of good-quality embryos available for transfer/cryopreservation (3.7 ± 0.6 vs 5.7 ± 0.5, $p = 0.01$). While embryo quality was similar between the two groups, endometrial thickness was significantly lower in the group receiving CC/CFA. PRs were significantly lower in the CC/CFA cohort compared to GPCC (31.8 vs 57.1%, $p = 0.04$) and 44% of CC/CFA participants required supplemental rFSH in order to achieve the hCG trigger criteria. Sequential clomiphene CFA protocol does not appear to be an optimal regime for low-impact IVF treatment, as it does not provide adequate COH from a single CFA injection and results in lower fresh embryo transfer PRs and fewer embryos for cryopreservation.

NEONATAL OUTCOME AFTER MINIMAL STIMULATION

Kato et al. compared neonatal outcome between children born after vitrified versus fresh SET. This was a retrospective, single-center cohort study of 6,623 delivered singletons following 29,944 SETs. Patients underwent minimal ovarian stimulation/natural cycle IVF followed by SET of fresh or vitrified-warmed cleavage-stage embryos or blastocysts. Gestational age (38.6 ± 2 weeks vs 38.7 ± 1.9 weeks) and preterm delivery rate (6.9% vs 6.9%, aOR: 0.96 95% CI: 0.76–1.22) in singletons born after the transfer of vitrified embryos were comparable to those born after the transfer of fresh embryos. Children born after the transfer of vitrified embryos had a higher birth weight (3,028 ± 465 vs 2,943 ± 470 g, $p < 0.0001$) and lower LBW (8.5% vs 11.9%, aOR: 0.65, 95% CI: 0.53–0.79) and SGA (3.6% vs 7.6% aOR: 0.43, 95% CI: 0.33–0.56) rates. Total birth defect rates (including minor anomalies) (2.4% vs 1.9%, aOR: 1.41, 95% CI: 0.96–2.10) and perinatal mortality rates (0.6% vs 0.5%, aOR: 1.02, 95% CI: 0.21–4.85) were comparable between the vitrified and fresh groups. Vitrification of embryos/blastocysts did not increase the incidence of adverse neonatal outcomes or birth defects following SET.

PREIMPLANTATION GENETIC SCREENING

The aim of a Russian study was to investigate, with FISH, the frequency of aneuploidies of the PB-I and PB-II of oocytes in women participating in IVF programs. The study included 93 women, 82 of them were after COS and 11 in natural cycles. FISH in 238 PB-I and PB-II was done. The study revealed that the frequency of aneuploidies in oocytes after COS was higher than in the natural cycle and also was higher after COS in women with infertility compared to women stimulated because of male infertility and egg donors. Aneuploidies of oocytes after COS are more common in patients after 35 years old.

De Sutter et al. compared fertilization and aneuploidy rates after two stimulation protocols in an IVF program. In 349 treatment cycles, CC and human menopausal gonadotropin (hMG) were used in one group ($n = 233$) and hMG after treatment with a GnRHa in two other groups (long protocol): goserelin ($n = 73$) and buserelin ($n = 43$). Cytogenetic analysis was performed on all unfertilized oocytes in both groups. Fertilization rates were significantly higher in the GnRHa/hMG group than in the CC/hMG group, but cleavage rates and embryo quality were not different. Out of 736 oocytes prepared for cytogenetic analysis, 256 were karyotyped—172 were found to be euploid and 84 were aneuploid. More oocytes were aneuploid in the GnRHa/hMG group than in the CC/hMG group and this difference was statistically significant.

A study by Rubio et al. aimed to test the influence of gonadotropin doses on embryo aneuploidy rates. A total of 32 young oocyte donors with a high response to ovarian stimulation were included in the study. Two subsequent stimulation treatments were performed in each donor: first, a standard dose cycle using a 225 IU starting dose of recombinant FSH (r-FSH) and second, a reduced dose cycle with a starting dose of 150 IU r-FSH. In both cycles, GnRHa cotreatment was used for downregulation. Ovarian response, embryo development, and aneuploidy for chromosomes 13, 15, 16, 17, 18, 21, 22, X, and Y were the main outcomes of the study. A total of 22 donors completed both treatments with different gonadotropin doses. In the remaining 10 donors, the reduced dose cycle was canceled due to low-ovarian response. In those donors who completed both regimens, significant increases in rates of fertilization and chromosomally normal blastocysts were observed in the reduced dose cycle. No differences were observed in pregnancy and implantation rates in recipients who received oocytes from standard and reduced doses cycles. Despite the limited numbers in the study, the authors concluded that in high responder donors, a decrease in the gonadotropin dose could improve fertilization rates and embryo quality.

To test whether ovarian stimulation for IVF affects oocyte quality and thus chromosome segregation behavior during meiosis and early embryo development, PGS of embryos was employed in a prospective, randomized controlled trial, comparing two ovarian stimulation regimens by Baart et al. in 2007. Infertile patients under 38 years of age were randomly assigned to undergo either a mild-stimulation regimen using GnRH antagonist cotreatment (67 patients), which does not disrupt secondary follicle recruitment, or a conventional high-dose exogenous gonadotropin regimen and GnRHa cotreatment (44 patients). Following IVF, embryos were biopsied at the eight-cell stage and the copy number of

10 chromosomes was analyzed in one or two blastomeres. The study was terminated prematurely after an unplanned interim analysis (which included 61% of the planned number of patients) found a lower embryo aneuploidy rate, following mild stimulation. Compared with conventional stimulation, significantly fewer oocytes and embryos were obtained following mild stimulation ($p < 0.01$ and < 0.05, respectively). Consequently, both regimens generated on average a similar number (1.8) of chromosomally normal embryos. Differences in rates of mosaic embryos suggest an effect of ovarian stimulation on mitotic segregation errors. The authors summarized that future ovarian stimulation strategies should avoid maximizing oocyte yield but aim at generating a sufficient number of chromosomally normal embryos by reduced interference with ovarian physiology.

INTERESTING CASE REPORTS

Xu and Li reported a novel strategy of continuous ovarian stimulation in a poor responder with two oocyte retrievals within the follicular and luteal phases of the same menstrual cycle. A patient, aged 41 years, diagnosed as infertile with low ovarian reserve sought IVF treatment. A minimal ovarian stimulation protocol was commenced with use of low-dose urinary FSH (150 IU/day) from Day 3, combined with using CC (50–100 mg) when the biggest follicle reached 10 mm in diameter to prevent ovulation. GnRH agonist was administered on Day 15 when the lead follicles reached 18 mm in diameter. The first ultrasound-guided oocyte retrieval was performed 21 hours later; however, no ovum was obtained. Luteal-phase ovarian stimulation was started 2 days later. The second oocyte retrieval was performed 25 hours after hCG administration. Finally, one mature oocyte resulting in a cleavage embryo (8-cell, grade 2) was obtained. The case demonstrates that it is feasible to obtain mature oocytes and good embryos from luteal-phase stimulation. Continuous stimulation during the follicular and luteal phase can be a solution for poor ovarian response. Ovarian stimulation may be performed flexibly in special circumstances. This was the first report on a novel strategy of continuous ovarian stimulation on a poor responder during the follicular and luteal phases of the same menstrual cycle with two oocyte retrievals. In the reported case, a patient, aged 41 years, who was diagnosed with very poor ovarian function, sought therapy for IVF. Antral follicles and basic hormones were evaluated on Day 2 of the menstrual cycle. The stimulation cycle was commenced with use of 150 IU/day urinary FSH from Day 3, combined with CC and ibuprofen in the late follicular and luteal phases to prevent ovulation. Oocyte retrieval was attempted twice. The authors performed luteal-phase ovarian stimulation continuously 2 days after the first failed oocyte retrieval during the follicular phase. Finally, one mature oocyte resulting in a cleavage embryo (8-cell, grade 2) was obtained after the luteal phase stimulation and retrieval, redeeming the previous unsuccessful oocyte retrieval. The case demonstrates that it is practical to obtain mature oocytes and good embryos from maintaining luteal-phase stimulation. For poor ovarian response, continuous stimulation during the follicular and luteal phases can be a solution.

In vitro fertilization–embryo transfer with ICSI was performed for a 45-year-old woman with a peak serum FSH level of 29 mIU/mL and a history of failing to conceive in five previous IVF-ET cycles at a younger age. A minimal FSH stimulation protocol was used. A fresh transfer of a 7-cell embryo was performed on Day 3. A successful pregnancy and delivery ensued. This case report establishes a precedent that a successful pregnancy following IVF-ET is possible in a woman whose serum FSH is >15 mIU/mL and is age of 45 years.

RECENT ADVANCES

There is an ever-increasing trend in ARTs to reduce the intensity of ovarian stimulation for IVF and to restrict the number of embryos that are transferred into the uterine cavity. Recent findings suggest that the magnitude of ovarian stimulation affects the proportion of euploid embryos. Ovarian stimulation regimens for IVF seem to have a deleterious effect on oocyte quality and embryo aneuploidy in a dose-dependent manner. We are moving to a global era of SET and now it becomes more important than ever before to ensure that this single embryo has the highest implantation potential. Strategies are being adopted to improve the accuracy for selecting euploid, viable embryos for transfer.

One such strategy involves further refinement of morphological criteria associated with improved viability by considering, for example, pronuclei disposition, nucleolar organization, and identification of the fast-cleaving embryos, with only mononucleated blastomeres and trying to correlate morphokinetics with cytogenetics. Another strategy employs preimplantation genetic diagnosis whereby a biopsied blastomere is tested for ploidy using next-generation sequencing. Even in older patients, lower oocyte yields may represent a more appropriate response to ovarian stimulation, allowing the most competent follicles and oocytes to develop and thereby reducing the occurrence of embryo aneuploidy. IVF Lite plus ACCU-VIT by repeated mild-stimulation cycles with subsequent vitrification of blastocysts, combined with PGS, is a promising new approach for poor responders as well as women of advanced maternal age.

CONCLUSION

Mild ovarian stimulation for IVF minimizes OHSS and multiple gestations without compromising the PR. Gentle ovarian stimulation protocols, such as "mini-IVF", have several potential advantages over conventional IVF protocols, including less medication and fewer injections, producing fewer eggs, but eggs of higher quality. IVF Lite involves a soft stimulation protocol with lesser amount of fertility drugs. When combined with Embryo ACCU-VIT, it provides a very efficient and cost-effective alternative to conventional IVF. It is designed to retrieve only a few eggs in each ovarian stimulation cycle. Stimulation in this manner has been associated with better quality eggs and hence better quality embryos. In other words, it is a simpler treatment schedule with lower doses of drugs, fewer risks (from multiple pregnancy and overstimulation), and consequently reduced cost.

During ART interventions, COS is used to obtain several oocytes in attempts to increase the likelihood of having at least one developmentally competent embryo available for transfer. Conventional ovarian stimulation regimens for IVF seem to have a deleterious effect on oocyte quality and embryo aneuploidy in a dose-dependent manner. Chromosome abnormalities are common in oocytes derived from patients undergoing IVF treatment. Future ovarian stimulation strategies should avoid maximizing oocyte yield but aim at generating a sufficient number of chromosomally normal embryos by reduced interference with ovarian physiology.

The proportion of oocytes displaying aneuploidy is closely related to maternal age and may exceed 80% in patients over 40 years old. Even in older patients, lower oocyte yields may represent a more appropriate response to ovarian stimulation, allowing the most competent follicles and oocytes to develop and thereby reducing the occurrence of embryo aneuploidy.

EDITORS' COMMENTS

1. The IVF Lite protocol consisting of msIVF + ACCU-VIT + remote embryo transfer (rET) may be explored as an approach to poor responders, larger study groups and more number of studies will land confidence to this form of IVF.
2. The IVF Lite protocols may be consecutively used without a testing cycle. The back-to-back stimulations may give a favorable pregnancy rate per time spent by the patient.
3. Due to the lesser amounts of fertility drugs used in this soft stimulation, cost-effectiveness is a major advantage in low-dose protocol.
4. Minimal stimulation protocols are also gaining momentum in patients with PCO and even normoresponders these days.

SUMMARY

The IVF Lite involves a soft stimulation protocol with lesser amount of fertility drugs. When combined with embryo Accumulation using the Cryotech™ Vitrification Technology (ACCU-VIT), it provides a very efficient and cost-effective alternative to conventional IVF. It is designed to retrieve only a few eggs in each ovarian stimulation cycle. Stimulation in this manner has been associated with better quality eggs and, hence, better quality embryos. In other words, it is a simpler treatment schedule with lower doses of drugs, fewer risks (from multiple pregnancy and overstimulation), and consequently reduced cost. Today, we can offer IVF Lite to almost everyone requiring IVF. The groups, which traditionally benefited from minimal stimulation IVF (msIVF), are poor responders, older patients (above age of 40), women with multiple previous conventional IVF failures, and hyper-responders [like patients with polycystic ovarian syndrome (PCOS) who go repeatedly into ovarian hyperstimulation]. Today, because of the cost advantages and much higher success rates, we have extended the indications of IVF Lite to almost all patients requiring IVF/intracytoplasmic sperm injection (ICSI).

SUGGESTED READING

1. Allahbadia GN. Getting older women pregnant: contemporary thoughts. J Obstet Gynaecol India. 2016;66(5):305-9.
2. Allahbadia GN. Have we finally written the obituary for conventional IVF? IVF Lite. 2014;1(1):1-5.
3. Allahbadia GN. IVF Lite: Is this the future of assisted reproduction? J Obstet Gynecol India. 2013;63(1):1-4.
4. Allahbadia GN. Stimulation and aneuploidy: Why are milder stimulation protocols better? IVF Lite. 2016;3(2):41-5.
5. Baart EB, Martini E, Eijkemans MJ, et al. Milder ovarian stimulation for in-vitro fertilization reduces aneuploidy in the human preimplantation embryo: A randomized controlled trial. Hum Reprod. 2007;22(4):980-8.

6. Baker VL, Brown MB, Luke B, et al. Gonadotropin dose is negatively correlated with live birth rate: analysis of more than 650,000 assisted reproductive technology cycles. Fertil Steril. 2015;104(5):1145-52.e1-5.
7. Blumenfeld Z. Why more is less and less is more when it comes to ovarian stimulation. J Assist Reprod Genet. 2015;32(12):1713-9.
8. Bodri D, Kawachiya S, De Brucker M, et al. Cumulative success rates following mild IVF in unselected infertile patients: a 3-year, single-centre cohort study. Reprod Biomed Online. 2014;28(5):572-81.
9. Bos AM, Pelinck MJ, Dumoulin JC, et al. IVF in a modified natural cycle. Ned Tijdschr Geneeskd. 2010;154(45):A2519.
10. Check JH, Choe JK, Cohen R. Successful pregnancy following a single fresh embryo transfer in a 45-year-old woman whose early follicular phase serum follicle stimulating hormone was 29 mIU/ml. Clin Exp Obstet Gynecol. 2011;38(4):335-7.
11. Chen Q, Wang Y, Sun L, et al. Controlled ovulation of the dominant follicle using progestin in minimal stimulation in poor responders. Reprod Biol Endocrinol. 2017;15(1):71.
12. De Sutter P, Dhont M, Vandekerckhove D. Hormonal stimulation for in vitro fertilization: A comparison of fertilization rates and cytogenetic findings in unfertilized oocytes. J Assist Reprod Genet. 1992;9(3):254-8.
13. Gandhi G, Allahbadia G, Kagalwala S, et al. ACCU-VIT: A new strategy for managing poor responders. Hum Reprod. 2013;28:i149-206.
14. Gandhi GN, Allahbadia GN, Kagalwala S, et al. IVF Lite—A new strategy for managing poor ovarian responders. IVF Lite. 2014;1(1):22-8.
15. Grabar VV, Stefanovich AV. Aneuploidies in oocytes used in IVF programs. Georgian Med News. 2014;23:7-12.
16. Haas J, Casper RF. In vitro fertilization treatments with the use of clomiphene citrate or letrozole. Fertil Steril. 2017;108(4):568-71.
17. Herrero L, Pareja S, Aragonés M, et al. Oocyte versus embryo vitrification for delayed embryo transfer: an observational study. Reprod Biomed Online. 2014;29(5):567-72.
18. Ho JR, Paulson RJ. Modified natural cycle in in vitro fertilization. Fertil Steril. 2017;108(4):572-6.
19. Kato K, Takehara Y, Segawa T, et al. Minimal ovarian stimulation combined with elective single embryo transfer policy: age-specific results of a large, single-centre, Japanese cohort. Reprod Biol Endocrinol. 2012;10:35.
20. Kato O, Kawasaki N, Bodri D, et al. Neonatal outcome and birth defects in 6,623 singletons born following minimal ovarian stimulation and vitrified versus fresh single embryo transfer. Eur J Obstet Gynecol Reprod Biol. 2012;161(1):46-50.
21. Kim CH, Kim SR, Cheon YP, et al. Minimal stimulation using gonadotropin-releasing hormone (GnRH) antagonist and recombinant human follicle-stimulating hormone versus GnRH antagonist multiple-dose protocol in low responders undergoing in vitro fertilization/intracytoplasmic sperm injection. Fertil Steril. 2009;92(6):2082-4.
22. Lazer T, Dar S, Shlush E, et al. Comparison of IVF outcomes between minimal stimulation and high-dose stimulation for patients with poor ovarian reserve. Int J Reprod Med. 2014;2014:581451.
23. Mendez Lozano DH, Brum Scheffer J, Frydman N, et al. Optimal reproductive competence of oocytes retrieved through follicular flushing in minimal stimulation IVF. Reprod Biomed Online. 2008;16(1):119-23.
24. Mohsen IA, El Din RE. Minimal stimulation protocol using letrozole versus microdose flare up GnRH agonist protocol in women with poor ovarian response undergoing ICSI. Gynecol Endocrinol. 2013;29(2):105-8.
25. Nargund G, Datta AK, Fauser BCJM. Mild stimulation for in vitro fertilization. Fertil Steril. 2017;108(4):558-67.
26. Pilehvari S, Shahrokh Tehraninejad E, Hosseinrashidi B, et al. Comparison pregnancy outcomes between minimal stimulation protocol and conventional GnRH antagonist protocols in poor ovarian responders. J Family Reprod Health. 2016;10(1):35-42.
27. Roque M, Valle M, Guimarães F, et al. Freeze-all policy: fresh vs. frozen-thawed embryo transfer. Fertil Steril. 2015;103(5):1190-3.
28. Rose BI, Laky DC, Rose SD. A comparison of the use of clomiphene citrate and letrozole in patients undergoing IVF with the objective of producing only one or two embryos. Facts Views Vis Obgyn. 2015;7(2):119-26.
29. Rubio C, Mercader A, Alamá P, et al. Prospective cohort study in high responder oocyte donors using two hormonal stimulation protocols: Impact on embryo aneuploidy and development. Hum Reprod. 2010;25(9):2290-7.
30. Xu B, Li Y. Flexible ovarian stimulation in a poor responder: a case report and literature review. Reprod Biomed Online. 2013;26(4):378-83.
31. Yan G, Xie X, Wang Y, et al. Twin pregnancy after intracytoplasmic sperm injection in woman aged 49 using autologous oocytes by mild ovarian stimulation: a case report. Int J Clin Exp Med. 2015;8(11):21707-9.
32. Zander-Fox D, Lane M, Hamilton H, et al. Sequential clomiphene/corifollitrophin alpha as a technique for mild controlled ovarian hyperstimulation in IVF: a proof of concept study. J Assist Reprod Genet. 2018;35(6):1047-52.
33. Zhang J, Chang L, Sone Y, et al. Minimal ovarian stimulation (mini-IVF) for IVF utilizing vitrification and cryopreserved embryo transfer. Reprod Biomed Online. 2010;21(4):485-95.
34. Zhang JJ, Choo S, Yang M. Autologous oocyte cryopreservation in women aged 40 and older using minimal stimulation IVF. Reprod Biol Endocrinol. 2015;13:112.
35. Zhang JJ, Merhi Z, Yang M, et al. Minimal stimulation IVF vs conventional IVF: a randomized controlled trial. Am J Obstet Gynecol. 2016;214(1):96.e1-8.
36. Zhang JJ, Yang M, Merhi Z. Efficiency of metaphase II oocytes following minimal/mild ovarian stimulation in vitro fertilization. Fertil Res Pract. 2016;2:2.

5

CHAPTER

Luteal Phase Stimulation

Markus Eckart Nitzschke, Nisha Bhatnagar, Payal Bajaj

INTRODUCTION

Since its inception, assisted reproductive technology (ART) has faced variety of challenges and has come up with numerous innovations. The percentage of infertility patients with low-ovarian reserve is growing in all infertility practices in the developed world because of a growing older population and the decisions of many women to start reproduction in their mid-30s. In some areas, especially in bigger cities, the percentage of patients with low-ovarian reserve exceeds 50% in most infertility practices.

Treating infertility patients with low-ovarian reserve is one of the most frustrating and challenging tasks that infertility specialists can encounter in their practice. These patients usually show strange menstrual cycle patterns, they do not respond normally to ovarian stimulation regimens and they often develop treatment-resistant ovarian cysts. Despite the urgent need for new treatment regimens for this patient population, very few groups are undertaking serious research in this field. Due to lack of better options, many infertility specialists simply refer those patients to egg donation. Although many stimulation protocols have been established to improve clinical outcomes in poor ovarian reserve patients, the most effective protocol remains controversial.

This Chapter aims to tell the efficacy of luteal phase ovarian stimulation (LPOS) protocol in poor ovarian reserve patients.

What is Already Known?

It has been proven beyond doubt by various studies that small antral follicles observed during the luteal phase may not undergo atresia but instead remain in the earlier stages of follicular development. It has also been proven by various studies that oocytes retrieved during luteal phase are mature and can get fertilized, which implicate that follicles are continuously available for stimulation by gonadotropins during menstrual cycle and that there is no difference in the quality of embryos produced in the follicular and the luteal phases.

LUTEAL PHASE OVARIAN STIMULATION

Luteal phase is defined as the period between ovulation/ovum pick-up and either the onset of menstruation or occurrence of pregnancy 2 weeks later (Fatemi et al.).

Poor Ovarian Reserve

In order to get the maximum benefit from the luteal phase stimulation protocol, it is very important to understand what poor ovarian reserve means and how it can be classified.

After a detailed observation of patients' cycles and understanding their individual hormonal pattern in hundreds of menstrual cycles, we were able to classify four different types of ovulation in women with low-ovarian reserve. We called them:

1. Compensated stage
2. Stage of desynchronized menstrual cycle
3. Stage of pathologic premature luteinizing hormone (LH) rise
4. Stage of suppressed follicle growth.

Below is a brief description of the hormonal pattern and changes seen in the stages and the treatment options best suitable for that group of patients.

1. *Compensated stage*: In this stage, the endocrine compensation mechanisms are still working and the women still have long and regular cycle of 26–33 days. Nevertheless, the anti-Mullerian hormone (AMH) or the antral follicle count (AFC) can be low and in some cycles, the early follicular phase follicular-stimulating hormone (FSH) can be elevated. As long as the menstrual cycle stays long and regular, the low-ovarian reserve probably does not reduce the fertility. In most cases, there is another explanation for the infertility of the couple, if they are seeking treatment. These patients are the typical low responders, if they are treated with a classical hyperstimulation protocol, such as the long agonist protocol or antagonist protocol. This group of patients can benefit most with LPOS with better quality and number of oocytes.
2. *The second stage of ovarian insufficiency or stage of desynchronized menstrual cycle*: Probably due to a lower number of antral follicles in the ovaries, serum inhibin levels and other inhibiting hormones fall under a certain limit and as a consequence, basal FSH levels rise (Welt et al., 2005). Without the stabilizing effect of these hormones, the estrogen and progesterone producing corpus luteum is not strong enough to completely block FSH production in the second half of the cycle. Due to these higher basal FSH levels in the luteal phase, follicular development starts too early, already in the middle of the luteal phase. On the onset of menses, a dominant follicle has already been recruited, which under normal circumstances would only happen on Day 6 of menstrual cycle. Because of the early follicular recruitment during the luteal phase of the previous cycle, ovulation will occur earlier, and the whole cycle becomes shorter. However, a shorter follicular phase may have negative effects on endometrium maturation and implantation of the embryo.

   Often in patients with short menstrual cycles, less than 26 days, a present dominant follicle of 12–14 mm or more can be detected in vaginal ultrasound at the beginning of the cycle. These patients often have a normal early follicular FSH, but high early follicular estradiol levels over 60 pg/mL. In order to resynchronize the cycle again, this subgroup of patients should be given combined oral contraceptive pills for at least 10 days during the luteal phase, for example from Day 16 to Day 26 of menstrual cycle. The additional effect of the combined oral contraceptive pills together with the hormones produced by the corpus luteum suppresses FSH and avoids follicle formation during the luteal phase. After discontinuation of combined oral contraceptive pills, the withdrawal bleeding marks the beginning of the new, resynchronized cycle.
3. *The third stage of ovarian insufficiency or stage of pathologic premature LH rise*: The progression of antral follicle loss and the lack of inhibiting hormones produced by the ovaries seem to destabilize the hypothalamus-pituitary system even further in this stage. In addition to higher baseline FSH levels, the system seems to be more sensitive to estrogen when it comes to the triggering of LH for ovulation. Under normal circumstances, the LH rise is triggered by estrogen on the hypothalamus level, once the follicle is mature. In this stage of ovarian insufficiency, LH rise is triggered too early, when estrogen levels are still low and the follicle is still small and immature. The eggs ovulated from these small and immature follicles are of a bad quality and may not lead to a pregnancy. The typical pattern in this stage is short menstrual cycles of less than 26 days, high early follicular phase FSH up to 25–30 IU/L, and normal or low early follicular estradiol levels.

   Normally, there is no dominant follicle at the beginning of the cycle, but nevertheless, ovulation occurs too early, due to the premature LH rise, which leads to a shorter follicular phase. The small and immature follicles seem to produce a weak corpus luteum, as we measured low progesterone during the luteal phase. The resulting luteal phase insufficiency also leads to a shorter second half of the cycle. Our way to treat the pathologic premature LH rise is to use the anti-estrogenic effect of clomiphene citrate around ovulation. As a competitive inhibitor of estrogen receptors on the hypothalamus level, the system is tricked to "think" that the follicle is still not mature enough to trigger LH surge. Depending on the dosage, clomiphene citrate is able to delay LH surge or to block it completely (Teramoto and Kato, 2007). In this case, it is necessary to trigger LH surge and ovulation artificially with gonadotropin-releasing hormone (GnRH) analogs, once the follicle has reached maturity.

   It is very difficult to differentiate between 2nd and 3rd stage unless repeat blood investigations are done. Usually, there is some kind of overlap between these two stages.
4. *The fourth stage of ovarian insufficiency or stage of suppressed follicle growth*: In this stage, either very high FSH levels of over 30 IU/L or high LH levels seem to block

follicle growth, probably due to the downregulation of the respective receptors on the follicle itself. These patients have long and irregular cycles. Most of the time, the follicular growth is inhibited by the high-serum FSH or LH levels, but from time to time, the ovaries seem to recover. FSH and LH levels fall to a certain limit and a follicle may grow again. Once a progesterone producing corpus luteum has developed, the ovary may enter into a dynamic phase with several ovulations during the luteal phase, as it was already described in the second stage of ovarian insufficiency. This is possible because progesterone has a negative feedback on the hypothalamus, so FSH and LH are kept relatively low. This phenomenon of luteal phase ovulations may also lead to longer periods of amenorrhea. Every time, a corpus luteum becomes weaker and is about to vanish, another one appears and progesterone production continues without withdrawal bleeding.

This knowledge opens new space for development of alternative protocols respecting the patients' own physiology with no need for heavy stimulation. Patients with ovarian insufficiency may benefit from this approach, which can be offered before referring them to egg donation.

LUTEAL PHASE STIMULATION PROTOCOL

Since the ovaries and the FSH receptors of the antral follicles in poor ovarian reserve patient are used to constantly high endogenous FSH levels and, therefore, even higher endogenous FSH levels are required in order to give a multifollicular response in normal follicular phase stimulation.

In case of antagonist protocol, the blood FSH levels of over 25–30 IU/mL are easily attained during usual stimulation and this usually blocks the ovarian response either completely or partially. Therefore, either no follicle grows or gives a suboptimum quality oocyte, which is not capable of giving a live pregnancy. On the other hand, if a long GnRH agonist protocol is used and all endogenous FSH is suppressed, very high dosages are needed to provoke the desired follicular growth, which again leads to poor egg quality and subsequently very low birth rates.

The best solution for these patients is the luteal phase stimulation. Here, the progesterone produced by the corpus luteum during the luteal phase stimulation is utilized, which has a protective effect on the growing follicle. It has been seen that the FSH levels during the luteal phase in women with poor ovarian reserve are similar to the FSH levels during follicular phase in women with normal ovarian reserve. Therefore, normal dosage of FSH between 150 IU/day and 225 IU/day administered during the luteal phase after ovulation results in optimal ovarian response for the patients.

Even if the number of dominant follicles might stay low during ovarian stimulation due to initial less number of antral follicles, the quality of oocytes will be better.

Another advantage of luteal phase stimulation is that no additional drug is needed to control the LH surge. The progesterone from the corpus luteum has strong inhibitory effect on the LH; and in the presence of significant progesterone levels in the body, LH surge and ovulation will not happen.

In case the stimulation is initiated too late, there is a small risk that the corpus luteum will disintegrate during stimulation and as progesterone level drops, menstrual bleeding might happen. This problem can be overcome by adding medroxyprogesterone acetate 10 mg daily at first sign of onset of spotting.

However, it is quite evident that, as endometrium is out of phase, there is no option of a fresh embryo transfer and all embryos need to be frozen and transferred in the next menstrual cycle.

The usual luteal phase stimulation protocols that we use are as follows:

- Day 2 scan
- Follow-up scan after 5–6 days to check for follicular growth or ovulation
- The scan is repeated in 2–3 days still spontaneous ovulations
- Usually, there is premature LH surge and ovulation occurs by Day 8 or 9 in LOR patients.

If there is no spontaneous ovulation, trigger can be given to induce ovulation.

- Patient is called after 48 hours later and a repeat scan done.
- LPOS is started, if 1–2 follicles are present between 8–10 mm.

Protocol 1 (Flowchart 1)

- Depending upon FSH, LH, estradiol, progesterone levels, clomiphene citrate 50–100 mg can be started with or without gonadotropins (Gn) depending on the values of FSH, LH.
- Usually, if FSH levels are between 8 and 12, Gn are added; but if FSH levels >12, only clomiphene citrate can be given.
- Trigger can be given at 18 mm of follicle size

Flowchart 1: Protocol 1 of luteal phase ovarian stimulation.

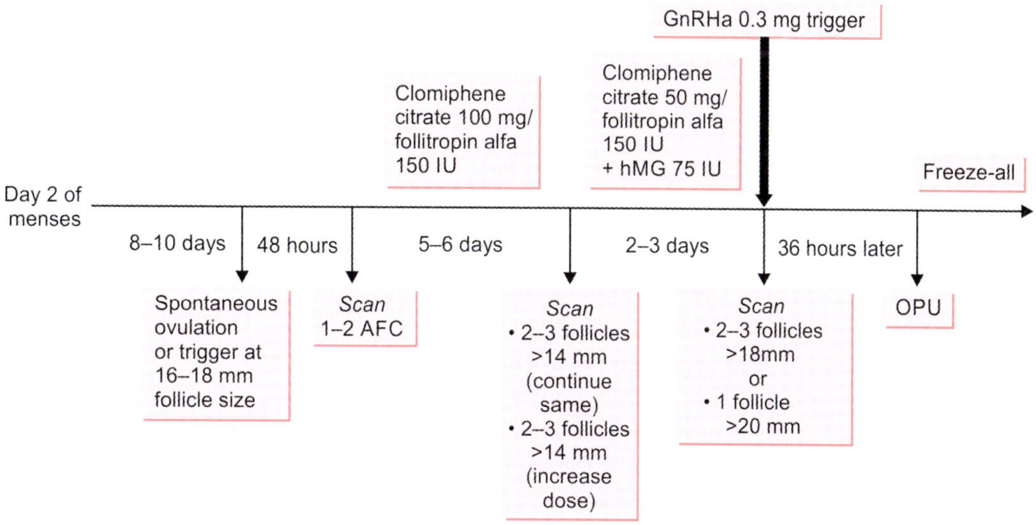

(AFC: antral follicle count; GnRHa: gonadotropin-releasing hormone agonist; hMG: human menopausal gonadotropin; OPU: oocyte pick-up)

Flowchart 2: Protocol 2 of luteal phase ovarian stimulation.

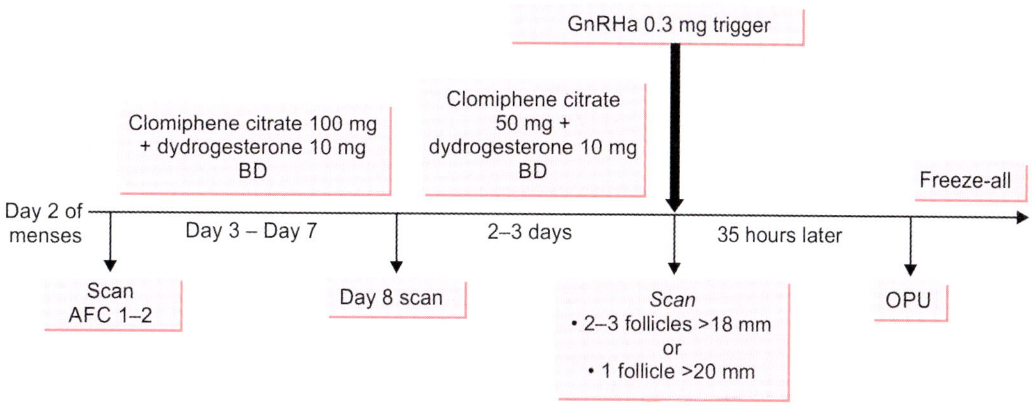

(AFC: antral follicle count; GnRHa: gonadotropin-releasing hormone agonist; hMG: human menopausal gonadotropin; OPU: oocyte pick-up)

- Transvaginal ultrasonography (TVS)-guided oocyte retrieval can be done 35–36 hours later.

Modified luteal phase stimulation:

- After having good results in the form of better egg quality, we tried to use this concept of luteal phase stimulation in follicular phase.
- The only difference was that instead of corpus luteum, the progesterone was given orally in the form of dydrogesterone tablets twice a day.

Here is the alternative protocol that we use.

Protocol 2 (Flowchart 2)

- Clomiphene citrate 100 mg can be started along with dydrogesterone 10 mg BD.
- Follicular monitoring can be done.
- Clomiphene citrate and dydrogesterone can be continued till trigger.
- Trigger can be given at 2–3 follicles >18, or 1 follicle at 20 mm.
- TVS-guided oocyte retrieval can be done 35–36 hours later.

CASE STUDY

A patient of 38 years with a history of a spontaneous conception and live birth 7 years ago comes to our clinic, because she is looking for a second child. Her left ovary was removed around 10 years ago because of a teratoma. Otherwise, she is healthy, her fallopian tubes are patent, and her husband's sperm parameters are. Her menstrual cycle is regular, but her cycle length, that has always been around 28/29 days, has become shorter in the last 2 years and is now around 24/25 days. 1 year before, the couple has done IVF stimulation in another clinic with a long agonist protocol and 300 IU recombinant FSH per day, but the cycle was canceled because of low ovarian response. A vaginal ultrasound on her 3rd day of cycle shows a dominant follicle of 14 mm together with three antral follicles below 10 mm in her remaining ovary. Her estradiol is 71 pg/mL, FSH is 14.3 IU/mL, and LH is 6.5 IU/mL. The patient's ovarian reserve is clearly reduced and her menstrual cycle is advanced with a dominant follicle already present on Day 3 of cycle. We decide to do luteal phase stimulation and ask the patient to come back to the clinic for a blood test on her cycle Day 15. On this day, her estradiol is 91 pg/mL, progesterone is 4.5 ng/mL, FSH is 6,7 IU/mL, and LH is 8.1 IU/mL. Having confirmed ovulation through positive progesterone, we instruct the patient to start stimulation with daily injections of 150 IU recombinant FSH, starting from that same day. We ask her to come back to the clinic for vaginal ultrasound and blood test after 5 days of stimulation, and then again after 3 days. We find two follicles of 17 mm, two follicles of 16 mm, and one follicle of 14 mm in her right ovary. Her estradiol is 1,134 pg/mL, progesterone is 7.2 ng/mL, FSH is 12.2 IU/mL, and LH is 4.3 IU/mL. We decide to trigger her ovulation with 0.3 mg decapeptyl subcutaneously after 2 more days of stimulation. Oocyte retrieval is done 36 hours after the trigger and five mature oocytes are retrieved. All oocytes are injected through intracytoplasmic sperm injection (ICSI) with her husband's sperm. On Day 3, we find three grade-A embryos and one grade-C embryo. We agree with the couple to culture 2 more days in order to reach blastocyst stage. On Day 5, we have two grade-A blastocysts, which are frozen. In the next cycle, the endometrium is prepared in an artificial cycle using GnRH agonist downregulation, oral estradiol valerate, and vaginal progesterone. One blastocyst is transferred 120 hours after beginning of vaginal progesterone. 12 days after the transfer, the patient is pregnant with a beta-hCG value of 476 IU/mL. Follow-up is done after 2 weeks and good cardiac activity is noted along with good choriodecidual reaction.

KEYNOTE

The concept of ovarian stimulation in the luteal phase was first introduced by a group from China (Yanping Kuang, Shanghai). Many groups around the world were inspired by the genius of this idea and started to try this concept with different patient groups that were difficult to treat with the traditional follicular phase stimulation regimens, such as low reserve patients, polycystic ovarian syndrome (PCOS) patients, or patients with endometriosis. Now, it is clinically proven without any doubts that the presence of progesterone during ovarian stimulation is not affecting egg quality, embryo quality, or pregnancy rates in any negative way. In some cases, results can even be improved compared with the traditional protocols. The use of progesterone to inhibit LH surge and ovarian ovulation as "oral antagonist" will revolutionize the way, we stimulate our patients in the future. With the introduction of embryo vitrification a few years ago, more and more groups are leaving fresh embryo transfers and apply a freeze-all concept with only frozen embryo transfers in the cycles after ovarian stimulation. This means we can separate ovarian stimulation and embryo transfer; and as a consequence, we do not need to pay attention to the endometrial lining during ovarian stimulation anymore. Knowing that the presence of progesterone during ovarian stimulation is not harmful to the egg quality and the fact that we do not need the endometrium after stimulation gives us new freedom to plan ovarian stimulation. Now, we can start stimulation any time during the cycle, except when a dominant follicle is present, so during the first 4–5 days of cycle, before the dominant follicle gets selected or any time during the luteal phase. If natural progesterone is present during the luteal phase, no additional progesterone is needed. If stimulation starts in the follicular phase, then some oral progesterone such as medroxyprogesterone 10 mg per day or dydrogesterone 20 mg per day can be added. This will also reduce the costs of stimulation and the patient comfort, because progesterone can be given orally and it is much cheaper than GnRH antagonist injections to control ovulation during ovarian stimulation.

KEY POINTS

- Follicles are always available in wave-like pattern for recruitment.
- The implantation rates and pregnancy rates of fresh and frozen cycles are comparable, especially with the advancements in cryopreservation techniques.
- Poor ovarian reserve can be divided into four stages as discussed.

- With luteal phase stimulation, it is important to see at least 1–2 AFC on scan after ovulation.
- Progesterone acts as perfect antagonist.
- To make the treatment cost-effective, we can use tablet clomiphene citrate for stimulation, which gives equally good results.

FUTURE PROSPECTS

The concept of using progesterone for lowering LH can be used with lots of benefits in PCOS patients too, despite various stimulation protocols we are still struggling with effective means of lowering LH, optimizing egg quality and embryo quality, as well as still keeping the cycle cost-effective and no risk of OHSS (ovarian hyperstimulation syndrome). Luteal phase stimulation might just be the thing in near future in solving the enigma of COS (controlled ovarian stimulation) in such patients.

EDITORS' COMMENTS

1. Luteal phase stimulation is a novel form of stimulation with an interesting science behind it. A thorough knowledge of endocrinology of female menstrual cycle is required to understand luteal phase stimulation.
2. It was developed as a part of dual stimulation for oocyte/embryo banking in poor responder patients to cut short the duration of ART treatment where the dual phase of stimulation would start in the luteal phase without withdrawal. In spite of the initial interest with which it was developed, its efficacy still remains to be proven.
3. Luteal phase support is important part of protocols that involve back-to-back stimulation.
4. Agonist trigger is a must for luteal poststimulation in dual stimulation.
5. Though the number of oocyte retrieved has been significantly higher, but the fertilization rates, blastocyst rate, and pregnancy rate have yet to show significant improvement.

SUGGESTED READING

1. Chian RC, Chung JT, Downey BR, et al. Maturational and developmental competence of immature oocytes retrieved from bovine ovaries at different phases of folliculogenesis. Reprod Biomed Online. 2002;4(2):127-32.
2. Cummins JM, Breen TM, Harrison KL, et al. A formula for scoring human embryo growth rates in in vitro fertilization: its value in predicting pregnancy and in comparison with visual estimates of embryo quality. J In Vitro Fert Embryo Transf. 1986;3(5):284-95.
3. Gougeon A. Dynamics of follicular growth in the human: a model from preliminary results. Hum Reprod. 1986;1(2):81-7.
4. Hu L, Bu Z, Guo Y, et al. Comparison of different ovarian hyperstimulation protocols efficacy in poor ovarian responders according to the Bologna criteria. Int J Clin Exp Med. 2014;7(4):1128-34.
5. Kuang Y, Chen Q, Hong Q, et al. Double stimulations during the follicular and luteal phases of poor responders in IVF/ICSI programmes (Shanghai protocol). Reprod Biomed Online. 2014;29(6):684-91.
6. Kuang Y, Hong Q, Chen Q, et al. Luteal-phase ovarian stimulation is feasible for producing competent oocytes in women undergoing in vitro fertilization/intracytoplasmic sperm injection treatment, with optimal pregnancy outcomes in frozen-thawed embryo transfer cycles. Fertil Steril. 2014;101(1):105-11.
7. Liu XY, Xue SG, Jin W. Impact of incubation time of vitrification-warming embryos on frozen-thawed embryo transfer outcomes. J Reprod Med. 2010;19:104-7.
8. Macklon NS, Stouffer RL, Giudice LC, et al. The science behind 25 years of ovarian stimulation for in vitro fertilization. Endocr Rev. 2006;27(2):170-207.
9. Madani T, Ashrafi M, Yeganeh LM. Comparison of different stimulation protocols efficacy in poor responders undergoing IVF: a retrospective study. Gynecol Endocrinol. 2012;28(2):102-5.
10. Ubaldi FM, Capalbo A, Vaiarelli A, et al. Follicular versus luteal phase ovarian stimulation during the same menstrual cycle (DuoStim) in a reduced ovarian reserve population results in a similar euploid blastocyst formation rate: new insight in ovarian reserve exploitation. Fertil Steril. 2016;105(6):1488-95.e1.
11. Wei LH, Ma WH, Tang N, et al. Luteal-phase ovarian stimulation is a feasible method for poor ovarian responders undergoing in vitro fertilization/intracytoplasmic sperm injection-embryo transfer treatment compared to a GnRH antagonist protocol: A retrospective study. Taiwan J Obstet Gynecol. 2016;55(1):50-4.
12. Weinerman R, Mainigi M. Why we should transfer frozen instead of fresh embryos: the translational rationale. Fertil Steril. 2014;102(2):10-8. (LH Wei and WH Ma contributed equally to this study).
13. Zhang J. Luteal phase ovarian stimulation following oocyte retrieval: Is it helpful for poor responders? Reprod Biol Endocrinol. 2015;13:76.

6

CHAPTER

Downregulation in IVF Cycles

Pratap Kumar

INTRODUCTION

The steps for a successful assisted reproduction involve a series of highly coordinated steps starting with gonadotropins and following the principle of controlled ovarian hyperstimulation (COHS). This is followed by oocyte pick-up from the ovaries under transvaginal ultrasound guidance, followed by fertilization of the gametes, and finally embryo transfer into the uterus. To have low cancellation rate with less side effects and lower incidence of multiple pregnancies is the ideal protocol. Luteinizing hormone (LH) levels can rise prematurely without control and hence ovulation may occur before oocyte pick-ups are done or there may be premature luteinization and poor implantation. If there is increased LH in the beginning of graafian follicle development, oocytes will be affected and gives reduced pregnancy rates. Hence, it is important to understand the role of gonadotropin-releasing hormone (GnRH) analogs with agonist and antagonist protocol for better outcome.

AGONIST PROTOCOL BY LONG SUPPRESSION METHOD (FIG. 1)

The GnRH agonist long protocol was introduced in 1980, thereby premature LH surge was tackled. Hence, frequent estimation of serum LH was not needed. This brought down the incidence of premature LH surge from 20% to 2%. This brought in flexibility of oocyte recovery.

Disadvantages

The GnRH agonist treatment suppresses the ovaries too much in certain women, thus, the dose of gonadotropins may have to be increased. Sometimes, there may be

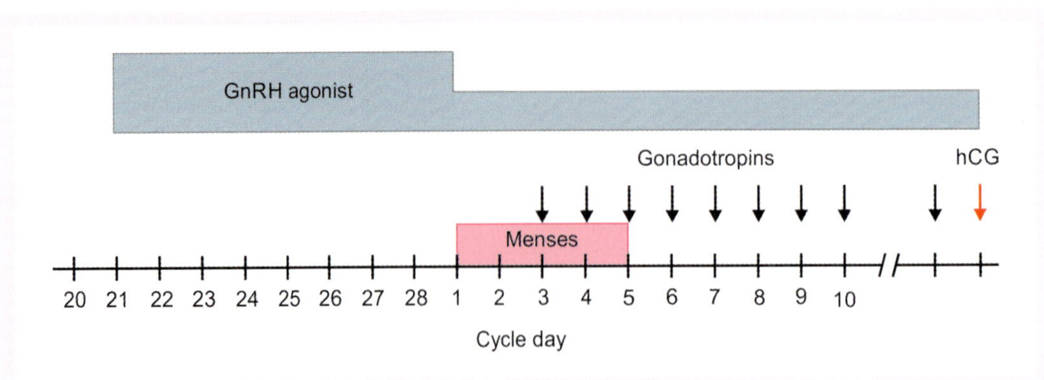

Fig. 1: Agonist protocol by long suppression method.
(GnRH: gonadotropin-releasing hormone; hCG: human chorionic gonadotropin)

a development of a cyst in the ovaries at the time of menstruation due to the flare up action of the GnRH analog.

Usually 1 week before the menses, GnRH analog is started, which will be mid-luteal phase. However, though the same can also be started in the early follicular phase, it takes a longer time to achieve pituitary downregulation. It is observed that more follicles and oocytes are obtained when GnRH analog is started in the luteal phase. This is due to circulating androgen levels, which are reduced throughout follicular phase.

The two GnRH agonists in common use are leuprolide acetate, decapeptyl (administered by subcutaneous injection), and nafarelin acetate (administered by intranasal spray). Elsewhere, buserelin acetate or decapeptyl (administered by subcutaneous injection or intranasal spray) and triptorelin (administered subcutaneously) are also commonly used, and all appear equally effective. For leuprolide, the usual treatment is with 0.5 mg daily, which usually is for 10 days or until the onset of menses or gonadotropin stimulation. Thereafter, the dose can be decreased to 0.25 mg daily. This is continued until human chorionic gonadotropin (hCG) administration. In women who respond poorly to stimulation using the standard daily GnRH agonist treatment regimens, it is ideal to decrease the doses of agonist by half or more or discontinue agonist treatment early (after 5 days of gonadotropin stimulation) or completely (when stimulation begins), which helps to improve response and overall results.

Ideally, if the estradiol is less than about 40 pg/mL, it seems to be ideal suppression. There should not be any cyst more than 10–15 mm in the ovary. Some may take longer time to achieve suppression or may develop a follicular cyst. Although the outcomes observed in completed cycles may be similar in women with and without baseline cysts; cycle cancellation rates are higher and the total dose of gonadotropins required is generally greater in those with cysts.

The response to gonadotropins is not good in those who take longer time suppression. In the beginning of ovarian follicular development, the starting dose of gonadotropins varies after downregulation according to estradiol levels and the antral follicles. The starting doses range between 150 IU and 450 IU of urinary follicle stimulating hormone (uFSH), recombinant FSH (rFSH), or urinary menotropins (hMG) daily.

It is necessary that only about 1% of LH receptors must be occupied to support normal follicular steroidogenesis. Hence with GnRHa downregulation, LH, mostly, is within the range. If the suppression is less than 1 IU/L, the dose and duration of gonadotropins will be higher. When LH levels are extremely low, there is evidence suggesting that outcome may be adversely affected. These women could be benefitted from supplemental hMG or rLH during ovarian stimulation.

Sequential Stimulation with a GnRH Agonist and Exogenous Gonadotropins the "Short" or "Flare" Protocols

In a short flare protocol, leuprolide acetate (1.0 mg daily) is given 2nd–4th day of menses. This is continued at a reduced dose (0.5 mg daily), and gonadotropin stimulation (150–450 IU daily) begins on the 3rd day of cycle. Further on adjustments in the dose of gonadotropin, stimulation is done depending on the response. The pregnancy rate remains relatively low. Oocyte quality, fertilization, and pregnancy rates are affected because there is a rise of progesterone and androgens. The "ultrashort" GnRH agonist protocol is a variation of the short protocol in which an agonist is administered for 3 days to stimulate the flare response, later same is discontinued. Exogenous gonadotropin alone is continued. Premature LH surges are more prevalent. However with ultrashort GnRH agonist, stimulation protocol results are not good.

ANTAGONIST PROTOCOL (FIG. 2)

The GnRH antagonists have provided good option for controlled ovarian stimulation in ART. GnRH receptors are affected and preventing the action of endogenous GnRH pulses on the pituitary. The secretion of gonadotropins is decreased by few hours of giving antagonist and has no flare-up effect. When the same is discontinued, the recovery of the hypothalamic-pituitary-ovarian (HPO) axis is rapid.

When the GnRH antagonist is administered LH is blocked within 6–8 hours of administration.

GnRH Antagonist and its Advantages

- Compared to agonist, the duration is much shorter.
- It is usually started after 4–5 days of gonadotropin stimulation, when the follicle is 12–14 mm and E2 is more than 400 pg/mL.
- The total dose and duration of gonadotropin needed is decreased.
- Cyst formation is not seen as in GnRH analog treatment.
- Ovarian hyperstimulation syndrome (OHSS) is less specially the severe type.

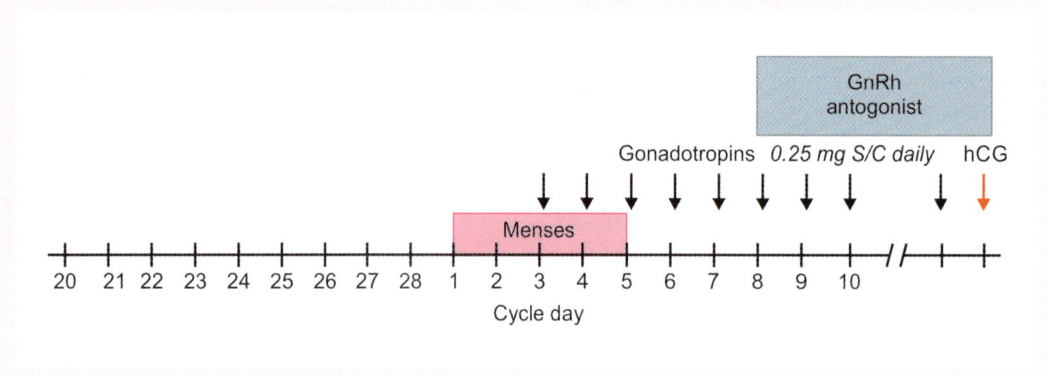

Fig. 2: Antagonist protocol.
(GnRH: gonadotropin-releasing hormone; hCG: human chorionic gonadotropin)

Disadvantages of GnRH Antagonists

It is reported that there is a slight reduction of pregnancy rates. This may be due to the changes of mitosis program, which controls follicle development.

The two GnRH antagonists available are ganirelix and cetrorelix. Both are potent and effective. The ideal effective dose to prevent premature LH surge is 0.25 mg daily, subcutaneously. The treatment protocol can be fixed on Day 5 or variable at around Day 5 or 6 when the biggest follicle reaches approximately 12–14 mm in diameter.

A depot of 3.0 mg can also be given with 13–14 mm in diameter.

This type of antagonists is good for those who had not responded well to agonist protocol and in those polycystic ovarian syndrome (PCOS) women with elevated LH levels.

REVIEW OF LITERATURE

Twenty-one randomized controlled trials (RCTs) have been studied, which included 3,865 participants. The pooled data showed that number of oocytes retrieved was less with GnRH antagonist. But the lower amount of gonadotropin used and the shorter duration of stimulation are mentioned as a positive note in all the studies. Though pregnancies were lower, the biggest advantage is that there was reduction in incidence of OHSS.

One of the studies done previously showed fewer numbers of follicles with antagonist on comparison to the agonist group. A recent review proved the reduction of OHSS.

On analyzing the live birth rate, the publication, a meta-analysis of 22 published RCTs was not significantly different. Hence, there seems to be a variation in literature. Cochrane analysis showed slightly lower results for the GnRH antagonist treatment group when the same was compared to GnRH agonist group. However, clinically antagonist protocol seems good for so many advantages. Changes related to mitochondria are unclear. The lower pregnancy and implantation rates are due to the fact when LH surge is not suppressed on time.

Earlier studies were done with poor responders and antagonist and hence, the disparity in the views. Hence, to get better results with antagonists, several methods have been suggested like pretreatment with OCP (oral contraceptive pills). This brings in good follicular synchrony. Several authors suggest flexible protocols. Premature LH surge is connected to serum progesterone levels. Hence, the control of LH surge is important. It was seen that the endometrial development after GnRH antagonist appears very close to the natural endometrium than after GnRH agonist.

The biggest advantage of not having severe OHSS together with the reduction in the amount of gonadotropins along with much shorter duration of analog treatment makes antagonist protocol favorable.

CONCLUSION

Understanding the long protocol with GnRH analog and the GnRH antagonist is important for a better outcome thereby reducing the cost, duration, and OHSS. It is important to know the time of starting the antagonist in the stimulated cycle with gonadotropins for a better outcome. However, certain times analog may be chosen as well depending upon the various hormonal parameters and the conditions.

KEY POINTS

Downregulation of the hypothalamic-pituitary axis is required in assisted reproduction:

- To allow multifollicular development uninfluenced by the endogenous HP hormones.
- For LH surge prevention.
- To conveniently time the oocyte pick-up after appropriate follicular development.
- To synchronize the cohort of follicles that will be responding to COHS.
- To suppress endometriosis prior to COHS to improve ART outcomes.
- To suppress very-high LH and/or FSH levels prior to ART cycles to improve ovarian response:
  - In diminishing ovarian reserve
  - In PCOD cycles.

Downregulation to prevent premature LH surge:

- GnRHa various protocols
- GnRH antagonist—fixed and flexible protocols.

Downregulation to synchronize cohort of follicles to be stimulated and can be done by:

- GnRHa
- OCP suppression prior to IVF.

Downregulation to suppress very high LH and or FSH levels prior to ART cycles:

- GnRHa
- Antagonist pretreatment
- Estradiol pretreatment

Prevention of OHSS:

- GnRH trigger causes a profound downregulation after the initial LH surge that mitigates the risk of OHSS.

EDITORS' COMMENTS

1. The GnRH before IVF/ICSI may be beneficial in patients with adenomyosis, severe endometriosis, idiopathic RIF, and now emerging "BATCH" IVF practice.
2. The impact of OCP for downregulation on pregnancy results in IVF/ICSI, which remains a controversy.
3. Modified ultra-long pituitary downregulation protocol is known to significantly improve endometrial thickness, morphology, blood flow, and clinical pregnancy rates.

SUGGESTED READING

1. Al-Inany HG, Abou-Setta AM, Aboulghar M. Gonadotrophin-releasing hormone antagonist for assisted conception (review). Cochrane Database Syst Rev. 2006;(3):CD001750.
2. Badrawi A, Al-Inany H, Hussein M, et al. Agonist versus antagonist in ICSI cycles: a randomized trial and cost effectiveness Analysis. Middle East Fertil Soc J. 2005;10(1): 49-54.
3. Balasch J, Vidal E, Penarrubia J, et al. Suppression of LH during ovarian stimulation: analysing threshold values and effects on ovarian response and the outcome of assisted reproduction in down-regulated women stimulated with recombinant FSH. Hum Reprod. 2001;16(8):1636-43.
4. Bosch E, Valencia I, Escudero E, et al. Premature luteinization during gonadotropin-releasing hormone antagonist cycles and its relationship with in vitro fertilization outcome. Fertil Steril. 2003;80(6):1444-9.
5. Daya S. Gonadotropin releasing hormone agonist protocols for pituitary desensitization in in vitro fertilization and gamete intrafallopian transfer cycles. Cochrane Database Syst Rev. 2000;(2):CD001299.
6. Faber BM, Mayer J, Cox B, et al. Cessation of gonadotropin-releasing hormone agonist therapy combined with high-dose gonadotropin stimulation yields favorable pregnancy results in low responders. Fertil Steril. 1998;69(5):826-30.
7. Felberbaum RE, Diedrich K. Gonadotrophin-releasing hormone antagonists: will they replace the agonists? RBM Online. 2002;6(1):43-53.
8. Goldberg JM, Miller FA, Friedman CI, et al. Effect of baseline ovarian cysts on in vitro fertilization and gamete intrafallopian transfer cycles. Fertil Steril. 1991;55(2):319-23.
9. Gordon UD, Harrison RF, Fawzy M, et al. A randomized prospective assessor-blind evaluation of luteinizing hormone dosage and in vitro fertilization outcome. Fertil Steril. 2001; 75(2):324-31.
10. Hernández ER. Embryo implantation and GnRH antagonists: the Rubicon for GnRH antagonists. Hum Reprod. 2000; 15(6):1211-6.
11. Karande V, Morris R, Rinehart J, et al. Limited success using the "flare" protocol in poor responders in cycles with low basal follicle-stimulating hormone levels during in vitro fertilization. Fertil Steril. 1997;67(5):900-3.
12. Kolibianakis EM, Collins J, Tarlatzis BC, et al. Among patients treated for IVF with gonadotrophins and GnRH analogues, is the probability of live birth dependent on the type of analogue used? A systematic review and meta-analysis. Hum Reprod Update. 2006;12(6):651-71.
13. Meldrum D. GnRH agonists as adjuncts for in vitro fertilization. Obstet Gynecol. 1989;44(5):314-6.
14. Meldrum DR, Wisot A, Hamilton F, et al. Timing of initiation and dose schedule of leuprolide influence the time course of ovarian suppression. Fertil Steril. 1988;50(3):400-2.
15. Simon C, Oberye J, Bellver J, et al. Similar endometrial development in oocyte donors treated with either high- or standard-dose GnRH antagonist compared to treatment with a GnRH agonist or in natural cycles. Hum Reprod. 2005;20(12):3318-27.
16. The Ganirelix Dose-Finding Study Group. A double-blind, randomized, dose-finding study to assess the efficacy of the gonadotrophin-releasing hormone antagonist ganirelix (Org 37462) to prevent premature luteinizing hormone surges in women undergoing ovarian stimulation with recombinant follicle stimulating hormone (Puregon). Hum Reprod. 1998;13(11):3023-31.

7

CHAPTER

Role of Adjuvants in Controlled Ovarian Hyperstimulation: Recent Evidences

Purnima Nadkarni, Aditi Nadkarni, Anuradha Rathi, Urmila Sunda

INTRODUCTION

Adjuvant is the treatment that is given in addition to normal treatment in infertility; to increase chances of success and to decrease complications. Use of adjuvants helps in improving oocyte quality, endometrial vascularity as well as endometrial receptivity, and thus increases pregnancy rate in IVF cycle.

It can be divided into three subgroups (Flowchart 1):

1. *Adjuvants for improving ovarian follicular output*:
   - Adjuvants in poor responders
   - Adjuvants in hyper-responders
   - Adjuvants in normal responders
2. Adjuvants to enhance endometrial receptivity
3. Adjuvants to prevent complications.

ADJUVANTS IN POOR RESPONDERS

- *Growth hormone (GH)*: GH has a role in ovarian folliculogenesis and steroidogenesis by increasing synthesis of insulin-like growth factor 1 (IGF-1) as well as enhancing action of follicle-stimulating hormone (FSH). Recent evidence has shown that GH significantly affects DNA repair capacity of oocyte which might be instrumental in age reversing changes with GH use. *Dose*: 4–12 IU SC from the day of stimulation.

Flowchart 1: Different groups of adjuvants.

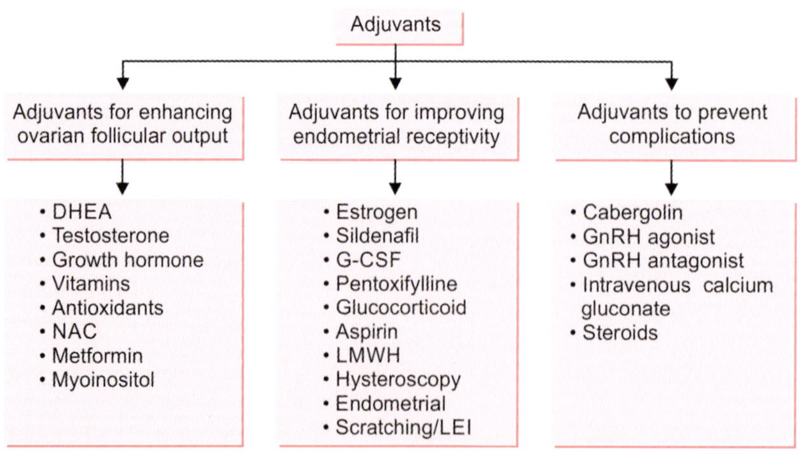

(DHEA: dehydroepiandrosterone; G-CSF: granulocyte colony-stimulating factor; GnRH: gonadotropin-releasing hormone; LMWH: low-molecular-weight heparin; NAC: N-acetyl cysteine; LEI: local endometrial injury)

- *Dehydroepiandrosterone (DHEA)*: This helps in ovarian steroidogenesis. It is a prohormone for follicular testosterone which is in turn source of estradiol (E2). It also increases IGF-1 and decreases dose of gonadotropins required for stimulation. Recent evidences support use of DHEA has increased anti-Müllerian hormone (AMH) concentration, antral follicle count (AFC), peak E2 levels, number of oocytes retrieved, and high quality embryos. DHEA suppresses apoptosis in granulosa cells.
  Dose: 75 mg daily for 2–4 months.
- *Testosterone*: It increases FSH receptor activity and synthesis of IGF-1. Use of transdermal testosterone patches in poor responders has increased number of oocyte retrieved, increased implantation rates, increased pregnancy rates, and reduced cycle cancellation. However, definitive use of androgens is still ambiguous as per recent studies and needs more trials.
- *L-arginine*: It helps in follicular maturation and growth by increasing periovulatory vascularity. Nitric oxide (NO) is synthesized by NO synthase from L-arginine.

ADJUVANTS IN HYPER-RESPONDERS

- *Metformin*: Metformin improves intraovarian hyperandrogenism. It increases peripheral utilization of glucose and decreases insulin resistance. It decreases number of non-periovulatory follicles and thereby E2 levels; thus, preventing complications. Evidence says, metformin in controlled ovarian hyperstimulation (COH)-intrauterine insemination (IUI), COH-assisted reproductive technology (ART) cycles increases pregnancy rates and reduces moderate/severe ovarian hyperstimulation syndrome (OHSS) by 80%. Use of metformin in older polycystic ovary (PCO) patients and those with FSH ≥10 yields poor response.
  Dose: 500 mg BD can be increased to 850 BD, if body mass index (BMI) is high.
- *Myoinositol + D-chiro-inositol*: It improves oocyte quality. It improves insulin resistance and thereby also prevents complications by decreasing vascular endothelial growth factor (VEGF), main causative agent of OHSS. It also decreases total androgen levels in patients with polycystic ovary syndrome (PCOS).
  Dose: 1,200 mg daily.

ADJUVANTS IN NORMAL RESPONDERS AND CLOMIPHENE CITRATE RESISTANCE

- *Antioxidants (Fig. 1)*: It includes enzymatic and nonenzymatic forms like superoxide dismutase, catalase, glutathione peroxidase, zinc, selenium, taurine, carotene, and beta carotene. It helps in reducing reactive oxygen species (ROS) which are responsible for decreased pregnancy rates.
- *Vitamins*: Folate improves oocyte quality and maturation. Hyper-homocysteinemia yields poor quality of embryos and is one of the causes of recurrent pregnancy loss (RPL). Pre-conceptional folic acid supplementation alters folate and B12 concentration in follicular fluids, yields good quality embryos and higher pregnancy rates.
- *Combined OC pills*: These are used in suppressing endogenous gonadotropins and sensitizing estrogen receptors. Combined oral contraceptives (COCs) help in synchronization of follicular development by downregulation, no cyst formation, avoidance of premature luteinizing hormone (LH) surge, and shorten duration of gonadotropin-releasing hormone (GnRH) analogs. Cochrane Review reveals fewer pregnancies, increased gonadotropins, and increased rates of miscarriage by prior use of COC pills in antagonists cycle.
- *N-acetyl cysteine (NAC)*: It is an acetylated variant of amino acid L-cysteine. It is an excellent source of sulfhydryl groups and is converted *in vivo* into metabolites that stimulate glutathione production, promote detoxification, and act directly as free radical scavengers, powerful antioxidant, has activity on insulin secretion in pancreatic cells and on insulin receptors on human erythrocytes. It has antiapoptotic effects also.
- Salehpour et al., 2009 and Badawy et al., 2007 conducted studies in PCOS patients with clomiphene citrate (CC) resistance. Results showed significant improvement in ovulation rate (55.6% as compared to placebo) with use of NAC.

ADJUVANTS FOR ENDOMETRIAL RECEPTIVITY

- *Estrogens*: It can be used for synchronization of endometrium with follicular growth. Luteal phase estrogen in previous cycles has shown increase in pregnancy and implantation rates. Estradiol valerate 2–4 mg is used. It can be used in form of tablets, gel, creams, and transdermal patches. Dosing is adjusted as per endometrial response.

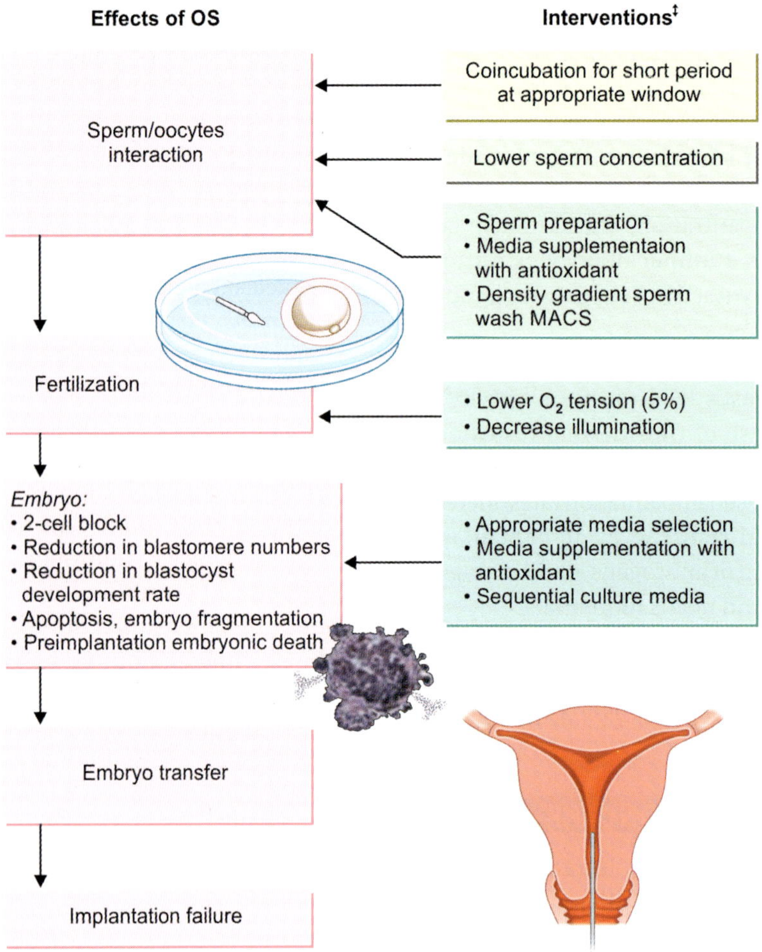

Fig. 1: Effects of oxidative stress (OS) and interventions to overcome its effects at different ART steps.
‡Interventions enhance gamete/embryo quality and fertility outcomes such as fertilization and implantation.
(MACS: magnetic cell separation; ART: assisted reproductive technology)
Source: Agarwal A, Durairajanayagam D, du Plessis SS. Utility of antioxidants during assisted reproductive techniques: an evidence based review. Reprod Biol and Endocrinol. 2014;12(1):112.

- *Vaginal sildenafil*: It is phosphodiesterase 5 (PDE 5) inhibitor. It increases vascularity of endometrium and uterus by vasodilatation. It is used when endometrial thickness (ET) is <9 mm on Day 10 or 11 and in recurrent implantation failure (RIF).
  Dose: 25 mg four times daily intravaginally.
- *Pentoxifylline*: It has anti-inflammatory, anti-platelet, and vasodilator effect. It improves blood flow to endometrium. It is used in combination with vitamin E which is the main antioxidant.
  Dose: 800 mg/day and vitamin E 1,000 IU/day for 6 months have improved pregnancy and live birth rates in patients with poor endometrial response.
- *Glucocorticoids*: It acts as an immunomodulator. It decreases NK cells activity, cytokines, and endometrial inflammation. It stimulates GH and IGF-1 synthesis. It increases uterine receptivity by suppressing adrenal androgens Dexamethasone, prednisolone, or methyl prednisolone can be used. Empirical use in all cases is not promoted. Recent evidence justifies its use in patient with thrombophilias [antinuclear antibody (ANA)/ATA/ antiphospholipid antibody (APLA) positive] and RIF.
  Doses: Dexamethasone—1 mg, prednisolone—10 mg, methyl prednisolone—16 mg, from the day of stimulation till 12–14 weeks.
- *Low dose aspirin*: It increases uterine blood flow by maintaining equilibrium between vasodilating prostacyclin and vasoconstricting thromboxane. It also prevents platelet aggregation and has anti-inflammatory effect. It is to be begun with the onset of mid luteal

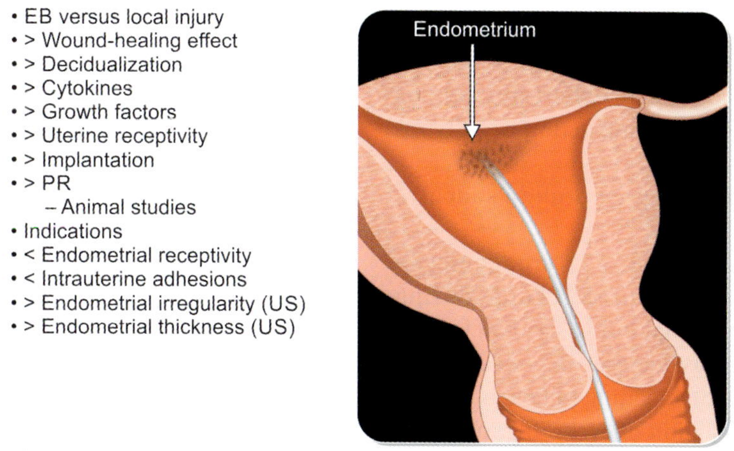

Fig. 2: Endometrial biopsy (Pipelle).

agonist and continued through early pregnancy. It increases uterine and ovarian blood flow implicated in implantation and good ovarian response. Recent Cochrane review updates do not promote use of aspirin empirically in all patients of ART.
Dose: 75/150 mg daily depending on BMI.

- *Low-molecular-weight heparin (LMWH)*: It helps to improve implantation by increasing growth factors like IGF-1, interleukin-2 and 6, and heparin binding epidermal factors. It helps in adhesion and invasion of blastocyst to endometrium. It takes care of many undiagnosed thrombophilias. Recent evidence s/o heparin protective against trophoblastic apoptosis.
Dose: 40 mg daily SC (1 mg/kg/day).
- *Granulocyte colony stimulating factor (G-CSF)*: It enhances cytokines promoting leukocyte growth and also trophoblast development.
Intrauterine G-CSF application significantly decreases CD16-CD56 dim/CD16-CD56 bright and NK cells subpopulation ratio, and increases leukemia inhibitory factor (LIF) expression in the endometrium.
Dose: 1.5 mg/kg SC daily from the day of transfer till positive beta-human chorionic gonadotropin (β-hCG) test.
- *Endometrial scratching*: It is proven that local endometrial injury to endometrium alters gene expression, increases decidualization and synthesis of growth factors. Endometrial biopsy (EB) is taken twice firstly on Day 7 or 8 and again on Day 24/28 of preceding cycle (Fig. 2). Gnainsky et al. have demonstrated increase in dendritic cells and macrophages after local endometrial injury that in turn increases decidualization and implantation. Recent Cochrane study says that local endometrial injury in previous cycle is associated with high pregnancy and implantation rates in patients with RIF.

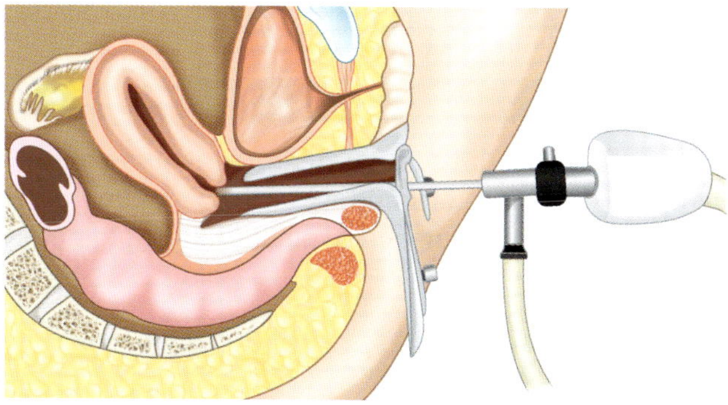

Fig. 3: Treatment with hysteroscopy.

- *Hysteroscopy*: Hysteroscopy is the gold standard for diagnosis of intrauterine pathology; which may be responsible for RIF. Local endometrial injury following hysteroscopy also increases implantation rates by increasing growth factors. It has proven as adjuvant in patients with RIF (Fig. 3).
- *Acupuncture*: It increases uterine blood flow, neurotransmitters, GnRH, E2, and FSH levels; decreases stress and thereby ROS and thus improves implantation rates. Studies are inadequate to prove this as a definitive adjuvant.

ADJUVANTS TO PREVENT COMPLICATIONS

- *Cabergoline*: It is dopamine agonist and decreases VEGF receptors which are the main causative agent for OHSS. It is started before trigger to prevent OHSS in patients prone to hyperstimulation.
Dose: 0–0.5 mg BD for 8 days.

- *GnRH agonist*: Agonist as a trigger, an antagonist protocol, in hyper-responders helps in preventing OHSS. Agonist has short ascending phase of 4 hours and long descending phase of 20 hours; hence short endogenous LH surge compared to long acting action of hCG for 7–10 days.
  Dose: 0.2 mg triptorelin, 1 mg leuprolide subcutaneously.
- *GnRH antagonist*: Main purpose of antagonist in ART cycles is to avoid premature LH surge during gonadotropin stimulation. It has temporary blockage of GnRH receptors that causes decrease in gonadotropin secretions. It is started when leading follicle is 14 mm or on Day 6 or 7 of stimulation of cycle. The luteolytic effect of the GnRH antagonist has been proposed as the main theory to explain the mode of action of this drug to prevent OHSS.
  Dose: 0.25 mg cetrorelix.

KEYNOTE

Adjuvants along with normal treatment course help in increasing pregnancy rates and live birth rates by improving ovarian follicular output, oocyte quality, and endometrial receptivity.

EDITORS' COMMENTS

1. Poor responders can benefit with prior DHEA, androgen gel, estradiol tablets, steroid tablets, and coenzyme to increase the quantity and quality of eggs.
2. Ovarian hyperstimulation syndrome can be reduced in PCOS by starting metformin for 2 months before IVF and confirm it.
3. Selected patients may benefit with the adjuvant therapy along with controlled ovarian stimulation.

SUGGESTED READING

1. Adashi EY, Resnick CE, Hurwitz A, et al. Insulin-like growth factors: the ovarian connection. Hum Reprod. 1991;6(9):1213-9.
2. Bohlmann MK. Effects and effectiveness of heparin in assisted reproduction. J Reprod Immunol. 2011;90(1):82-90.
3. Boomsma CM, Keay SD, Macklon NS. Peri-implantation glucocorticoid administration for assisted reproductive technology cycles. Cochrane Database Syst Rev. 2012;(6):CD005996.
4. FalboA, Russo T, Rocca M, et al. Serum and follicular anti-Mullerian hormone levels in women with polycystic ovary syndrome (PCOS) under metformin. J Ovarian Res. 2010;3:16.
5. Fanchin R, Salomon L, Castelo-Branco A, et al. Luteal estradiol pre-treatment coordinates follicular growth during controlled ovarian hyperstimulation with GnRH antagonists. Hum Reprod. 2003;18(12):2698-703.
6. Frattarelli JL, Hill MJ, McWilliams GDE, et al. A luteal estradiol protocol for expected poor responders improves embryo number and quality. Fertil Steril. 2008;89:1118-22.
7. Genazzani AD, Lanzoni C, Ricchieri F, et al. Myo-inositol administration positively affects hyperinsulinemia and hormonal parameters in overweight patients with polycystic ovary syndrome. Gynecol Endocrinol. 2008;24(3):139-44.
8. Gnainsky Y, Granot I, Aldo P, et al. Local injury of the endometrium induces an inflammatory response that promotes successful implantation. Fertil Steril. 2010; 94(6): 2030-6.
9. Hammadeh ME, Huquki M, Solomayer EF. Correlation between total homocysteine (tHcy), folic acid, vitamin B12 concentration in serum, follicular fluid (FF) and their effect on ICSI outcome. Fertil Steril. 2011;96(3):S93-4.
10. Haning RV, Hackett RJ, Flood CA, et al. Plasma dehydroepiandrosterone sulfate serves as a prehormone for 48% of follicular fluid testosterone during treatment with menotropins. J Clin Endocrinol Metab. 1993;76(5):1301-7.
11. Humaidan P, Papanikolaou EG, Tarlatzis BC. GnRHa to trigger final oocyte maturation: a time to reconsider. Hum Reprod. 2009;24(10):2389-94.
12. Lewicka S, von Hagens C, Hettinger U, et al. Cortisol and cortisone in human follicular fluid and serum and the outcome of IVF treatment. Hum Reprod. 2003;18:1613-7
13. Ludwig M, Katalinic A, Banz C, et al. Tailoring the GnRH antagonist cetrorelix acetate to individual patients' needs in ovarian stimulation for IVF: results of a prospective, randomized study. Hum Reprod. 2002;17(11);2842-5.
14. Nelson SM, Greer IA. The potential role of heparin in assisted conception. Hum Reprod Update. 2008;14(6):623-45.
15. Nielsen ME, Rasmussen IA, Kristensen SG, et al. In human granulosa cells from small antral follicles, androgen receptor mRNA and androgen levels in follicular fluid correlate with FSH receptor mRNA. Mol Human Reprod. 2011;17(1):63-70.
16. Palomba S, Orio F Jr, Falbo A, et al. Clomiphene citrate versus metformin as first-line approach for the treatment of anovulation in infertile patients with polycystic ovary syndrome. J Clin Endocrinol Metab. 2007;92(9):3498-503.
17. Sher G, Fisch JD. Effect of vaginal sildenafil on the outcome of in vitro fertilization (IVF) after multiple IVF failures attributed to poor endometrial development. Fertil Steril. 2002;78:1073-6.
18. Sher G, Fisch JD. Vaginal sildenafil (Viagra): A preliminary report of a novel method to improve uterine artery blood flow and endometrial development in patients undergoing IVF. Hum Reprod. 2000;15:806-9.
19. Siristatidis CS, Dodd SR, Drakeley AJ. Aspirin for in vitro fertilisation. Cochrane Database Syst Rev. 2011;(8):CD004832.
20. Soares SR. Etiology of OHSS and use of dopamine agonists. Fertil Steril. 2012;97:517-22.
21. Tso LO, Costello MF, Albuquerque LE, et al. Metformin treatment before and during IVF or ICSI in women with polycystic ovary syndrome. Cochrane Database Syst Rev. 2009;(2):CD006105.
22. Vendola K, Zhou J, Wang J, et al. Androgens promote oocyte insulin-like growth factor I expression and initiation of follicle development in the primate ovary. Biol Reprod. 1999;61(2):353-7.

8

CHAPTER

Ovarian Hyperstimulation Syndrome

Asha Baxi, Dhaval Baxi

INTRODUCTION

The first *in vitro* fertilization (IVF) baby, Louise Brown, was born with a single embryo transfer in a natural cycle; however with time, in the race of improving results, protocols of superovulation were introduced. The aim of these protocols was to increase the number of oocytes available for fertilization and these protocols were termed as controlled ovarian hyperstimulation protocols. This introduced a new iatrogenic problem of ovarian hyperstimulation syndrome (OHSS). The seriousness of OHSS in the form of morbidity and mortality was identified and measures were developed to reduce its incidence. The syndrome is characterized by fluid shift into the third space due to either increased capillary permeability or ovarian neoangiogenesis.

Ovarian hyperstimulation syndrome is one of the most common but at the same time one of the most serious issues faced in an IVF clinic with mild OHSS occurring in almost a third of IVF cycles and the incidence of moderate to severe OHSS ranging from 1.1% to 8% with a hospitalization rate of 0.3%.

PATHOPHYSIOLOGY

The clinical manifestations of OHSS are a cascade of pathophysiologic events resulting from a global increase in vascular permeability. This increased vascular permeability causes a decrease in the colloid oncotic pressure, which results in a change in extracellular fluid equilibrium. Fluid consequently shifts into the extravascular or "third" space, depleting intravascular volume and causing hypotension. "Third spacing" causes abdominal ascites, pleural and pericardial effusions, and dependent edema. Cardiac preload falls due to a combination of hypovolemia caused by fluid shifts and compression of the inferior vena cava from the increasing intraperitoneal pressure due to ascites accumulation. Falling cardiac preload reduces cardiac output, which, together with a decrease in peripheral vascular resistance due to an arterial vasodilatation, in turn leads to a decrease in renal perfusion. Decreasing renal perfusion increases proximal tubule reabsorption of salt and water, leading to decreased urinary sodium excretion and oliguria. The proximal sodium reabsorption, and consequently diminished exposure of the distal tubule to sodium, impairs the sodium-hydrogen/potassium exchange in the distal tubule, causing hyperkalemic acidosis. Decreasing renal perfusion also decreases glomerular filtration rate, which can result in oliguria or anuria and a full-blown prerenal azotemia. OHSS also produces a hypercoagulable state, possibly due to a combination of hemoconcentration, high levels of ovarian steroids, and changes in liver perfusion, resulting in decreased hepatic protein synthesis with consequent depletion of circulating antithrombotic factors.

Although the exact mechanism for OHSS is not known, the strongest single factor seems to be human chorionic gonadotropin (hCG). OHSS is not seen when hCG trigger is not administered and the persistent production of hCG in early pregnancy is a significant risk factor for severe OHSS. hCG leads to the expression of vascular endothelial growth factor (VEGF) mRNA (messenger ribonucleic acid) from the luteinized granulosa cells. Insulin and insulin-like growth factor levels in women with polycystic ovarian syndrome (PCOS) also have a synergistic action on VEGF mRNA production. VEGF is a protein which is involved in angiogenesis. There are five types A, B, C, D, and E of which A is the most active form. It acts via tyrosine kinase receptors (VEGFR) of which VEGFR-2 is responsible for most of the known actions of VEGF. VEGF levels have been shown to directly correlate with the severity of OHSS, and anti-VEGF serum has been shown to reduce the severity of OHSS which makes it an important mediator in OHSS.

Ovarian hyperstimulation syndrome has also been seen in women with spontaneous singleton pregnancies. Mutations in FSH receptors causing a loss in ligand specificity allow activation by hCG leading to a prolonged and increased response by the high amount of endogenous hCG resulting in late-onset OHSS.

CLASSIFICATION

Ovarian hyperstimulation syndrome is a disease with a wide spectrum of clinical features depending upon the severity of the disease. Classification is important as it helps in directing the management strategies and for standardization of the disease which will then simplify application of results from research into clinical practice. OHSS can be classified based on timing of onset and on disease severity.

On the basis of severity, the earliest classification was proposed by Rabau et al. in 1967. He classified OHSS into six different grades based on clinical and laboratory parameters. Rabau considered grade 1 and 2 to be natural features of a stimulation cycle and grade 3 and beyond as OHSS (Table 1).

Schenker and Weinstein in 1978 simplified Rabau's classification into three distinct entities being mild (grade 1 and 2), moderate (grade 3 and 4), and severe (grade 5 and 6) OHSS, while retaining the original definitions proposed by Rabau.

With the evolution of assisted reproductive techniques (ARTs), many drawbacks of the above system were pointed out, being that they were more focused on ovarian response rather than the clinical syndrome, they used cumbersome and sparingly used laboratory tests (24 hour urinary hormone collection), and that early grades of the classification were routinely observed in patients undergoing controlled ovarian stimulation and a need for a new system was felt. Golan et al. in 1989 classified the disease into three broad categories being mild, moderate, and severe which were subdivided into five grades viz., grade 1 and 2 (mild), grade 3 (moderate), and grade 4 and 5 (severe) (Table 2). The most distinguishing feature of the syndrome was the inclusion of ultrasound findings into the classification.

Navot et al. in 1992 modified Golan's classification by dividing severe OHSS into severe and critical categories (Table 3).

Rizk and Aboulghar in 1999 omitted mild OHSS as they believed it to be a normal finding in the ART cycle and divided Golan's severe category into three grades A, B, and C (Table 4).

Early and Late OHSS

Based on the timing of onset, OHSS has been classified into two different entities, early OHSS and late OHSS. Early OHSS typically occurs within 7 days of ovulation triggering and is related to an exaggerated ovarian response to gonadotropin stimulation which is precipitated by the exogenous hCG trigger. As it is directly related to the stimulation parameters, it can be predicted and corrective measures can be taken early.

Late OHSS is seen in patients after 10 days of the trigger and is seen in patients who get pregnant and is due to excessive endogenous hCG production. It occurs only in the setting of pregnancy and most cases tend to be severe. It can occur with singleton and multiple pregnancies with an equal incidence.

TABLE 1 Rabau's classification.

Category	*Features*
Grade 1	Only laboratory evidence of ovarian hyperstimulation syndrome (OHSS) exists: Total urinary estrogens above 150 μg/24 hr and pregnanediol excretion above 10 mg/24 hr
Grade 2	The features of grade 1 plus enlargement of the ovaries. Ovaries not enlarged beyond 5 cm in diameter
Grade 3	The features of Grade 1 and 2 plus abdominal distension
Grade 4	The features of grade 3 plus nausea, vomiting, and/or diarrhea. (In moderate OHSS, there is a considerable degree of abdominal discomfort with symptoms of gastrointestinal irritation.) Ovaries usually 5–12 cm in diameter
Grade 5	The features of moderate OHSS plus ascites and/or hydrothorax
Grade 6	All of the above plus a change in blood volume and increased blood viscosity due to hemoconcentration, resulting in coagulation abnormalities and diminished renal perfusion complicated by anuria and renal failure

TABLE 2 Golan's classification.

Category	*Features*
Mild	
Grade 1	Abdominal distension and discomfort
Grade 2	Features of grade 1 plus nausea, vomiting, and/or diarrhea. Ovaries are enlarged to 5–12 cm
Moderate	
Grade 3	Features of mild OHSS plus ultrasonic evidence of ascites
Severe	
Grade 4	Features of moderate OHSS plus clinical evidence of ascites and/or hydrothorax or breathing difficulties
Grade 5	All of the above plus change in blood volume, increased blood viscosity due to hemoconcentration, coagulation abnormalities, and diminished renal perfusion and function

TABLE 3 Navot's classification.

Severe OHSS	*Critical OHSS*
Variably enlarged ovary	Variably enlarged ovary
Tense ascites ± hydrothorax	Tense ascites ± hydrothorax ± pericardial effusion
Hematocrit >45% (or >30% increase over baseline)	Hematocrit >55%
WBC >15,000 cells/mm^3	WBC ≥25,000 cells/mm^3
Oliguria	Oligo/anuria
Creatinine 1.0–1.5 mg/dL	Creatinine ≥1.6 mg/dL
Creatinine clearance >50 mL/min	Renal failure
Liver dysfunction	Thromboembolic phenomena
Anasarca	Adult respiratory distress syndrome

TABLE 4 Rizk and Aboulghar's classification.

Category	*Features*
Moderate OHSS	Discomfort, pain, nausea, distension, ultrasonic evidence of ascites and enlarged ovaries, and normal hematological and biological profiles
Severe OHSS	
Grade A	Dyspnea, oliguria, nausea, vomiting, diarrhea, abdominal pain, clinical evidence of ascites, marked distension of abdomen or hydrothorax, ultrasound showing large ovaries and marked ascites, and normal biochemical profile
Grade B	Grade A plus massive tension ascites, markedly enlarged ovaries, severe dyspnea and marked oliguria, increased hematocrit, elevated serum creatinine, and liver dysfunction
Grade C	Complications such as respiratory distress syndrome, renal shut-down or venous thrombosis

RISK FACTORS AND PREDICTION OF OVARIAN HYPERSTIMULATION SYNDROME

Identification of patients at risk of hyper-response to treatment and subsequently OHSS is one of the most important steps in prevention of the syndrome. A hyper-response is defined as the retrieval of >15 oocytes from a patient following a standard ovarian stimulation protocol.

Risk factors can be divided into primary (patient related) risk factors and secondary (ovarian response related) risk factors.

Primary Risk Factors

Anti-Müllerian hormone (AMH) levels: AMH levels are a marker of the ovarian reserve. Patients with a high ovarian reserve have a larger follicular pool which is available for stimulation and puts them at a higher risk for hyper-response. An AMH level of 3.36 independently predicts OHSS with a sensitivity of 90.5% and specificity of 81.3%.

Young age: Age of the patient below 33 years predicts OHSS with a sensitivity of 76% and specificity of 59%.

Body weight: There have been contradictory reports regarding the effect of BMI on the incidence of OHSS. As of now there is no conclusive evidence that body weight influences OHSS incidence/severity.

Previous history of OHSS: Patients with previous history of OHSS, especially those requiring hospitalization, have an increased risk of developing OHSS.

History of allergies: Patients with OHSS tend to have a higher prevalence of pre-existing allergies (56% vs. 21% in controls). The link between the two is feasible as the changes in the hyperstimulated ovary are similar to those seen in an inflammatory response.

Antral follicular count: Patients with >24 antral follicles have a risk of moderate/severe OHSS (8.6% vs. 2.2% in controls). The risk rose to 11% in patients who had polycystic ovaries.

Secondary Risk Factors

Pretrigger: High number of medium/large follicles 13 or more follicles >11 mm is predictive of OHSS with 85.5% sensitivity and 69% specificity. This number had a highly significant negative likelihood ratio of <0.001 which indicates that development of OHSS in patients with less than 13 follicles is highly unlikely.

High or rapidly rising E2 levels and high number of follicles: Poorly predictive for OHSS; however, the combination of E2 and number of follicles (≥18 follicles and/or E2 of 5,000 ng/L) with a significant positive-likelihood ratio (LR = 5.19) can predict 83% of the severe OHSS cases, including both early and late cases, with an acceptable specificity of 84%.

On the day of pickup: Number of oocytes retrieved. Retrieval of more than 11 oocytes is a predictor of OHSS with a sensitivity of 90.5% and sensitivity of 66%. The negative predictive value of this is 98.8% which would mean that it is highly unlikely that a patient would develop OHSS below this number.

Proteomic analysis of serum and follicular fluid: When proteomic analysis of follicular fluid of patients with OHSS was performed, 57 proteins were found to have a difference of which 29 were upregulated and 28 proteins were downregulated. Three biomarkers namely haptoglobin, fibrinogen, and lipoprotein lipase were identified to have a strong correlation.

Post-transfer: Human chorionic gonadotropin for luteal phase support. IVF cycles are dependent on luteal phase support owing to the negative feedback on the pituitary due to the supraphysiological levels of estrogen and progesterone after controlled ovarian hyperstimulation. When hCG and progesterone are compared, there is no difference in live birth or ongoing pregnancy rates but the risk of OHSS is twice when hCG is used.

PREVENTION OF OVARIAN HYPERSTIMULATION SYNDROME

Prevention is better than cure. Once the "at risk" patient is identified, strategies need to be planned to reduce the development of OHSS in the patient while at the same time not compromising on the results. Commonly employed strategies have been mentioned below.

Choice of Stimulation Protocol

Multiple studies have shown the efficacy of an antagonist protocol in reducing the incidence of OHSS when compared to agonist protocol. The mechanism at work here may be related to the lower levels of E2 seen due to gonadotropin-releasing hormone (GnRH) suppression. In a large randomized controlled trial (RCT) involving 1,050 patients, the incidence of severe OHSS was significantly lower in the antagonist group (5.1% vs 8.9%) with no difference in live birth rates. A Cochrane review evaluated data from 29 RCTs and demonstrated a statistically significant lower incidence of OHSS in the GnRH antagonist group [odds ratio (OR) 0.43; 95% confidence interval (CI) 0.33–0.57] and no difference in live-birth rates when compared with patients receiving GnRH agonist.

An oocyte donor-based study reported that doubling the dose of the antagonist and reducing the dose of stimulation was effective in reducing the incidence of OHSS without having to coast and without affecting the egg retrieval rate and quality.

Use of a clomiphene citrate-based low dose protocol has shown to decrease the incidence of OHSS (OR 0.23; 95% CI 0.10–0.52) but this may be due to the low dose of gonadotropins used and not the effect of clomiphene citrate per se.

The authors recommend using a low dose antagonist-based protocol for reducing the incidence of OHSS with a starting dose of not more than 150 IU in patients at high risk of hyper-response.

Type of Gonadotropin

With a variety of gonadotropin preparations available to choose from the market, various preparations have been compared with each other to identify which one is more effective and also the safety profiles. On comparing urinary gonadotropins with recombinant follicle-stimulating hormone (rFSH), there was no difference in the rates of OHSS between the two groups as observed in the MEGASET trial (3% in both groups).

Corifollitropin alpha is a long-acting gonadotropin which has a half-life of 65 hours and a single injection can replace 7 of rFSH. When the data of two large RCTs (Engage and Ensure) were pooled, the incidence of OHSS was similar to that in patients receiving rFSH (6.9% vs 6.0%).

Another new gonadotropin, corifollitropin delta, has an AMH-based dosage algorithm and may be promising in the prevention/reduction in severity of OHSS in high risk patients.

Coasting

Coasting involves withholding exogenous gonadotropins and postponing the hCG trigger until a patient's E2 level has declined to a safer predefined level (usually ~3,000 pg/nL). Coasting leads to the selective regression of the pool of immature (small/medium) follicles, which reduces the functioning granulosa cell mass available for luteinization and results in a decline in vasoactive substances involved in the pathogenesis of OHSS. Coasting has been shown to reduce the incidence of OHSS in high-risk patients without affecting cycle outcome.

However, coasting for more than 3–4 days results in lower than anticipated pregnancy and implantation rates.

Accelerated coasting involves continuation of the antagonist up to and beyond the day of the agonist trigger. This helps is reducing OHSS and cycle cancellation without affecting oocyte maturation.

Individualized Human Chorionic Gonadotropin Trigger

With the concept of hCG being the final trigger to the development of OHSS, reducing the dose of hCG may be an option to reduce the incidence of OHSS. Use of a sliding scale concept with the dose of the trigger adjusted to the E2 levels on the day of trigger has shown that doses as low as 3,300 IU of hCG can be used as a trigger is effective to reduce the incidence of OHSS without adversely affecting the pregnancy rates.

Use of an Agonist Trigger

The use of a GnRH agonist as an alternative to hCG for triggering ovulation and prevention of OHSS can be made in GnRH antagonist cycles. The oocyte yield and oocyte maturation is similar to that of an hCG trigger with a significant decrease in OHSS. However the corpus luteum formed after a GnRH trigger produces significantly less progesterone and undergoes early luteolysis leading to poor pregnancy rates and high miscarriage rates in fresh transfers but not in donor-recipient cycles. To overcome this dilemma of poor pregnancy rates, segmentation of the IVF cycle into four parts viz., stimulation with antagonist protocol, GnRH analogue trigger, oocyte/embryo vitrification and thawing with transfer in an unstimulated cycle can be done. Segmentation is an effective strategy and the concept of an OHSS-free clinic is based on it.

Kisspeptin Trigger

Kisspeptin-54 is a hormone that offers a novel approach to trigger oocyte maturation during IVF treatment. It stimulates the release of endogenous GnRH from the hypothalamus and the consequent release of LH and FSH. Hence, kisspeptin induces an LH surge that is dependent upon the patient's individual endogenous GnRH/gonadotropin reserves and thus should prevent excessive stimulation of the ovaries and therefore reduce the incidence of OHSS. However studies comparing kisspeptin to standard triggers are lacking and the use of kisspeptin as a trigger may still take some time to enter routine clinical practice.

Freeze-all Strategy

Elective cryopreservation of all embryos and their subsequent transfer in nonstimulated cycles may be used to avoid the endogenous hCG rise in fresh transfer cycles, which can exacerbate late-onset OHSS symptoms and duration. Two RCTs have concluded that elective cryopreservation prevents OHSS. With this strategy there is a significantly reduced incidence of OHSS and no difference or a higher live birth rate when compared with transfers in the same cycle with or without intravenous (IV) albumin.

Metformin

Metformin is a commonly used insulin sensitizer used to treat type 2 diabetes. It also improves the intraovarian androgenism and thereby leads to a reduction in the number of nonperiovulatory follicles and granulosa cells which in turn reduces estrogen production. Metformin 1,500 mg daily when started with downregulation leads to a reduction in OHSS in PCOS patients vs. placebo (3.8% vs. 20.4%) in GnRH agonist cycles. A Cochrane review found that the use of metformin increased clinical pregnancy rates (OR 1.52; 95% CI 1.07–2.15) and decreased the risk of OHSS (OR 0.29; 95% CI 0.18–0.49). A recent meta-analysis included 12 studies of 1,516 participants and showed that there were no differences in pregnancy rates, live-birth rates, and spontaneous abortion rates between the metformin group and placebo group, but that OHSS risk was significantly lower with metformin use [relative risk (RR) 0.44; 95% CI 0.26–0.77).

Aspirin

Aspirin is a nonsteroidal anti-inflammatory drug. Low dose aspirin (100 mg/day) has shown to reduce the incidence of OHSS (0.25% vs. 8.4% in control group) in a large RCT with no effect on the pregnancy rates.

Corticosteroids

Glucocorticoids have an inhibitory effect on VEGF expression and also have a strong anti-inflammatory action which prevents capillary leakage. Initial studies showed a benefit of methylprednisolone when 16 mg/day starting on Day 6 of the stimulation and tapered after the first pregnancy test (Day 13 after embryo transfer), but new studies report no effect on the incidence of OHSS.

Calcium

Calcium acts by inhibition of cyclic adenosine monophosphate-stimulated renin secretion, which reduces angiotensin II synthesis and its subsequent effect on VEGF production. 10 mL of 10% calcium gluconate (in 200 mL normal saline) on the day of oocyte retrieval and Days 1, 2, and 3 after oocyte retrieval has shown to decrease the risk for developing OHSS (7% vs. 23% in controls).

Volume Expanders

Albumin is a plasma protein which acts by acting as a binding protein to vasoactive substances leading to their inactivation and secondly by increasing the oncotic pressure and preventing capillary leakage. Albumin administration has shown to lower the incidence of OHSS (OR 0.67; 95% CI 0.47–0.95), but it is associated with a detrimental effect on the pregnancy rates (OR 0.75; 95% CI 0.55–0.94). Apart from being expensive, it has a side effect profile which includes viral transmission, nausea, vomiting, and febrile allergic reactions, and pulmonary edema in patients with an impaired cardiac reserve, the role of albumin administration is limited in the prevention of OHSS.

Mannitol is an osmotic diuretic which acts by increasing the oncotic pressure and prevents leakage into the third space. Mannitol administration decreases the incidence of OHSS (OR 0.38; 95% CI 0.22–0.64) without any effect on the pregnancy rates. It is a more cost-effective drug to use when compared with albumin. The use of mannitol should however be restricted as it may cause electrolyte disturbances, dehydration, and the effect on pregnancy is not known.

Hydroxyethyl starch (HES) is a starch derivative used as a volume expander and has been suggested as an alternative to albumin. HES administration reduces the incidence of OHSS (OR 0.27; 95% CI 0.12–0.59) without affecting pregnancy rates (OR 1.20; 95% CI 0.49–2.93). It was thought that, as a cheaper, potentially safer alternative to albumin, HES should be the first-line treatment. However, recently the US Food and Drug Administration (US-FDA) has discouraged the use of HES in critically ill patients, due to the increased incidence of renal failure, septic shock and death. The European Medical Agency (EMA) has called for a withdrawal of all HES-containing products across Europe.

Dopamine Agonists

Cabergoline is a dopamine agonist which also has a VEGF-2 receptor blocking action. It is postulated that through its VEGF receptor blocking action, cabergoline should reduce the incidence and severity of OHSS. The typical dose of cabergoline is 0.5 mg started on the day of trigger and continued for 7 days. A study examined the effect of timing of cabergoline and its effectiveness in preventing OHSS. They found that there was no difference in the incidence of OHSS when cabergoline was started on the day of hCG vs. the day of oocyte retrieval. A Cochrane review suggested that dopamine agonists appeared to reduce the incidence of moderate or severe OHSS in women at high risk of OHSS. However, there are no effects on the pregnancy outcome (live birth rate, clinical pregnancy rate, and miscarriage rate) in fresh transfers.

Cycle Cancellation

Cycle cancellation by withholding the hCG trigger is an effective to prevent OHSS. However, it is a costly option both in financial and emotional terms for the patient and is therefore reserved only for those patients who are at a high risk of developing OHSS and in whom control over the cycle is lost. Once the cycle is cancelled, a review of the stimulation protocol and gonadotropin dose must be done and the subsequent stimulation should be planned accordingly.

In vitro Maturation

In vitro maturation (IVM) may be used as an alternative to conventional IVF for patients with a high risk of developing OHSS or in those who have had a history of severe or critical OHSS in the past. IVM involves no or minimal stimulation and aspiration of immature follicles which are then matured in-vitro and then fertilized. Live birth rates with IVM have been reported to be similar to that of IVF cycles (37.78% vs.

41.39%). However IVM is being performed only in a few centers globally and results may vary from center to center.

CLINICAL FEATURES

Abdominal Pain, Nausea, and Vomiting

Abdominal pain, nausea, and vomiting are seen secondary to ovarian enlargement. The enlargement is sometimes as much as 25 cm and patients have abdominal distension and palpable masses in the lower abdomen. Acute abdominal pain may be due to ovarian torsion, intraperitoneal hemorrhage or rupture of cysts.

Ascites and Tense Distention

Leakage of fluid from follicles and increased capillary permeability lead to extravasation of fluid into the third space. Frank rupture of follicles may also occur. Both of these phenomena may cause ascites. The increased intra-abdominal pressure secondary to ascites also contributes to the abdominal distention and discomfort.

Localized or Generalized Peritonitis

Localized or generalized peritonitis is caused by peritoneal irritation secondary to blood, protein-rich fluid, and inflammatory mediators from ruptured cysts.

Hypotension and/or Hypovolemia

Leakage of fluid through the impaired blood vessels both within and outside the ovary causes a massive fluid shift from the intravascular compartment into the third compartment. This results in intravascular hypovolemia with concomitant development of edema, ascites, hydrothorax, and/or pericardial effusion.

Dyspnea

Enlarged ovaries and ascites restrict diaphragmatic movement which may compromise pulmonary function. Dyspnea may also occur due to the relatively rare manifestations of OHSS, such as pleural effusion, pulmonary edema, atelectasis, pulmonary embolism, acute respiratory distress syndrome (ARDS), and pericardial effusion.

Hypercoagulable State

Hemoconcentration and hypovolemia resulting from third space shift of fluid lead to a state of hypercoagulability. Patients have an increased risk of developing deep venous thrombosis and pulmonary embolism. Both venous (65.7%) and arterial thromboses have been described and 83% of these occur in the veins of neck, arm or head (60%). Thrombosis also occurs in arteries and veins of the lower body. Pulmonary embolism occurs in 4–12%. Microthrombi in the renal tubules may lead to decreased renal perfusion and may result in acute renal failure.

Electrolyte Imbalance

Extravasation of fluid and resultant renal dysfunction resulting from decreased perfusion leads to oliguria. Increased reabsorption of sodium and water which occurs in the proximal tubule, leads to low urinary sodium excretion. The exchange of hydrogen and potassium for sodium in the distal tubule is reduced causing, hyperkalemia and a tendency to develop acidosis.

MANAGEMENT

Owing to the broad spectrum of presentation of OHSS, patients can be managed on an inpatient or outpatient basis depending upon the severity. These patients should be managed by an experienced ART clinician. The first step involves counseling the patients about the disease and to emphasize the importance of monitoring.

Patients should be examined daily for weight, abdominal palpation including abdominal girth (at the level of umbilicus), chest auscultation to rule out pulmonary edema/pleural effusion, enquire regarding urine output and to look for development of any new signs/symptoms like tachycardia, hypotension, reduced urine output, shortness of breath, and worsening of abdominal pain.

INVESTIGATIONS

Baseline investigations include:

- Full blood count
- Hematocrit (hemoconcentration)
- Urea and electrolytes (hyponatremia and hyperkalemia)
- Liver function tests (elevated enzymes and reduced albumin)
- *Ultrasound scan*: Ovarian size, pelvic and abdominal free fluid. Consider ovarian Doppler to rule out torsion.

Other tests that may be indicated:

- Human chorionic gonadotropin (to determine outcome of treatment cycle) if appropriate
- Coagulation profile (elevated fibrinogen and reduced antithrombin)
- Serum osmolality (hypo-osmolality)
- Arterial blood gases (hypoxia)
- C-reactive protein (severity)
- D-dimers (thromboembolism)

- Electrocardiogram (ECG)/echocardiogram
- Chest X-ray (pleural effusion/pulmonary edema)
- Computerized tomography pulmonary angiogram (CTPA) or ventilation-perfusion (V-Q) scans.

TREATMENT

Mild OHSS

Treatment for OHSS is supportive. Mild ovarian hyperstimulation can develop into moderate or severe disease, especially if the patient becomes pregnant. Baseline investigations should be sent. Therefore, women with mild disease should be observed for enlarging abdominal girth, acute weight gain, and abdominal discomfort on an ambulatory basis for at least 2–3 weeks or until menstrual bleeding occurs.

Moderate OHSS

Treatment of moderate OHSS consists of observation, bed rest, provision of adequate fluids, and sonographic monitoring of the size of cysts. Serum electrolyte concentrations, hematocrit, and creatinine levels should also be evaluated.

Patients should be advised to drink water as per thirst and avoid excessive water intake. Fluid input of <1,000 mL/day, output <1,000 mL/day or a difference in fluid balance >1,000 mL/day is a cause for concern.

Paracetamol and oral opiates should be given to patients for pain relief. Nonsteroidal anti-inflammatory drugs should be avoided as they may cause renal injury.

Resolution of OHSS is apparent when a decreasing trend in the ovarian size is noted on two consecutive ultrasound examinations, and when a clinical improvement in the symptoms is seen. In contrast, early detection of progression to the severe form of the syndrome is marked by continuous weight gain (>2 lb/day), increased severity of existing symptoms, or appearance of new symptoms (e.g. vomiting, diarrhea or dyspnea).

Patients with moderate OHSS can be managed on an outpatient basis with daily follow-up. However, some patients may need admission when there is:

- Inability to achieve satisfactory pain control
- Inability to maintain adequate fluid intake due to nausea
- Signs of worsening of OHSS despite outpatient management
- Patients unable to attend for regular outpatient follow-up
- Severe/Critical OHSS.

Severe OHSS

Patients with severe OHSS should be managed on an inpatient basis with access to radiology, laboratory, and intensive care facilities. Management aims at control of disease progression, complication prevention, and symptomatic relief.

Use of diuretics should be avoided on a routine basis as they will lead to further depletion of intravascular volume and exacerbate hypovolemia, but may be used in a multidisciplinary setup to manage oliguria which persists even after adequate fluid replacement.

Ovarian enlargement and increasing ascites may lead to abdominal tightening, discomfort, and dyspnea for which paracentesis must be done. Paracentesis is done vaginally with a setup resembling that of an oocyte retrieval and should be performed by an experienced clinician owing to the risk of injury to bowel, rupture of cysts, and vascular injury associated with the procedure. Multiple paracentesis (>3) have shown to reduce the duration of hospitalization, increase the pregnancy rate and reduce the abortion rate. In patients with large ascites, an alternative to repeated paracentesis is the placement of a pigtail catheter which can be kept for 3–12 days. Paracentesis may also aid in the management of oliguria. Rarely some patients may need a pleural tap due to dyspnea secondary to hydrothorax.

Prophylactic anti-coagulation must be started when the patient's hematocrit is >45% with unfractionated heparin 5,000 IU twice daily. Alternatively, low-molecular-weight heparin may be used with the benefit of once daily dosage. Compression stockings can be used as an alternative to chemical thromboprophylaxis when the latter is contraindicated. In patients who conceive thromboprophylaxis should be continued till the end of the first trimester.

Gonadotropin-releasing hormone antagonist administration in women with established severe early OHSS may result in quicker regression of the syndrome. Studies also suggest that dopamine agonists may have a beneficial role in the treatment of established OHSS.

Transfusion of fresh thawed plasma may be a useful therapeutic option in patients not responding to conventional therapy and has shown to provide rapid resolution of symptoms.

Critical OHSS

Critical OHSS may include renal failure, hepatic damage, thromboembolic phenomena, ARDS, and multiorgan failure. They should be managed in an intensive care unit by a multidisciplinary team which may include a nephrologist, chest physician, intensivist, and a clinician with expertise in managing OHSS patients. In some patients with late onset OHSS with pregnancy, who do not respond to any treatment, a therapeutic abortion may have to be performed as a last resort measure. Some cases of bilateral oophorectomy have been reported but it is not recommended.

Surgical Treatment

Surgical treatment is rarely required and limited to management of ovarian torsion, ovarian rupture, and ectopic pregnancy. Surgery must be performed by an experienced surgeon keeping in mind the presence of ascites and the delicate nature of the ovaries.

OVARIAN HYPERSTIMULATION SYNDROME AND PREGNANCY OUTCOME

There is no evidence of an increased risk of miscarriage in women with OHSS when compared to those without it. A higher incidence of pre-eclampsia (21.2% vs 9.2%) and prematurity (36% vs 10.7%) has been reported in pregnancies with OHSS.

KEY POINTS

- Early identification of potential hyper-responders is vital for prevention of OHSS.
- Use of an antagonist-based protocol with a low starting dose should be employed for ovarian stimulation.
- Individualization of hCG trigger can help in reducing OHSS.
- Use of GnRH agonists as trigger with cryopreservation of embryos and transfer in an unstimulated cycle is an effective strategy to reduce OHSS.
- Management of patients with OHSS should be under an experienced ART clinician.
- Multidisciplinary care may be needed for patients with severe/critical OHSS.
- Thromboprophylaxis should be started when there is an increase in hematocrit.
- Use of HES should be avoided in patients with severe disease.
- The experience with newer modalities like IVM is still lacking to consider it as a reliable alternative to conventional IVF.

CONCLUSION

Ovarian hyperstimulation syndrome is an iatrogenic problem, which in its severe form can be life-threatening. Identification of patients at a high risk, using soft protocols, GnRH agonist triggers, and cryopreservation have helped in reducing the incidence of OHSS. Early identification and close monitoring of patients are essential to prevent disease progression. The use of newer modalities like Kisspeptin trigger and analysis of proteins in the serum and follicular fluid seem to be promising but are yet to be available for routine practice. Further research into understanding the exact pathophysiology is required to develop more effective, preventive, and management strategies to achieve the dream of an OHSS-free clinic.

EDITORS' COMMENTS

1. Ovarian hyperstimulation syndrome is one of the most severe and preventable complication in ART; which every practicing clinician wants to stay away from.
2. Every clinic in the world aims to become OHSS-free clinic, which is one of the benchmarks today for safe and evidence-based ART practices.
3. With advent of agonist trigger and freeze all policy OHSS has almost been eradicated. Various treatment and preventions options are recommended but, segmentation of cycle with agonist triggers remains the best option.

SUGGESTED READING

1. Abbara A, Jayasena CN, Christopoulos G, et al. Efficacy of kisspeptin-54 to trigger oocyte maturation in women at high risk of ovarian hyperstimulation syndrome (OHSS) during in vitro fertilization (IVF) therapy. J Clin Endocrinol Metab. 2015;100(9):3322-31.
2. Abdallah R, Kligman I, Davis O, et al. Withholding gonadotropins until human chorionic gonadotropin administration. Semin Reprod Med. 2010;28:486-92.
3. Abramov Y, Elchalal U, Schenker JG, et al. Pulmonary manifestations of severe ovarian hyperstimulation syndrome: a multicenter study. Fertil Steril. 1999;71(4):645-51.
4. Abuzeid M, Warda H, Joseph S, et al. Outpatient management of severe ovarian hyperstimulation syndrome (OHSS) with placement of pigtail catheter. Facts Views Vis ObGyn. 2014;6(1):31-7.
5. Amarin ZO. Bilateral partial oophorectomy in the management of severe ovarian hyperstimulation syndrome. An aggressive, but perhaps life-saving procedure. Hum Reprod. 2003;18:659-64.
6. Asch RH, Ivery G, Goldsman M, et al. The use of intravenous albumin in patients at high risk for severe ovarian hyperstimulation syndrome. Hum Reprod. 1993;8:1015-20.
7. Balasch J, Arroyo V, Fábregues F, et al. Neurohormonal and hemodynamic changes in severe cases of ovarian hyperstimulation syndrome. Ann Intern Med. 1994;121:27-33.

8. Balasch J, Carmona F, Llach J, et al. Acute prerenal failure and liver dysfunction in a patient with severe ovarian hyperstimulation syndrome. Hum Reprod. 1990;5:348-51.
9. Baumgarten M, Polanski L, Campbell B, et al. Do dopamine agonists prevent or reduce the severity of ovarian hyperstimulation syndrome in women undergoing assisted reproduction? A systematic review and meta-analysis. Hum Fertil (Camb). 2013;16:168-74.
10. Beerendonk CC, van Dop PA, Braat DD, et al. Ovarian hyperstimulation syndrome: facts and fallacies. Obstet Gynecol Surv. 1998;53(7):439-49.
11. Bellver J, Escudero E, Pellicer A. Bilateral partial oophorectomy in the management of severe ovarian hyperstimulation syndrome (OHSS): ovarian mutilating surgery is not an option in the management of severe OHSS. Hum Reprod. 2003;18:1363-7.
12. Ben-Chetrit A, Eldar-Geva T, Gal M, et al. The questionable use of albumin for the prevention of ovarian hyperstimulation syndrome in an IVF programme: a randomized placebo-controlled trial. Hum Reprod. 2001;16:1880-4.
13. Courbiere B, Oborski V, Braunstein D, et al. Obstetric outcome of women with in vitro fertilization pregnancies hospitalized for ovarian hyper stimulation syndrome: a case-control study. Fertil Steril. 2011;95:1629-32.
14. Cupisti S, Emran J, Mueller A, et al. Course of ovarian hyperstimulation syndrome in 19 intact twin pregnancies after assisted reproduction techniques, with a case report of severe thromboembolism. Twin Res Hum Genet. 2006;9:691-6.
15. Dart AB, Mutter TC, Ruth CA, et al. Hydroxyethyl starch (HES) versus other fluid therapies: effects on kidney function. Cochrane Database Syst Rev. 2010;20(1):CD007594.
16. De Neubourg D, Mangelschots K, Van Royen E, et al. Singleton pregnancies are as affected by ovarian hyperstimulation syndrome as twin pregnancies. Fertil Steril. 2004;82:1691-3.
17. Delvigne A, Rozenberg S. Epidemiology and prevention of ovarian hyperstimulation syndrome (OHSS): a review. Hum Reprod Update. 2002;8:559-77.
18. Devroey P, Pellicer A, Nyboe Andersen A, et al. A randomized assessor-blind trial comparing highly purified hMG and recombinant FSH in a GnRH antagonist cycle with compulsory single-blastocyst transfer. Fertil Steril. 2012;97(3):561-71.
19. El-Khayat W, Elsadek M. Calcium infusion for the prevention of ovarian hyperstimulation syndrome: a double-blind randomized controlled trial. Fertil Steril. 2015;103:101-5.
20. Enskog A, Henriksson M, Unander M, et al. Prospective study of the clinical and laboratory parameters of patients in whom ovarian hyperstimulation syndrome developed during controlled ovarian hyperstimulation for in vitro fertilization. Fertil Steril. 1999;71:808-14.
21. Erstad BL, Gales BJ, Rappaport WD. The use of albumin in clinical practice. Arch Intern Med. 1991;151:901-11.
22. ESHRE Capri Workshop Group. Venous thromboembolism in women: a specific reproductive health risk. Hum Reprod Update. 2013;19:471-82.
23. Evbuomwan I. The role of osmoregulation in the pathophysiology and management of severe ovarian hyperstimulation syndrome. Hum Fertil (Camb). 2013;16:162-7.
24. Fábregues F, Balasch J, Gìnès P, et al. Ascites and liver test abnormalities during severe ovarian hyperstimulation syndrome. Am J Gastroenterol. 1999;94:994-9.
25. Ferraretti AP, Gianaroli L, Magli C, et al. Elective cryopreservation of all pronucleate embryos in women at risk of ovarian hyperstimulation syndrome: efficiency and safety. Hum Reprod. 1999;14:1457-60.
26. Galal AF, Abbassy HA, AbdElrahman AH, et al. Accelerated coasting does not affect oocyte maturation. Gynecol Obstet Invest. 2018;83:145-50.
27. García-Velasco JA, Zúñiga A, Pacheco A, et al. Coasting acts through downregulation of VEGF gene expression and protein secretion. Hum Reprod. 2004;19:1530-8.
28. Gibreel A, Maheshwari A, Bhattacharya S. Clomiphene citrate in combination with gonadotropins for controlled ovarian stimulation in women undergoing in vitro fertilization. Cochrane Database Syst Rev. 2012;11:CD008528.
29. Golan A, Ron-El R, Herman A, et al. Ovarian hyperstimulation syndrome: An update review. Obstet Gynecol Surv. 1989;44:430-40.
30. Griesinger G, Diedrich K, Devroey P, et al. GnRH agonist for triggering final oocyte maturation in the GnRH antagonist ovarian hyperstimulation protocol: A systematic review and meta-analysis. Hum Reprod Update. 2006;12(2):159-68.
31. Gunnala V, Melnick A, Irani M, et al. Sliding scale hCG trigger yields equivalent pregnancy outcomes and reduces ovarian hyperstimulation syndrome: Analysis of 10,427 IVF-ICSI cycles. PLoS One. 2017;12(4):e0176019.
32. Herr F, Baal N, Reisinger K, et al. hCG in the regulation of placental angiogenesis. Results of an in vitro study. Placenta. 2007;28(Suppl A):S85-93.
33. Huang X, Wang P, Tal R, et al. A systematic review and meta-analysis of metformin among patients with polycystic ovary syndrome undergoing assisted reproductive technology procedures. Int J Gynaecol Obstet. 2015;131:111-6.
34. Humaidan P, Quartarolo J, Papanikolaou EG. Preventing ovarian hyperstimulation syndrome: guidance for the clinician. Fertil Steril. 2010;94:389-400.
35. Insler V, Lunenfeld B. Pathogenesis of ovarian hyperstimulation syndrome. In: Gomel V, Leung PC (Eds). In vitro fertilization and assisted reproduction. Bologna Italy: Monduzzi Editore; 1997. pp. 433-9.
36. Jayaprakasan K, Chan Y, Islam R, et al. Prediction of in vitro fertilization outcome at different antral follicle count thresholds in a prospective cohort of 1,012 women. Fertil Steril. 2012;98(3):657-63.
37. Kamath MS, Joshi A, Kamath AM, et al. Management of severe ovarian hyperstimulation syndrome with thawed plasma. J Hum Reprod Sci. 2013;6(1):82-5.
38. Kawwass JF, Kissin DM, Kulkarni AD, et al.; National ART Surveillance System (NASS) Group. Safety of assisted reproductive technology in the United States, 2000-2011. JAMA. 2015;313:88-90.
39. König E, Bussen S, Sütterlin M, et al. Prophylactic intravenous hydroxyethyl starch solution prevents moderate-severe

ovarian hyperstimulation in in-vitro fertilization patients: a prospective, randomized, double-blind and placebo-controlled study. Hum Reprod. 1998;13(9):2421-4.
40. Kupka MS, Ferraretti AP, de Mouzon J, et al.; European IVF-Monitoring Consortium, for the European Society of Human Reproduction and Embryology (ESHRE). Assisted reproductive technology in Europe, 2010: results generated from European registers by ESHRE. Hum Reprod. 2014;29:2099-113.
41. Lainas GT, Kolibianakis EM, Sfontouris IA, et al. Outpatient management of severe early OHSS by administration of GnRH antagonist in the luteal phase: an observational cohort study. Reprod Biol Endocrinol. 2012;10:69.
42. Lainas T, Petsas G, Stavropoulou G, et al. Administration of methylprednisolone to prevent severe ovarian hyperstimulation syndrome in patients undergoing in vitro fertilization. Fertil Steril. 2002;78(3):529-33.
43. Lan Wu, Yazhou Sun, Jun Wan, et al. A proteomic analysis identifies candidate early biomarkers to predict ovarian hyperstimulation syndrome in polycystic ovarian syndrome patients. Mol Med Rep. 2017;16(1):272-80.
44. Lee TH, Liu CH, Huang CC, et al. Serum anti-Müllerian hormone and estradiol levels as predictors of ovarian hyperstimulation syndrome in assisted reproduction technology cycles. Hum Reprod. 2008;23:160-7.
45. Levinsohn-Tavor O, Friedler S, Schachter M, et al. Coasting-what is the best formula?. Hum Reprod. 2003;18:937-40.
46. Maslovitz S, Jaffa A, Eytan O, et al. Renal blood flow alteration after paracentesis in women with ovarian hyperstimulation. Obstet Gynecol. 2004;104:321-6.
47. Mathur RS, Akande VA, Keay SD, et al. Distinction between early and late ovarian hyperstimulation syndrome. Fertil Steril. 2000;73:901-7.
48. Mathur RS, Jenkins JM. Is ovarian hyperstimulation syndrome associated with a poor obstetric outcome? BJOG. 2000;107:943-6.
49. McClure N, Healy DL, Rogers PA, et al. Vascular endothelial growth factor as capillary permeability agent in ovarian hyperstimulation syndrome. Lancet. 1994;344(8917):235-6.
50. Miele C, Rochford JJ, Filippa N, et al. Insulin and insulin-like growth factor-I induce vascular endothelial growth factor mRNA expression via different signaling pathways. J Biol Chem. 2000;275(28):21695-702.
51. Mohammadi Yeganeh L, Moini A, Shiva M, et al. Methylprednisolone for prevention of ovarian hyper-stimulation syndrome in patients with polycystic ovarian syndrome undergoing in-vitro fertilisation: a randomised controlled trial. J Obstet Gynaecol. 2018;38(2):241-6.
52. Navot D, Bergh PA, Laufer N. Ovarian hyperstimulation syndrome in novel reproductive technologies: Prevention and treatment. Fertil Steril. 1992;58:249-61.
53. Papanikolaou EG, Pozzobon C, Kolibianakis EM, et al. Incidence and prediction of ovarian hyperstimulation syndrome in women undergoing gonadotropin-releasing hormone antagonist in vitro fertilization cycles. Fertil Steril. 2006;85(1):112-20.
54. Park EA , Kim MK, Kim BY, et al. Analysis of clinical outcome of IVM-IVF-ET and IVF-ET cycles. Fertil Steril. 2012;98(3 Suppl):S262.
55. Polishuk WZ, Schenker JG. Ovarian overstimulation syndrome. Fertil Steril. 1969;20(3):443-50.
56. Practice Committee of the American Society for Reproductive Medicine. Ovarian hyperstimulation syndrome. Fertil Steril. 2008;90 Suppl 5:S188-93.
57. Prapas Y, Panagiotidis I, Kalogiannidis I, et al. Double GnRH-antagonist dose before HCG administration may prevent OHSS in oocyte-donor cycles: A pilot study. Reproductive BioMed Online. 2010;21(2):159-65.
58. Rabau E, David A, Serr DM, et al. Human menopausal gonadotropin for anovulation and sterility: Results of 7 years of treatment. Am J Obstet Gynecol. 1967;98:92-8.
59. RCOG (2016). The Management of Ovarian Hyperstimulation Syndrome. Green-top guidelines No. 5. [online] Available from https://www.rcog.org.uk/globalassets/documents/guidelines/green-top-guidelines/gtg_5_ohss.pdf [Last accessed July, 2019].
60. Rizk B, Aboulghar MA. Classification, pathophysiology, and management of ovarian hyperstimulation syndrome. In: In-vitro Fertilization and Assisted Reproduction. Brinsden P (Ed.). New York, NY and London, U.K.: The Parthenon Publishing Group; 1999. pp. 131-55.
61. Rollene NL, Amols MH, Hudson SB, et al. Treatment of ovarian hyperstimulation syndrome using a dopamine agonist and gonadotropin releasing hormone antagonist: a case series. Fertil Steril. 2009;92:1169.e15-7.
62. Royal College of Obstetricians and Gynaecologists. Reducing the risk of venous thromboembolism during pregnancy and the puerperium. Green-top Guideline No. 37a. London: RCOG; 2015.
63. Schenker JG, Weinstein D. Ovarian hyperstimulation syndrome: A current survey. Fertil Steril. 1978;30:255-68.
64. Seow KM, Lin YH, Bai CH, et al. Clinical outcome according to timing of cabergoline initiation for prevention of OHSS: a randomized controlled trial. Reprod Biomed Online. 2013;26(6):562-8.
65. Shaker AG, Zosmer A, Dean N, et al. Comparison of intravenous albumin and transfer of fresh embryos with cryopreservation of all embryos for subsequent transfer in prevention of ovarian hyperstimulation syndrome. Fertil Steril. 1996;65:992-6.
66. Shrivastav P, Nadkarni P, Craft I. Day care management of severe ovarian hyperstimulation syndrome avoids hospitalization and morbidity. Hum Reprod. 1994;9:812-4.
67. Smits G, Olatunbosun O, Delbaere A, et al. Ovarian hyperstimulation syndrome due to a mutation in the follicle-stimulating hormone receptor. N Engl J Med. 2003;349:760-6.
68. Soares SR, Gómez R, Simón C, et al. Targeting the vascular endothelial growth factor system to prevent ovarian hyperstimulation syndrome. Hum Reprod Update. 2008;14(4):321-33.
69. Speroff L, Fritz M. Clinical Gynecological Endocrinology and Infertility, 7th edition. Philadelphia, Pa: Lippincott Williams and Wilkins; 2004. pp. 1999-200.

70. Tang H, Mourad S, Zhai S, et al. Dopamine agonists for preventing ovarian hyperstimulation syndrome. Cochrane Database Syst Rev. 2016;11:CD008605.
71. Tang T, Glanville J, Orsi N, et al. The use of metformin for women with PCOS undergoing IVF treatment. Hum Reprod. 2006;21:1416-5.
72. Tarlatzis BC, Griesinger G, Leader A, et al. Comparative incidence of ovarian hyperstimulation syndrome following ovarian stimulation with corifollitropin alfa or recombinant FSH. Reprod Biomed Online. 2012;24(4):410-9.
73. Toftager M, Bogstad J, Bryndorf T, et al. Risk of severe ovarian hyperstimulation syndrome in GnRH antagonist versus GnRH agonist protocol: RCT including 1050 first IVF/ICSI cycles. Hum Reprod. 2016;31(6):1253-64.
74. Tollan A, Holst N, Forsdahl F, et al. Transcapillary fluid dynamics during ovarian stimulation for in vitro fertilization. Am J Obstet Gynecol. 1990;162:554-8.
75. Tozer AJ, Iles RK, Iammarrone E, et al. The effects of 'coasting' on follicular fluid concentrations of vascular endothelial growth factor in women at risk of developing ovarian hyperstimulation syndrome. Hum Reprod. 2004; 19:522-8.
76. Tso LO, Costello MF, Albuquerque LT, et al. Metformin treatment before and during IVF or ICSI in women with polycystic ovary syndrome. Cochrane Database Syst Rev. 2014;(11):CD006105.
77. van der Linden M, Buckingham K, Farquhar C, et al. Luteal phase support for assisted reproduction cycles. Cochrane Database Syst Rev. 2015;7:CD009154.
78. Várnagy A, Bódis J, Mánfai Z, et al. Low-dose aspirin therapy to prevent ovarian hyperstimulation syndrome. Fertil Steril. 2010;93(7):2281-4.
79. Whelan JG 3rd, Vlahos NF. The ovarian hyperstimulation syndrome. Fertil Steril. 2000;73(5):883-96.
80. Wiedermann CJ, Eisendle K. Comparison of hydroxyethyl starch regulatory summaries from the Food and Drug Administration and the European Medicines Agency. J Pharm Policy Pract. 2017;10:12.
81. Xiao JS, Su CM, Zeng XT. Comparisons of GnRH antagonist versus GnRH agonist protocol in supposed normal ovarian responders undergoing IVF: a systematic review and meta-analysis. PLoS One. 2014;9:e106854.
82. Youssef MA, Mourad S. Volume expanders for the prevention of ovarian hyperstimulation syndrome. Cochrane Database Syst Rev. 2016;8:CD001302.

9

CHAPTER

Luteal Phase Support: Current Evidence

Sadhana Desai, Partha Guha Roy

INTRODUCTION

In the normal menstrual cycle, following ovulation the luteal phase starts. This phase varies between 14 and 15 days and ends with the onset of next menstruation or pregnancy. Progesterone is the main hormone that is secreted by corpus luteum (CL). This maintains the luteal phase and induces secretory changes in the endometrium.

Currently in assisted reproductive technique (ART) cycles, LPS is routinely prescribed. In intrauterine insemination (IUI) and in unexplained recurrent pregnancy loss (RPL), the LPS is also given. For luteal supplementation the hormone progesterone is mainly used as a sole preparation for the support (Box 1).

LUTEAL PHASE DEFICIENCY

In luteal phase defect the endometrium is exposed to insufficient progesterone leading to inadequate secretory changes in the endometrium. This leads to difficulty in implantation and growth of the normal embryo. Diagnosis of luteal phase deficiency (LPD) by clinical symptoms of short luteal phase, irregular bleeding, and histological dating of endometrium and midluteal progesterone level is not precise.

Clinically over multiple cycles, LPD may be suspected as a cause of infertility and miscarriage. This can be corrected by empirical treatment with progesterone and improving follicular development. It is acknowledged that the empirical treatment with progesterone in LPD is based not on strong evidence but on clinical interpretations of underlying physiology.

BOX 1 Indications for luteal phase support

- *In vitro* fertilization/intracytoplasmic sperm injection (IVF-ICSI) cycles
- Frozen embryo transfer cycles
- Donor oocyte cycles
- Luteal phase deficiency
- Recurrent pregnancy loss
- Gonadotropins + intrauterine insemination (IUI) cycles

LUTEAL PHASE SUPPORT IN ART CYCLES

Treatment that encompasses ART includes: (1) Fresh embryo transfer in a woman who underwent controlled ovarian stimulation (COS) and oocytes retrieval. (2) Frozen embryo replacement in hormone replacement therapy (HRT) cycles. (3) Fresh embryo transfer in a recipient following donor oocytes programme. In these situations, there is an effective LPD.

It was observed from the early stages of IVF program that the luteal phase for COS and oocytes aspiration is dysfunctional. Controversy exists till date concerning the reason for this deficiency. Initially, it was believed that there is destruction of granulous cells during oocytes aspiration resulting in damage of CL and thereby causing LPD. This theory was challenged when the progesterone levels or the luteal phase length showed no changes following aspiration of a single matured follicle in an unstimulated cycle.

Endogenous suppression of luteinizing hormone: The administration of hCG in IVF cycle is said to be a cause of LPD. It inhibits endogenous secretion of luteinizing hormone (LH) from the pituitary. The success rate has improved with the use of GnRH agonist in IVF for downregulation but it causes LPD as the LH secretion is suppressed well into the luteal phase.

GnRH antagonist has been incorporated lately in ART cycles for LH suppression. It does not cause long-term pituitary LH suppression and has a short half-life with quick clearances. But premature luteolysis and poor pregnancy rates were observed in IVF antagonist cycles without progesterone support.

In early luteal phase following oocytes retrieval in IVF cycles multiple CL comes into existences. Currently, it is believed that these CL via negative feedback on the hypothalamic-pituitary axis causes direct inhibition of LH secretion.

The success rate in ART is influenced by quality of the embryos and a receptive endometrium. In the luteal phase of IVF and FET cycles, the ideal supplementation would be one that increases live birth rate while minimizing patient discomfort and inconvenience. Significant research in search of optimum supplement has been done since last 40 years.

In the luteal phase following IVF not only progesterone, but also hCG and GnRH agonist, has been used as a supplement. One of the study had surveyed 408 centers acrossed 82 countries. They observed the use of some form of progesterone for LPS. However none of the centers were using solely hCG as an LPS. In contrast an earlier survey had observed that 5% of the clinics were using hCG alone as LPS. Luteal supplementation with progesterone and hCG has same pregnancy outcome, but hCG is avoided due to increased risk of ovarian hyperstimulation syndrome (OHSS).

Progesterone supplementation is available in the form of intramuscular, vaginal, oral and subcutaneous preparation. The choice of progesterone as a luteal phase supplementation depends upon regional difference. A survey was conducted in 2014 involving 82 different centers having 284,600 IVF cycles. The LPS was by vaginal progesterone only in 77% of the cycle, while progesterone in combination with oral or intramuscular progesterone was used in additional 17% (Box 2).

BOX 2 Different types of luteal support.

- Oral progesterone tablets
- Intramuscular progesterone injections
- Vaginal pessary
- Vaginal gel
- Subcutaneous progesterone injection

Earlier the luteal support of choice was oral micronized progesterone. However, its bioavailability was inconsistent and poor, due to the first past effect of liver. The bioavailability was only 10% by that of intramuscular progesterone. Following frequent dosing the serum level of oral micronized progesterone reaches maximum in 2–4 hours, and remains elevated significantly for 6–7 hours. In a randomized, controlled trial, comparing oral micronized progesterone to intramuscular progesterone the implantation rate was significantly reduced with oral preparation.

As compared to oral micronized progesterone, dydrogesterone, an oral progestin showed improved bioavailability. Increased pregnancy rate was observed in women undergoing IVF who had oral dydrogesterone as LPS as compared to vaginal micronized progesterone. Same agents when compared showed similar pregnancy rates in another randomized controlled trial (RCT). Similar pregnancy rates were observed in a trial comparing oral dydrogesterone to progesterone vaginal gel. No changes in pregnancy or implantation was observed when chlormadinone acetate, was compared to intramuscular progesterone. For clinical pregnancy the use of synthetic progesterone was favored against micronized progesterone in the 2011 Cochrane review analysis. As a LPS following IVF, intramuscular progesterone was first described in the year 1985. The use of intramuscular progesterone causes pain in the site, irritation, allergic reaction, and rarely abscess formation. In a meta-analysis in 2009, no difference was observed in pregnancy and live birth when intramuscular progesterone was compared to vaginal progesterone. In 2011 Cochrane review, no difference in pregnancy or live birth rate were observed. However, in the ongoing pregnancies intramuscular progesterone was favored. The outcome of IVF pregnancy is considered to be same when intramuscular or vaginal progesterone is used as LPS. Vaginal progesterone is currently the main stay of LPS. This is due to relative ease of use and its efficacy is same as that of intramuscular progesterone.

Vaginal progesterone preparations are available in the form of tablet, suppository, and 8% gel. The progesterone concentration in the endometrium is much higher as compared to that of serum when vaginal progesterone is used. This is due to the first pass uterine effect. Majority of the patients tolerate vaginal progesterone well. The drawback is its higher cost, difficulty in inserting, and presence of irritant vaginal discharge. Latest addition to LPS is a water-soluble progesterone complex and it can be administered intramuscularly as well as subcutaneously.

BOX 3 Different route and dose of administrations.

- Oral tablets (10 mg thrice a day)
- Intramuscular (50–100 mg IM)
- Vaginal pessary (400–600 mg/day)
- Vaginal gel (0.9% twice a day)
- Subcutaneous (25 mg once a day)
- Intranasal gonadotropin-releasing hormone agonist (200 µg twice a day)

The water-soluble progesterone complex when compared to 8% gel and vaginal progesterone did not show any difference as far as ongoing pregnancy rate was concerned. Pain at the site of injection, bruise, inflammation, and edema are some of the common side effects of subcutaneous progesterone injection (Box 3).

During an IVF cycle the timing of onset of progesterone supplementation is debatable. Pregnancy rates remain unaltered when progesterone was administrated between the day of retrieval to 2 days after retrieval. Most of the clinics start progesterone supplementation on the day of oocytes retrieval. Consensus on duration of progesterone supplementation is debatable. In a recent meta-analysis it was observed that there is no extra benefit of progesterone supplementation beyond the first positive β-hCG value as well as no difference in live birth was observed. 15% of the clinics discontinue progesterone after the first positive β-hCG report. Majority of the clinic continue till 8 weeks or more.

ADJUVANTS IN LUTEAL PHASE SUPPORT

Role of Estradiol

Estradiol has a role in luteal support in ART cycles. Though the major source of progesterone is the CL yet it also secretes estradiol along with many nonsteroidal hormones. In a meta-analysis it was observed that estradiol supplementation did not make any difference between clinical pregnancy and live birth rate. When compared to progesterone alone, progesterone + estradiol did not perform better than progesterone in terms of biochemical pregnancy, clinical pregnancy or live birth. In a subgroup analysis concerning clinical pregnancy it was observed that progesterone together with transdermal estradiol performed better as compared to progesterone alone. This suggests that the route of estradiol administration has a role.

Role of GnRH Agonist

In various IVF protocol GnRH administration in single or multiple doses in midluteal phase is getting popular. The GnRH agonist trigger induces final follicular maturation which leads to endogenous surge of both LH and follicle-stimulating hormone from the pituitary. The GnRh agonist trigger causes a lower pregnancy rate. This is due to its short half-life and luteolytic effect on the CL unlike hCG which provides prolonged stimulation of the CL. To overcome this disadvantage and to rescue the luteal phase, supplementation with mini hCG doses, intensive supplementation, and freeze-all approach has been described in the literature.

In non-downregulated cycles of intrauterine insemination, Pirard et al. in 2005 used GnRH agonist (buserelin) 100 µg intranasal per day. At this dose the luteal phase was of more than 14 days consistently and the serum level of progesterone was significantly increased. They observed that GnRH agonist did not shorten the luteal phase and a good pregnancy rate was also observed. In a pilot study it was observed that the results were same when GnRH agonist was used as LPS in an antagonist cycle triggered by GnRH agonist and hCG triggering followed by progesterone support. In a prospective trial of normal responding patients with antagonist protocol 20 patients were triggered with and luteal support was with intranasal GnRH agonist. Another 20 patients were triggered with hCG followed by luteal support with intravaginal progesterone. Clinical pregnancy rate did not differ in the study groups. It shows that repeated administration of GnRH agonist all through the luteal phase maintains the LH secretion and overcomes the GnRH agonist trigger induced luteolysis.

To avoid OHSS in non-downregulated cycles in a retrospective study of high responders patients, triggering was done by GnRH agonist. The luteal phase was supported by intranasal GnRH 200 µg twice daily. This enabled successful LPS resulting in fresh embryo transfer with excellent ongoing pregnancy rate. GnRh agonist administration was discontinued 2 weeks after the ovum pickup (OPU). No additional luteal support was provided in case with positive serum hCG results. In a retrospective study of non-downregulated cycles in normo-ovulatory women, triggering with hCG and intravaginal progesterone support was compared with GnRH agonist trigger and LPS with only GnRH agonist. The results showed higher live birth rate in the group which had daily repeated intranasal GnRH agonist as LPS. Midluteal progesterone and estradiol levels were higher among the GnRH agonist group.

Five to six days after oocyte retrieval, a single dose of triptorelin acetate (0.1 mg) has been suggested as adjuvant to progesterone supplementation. A meta-analysis evaluated five RCT investigating GnRH agonist in both long and antagonist protocol. On analyzing the data it was found that higher pregnancy rates were reported when a single dose of GnRH agonist was given as LPS after 5–6 days of oocytes retrieval. Another subgroup analysis observed that when luteal GnRH agonist was used the pregnancy rate was significantly higher in antagonist protocol as compared to long protocol. The recent Cochrane review involving subjects receiving luteal GnRH agonist showed increased pregnancy, ongoing pregnancy, and live birth rates.

Frozen Embryo Transfer, Donor and Recipient Cycles—Luteal Phase Progesterone

In FET and in donor-recipient cycles, endometrium is prepared for implantation with exogenous estradiol and addition of exogenous progesterone later. When intramuscular progesterone was compared to vaginal progesterone in recipient and donor oocytes, it was observed that there was no difference in ongoing pregnancy rates. No difference was observed in implantation, clinical pregnancy or live birth rates in a retrospective study of donor oocyte recipient's and in subjects receiving donor and autologous frozen blastocysts. However in women undergoing FET a decreased live birth rate was observed in subjects who were using vaginal progesterone as reported in two other retrospective studies. In a review of luteal progesterone during FET cycles it was concluded that cleavage-stage embryos should not be transferred before 3–4 days of progesterone treatment and blastocysts to be transferred on 6th day of progesterone exposure.

Mild Ovarian Stimulation and Intrauterine Insemination—Luteal Phase Support

It is a well-known fact that deficient luteal phase exists in stimulated IVF/ICSI (intracytoplasmic sperm injection) cycles. LPD is doubtful in mildly stimulated cycles with gonadotropin where two or three corpora lutea are present. One of the study found a short luteal phase in 20% of the mild stimulated cycles in women while another study found a luteal phase defect in 11.9% of the mildly stimulated cycles. No large prospective trial exists that has investigated luteal phase defects in mild ovarian stimulations/IUI program. Thus the question of luteal phase defects existing in cycles with only 2–3 follicles remains unanswered.

First randomized trial investigating the efficiency of luteal support in couples with unexplained infertility undergoing IUI in cycles with ovarian stimulations was recently published. The study observed that live birth rate per couple was 45% in the study group and 31% in control group which was statistically significant and thereby favoring luteal support. In gonadotropins stimulated IUI cycles a strong suggestion is thereby raised that the luteal support might be beneficial.

IUI Cycles Stimulated with Clomiphene Citrate and Letrozole—Luteal Phase Support

Superovulation and IUI have a beneficial role in patients with unexplained infertility. One of the popular drug for superovulation in women undergoing IUI is clomiphene citrate (CC).

It is a well-established clinical practice to add progesterone in the luteal phase. However, review of literature shows lack of evidence in justifying the need for LPS in CC stimulated IUI cycles.

Luteal phase support with vaginal progesterone is sometimes offered in normo-ovulatory patients stimulated with CC for IUI. However, it is not associated with higher ongoing pregnancy rate as compared to patients without LPS.

In PCOS patients using letrozole for ovulation induction, LPS was strongly recommended. Those stimulated with CC showed no positive effect of progesterone as LPS.

Unexplained Recurrent Pregnancy Loss—Luteal Phase Support

The effect of vaginal and oral administration of progesterone has been studied in women with unexplained RPL. The conclusion of the study varies significantly. However the European Society of Human Reproduction and Embryology (ESHRE) guideline recommends not to prescribe progesterone in women with unexplained RPL based on the recently published PROMISE trial. There is insufficient evidence to recommend the use of progesterone/hCG to improve live birth rate in women with RPL and luteal phase insufficiency.

The use of luteal phase vaginal micronized progesterone in an observational cohort study was associated with improved pregnancy rate in a strictly defined cohort of women with unexplained RPL. Need of the hour is to organize a well-controlled study to determine if luteal phase vaginal progesterone can improve the subsequent live birth rate in women with RPL.

KEYNOTE

Gonadotropin-releasing hormone (GnRH) analogs are integral part of in vitro fertilization (IVF) cycles and require luteal phase support (LPS). Frozen embryo transfer (FET) or donor or recipient cycles also require LPS. Controversy exists worldwide concerning the type of hormone to be used for luteal support and its dose and duration. This chapter reviews the recent evidence on the LPS.

KEY POINTS

- In LPS, progesterone alone is the drug of choice. However no consensus exists in the best route of administration.
- Human chorionic gonadotropin can support luteal phase but there lies a high risk of OHSS.
- Gonadotropin-releasing hormone agonist can be used as a sole LPS.
- No benefit has been observed on addition of estradiol.
- Luteal phase support should start within 48 hours from hCG injection and lasts till BHCG assay or first ultrasound at 6–7 weeks of pregnancy.
- No convincing evidence exists that mild ovarian stimulation as applied in IUI programs influences the luteal phase negativity.

EDITORS' COMMENTS

The luteal phase of all stimulated cycles is defective mainly due to supraphysiological steroid levels resulting multifollicular development, which inhibits LH secretion. Low LH levels causes luteolysis, shortened luteal phase, and may result in implantation failure. Therefore, LPS is mandatory in IVF cycles when a fresh embryo transfer is planned.

In the most recent Cochrane systematic review and meta-analysis (van der Linden et al. Cochrane 2015) comparing different type of progesterone regimens for LPS in IVF cycles, including 45 trials and over 13,000 patients, it was concluded that no regimens is clearly superior than the other concerning the odds of achieving a pregnancy, but notably, the quality of the evidence was deemed low or very low. When asked about their personal preferences, patients clearly prefer the vaginal route as being the most convenient form of progesterone supplementation.

In fresh ET cycles, LPS regimen should be individualized according to trigger:

- *Human chorionic gonadotropin trigger*: Progesterone alone is enough
- *Gonadotropin-releasing hormone- agonist trigger*: Progesterone plus hCG (either bolus or low dose daily)
- Modified LPS in GnRHa trigger needs to be refined further
- Human chorionic gonadotropin trigger and conventional LPS method of choice for eligible patients.

SC Esteves, Campinas, Brazil

SUGGESTED READING

1. Ata B, Urman B. Single dose GnRH agonist administration in the luteal phase of assisted reproduction cycles: is the effect dependent on the type of GnRH analogue used for pituitary suppression? Reprod Biomed Online. 2010;20(1):165-6.
2. Ata B, Yakin K, Balaban B, et al. GnRH agonist protocol administration in the luteal phase in ICSI-ET cycles stimulated with the long GnRH agonist protocol: a randomized, controlled double blind study. Hum Reprod. 2008;23(3):668-73.
3. Baker VL, Jones CA, Doody K, et al. A randomized controlled trial comparing the efficacy and safety of aqueous subcutaneous progesterone with vaginal progesterone for luteal phase support of invitro fertilization. Hum Reprod. 2014;29:2212-20.
4. Bar Hava I, Blueshtein M, Ganer Herman H, et al. Gonadotropin-releasing hormone analogue as sole luteal support in antagonist-based assisted reproductive technology cycles. Fertil Steril. 2017;107(1):130-5.e1.
5. Bar-Hava I, Mizrachi Y, Karfunkel-Doron D, et al. Intranasal gonadotropin-releasing hormone agonist (GnRHa) for luteal phase support following GnRHa triggering, a novel approach to avoid ovarian hyperstimulation syndrome in high responders. Fertil Steril. 2016;106(2):330-3.
6. Baruffi R, Mauri AL, Petersen CG, et al. Effects of vaginal progesterone administration starting on the day of oocyte retrieval on pregnancy rates. J Assist Reprod Genet. 2003;20(12):517-20.
7. Beckers NG, Macklon NS, Eijkemans MJ, et al. Nonsupplemented luteal phase characteristics after the administration of recombinant human chorionic gonadotropins, recombinant luteinizing hormone, or gonadotropin-releasing hormone (GnRH) agonist to induce final oocyte maturation in In vitro fertilization patients after ovarian stimulation with recombinant follicle-stimulating hormone and GnRH antagonist cotreatment. J Clin Endocrinol Metab. 2003;88(9):4186-92.
8. Berger BM, Phillips JA. Pregnancy outcomes in oocyte donation recipients: vaginal gel versus intramuscular injection progesterone replacement. J Assist Reprod Genet. 2012;29(3):237-42.
9. Chakravarty BN, Shirazee HH, Dam P, et al. Oral Dydrogesterone versus intravaginal micronized progesterone as luteal phase support in assisted reproductive technology (ART) cycles: result of a randomized study. J Steroid Biochem Mol Biol. 2005;97(5):416-20.
10. Coelingh Bennink HJ, Boerrigter PJ. Use of Dydrogesterone as a progestogen for oral contraception. Steroids. 2003;68(10-13):927-9.
11. Coomarasamy A, Williams H, Truchanowicz E, et al. A randomized trial of progesterone in women with recurrent miscarriages. N Engl J Med. 2015;373:2141-8.
12. Daya S, Gunby J. Luteal phase support in assisted reproduction cycles. Cochrane Database Syst Rev. 2004;3:CD004830.

13. Duffy DA, Manzi D, Benadiva C, et al. Impact of leuprolide acetate on luteal phase function in women undergoing controlled ovarian hyperstimulation and intrauterine insemination. Fertil Steril. 2006;85:407-11.
14. Edwards RG, Steptoe PC, Purdy JM. Establishing full-term human pregnancies using cleaving embryos grown in vitro. Br J Obstet Gynaecol. 1980;87(9):737-56.
15. Erdem A, Erdem M, Atmaca S, et al. Impact of luteal phase support on pregnancy rates in intrauterine insemination cycles: a prospective randomized study. Fertil Steril. 2009;91(6):2508-13.
16. ESHRE. Guidelines on management of recurrent pregnancy loss 2017. [online] Available from https://www.eshre.eu/Guidelines-and-Legal/Guidelines/Recurrent-pregnancy-loss.aspx [Last accessed July, 2019].
17. Fatemi HM, Popovic-Todorovic B, Papanikolaou E, et al. An update of luteal phase support in stimulated IVF cycles. Hum Reprod Update. 2007;13(6):581-90.
18. Fatemi HM. The luteal phase after 3 decades of IVF: what do we know? Reprod Biomed Online. 2009;19:1-13.
19. Fauser BC, Devroey P. Reproductive biology and IVF: ovarian stimulation and luteal phase consequences. Trends Endocrinol Metab 2003;14(5):236-42.
20. Friedler S, Raziel A, Schachter M, et al. Luteal support with micronized progesterone following in-vitro fertilization using a down-regulation protocol with gonadotropin-releasing hormone agonist: a comparative study between vaginal and oral administration. Hum Reprod. 1999;14(8):1944-8.
21. Ganesh A, Chakravorty N, Mukherjee R, et al. Comparison of oral dydrogesterone with progesterone gel and micronized progesterone for luteal support in 1,373 women undergoing in vitro fertilization : a randomized clinical study. Fertil Steril 2011;95(6):1961-5.
22. Gibbons WE, Toner JP, Hamacher P, et al. Experience with a novel vaginal progesterone preparation in a donor oocyte program. Fertil Steril. 1998;69(1):96-101.
23. Isik AZ, Caglar GS, Sozen E, et al. Single-dose GnRH agonist administration in the luteal phase of GnRH antagonist cycles: a prospective randomized study. Reprod Biomed Online. 2009;19(4):472-7.
24. Iwase A, Ando H, Toda S, et al. Oral progesterone versus intramuscular progesterone for luteal support after assisted reproductive technology treatment: a prospective randomized study. Arch Gynecol Obstet. 2008;277(4):319-24.
25. Jobanputra K, Toner JP, Denoncourt R, et al. Crinone 8% (90 mg) given once daily for progesterone replacement therapy in donor egg cycles. Fertil Steril. 1999;72(6):980-4.
26. Kerin JF, Broom TJ, Ralph MM, et al. Human luteal phase function following oocyte aspiration from the immediately preovular graafian follicle of spontaneous ovular cycles. Br J Obstet Gynaecol. 1981:88(10):1021-8.
27. Kolibianakis EM, Venetis CA, Papanikolaou EG, et al. Estrogen addition to progesterone for luteal phase support in cycles stimulated with GnRH analogues and gonadotropins for IVF: a systematic review and meta-analysis. Hum Reprod. 2008;23(6):1346-54.
28. Leeton J, Trouson A, Jessup D. Support of the luteal phase in in vitro fertilization programs: results of a controlled trial with intramuscular Proluton. J In Vitro Fert Embryo Transf. 1985;2(3):166-9.
29. Licciardi FL, Kwiatkowski A, Noyes NL, et al. Oral versus intramuscular progesterone for in-vitro fertilization: a prospective randomized study. Fertil Steril. 1999;71(4):614-8.
30. Liu XR, Mu HQ, Shi Q, et al. The optimal duration of progesterone supplementation in pregnant women after IVF/ICSI: a meta-analysis. Reprod Biol Endocrinol. 2012;10(1):107.
31. Lockwood G, Griesinger G, Cometti B, 13 European Centers. Subcutaneous progesterone versus vaginal progesterone gel for luteal phase support in Invitro fertilization: a noninferiority randomized controlled study. Fertil Steril. 2014;101(1):112-9.e3.
32. Maxson WS, Hargrove JT. Bioavailability of oral micronized progesterone. Fertil Steril. 1985;44(5):622-6.
33. Miles RA, Paulson RJ, Lobo RA, et al. Pharmacokinetics and endometrial tissue levels of progesterone after administration by intramuscular and vaginal routes: a comparative study. Fertil Steril. 1994;62(3):485-90.
34. Miyake A, Aono T, Kinugasa T, et al. Suppression of serum levels of luteinizing hormone by short- and long-loop negative feedback in ovariectomized women. J Endocrinol. 1979;80(3):353-6.
35. Mochtar MH, Van Wely M, Van der Veen F. Timing luteal phase support in GnRH agonist down-regulated IVF/embryo transfer cycles. Hum Reprod. 2006;21(4):905-8.
36. Montville C, Khabbaz M, Aubuchon M, et al. Luteal support with intravaginal progesterone increase clinical pregnancy in women with polycystic syndrome using letrozole for ovulation induction. Fertil Steril. 2010;94:678-83.
37. Nawroth F, Ludwig M. What is the "ideal" duration of progesterone supplementation before the transfer of cryopreserved-thawed embryos in estrogen/progesterone replacement protocols? Hum Reprod. 2005;20(5):1127-34.
38. NICE, National Collaborating Center for Women's and Children's Health. Fertility: Assessment and Treatment for People with Fertility Problems. Clinical Guideline: London RCOG Press; 2004.
39. Oliveira JB, Baruffi R, Petersen CG, et al. Administration of single-dose GnRH agonist in the luteal phase in ICSI cycles: a meta-analysis. Reprod Biol Endocrinol. 2010;8(1):107.
40. Olson JL, Rebar RW, Schreiber JR, et al. Shortened luteal phase after ovulation induction with human menopausal gonadotropin and human chorionic gonadotropin. Fertil Steril. 1983;39:284-91.
41. Patki A, Pawar VC. Modulating fertility outcome in assisted reproductive technologies by the use of Dydrogesterone. Gynecol Endocrinol. 2007;23 (Suppl 1):68-72.
42. Pirard C, Donnez J, Loumaye E. GnRH agonist as luteal phase support in assisted reproduction techniques cycles: results of a pilot study. Hum Reprod. 2006;21:1894-900.
43. Pirard C, Donnez J, Loumaye E. GnRH agonist as novel luteal support results of a randomized, parallel group, feasibility study using intranasal administration of buserelin. Hum Reprod. 2005;20:1798-804.

44. Pirard C, Loumaye E, Laurent P, et al. Contribution to more patient-friendly ART treatment: efficacy of continuous low-dose GnRH agonist as the only luteal support-results of a prospective, randomized, comparative study. Int J Endocrinol. 2015;2015:727569.
45. Practice Committee of American Society for Reproductive Medicine in collaboration with Society for Reproductive Endocrinology and Infertility. Progesterone supplementation during the luteal phase and in early pregnancy in the treatment of infertility: an educational bulletin. Fertil Steril. 2008;90(5):S150-3.
46. Propst AM, Hill JA, Ginsburg ES, et al. A randomized study comparing Crinone 8% and intramuscular progesterone supplementation in In vitro fertilization-embryo transfer cycles. Fertil Steril. 2001;76(6):1144-9.
47. Razieh DF, Maryam AR, Nasim T. Beneficial effect of luteal-phase gonadotropin releasing hormone agonist administration on implantation rate after intracytoplasmic sperm injection. Taiwan J Obstet Gynecol. 2009;48(3):245-8.
48. Shapiro DB, Pappadakis JA, Ellsworth NM, et al. Progesterone replacement with vaginal gel versus IM injection: cycle and pregnancy outcomes in IVF patients receiving vitrified blastocysts. Hum Reprod. 2014;29(8):1706-11.
49. Simon JA, Robinson DE, Andrews MC, et al. The absorption of oral micronized progesterone: the effect of food, dose proportionality, and comparison with intramuscular progesterone. Fertil Steril. 1993;60(1):26-33.
50. Smitz J, Erard P, Camus M, et al. Pituitary gonadotropin secretory capacity during the luteal phase in superovulation using GnRH-agonists and HMG in a desensitization or flare-up protocol. Hum Reprod. 1992;7(9):1225-9.
51. Stephenson MD, McQueen D, Winter M, et al. Luteal start vaginal micronized progesterone improves pregnancy success in women with recurrent pregnancy loss. Fertil Steril. 2017;107(3):684-90.e2.
52. Tesarik J, Hazout A, Mendoza-Tesarik R, et al. Beneficial effect of luteal-phase GnRH agonist administration on embryo implantation after ICSI in both GnRH agonist-and antagonist-treated ovarian stimulation cycles. Hum Reprod. 2006;21(10):2572-9.
53. Vaisbuch E, de Ziegler D, Leong M, et al. Luteal-phase support in assisted reproduction treatment: real-life practices reported worldwide by an updated website-based survey. Reprod Biomed Online. 2014;28(3):330-5.
54. Vaisbuch E, Leong M, Shoham Z. Progesterone support in IVF: is evidence-based medicine translated to clinical practice? A worldwide web-based survey. Reprod Biomed Online. 2012;25(2):139-45.
55. van der Linden M, Buckingham K, Farquhar C, et al. Luteal phase support for assisted reproduction cycles. Cochrane Database Syst Rev. 2011;(10):CD009154.
56. Verhulst SM, Cohlen BJ, Hughes E, et al. Intrauterine insemination for unexplained subfertility. Cochrane Database Syst Rev. 2006;(9):CD001838.
57. Zarutskie PW, Phillips JA. A meta-analysis of the route of administration of luteal phase support in assisted reproductive technology: vaginal versus intramuscular progesterone. Fertil Steril. 2009;92(1):163-9.

10

CHAPTER

Endometrial Receptivity: Recent Advances

Diksha Goswami, Narendra Malhotra, Jaideep Malhotra, Neharika Malhotra, Shally Gupta, Rishabh Bora

INTRODUCTION

The field of infertility and assisted reproduction has been witness to significant advances in the last decade, but still the success rates remain stagnant. The main recipe behind successful implantation is the embryo quality and a receptive endometrium along with a successful dialogue between the two. Endometrial causes are implicated in two-thirds of the patients with implantation failure. There are still many lacunae in our understanding of endometrial receptivity, its measurement, and application of this knowledge to increase the implantation rates.

WHAT IS ENDOMETRIAL RECEPTIVITY?

The endometrium is a multilayered, dynamic organ overlaying the myometrium. It is one of the most dynamic target tissues in women which undergoes cyclic structural and metabolic changes during the menstrual cycle. The term "endometrial receptivity" can be described as the state of endometrium when it is most conducive for accepting a nascent embryo resulting in subsequent implantation and pregnancy. Several crucial events underlie the process of implantation which is regulated by various immune mechanisms including cellular apposition, adhesion, and invasion.

Before implantation, the trophoblastic cells of the blastocyst become closely attached to the luminal epithelium (LE) forming an unstable adhesion known as "Apposition". This is facilitated by decrease in uterine fluid volume, edema of the endometrium, and expansion of the embryo. This is followed by an intimate association between the two or "Adhesion". And finally during the process of "Invasion" the epithelial layer is penetrated by the blastocyst to invade the stroma (Fig. 1).

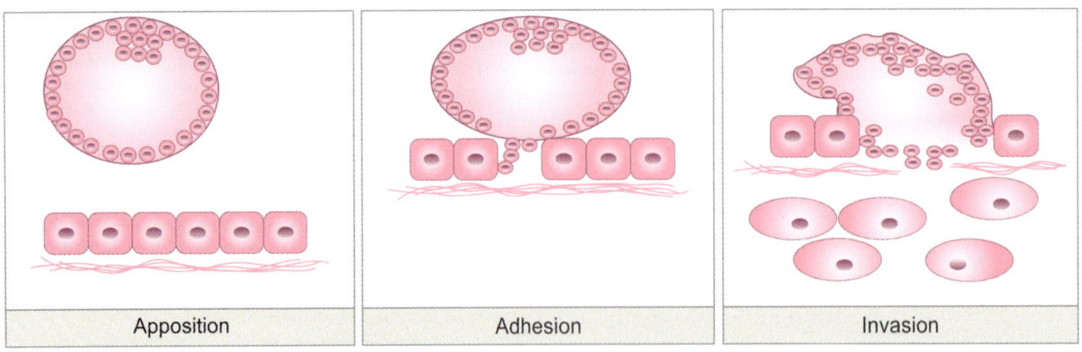

Fig. 1: Process of implantation of blastocyst.

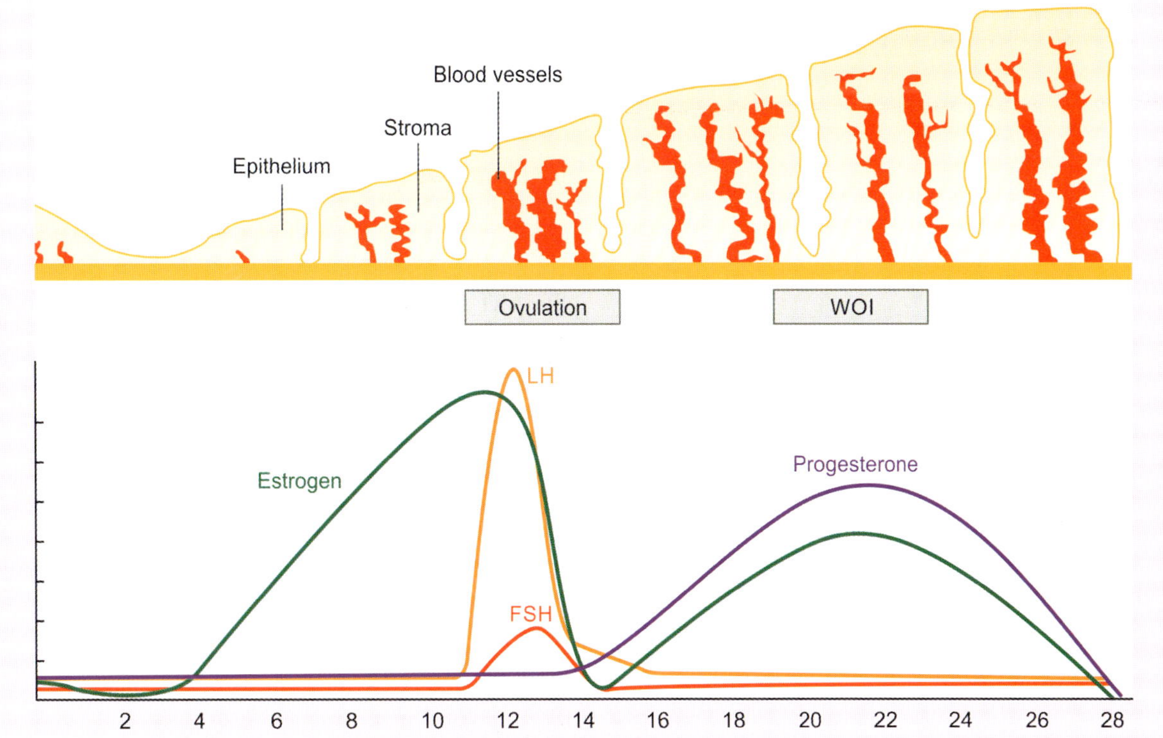

Fig. 2: Hormone pattern and its correlation with WOI.
(FSH: follicle-stimulating hormone; WOI: window of implantation; LH: luteinizing hormone)

This process of implantation of the fertilized embryo to a receptive endometrium can occur only during a regulated period 3–4 days after it enters into the uterine cavity, i.e. 5–7 days after fertilization.

"Window of implantation" (WOI) as first coined by Hertig and Rock in 1958 refers to this period of maximal receptivity of the endometrium for the blastocyst and corresponds with a time of peak progesterone secretion. In the natural human cycle, this period begins from day luteinizing hormone (LH) + 6 when and is completed by day LH +10, i.e. Day 20–24 of the cycle (Fig. 2).

Estrogen and progesterone facilitate the blastocyst-endometrium dialogue by acting through their nuclear receptors. Various growth factors, cytokines, vasoactive mediators, and adhesion molecules play a key role in mediating the signaling pathways for facilitating this dialogue.

During the prereceptive phase, in response to estrogenic environment, the stroma and luminal glandular epithelium undergo certain changes. The apical-basal polarity of LE cells becomes less marked with appearance of laterobasal markers in the apical membrane and during implantation desmosomal proteins density decreases in human LE. In humans at this time, the distribution and complexity of tight junction particle networks in the lateral membrane also change.

This brief period also corresponds to the maximal expression of "pinopodes" which are bleb-like projections protruding into the uterine lumen from the apical surface of endometrium first described by Nilsson in mice in the year 1958. Their expression seems to be linked to an increased progesterone levels and a decrease in progesterone receptor density in glandular and luminal cells. These pinopodes are believed to be preferred sites for blastocyst attachment and useful for assessment of endometrial receptivity. The process of implantation involves complex signaling mediated by upregulation of adhesion ligands and loss of inhibitory components for endometrial to become receptive to the blastocyst.

Flowchart 1: Events at implantation.

Endometrial cell proliferation (Estrogen)

↓

Differentiation of endometrium (Progesterone)

↓

Blastocyst enters uterine cavity (Day 4 after ovulation)

↓

Rolling phenomena of blastocyst (L-selectins, L-selectin ligands)

↓

Increased MUC1 (Mucin 1) expression over endometrium before implantation

↓

Apposition

↓

Increase in chemokines and growth factors attracting blastocyst to pinopodes

↓

Adhesion (Integrins and Cadherins)

↓

Invasion

IMPACT OF IVF STIMULATION ON ENDOMETRIAL RECEPTIVITY

Several factors influence the endometrial development in *in vitro* fertilization (IVF) cycles. Nowadays, most controlled ovarian stimulation protocols for IVF include use of gonadotropin-releasing hormone (GnRH) analogs (agonist or antagonist) to prevent premature LH surge along with high-dose gonadotropins. High supraphysiological concentrations of estradiol and progesterone in stimulated cycles can lead to asynchronous glandular and stromal changes. The early P4 rise has been implicated as a negative factor for embryo implantation. In cycles with increased and premature progesterone rise, there is early secretory transformation of the endometrium and subsequent midluteal glandular maturation arrest. Another factor implicated in disturbing luteal phase endometrial morphology is the human chorionic gonadotropin (hCG) injection used to achieve final oocyte maturation. *In vitro* experiments as well as studies in hormone replacement therapy (HRT) cycles have demonstrated a negative effect of hCG on endometrial maturation especially its advancement.

It is now well documented that the altered hormonal environment prevalent in assisted reproductive technique (ART) cycles can change the window of receptivity (regarding timing) or it can even be absent. Several new studies have demonstrated higher clinical pregnancy rates per transfer with cryopreserved embryos than with fresh embryo transfers (ETs). This new evidence proves the hypothesis that ovarian stimulation induces a state of impaired endometrial receptivity when compared with the artificial endometrial preparation required for frozen ET cycles.

Further it has been seen that the histological and immunohistochemical markers for WOI are altered in the controlled ovarian stimulation cycles compared with natural cycles. Histological, immunological, transcriptomic, proteomic, and secretomic studies have demonstrated that the ART endometrium presents a different environment to the blastocyst compared with normally cycling endometrium at the same stage of the menstrual cycle.

Various modes of modification of stimulation protocol have been investigated to overcome the effects of hormonal stimulation. Mild IVF protocols (lower estradiol levels), GnRH antagonist protocols, and earlier administration of hCG for final oocyte maturation (as soon as three follicles >17 mm are present) appear to beneficial in improving the pregnancy rates. However, the critical point to highlight is while stimulation, the derangements of hormones play a very crucial role in desynchronizing the endometrium.

IMPACT OF VARIOUS PATHOLOGIES ON ENDOMETRIAL RECEPTIVITY

Table 1 shows impact of various pathologies on endometrial receptivity.

TABLE 1 Impact of various pathologies on endometrial receptivity.

Endometriosis	• Reduced v3 integrin and LIF (leukemia inhibiting factor) expressions in window of implantation (WOI) • Lack of interleukin (IL)-II and IL-IR expressions in secretory phase • Absence of HOXA-10 and HOXA-2 peak in secretory phase • Progesterone resistance • Altered PR-A to PR-B ratio • Decreases HOXA-10 expression due to hypermethylation
Hydrosalpinx	• Reduced v3 integrin and LIF expressions • Decreased HOXA-10 expression
Leiomyoma	• Decreased HOXA-10 and BTEB1 expressions • Low insulin-like growth factor-binding protein 1 (IGFBP1) and osteopontin levels in secretory phase • Low PR levels in secretory phase
Polycystic ovarian syndrome	• Decreased IGFBP1, HOXA-10, and v3 during secretory phase • Failure to downregulate ER during WOI • Increased androgen receptors • Overexpression of steroid receptor coactivators AIB1 and TIF2

(PR-A: progesterone receptor isoform A; PR-B: progesterone receptor isoform B; HOXA: homeobox; BTEB1: basic transcription element-binding protein 1; ER: endometrial receptivity)

ASSESSMENT OF ENDOMETRIAL RECEPTIVITY

The monitoring of endometrial changes in practical settings is of paramount importance. Methods to evaluate endometrial receptivity can be invasive like endometrial biopsies and histological study of pinopodes which are expensive, sophisticated, and cannot be done in the treatment cycle.

Role of Ultrasound

It offers a noninvasive reliable tool to assess endometrial receptivity. Evaluation of endometrial thickness, morphology, volume, and endometrial blood flow act as surrogate markers of endometrial receptivity.

Endometrial thickness is measured in sagittal plane at maximum thickness including both endometrial layers placing the callipers at two opposite endometrial-myometrial interface. In case of fluid, thickness of both single layers is measured and is added. Assessment of the endometrial morphology should include endometrial echogenicity, endometrial midline, and endometrial-myometrial interface (Fig. 3A and B).

The cyclic histologic changes and changes in the thickening of the endometrium with hormonal stimulation can be imaged using transvaginal ultrasound during the different phases of the menstrual cycle. Sakamoto described the characteristic sonographic image noted during the menstrual cycle in 1985. The proliferative endometrium is characterized by:

- The presence of a well-defined three line sign
- A hypoechogenic functional layer
- A minimal or absent posterior acoustic enhancement.

The three line sign is formed by the central hyperechoic reflection representing the endometrial cavity and the additional hyperechoic reflection representing the thin developing layer of endometrium. There is also a surrounding hypoechoic halo.

Luteal phase endometrium is (A) hyperechoic; (B) posterior enhancement is present; (C) three line sign and halo are absent.

Various studies have compared endometrial thickness in predicting pregnancy outcome in ART cycles with varied results. Although an appropriate conclusion has not been made, it is accepted that a very thin endometrium below 7 mm negatively impacts implantation rates.

Color Doppler

Uterine artery resistive index (RI) remains around 0.88 ± 0.04 in the follicular phase, with an increase in uterine artery impedance 3 days after the LH peak (Day 16). This is due to the compression of vessels traversing the uterine wall, which decreases their diameter and consequently causes higher resistance to flow. The uterine artery impedance again declines to its lowest in the midluteal phase (RI = 0.84 ± 0.04) favoring implantation (Fig. 4).

Similarly, blood flow changes in the spiral arteries can be used to predict implantation more precisely than uterine artery waveforms. Blood flow velocity wave form changes in the spiral arteries during normal ovulatory cycles are characteristics of by lower velocity and lower impedance to blood flow than in the uterine arteries. Michael Applebaum in his study with transvaginal color Doppler divided the endometrium and periendometrial areas into four zones. In the study conducted by him no pregnancy was reported in IVF patients unless vascularity was demonstrated in Zone III or with in Zone III or IV prior to transfer.

- *Zone I*: 2 mm thick area surrounding the hyperechoic outer layer of the endometrium.

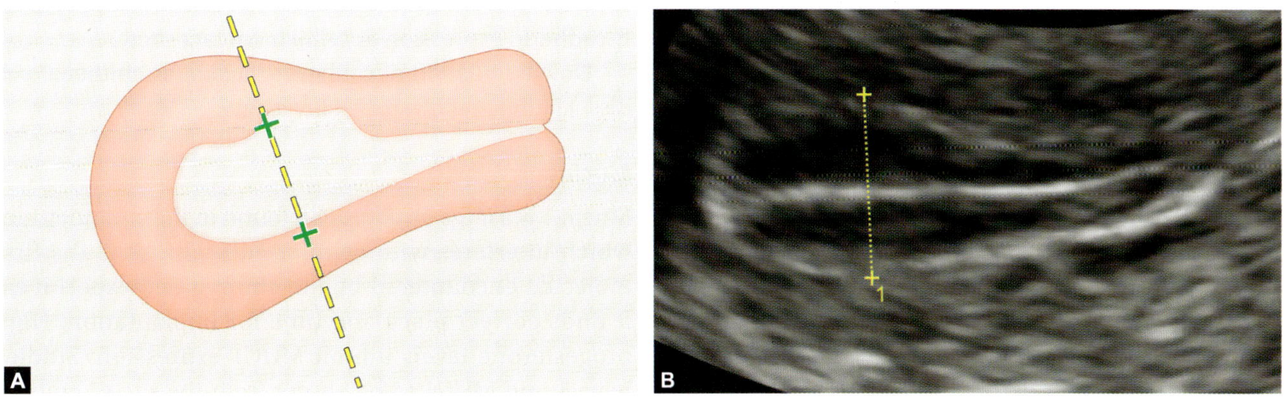

Figs. 3A and B: Assessment of endometrial morphology.

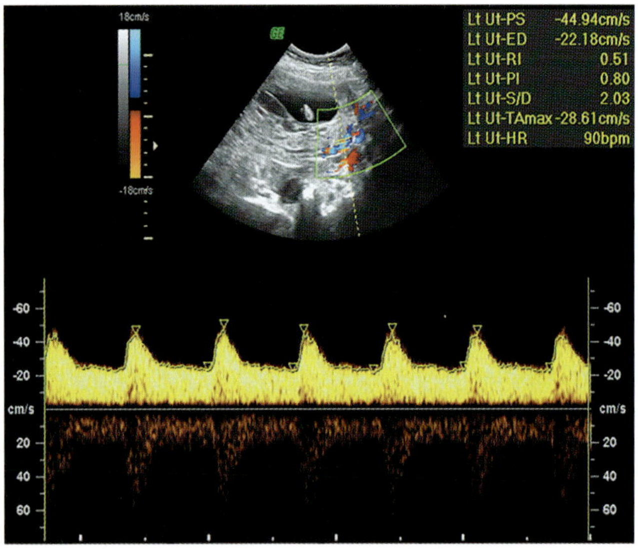

Fig. 4: Uterine artery Doppler in midluteal phase.

- *Zone II*: The hyperechoic outer layer of the endometrium.
- *Zone III*: The hypoechoic inner layer of the endometrium.
- *Zone IV*: The endometrial cavity.

Friedler et al. showed that the uterine artery impedance was different in the midluteal phase in women with subinfertility compared with those with normal fertility. They grouped the patients according to whether the pulsatility index (PI) was low (1–1.99), medium (2–2.99) or high (>3.0). There were no pregnancies in high PI group and the PI was significantly lower in women who become pregnant as compared with those who did not. The ability to predict implantation before the administration of hCG allows the clinician the option to delay giving hCG until the uterine artery PI improves.

Endometrial Volume

Advances in three-dimensional ultrasound, together with automated software for endometrial measurements, have resulted in more accurate and reproducible measures of endometrial volume which are less operator dependent than standard two-dimensional techniques. Kovachev et al. examined the predictive value of endometrial volume as assessed by 3D ultrasound on the day of ET and found that a volume of < 2 mL resulted in significantly lower implantation rates, whereas an endometrial volume of > 2 mL was a positive predictor for successful ART outcome. Kovachev et al. compared the predictive value of endometrial thickness on the day of ET to that of endometrial volume on the same day. Their results imply that volume is a better predictor of ART outcome.

Analysis of Biomarkers

Integrins

Integrins are a family of transmembrane glycoproteins some of which α1 β1, α4 β1, and αVβ3 are found to be increased during the midluteal phase and suggested as markers for WOI. αVβ3 has been proposed as a marker of embryonic attachment and is detected on the LE cells along with its ligand osteopontin. High levels of estrogen act via the estrogen receptor-α (ERα) to prohibit integrin expression at the time of proliferative phase.

The luteal progesterone rise inhibits this ER-α resulting in a net integrin increase. During the time of implantation integrins are expressed by trophoblast. The αVβ3 integrin appears on the apex of luminal and glandular cell surfaces, coinciding with the opening of the WOI and is operated by the transcription factor HOXA-10.

Integrin messenger RNA level on Day 21 found could predict IVF success rates as patients with normal levels had better pregnancy rates.

Selectins

Selectins belonging to the CAM family plays a cardinal role in the apposition of the blastocyst to the endometrium. L-selectin is expressed on the entire embryo surface while on maternal side, oligosaccharide ligands like MECA-79 and HECA-452 are upregulated during WOI. Interaction between L-selectins and their ligands on the LE helps blastocyst to find best site for implantation.

Cadherins

Cadherins play role in cell to cell adhesion, E-cadherins were found to be elevated during luteal phase by Fujimoto et al. suggesting a role in implantation. The rising level of progesterone affects calcitron expression which increases the concentration of intracellular calcium, suppressing E-cadherin expression at cellular contact sites.

Downregulation of cadherins facilitates epithelial cell dissociation and blastocyst invasion.

Mucins

Mucin 1 is a large glycoprotein found in the endometrium which interferes with cellular adhesion. It is the first molecule encountered by the embryo and expels it till it finds correct place and time for implantation. High progesterone levels inhibit MUC1 expression. Studies have found MUC1 to be absent from the site of embryo attachment.

Thathiah and Carson, 2004 suggest that factors expressed on the blastocyst cell surface or secreted by the blastocyst itself trigger the local loss of MUC1.

Leukemia Inhibiting Factor

It is an IL-6 family cytokine seen in the luminal and glandular epithelium as well as stroma peaking at day 20 of menstrual cycle. Abnormal leukemia-inhibitory factor (LIF) levels are seen in women with infertility esp RIF's. In woman with unexplained Infertility, levels of LIF were found to weakly increase from proliferative to secretory phase.

IL-1 and IL-6

Interleukins have an autocrine/paracrine role in implantation as suggested by an increase in immunoreactivity during the WOI. Supplementation of IL-1 in the culture media of EECs was found to increase integrin β3 expression and thereby to enhance blastocyst implantation (Simon et al., 1997).

Prostaglandins

Prostaglandins (PGs) play an important role in timing the WOI. Mice studies have demonstrated that deficiency of PG synthesis can lead to severe implantation defects. Murine blastocyst signals lead to local induction of cyclooxygenase-2 (Cox-2) enzyme in the LE and stroma adjacent to the embryo. Cox-2 is a key enzyme in PG and prostacyclin synthesis. PGI-2 has been shown to induce increased uterine vascular permeability, a key feature of the decidual reaction, this may be its prime target at implantation. PGI-2 may interact with the cellular machinery through activation of the nuclear PPARd receptor rather than through its membrane receptor.

Glycodelin A: (Placental Protein 14 or Progesterone-associated Endometrial Protein)

It is a very promising marker of implantation which protects embryo from maternal immune system. Its levels increase from day 18, and maximum at 8–10 weeks of pregnancy. Uterine flushing is very useful for its measurement rather than serum. Levels are low in unexplained infertility or recurrent pregnancy losses.

Endometrial Immune Markers

Patients with unexplained infertility are found to have lower levels of endometrial CD8+ (T suppressor) and CD56+ (natural killer) cells and higher levels of CD4+ (T-helper) cells. While CD56+ CD16+ cells in peripheral blood are higher in implantation failure. But there are no valid treatment options for these patients.

HOXA Genes

These act as regulators of embryonic morphogenesis and differentiation and are upregulated during the implantation period. HOXA-10 is reduced in endometriosis, hydrosalpinx, and polycystic ovary and implicated for implantation failure in these patients. Gene therapy modulating HOXA-10 has role in improving implantation rates.

Endometriomics: Proteomics and Secretomics

Some 32 proteins like stathmin 1 and annexin A2 have been identified with different expression between prereceptive endometrium and refractory. This new technology can be applied to search for new biomarkers to determine the endometrial receptivity and identify key molecules to improve implantation in infertile patients. Its drawback is the need for embryo biopsy

Secretomics of endometrial fluid is a potential nondisruptive diagnostic tool for human endometrial receptivity. Uterine secretions are aspirated prior to ET and electrophoresis of the material can be done for glycoproteins, chemokines, cytokines, growth factor, and signaling factors.

Endometrial Receptivity Array Test

Unlike the embryo, the transition from anatomical to molecular medicine in the diagnosis of the endometrial function just happened a decade ago. It is a customized microarray test array based on transcriptomic signature of human endometrial receptivity. It analyses 238 genes in the endometrial biopsy sample obtained on Day LH + 7 in natural cycle or P+5 in HRT cycle, i.e. during the WOI.

The endometrial receptivity array (ERA) is now performed by next generation sequencing that is coupled with a computational predictor and algorithm able to identify the receptivity of an endometrial sample, providing the personalized WOI (pWOI) of a given patient regardless of its histological appearance.

MEASURES TO IMPROVE ENDOMETRIAL RECEPTIVITY

- Treatment of underlying pathologies associated with impaired receptivity is a step towards improving implantation. Excision or ablation of endometrial implants prolonged suppression with 3–6 months of GnRH agonist therapies are believed to rectify the altered receptivity and increase pregnancy rates.

  Myomectomy should be done for submucous fibroids and large intramural or cavity distorting fibroids. Hysteroscopic polypectomy, salpingectomy for hydrosalpinges, and antibiotics for endometritis are some of the other proposed therapies to improve implantation.

- Mild stimulation protocols or cryopreservation of embryos as discussed earlier
- Endometrial injury has been proposed to improve the implantation and pregnancy rates in IVF cycles and also in patients with previous implantation failure. It is hypothesized that injury during the preceding luteal phase might induce endometrial decidualization, increase release of cytokines, growth factors, and also recruit stem cells to the endometrium. Evidence that endometrial injury performed in the cycle before ART increases the probability of live birth and clinical pregnancy is of moderate quality as reported by a recent Cochrane review.
- *Aspirin*: It inhibits the cyclooxygenase enzyme in platelets and decreases prostaglandin secretion thereby causing vasodilatation which is believed to improve uterine blood flow and uterine receptivity. Various meta-analyses have conflicting views but Cochrane review by Siristatidis et al. 2016, has concluded that the use of empirical aspirin in general IVF population cannot be recommended. This meta-analysis of 13 trials did not find any significant difference between aspirin and control group for live birth rate, clinical pregnancy rate, and miscarriage rate. These findings are in contrast to the recently published meta-analysis by Lipin Wang et al. stating that aspirin in 100 mg doses may improve pregnancy rates in IVF.
- *Low-molecular-weight heparin (LMWH) (Box 1)*: Heparin by its antithrombolytic activity potentially improves the implantation in women with thrombophilia. But observational studies have shown conflicting results regarding this effect. The effect of LMWH in women with recurrent implantation failure (RIF) was evaluated by Potdar et al. 2013 and found that it significantly improves live birth rate by 79% and reduced the risk of miscarriage by 78% compared with that in the control group. Subsequent studies in unselected population and in women with two previous failures.

BOX 1 Mechanism of action.

- Modulates endometrial receptivity and decidualization of endometrial stromal cells
- Inhibition of production of insulin-like growth factor-binding protein
- Blockage of complement activation and modulation of inflammatory responses
- Reduction in expression of adhesion molecules such as E-cadherin which promotes trophoblast invasion

- *Sildenafil citrate*: Type-5 phosphodiesterase inhibitor—hypothesized to improve the endometrial thickness and blood flow. Some studies like Takasaki et al. 2010, and Sher and Fisch 2002, found it to improve endometrial thickness and improve uterine artery RI while others like Check et al. 2004 did not find any improvements. Not recommended for routine use by British Fertility Society.
- Acupuncture, vitamin E, pentoxifylline, etc. have been tried by various scientist but the evidence still lacking.
- *Intrauterine therapies*: The logic is improving the intrauterine microenvironment. There are many suggestions like low volume hCG, autologous peripheral blood mononuclear cell, granulocyte-colony stimulation factor, and autologous stem cell therapy. However, the scientific data so far is inconclusive for the routine use and the clear-cut benefits is not proven with adequately powered studies.

EDITORS' COMMENTS

Endometrial receptivity is been in debate in the field of ART since long time, one cannot deny its vital role in implantation, the biggest challenge is the prediction and diagnosis of endometrial receptivity and the entire concept of WOI which is a major bone of contention amongst various ART clinicians on the time window, its diagnostic, and prognostic value.

Endometrial receptivity array test is the most widely used test for diagnosis but also has its own set of criticism. Different other tests such as EMMA (endometrial microbiome metagenomic analysis) and AHCF have also been developed. The molecular basis of endometrial receptivity is a fast developing field and hopefully will provide robust data which everyone can agree upon would come soon.

11

CHAPTER

Influence of Endometrial Preparation Protocols on Embryo Implantation in Frozen Embryo Transfer

Arunima Halder, Kamini A Rao

INTRODUCTION

The mechanism of implantation of the human embryo still remains an enigma. Researchers have devised various techniques to study the development of an optimum endometrium, but the intricacies are still elusive. However, from the current knowledge, one can deduce that the process of embryo implantation is a delicate choreography between the embryo and the endometrium, popularly termed as the "embryo-endometrial dialogue" which eventually leads to the attachment and invasion of the embryo into the endometrium.

Human reproduction is not an efficient process, be it assisted or unassisted. In her fertile age, a woman's chance of producing a live baby is approximately 15–20%.

Though the embryo might have a greater influence on the process of implantation, the endometrium whether in a natural or an assisted cycle does play a very crucial role.

In stimulated cycles, very high levels of sex hormones and pituitary desensitizing drugs leading to corpus luteal insufficiency may lead to asynchrony of the endometrium, ultimately causing implantation failure.

WINDOW OF IMPLANTATION

The window of implantation is a time bound interval of about 4–5 days in the mid-luteal phase, when the endometrium acquires a functional and transient steroid-dependent status that allows the attachment of the blastocyst and further supports the embryo by an array of paracrine activity.

Window of implantation opens on the 19–20 days of menstrual cycle, 7–10 days of luteinizing hormone (LH) surge or 4–5 days of progesterone exposure [in a frozen embryo transfer (FET) cycle].

ROLE OF ESTROGEN AND PROGESTERONE IN GENERATION OF THE ENDOMETRIUM

The temporal action of estrogen and progesterone on the endometrium and its manifestations has been well elucidated. The endometrium has two parts: (1) the epithelial and (2) the stromal components both of which express estrogen and progesterone receptors on them.

Estrogen causes endometrial proliferation, upregulation of the progesterone receptors as well as release of several growth factors like vascular endothelial growth factor (VEGF), insulin-like growth factor 1 (IGF1) and selectins. Whereas, progesterone induces decidualization, causes stromal edema, downregulates estrogen receptors and estrogen activity as well as leukemia inhibitory factor (LIF) and β_3-integrin levels. Overall, estrogen-primed progesterone activity enhances the receptivity of the endometrium for the embryo.

The response of the endometrium to these hormones depends upon:

- The concentration of these hormones
- The levels of receptors in the epithelial and stromal components (Table 1)
- Rate of metabolism of these hormones
- Presence of coactivators and repressors
- Associated paracrine signaling.

TABLE 1 Estrogen and progesterone receptors at various phases of the menstrual cycle.

Phase of menstrual cycle	*Epithelium*				*Stroma*			
	PR-A	*PR-B*	*ER-A*	*ER-B*	*PR-A*	*PR-B*	*ER-A*	*ER-B*
Proliferative phase	H	H	H	M	M (Predominant)	M	H	M
Early secretory phase	M	M	M	M	M (Predominant)	M	M	L
Mid secretory phase	A	L	A	M	M	L	A	L
Late secretory phase	A	A	A	M	M	A	A	L

(H: high; M: moderate; L: low; A: absent)

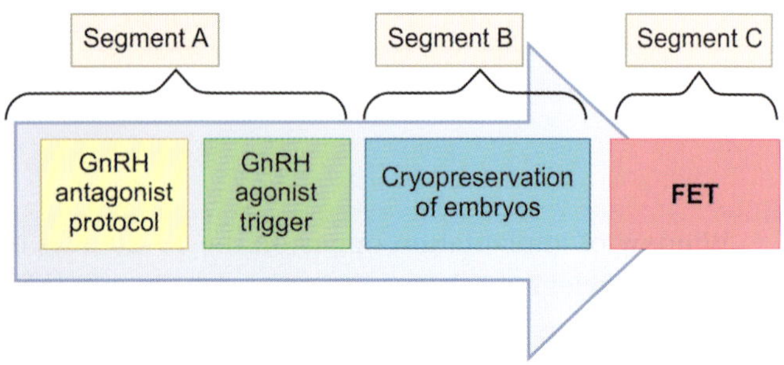

Fig. 1: OHSS-free clinic.
(GnRH: gonadotropin-releasing hormone; FET: frozen embryo transfer).

Flowchart 1: Endometrial preparation protocols.

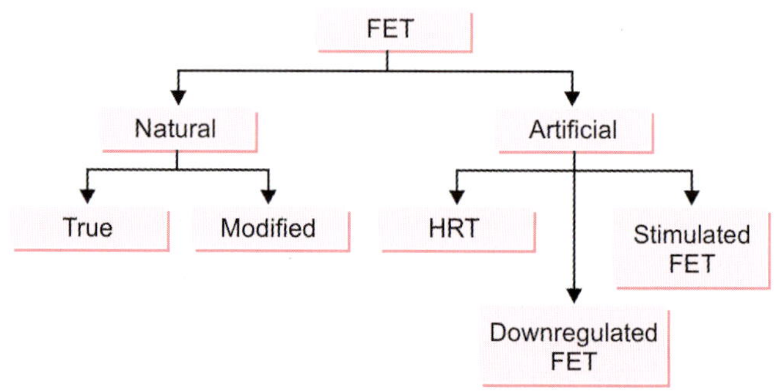

(HRT: hormone replacement therapy; FET: frozen embryo transfer)

The aim of FET is to emulate the estrogenic and the progesteronic effects on the endometrium such that the frozen embryo can be appropriately transferred during the window of implantation.

INDICATIONS FOR FROZEN EMBRYO TRANSFER

The advent of vitrification provided a much required boost to the cryopreservation techniques already available which not only met the rising requirements of embryo freezing, but also opened up news arenas in the field of infertility.

Devroey et al. came up with the concept of ovarian hyperstimulation syndrome (OHSS)-free clinic (Fig. 1) which involved segmentation of *in vitro* fertilization (IVF) into three segments: Segment A, Segment B and Segment C.

Frozen embryo transfer came into the limelight in cases requiring OHSS prevention. Other indications for the use of FET were in cases with supernumerary embryos, postponement of transfer due to asynchronous endometrium either too thick or too thin, premature rise of the progesterone or patient's desire. Embryo freezing and FET may also be offered to those undergoing donor-recipient cycles and those opting for medical or social freezing of embryos.

ENDOMETRIAL PREPARATION PROTOCOLS IN FROZEN EMBRYO TRANSFER

Endometrial preparation protocols can be classified into natural or artificial (Flowchart 1).

Natural Cycle Frozen Embryo Transfer

Natural cycle FET involves no medical intervention; however, it necessitates meticulous monitoring by transvaginal ultrasonography and endocrine profile (Figs. 2A and B).

A synchrony is desired between the embryo and the endometrium. This is achieved using the patient's endogenous hormones. Natural cycle tracking involves monitoring of the cycle with serial ultrasonography and serum LH levels, the advantage being lack of any medications. In a randomized control trial (RCT) conducted by Peeraer et al., it was observed that in women with regular menstrual cycles, gonadotropins in FET were not associated with improved implantation and live birth rates as compared to natural cycle FET.

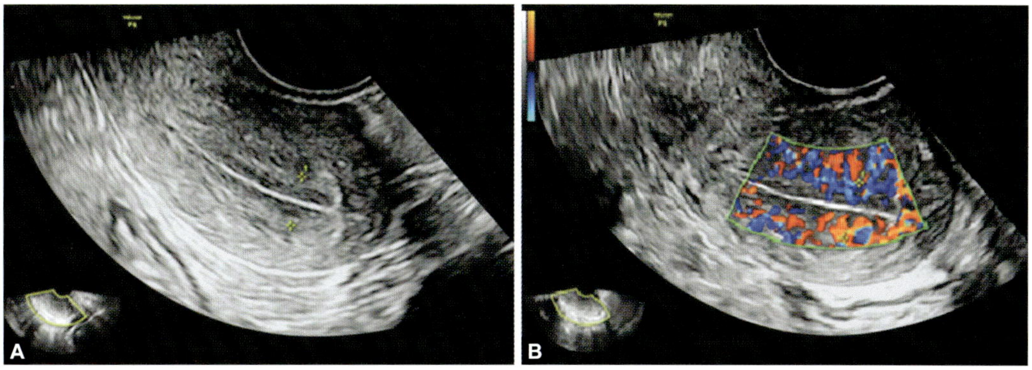

Figs. 2A and B: Ultrasonographic photographs showing a receptive endometrium. (A) A triple line endometrium >8 mm; (B) A Doppler image showing excellent subendometrial blood flow.

However, the obstacles in using the natural cycle FET are manifold:

- It involves stringent monitoring which increases the number of hospital visits.
- Number of scans and blood tests to measure the hormonal milieu, increases the cost of the treatment.
- Ovulation may not be under complete control as a result of which the cycle flexibility decreases.
- The urinary LH surge follows the serum LH surge by around 21 hours which should be kept in mind while monitoring these cycle.
- Also, there may be intercycle and interindividual variations in the LH surge.
- The LH kits may show a false-negative result in as high as 30% of the cases.
- The actual definition of LH surge is not clear. Some schools advocate it as a LH measurement of 180% of the basal value and others may consider a value of 10 ng/mL as adequate.
- In natural cycles, in view of the aforementioned reasons, the cycle cancellation may be approximately 10% due to missed ovulation.

Modified Natural Cycle Frozen Embryo Transfer (Fig. 3)

The aforementioned problems of natural cycle FET could be overcome by using the modified natural cycle (mNC) where human chorionic gonadotropin (hCG) is administered to obtain an artificially induced ovulation.

In these cycles, sonographic monitoring is done till the development of a follicle ≥17 mm. hCG is administered at this point and ovulation is expected to occur approximately 36 hours after the trigger. Once embryo transfer is done, progesterones are started as the luteal phase support.

The mNC provides a better control over the cycle and prevents untimely ovulation. Theoretically, the administration of hCG should be beneficial in supporting the luteal phase. However, in a study by Montagut et al., mNC showed a lower clinical performance as compared to natural cycles with or without luteal phase support.

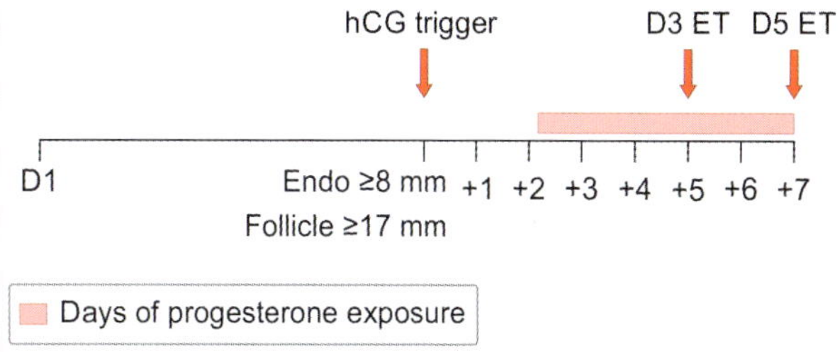

Fig. 3: Schematic representation of modified natural cycle. (hCG: human chorionic gonadotropin; ET: embryo transfer; D1: Day 1; D3: Day 3; D5: Day 5)

Meta-analysis done by Ghobara et al. and Groenewoud et al. however does not recommend the usage of one protocol over the other.

Frozen Embryo Transfer-Hormone Replacement Therapy (Fig. 4)

Hormone replacement therapy (HRT) cycles were first studied by Lutjen et al. as early as 1984. Embryo formed out of a donor oocyte and husband's sperm was transferred into an endometrium prepared by exogenous estrogen and progesterone supplementation in a woman with primary ovarian insufficiency. Later a healthy baby was born.

Younis et al. studied endometrial preparation in donor recipient cycle and used a sequentially incremental dose of estrogen for the same.

Hormone replacement therapy involves supplementing with estrogen in the follicular phase. Starting the estradiol

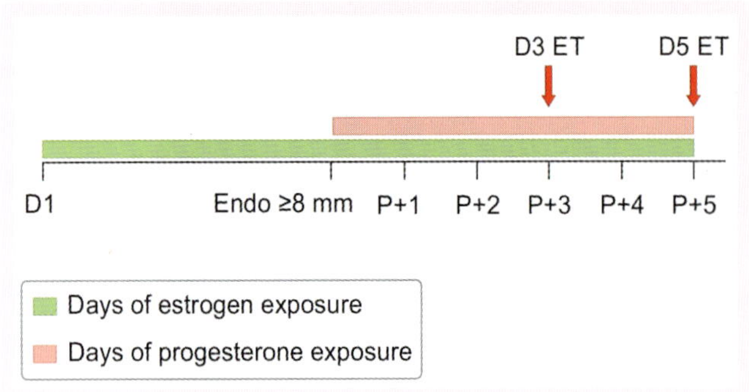

Fig. 4: Schematic representation of FET-HRT.

prior to the 4th day of the cycle prevents the development of a dominant follicle and escape ovulation in a later stage.

Estrogen replacement may be done in sequentially incremental doses (2 mg twice a day for 4 days followed by 2 mg thrice a day for the remaining days) or a steady dose of 2 mg thrice a day may be used.

The length of estrogen therapy did not have much effect on the implantation potential. It was seen that supplementation of estradiol for even a period of 36 days prior to the FET was not deleterious. However, decreasing length of estrogen may be beneficial in terms of cost and time to pregnancy. However, this requires further emphasis in the future studies.

Form of Estrogen Used

Estrogen is usually used in the form of estradiol valerate, estradiol hemihydrates or 17β-estradiol. It can be administered as oral, transdermal or transvaginal ring, oral being the most common form that is used.

Davar et al. conducted a randomized controlled trial where comparison was made between transdermal estrogen patches and oral estradiol valerate in FET cycles. Though there was no significant difference between the two groups as far as implantation rates, pregnancy rates or live birth rates were concerned. The cost of treatment and patient compliance was better in the transdermal estrogen group.

In another study conducted by Molina et al., usage of transdermal estrogen led to the development of thicker endometrium. However, there was no difference between the two groups with respect to clinical pregnancy rates and miscarriage rates.

Oral estrogen undergoes excessive first pass metabolism in the liver where the estradiol is converted to estrone such that its activity decreases by 30%. However, the transdermal form does not undergo breakdown in the liver and hence maintains a better estradiol:estrone ratio.

Monitoring the Estrogen Phase

Prior to starting the cycle, a transvaginal ultrasonography is mandatory. This is done to assess the thickness of the endometrium as well as absence of any dominant follicle or retained corpus luteal cyst.

The optimum endometrium is said to be between 9 mm and 14 mm. However, several studies have suggested an endometrium of at least 7 mm as optimum for planning embryo transfer. An endometrium of <7 mm was associated with poor pregnancy outcome.

On transvaginal sonography (TVS), bilateral ovaries should be assessed for presence of a dominant follicle as a functional follicle may interfere with the development of a synchronous endometrium.

Doppler monitoring has also been suggested while monitoring the FET cycle. Presence of subendometrial blood flow has been associated with higher implantation and pregnancy rates (*See* Fig. 2B).

Endocrine monitoring of the FET cycle is not suggested, though serum progesterone levels may be helpful in determining escape ovulation that may occur in about 1.9–7.4% of FET cycles with any previous downregulation.

Addition of Progesterone

Once the endometrium is satisfactorily prepared, progesterone can be supplemented in various modes. Vaginal and intramuscular routes are the most common routes used. Oral route for progesterone administration fails the acid test due to excessive first pass metabolism. In a meta-analysis conducted by Glujovsky et al., there was no significant difference found in between the vaginal or the intramuscular routes for progesterone administration.

Vaginal progesterone undergoes the first uterine pass effect and very high concentration of the drug can be achieved in the uterus within a short duration. However, the serum concentration seems to be very low in the vaginal preparation. On the other hand, in case of injectable progesterone, the serum concentration is higher. Vaginal progesterones are used in the dose of up to 400–800 mg/day and injectable progesterones are used at 25 mg/day, 50 mg/day or 100 mg/day.

Depending on the day of the embryo transfer, the progesterone may be administered for 3 days or 5 days prior to the embryo transfer.

Till date there is no unanimity in the duration of administration of progesterone. Few studies suggest stoppage of progesterone when a positive β-hCG is obtained. This has been especially elucidated in cases of fresh embryo transfers.

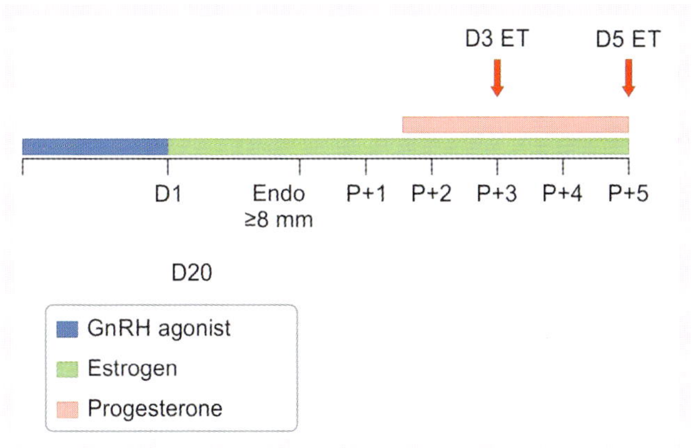

Fig. 5: Schematic representation of downregulated frozen embryo transfer.

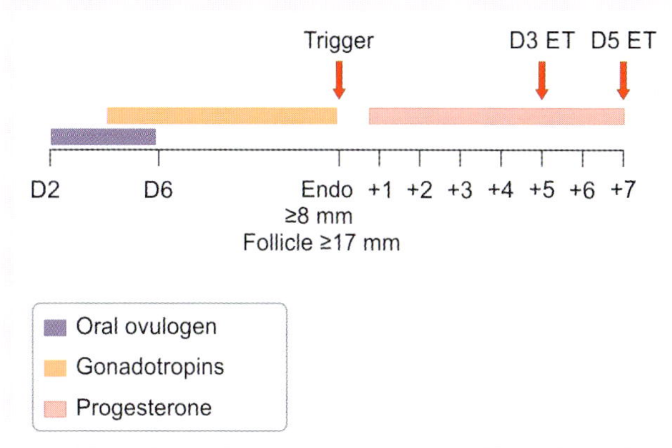

Fig. 6: Schematic representation of stimulated frozen embryo transfer.

However, in case of FET cycles, the absence of corpus luteum mandates the usage of progesterone till the luteo-placental shift occurs at around 7–8 weeks. Robust studies are needed to support this hypothesis.

Recently, Groenewoud et al. conducted the ANTARCTICA trial, wherein FET-HRT was compared with mNC-FET with regards to the live birth rates as the primary outcome. Nine hundred fifty-nine patients were included. It was found that FET-HRT was noninferior to mNC-FET as far as live birth rates, clinical pregnancy rates and ongoing pregnancy rates were concerned. However, it was noted that FET-HRT results in higher cancellation rates.

Downregulated Frozen Embryo Transfer (Fig. 5)

Problems with the HRT protocol:
- Higher chance of escape ovulation
- Inappropriate downregulation
- High cancellation rates.

Theoretically, in the aforementioned situations, gonadotropin-releasing hormone (GnRH) agonists would downregulate the cycle and prevent the development of a follicle. This has been validated especially in cases of adenomyosis and endometriosis where use of long-term pituitary suppression has led to improved pregnancy outcomes. On the other hand, in two meta-analysis by Ghobara et al., the author did not find any significant differences in the pregnancy rates between downregulated HRT (DR-HRT) versus stimulated or a natural cycle. Similar results were obtained in another systematic review by Groenewoud et al., wherein it was not possible to recommend one protocol to be more effective than the other.

Stimulated Cycles (Fig. 6)

When stimulated cycles are used, the protocol may help to overcome any defect in the follicular apparatus and may help to support the luteal phase. The contradictory school of thought could be that supraphysiological levels of estrogen may alter the receptivity of the endometrium and hinder implantation. This controversy remains unresolved in light of the meagre evidence available in literature. A pilot study conducted by Hu et al. on efficiency of letrozole for endometrial preparation for FET in polycystic ovarian syndrome (PCOS) patients suggested that letrozole may be associated with higher implantation rates, clinical and ongoing pregnancy rates when compared to FET-HRT or mNC-HRT. Peeraer et al. did not find stimulated cycles to be superior to mNCs as far as implantation rates and live birth rates were concerned. Moreover, it was suggested that mNCs were advantageous especially in women with regular menstrual cycles. Yarali et al. noted that stimulation with gonadotropins or aromatase inhibitors may be promising but the fact that mNCs are extremely patient-friendly shall not be discounted.

Comparison between various protocols has been shown in Table 2.

ADJUVANTS USED IN FROZEN EMBRYO TRANSFER CYCLES

1. *Aspirin*: It was hypothesized that low-dose aspirin enhances the blood flow to the uterine vessel leading to a decrease in impedance and low uterine artery pulsatility indices. Check et al. noted an increase in the endometrial thickness in luteal phase in those treated with aspirin. However, Weckstein et al. did not find

TABLE 2 Comparison between various protocols.

Sl no.	Protocol	Rationale	Drugs used	Advantages	Disadvantages	Evidences
1	Natural cycle	Development of a physiological synchrony between the embryo and endometrium	Nil	Patient-friendly No drugs used	Lack of flexibility High cancellation rates Stringent monitoring required	Peeraer et al.
2	Modified natural cycle	To have more control over the cycle, by controlling the time of ovulation	hCG for trigger	Better cycle control HCG used as a trigger may support in the luteal phase	Lack of evidence suggestive of mNC being better than NC with respect to pregnancy rates	Montagut et al. Ghobara et al. Groenewoud et al.
3	FET-HRT	To emulate the hormonal changes during the menstrual cycle	Estrogen and progesterone	Enormous cycle control Better flexibility Less monitoring	High cancellation rates Chances of escape ovulation	Molina et al. Montagut et al.
4	DR-FET	Prevention of development of a dominant follicle	GnRH with estrogen and progesterone	Less chances of escape ovulation Better in cases of endometriosis	Lack of evidence supporting it over other protocols	Ghobara et al.
5	Stimulated FET	To overcome problem with the follicular apparatus and support the luteal phase	Oral ovulogens with or without gonadotropins	May repair any faulty mechanism in the follicular apparatus Provides luteal phase support due to existing corpora lutea	May lead to asynchronous endometrium Lack of evidence supporting it	Peeraer et al. Yarali et al.

(FET: frozen embryo transfer; HRT: hormone replacement therapy; hCG: human chorionic gonadotropin; mNC: malified natural cycle)

any significant difference between the aspirin and the nonaspirin group. Interestingly, it was also noted that in those patients whose endometrium failed to reach above 8 mm, increased blood flow following Ecosprin improved pregnancy rates.

2. *Vaginal sildenafil*: Sildenafil is a phosphodiesterase inhibitor. It enhances nitric oxide-induced vasodilatation. This helps in increasing subendometrial blood flow. Sher et al. reported significant increase in the subendometrial blood flow and a fall in the pulsatility indices with the usage of vaginal sildenafil. Similar results were also seen by Takasaki et al. who found increased endometrial thickness and increased pregnancy rates in patients taking sildenafil. Eid et al. found a decrease in the pulsatility indices of uterine arteries after using vaginal sildenafil.
3. *Pentoxifylline*: Pentoxifylline is a methylxanthine derivative that acts a phosphodiesterase inhibitor. It decreases inflammation by decreasing the production and action of cytokines like tumor necrosis factor-alpha (TNF-α). Lédée-Bataille et al. noted a significant increase in the endometrial thickness and the blood flows when sildenafil was used with tocopherol. Vitamin E or tocopherol is an antioxidant that scavenges reactive oxygen species. Vitamin E induces angiogenesis and endometrial glandular proliferation.
4. *L-arginine*: It also acts as a nitric oxide donor which causes vasodilatation. In a pilot study conducted by Takasaki et al., it was observed that addition of vitamin E, arginine and sildenafil improved the uterine radial artery resistivity indices and was beneficial in cases of thin endometrium.
5. *Granulocyte colony-stimulating factor (G-CSF)*: It is a hematopoietic factor which has a role in endometrial growth. It is expressed by the decidual cells of the endometrium and is involved in neutrophilic proliferation, recruitment of dendritic cells and angiogenesis. Gleicher et al. conducted a pilot study in four women who had endometrial thickness of 3–6.5 mm after the usage of oral and vaginal estrogen. On addition of G-CSF, there was a significant increase in endometrial thickness reaching 7 mm in 2 days. Lucena et al. found a significant increase in the endometrial thickness following the use of 300 μg of G-CSF. Recent

study by Xu et al. is suggestive of increased endometrial thickness and increased pregnancy rates with the usage of 100 μg of G-CSF. However, studies by Check et al. and Li et al. failed to find any significant increase in the thickness of the endometrium.

6. *Endometrial scratching*: Endometrial injury prior to the FET cycle can lead to the production of several growth factors and chemokines. It causes the initiation of the process of wound repair and upregulation of certain genes expressed during the window of implantation. However to scratch the endometrium or not is a very controversial subject. Recently, Nastri et al. presented a meta-analysis including 14 trials where there was moderate quality evidence indicates that endometrial injury performed between Day 7 of previous cycle and Day 7 of present cycle was associated with better pregnancy and live birth rates.
7. *Stem cell therapy*: Regeneration of the endometrium occurs due to the presence of endometrium progenitor cells and bone marrow derived stem cells on the endometrium that may be hematopoietic or non-hematopoietic. Initial animal experiments were conducted by Cervello et al. and Zhao et al., increase in the endometrial thickness was noted in mice on infusion of bone marrow mesenchymal stem cells (BMSCs). The first human use of stem cells occurred in 2011. Nagori et al. transferred autologous stem cells in an endometrium of thickness 3.6 which along with estrogen and other adjuvants developed an endometrium of 7.1. Later three donor oocytes were transferred which resulted in a live birth.
8. *Platelet-rich plasma*: Platelet-rich plasma when infused into the endometrium causes the release of cytokines and growth factors like VEGF, epidermal growth factor (EGF), transforming growth factor (TGF), etc. Chang et al. found an increase in the endometrial thickness with the usage of platelet-rich plasma. Recently, Zadeh-modarres et al. also confirmed the same in their study.

CONCLUSION

There are several protocols for preparation of the endometrium in our armamentarium. However, evidence at present does not focus on appropriate outcomes and no conclusion is arrived to as far as recommending one protocol over the other is concerned. Quality of the evidences at hand is low and robust studies are needed to pinpoint toward a particular guideline. At the present date, individualization of the protocol could be the right step toward a successful FET.

KEY POINTS

- The window of implantation is a time bound interval of about 4–5 days in the mid-luteal phase.
- The aim of FET is to emulate the estrogenic and the progesteronic effects on the endometrium such that the frozen embryo can be appropriately transferred during the window of implantation.
- Indications for FET could be usage of supernumerary embryos, prevention of OHSS or asynchronous endometrium. It could also be for the purpose of pre-implantation genetic screening (PGS) or as requested by the patient.
- The endometrial preparation protocol can be broadly divided into natural and artificial. Studies have suggested that no particular method is superior over the others. Good quality studies are still lacking.

EDITORS' COMMENTS

With a steady increase in FET worldwide despite an overall early pregnancy loss of approximately 25% and delivery rates [single embryo transfer (SET)] of 20–25% (ESHRE report 2012), there is no consensus and conflicting evidence on optimal endometrium preparation. What seems clear though is that patients prefer vaginal route for progesterone administration (Levine 2000). However, the optimal mid-luteal progesterone levels, progesterone duration and dosage, and when to stop progesterone in HRT-FET cycles after implantation remains debatable. At present, decision is mainly based on clinician experience and patient preferences. Our current practices are based on the replacement of blastocysts in artificially prepared endometrium without suppression and vaginal progesterone; the embryo is replaced to the uterine cavity after 115 ± 3 hours of progesterone exposure. Further research is needed to elucidate these gaps of knowledge as a means to providing clinicians robust evidence for proper clinical decision making.

SC Esteves, Campinas, Brazil

SUGGESTED READING

1. Bardos J, Rodriguez-Purata J, Whitehouse MC, et al. Optimal endometrial preparation for frozen embryo transfer (FET) of screened embryos is independent of follicular phase length. Fertil Steril. 2015;104:e47-8.
2. Cervello I, Gil Sanchis C, Mas A, et al. Bone marrow-derived cells from male donors do not contribute to the endometrial side population of the recipient. PLoS One. 2012;7(1):e30260.
3. Chang Y, Li J, Chen Y, et al. Autologous platelet-rich plasma promotes endometrial growth and improves pregnancy outcome during in vitrofertilization. Int J Clin Exp Med. 2015;8(1):1286-90.

4. Check JH, Cohen R, Choe JK. Failure to improve a thin endometrium in the late proliferative phase with uterine infusion of granulocyte-colony stimulating factor. Clin Exp Obstet Gynecol. 2014;41(4):473-5.
5. Check JH, Diatterich C, Lurie D, et al. A matched study to determine whether low-dose aspirin without heparin improves pregnancy rates following frozen embryo transfer and/or affects endometrial sonographic parameters. J Assist Reprod Genet. 1998;15(10):579-82.
6. Dal Prato L, Borini A, Cattoli M, et al. Endometrial preparation for frozen-thawed embryo transfer with or without pretreatment with gonadotropin-releasing hormone agonist. Fertil Steril. 2002;77:956-60.
7. Davar R, Janati S, Mohseni F, et al. A comparison of the effects of transdermal estradiol and estradiol valerate on endometrial receptivity in frozen-thawed embryo transfer cycles: a randomized clinical trial. J Reprod Infertil. 2016;17(2):97-103.
8. De Ziegler D, Bulletti C, De Monstier, et al. The first uterine pass effect. Ann N Y Acad Sci. 1997;828:291-9.
9. Devroey P, Polyzos NP, Blockeel C. An OHSS-free clinic by segmentation of IVF treatment. Hum Reprod. 2011;26:2593-7.
10. Eid ME. Sildenafil improves implantation rate in women with a thin endometrium secondary to improvement of uterine blood flow; "pilot study". Fertil Steril. 2015;104:e342.
11. El-Toukhy T, Coomarasamy A, Khairy M, et al. The relationship between endometrial thickness and outcome of medicated frozen embryo replacement cycles. Fertil Steril. 2008;89:832-9.
12. Fatemi HM, Popovic-Todorovic B, Papanikolaou E, et al. An update of luteal phase support in stimulated IVF cycles. Hum Reprod Update. 2007;13:581-90.
13. Ghobara T, Gelbaya TA, Ayeleke RO. Cycle regimens for frozen-thawed embryo transfer. Cochrane Database Syst Rev. 2017;7:CD003414.
14. Ghobara T, Vanderkerchove P. Cycle regimens for frozen-thawed embryo transfer. Cochrane Database Syst Rev. 2008;1:CD003414.
15. Gleicher N, Vidali A, Barad DH. Successful treatment of unresponsive thin endometrium. Fertil Steril. 2011;95(6):2123.e13-7.
16. Glujovsky D, Pesce R, Fiszbajn G, et al. Endometrial preparation for women undergoing embryo transfer with frozen embryos or embryos derived from donor oocytes. Cochrane Database Syst Rev. 2010;(1):CD006359.
17. Groenewoud ER, Cantineau AE, Kollen BJ, et al. What is the optimal means of preparing the endometrium in frozen-thawed embryo transfer cycles? A systematic review and meta-analysis. Hum Reprod Update. 2013;19:458-70.
18. Groenewoud ER, Cohlen BJ, Al-Oraiby A, et al. A randomized controlled, non-inferiority trial of modified natural versus artificial cycle for cryo-thawed embryo transfer. Hum Reprod. 2016;31:1483-92.
19. Hardarson T, Hanson C, Sjogren A, et al. Human embryos with unevenly sized blastomeres have lower pregnancy and implantation rates: indications for aneuploidy and multinucleation. Hum Reprod. 2001;16:313-8.
20. Hjollund NH, Jensen TK, Bonde JP, et al. Spontaneous abortion and physical strain around implantation: a follow-up study of first-pregnancy planners. Epidemiology. 2000;11:18-23.
21. Hoozemans DA, Schats R, Lambalk CB, et al. Human embryo implantation: current knowledge and clinical implications in assisted reproductive technology. Reprod Biomed Online. 2004;9:692-715.
22. Hu Y-J, Chen Y-Z, Zhu Y-M, et al. Letrozole stimulation in endometrial preparation for cryopreserved-thawed embryo transfer in women with polycystic ovarian syndrome: A pilot study. Clin Endocrinol (Oxf). 2014;80:283-9.
23. Jones HW, Oehninger S, Bocca S, et al. Reproductive efficiency of human oocytes fertilized in vitro. Facts Views Vis Obgyn. 2010;2(3):169-71.
24. Juneau CR, Franasiak JM, Morin SJ, et al. Obstetric outcomes following frozen embryo transfer (FET) in patients with an endometrial thickness measuring <7 mm. Fertil Steril. 2016;106:e214-5.
25. Kalem Z, Kalem MN, Gürgan T. Methods for endometrial preparation in frozen-thawed embryo transfer cycles. J Turk Ger Gynecol Assoc. 2016;17(3):168-72.
26. Kasius A, Smit JG, Torrance HL, et al. Endometrial thickness and pregnancy rates after IVF: a systematic review and meta-analysis. Hum Reprod Update. 2014;20:530-41.
27. Lédée-Bataille N, Olivennes F, Lefaix J-L, et al. Combined treatment by pentoxifylline and tocopherol for recipient women with a thin endometrium enrolled in an oocyte donation programme. Hum Reprod. 2002;17(5):1249-53.
28. Li Y, Pan P, Chen X, et al. Granulocyte colony-stimulating factor administration for infertile women with thin endometrium in frozen embryo transfer program. Reprod Sci. 2014;21(3):381-5.
29. Liu X-R, Mu H-Q, Shi Q, et al. The optimal duration of progesterone supplementation in pregnant women after IVF/ICSI: a meta-analysis. Reprod Biol Endocrinol. 2012;10:1.
30. Lucena E, Moreno-Ortiz H. Granulocyte colony-stimulating factor (G-CSF): a mediator in endometrial receptivity for a patient with polycystic ovary (PCO) undergoing in vitro maturation (IVM). BMJ Case Rep. 2013;2013. pii: bcr2012008115.
31. Lutjen P, Trounson A, Leeton J, et al. The establishment and maintenance of pregnancy using in vitro fertilization and embryo donation in a patient with primary ovarian failure. Nature. 1984;307:174-5.
32. Molina PF, Lliso CC, Collado RC, et al. Prospective, randomized, clinical trial to compare two endometrial preparation protocols. Fertil Steril. 2016;106:e206.
33. Montagut M, Santos-Ribeiro S, De Vos M, et al. Frozen-thawed embryo transfers in natural cycles with spontaneous or induced ovulation: the search for the best protocol continues. Hum Reprod. 2016;31:2803-10.
34. Nagori CB, Panchal SY, Patel H. Endometrial regeneration using autologous adult stem cells followed by conception by in vitro fertilization in a patient of severe Asherman's syndrome. J Hum Reprod Sci. 2011;4(1):43-8.
35. Nastri CO, Lensen SF, Gibreel A, et al. Endometrial injury in women undergoing assisted reproductive techniques. Cochrane Database Syst Rev. 2015;3:CD009517.

36. Niu Z, Chen Q, Sun Y, et al. Long-term pituitary downregulation before frozen embryo transfer could improve pregnancy outcomes in women with adenomyosis. Gynecol Endocrinol. 2013;29:1026-30.
37. Peeraer K, Couck I, Debrock S, et al. Frozen-thawed embryo transfer in a natural or mildly hormonally stimulated cycle in women with regular ovulatory cycles: a RCT. Hum Reprod. 2015;30:2552-62.
38. Sardana D, Upadhyay AJ, Deepika K, et al. Correlation of subendometrial-endometrial blood flow assessment by two-dimensional power Doppler with pregnancy outcome in frozen-thawed embryo transfer cycles. J Hum Reprod Sci. 2014;7(2):130-5.
39. Sekhon L, Feuerstein J, Nazem TG, et al. Endometrial preparation for FET: does the duration of estradiol supplementation matter? Fertil Steril. 2017;108:e364.
40. Sher G, Fisch JD. Vaginal sildenafil (Viagra): a preliminary report of a novel method to improve uterine artery blood flow and endometrial development in patients undergoing IVF. Hum Reprod. 2000;15(4):806-9.
41. Takasaki A, Tamura H, Miwa I, et al. Endometrial growth and uterine blood flow: a pilot study for improving endometrial thickness in patients with a thin endometrium. Fertil Steril. 2010;93(6):1851-8.
42. Van Der Gaast MH, Beckers NG, Beier-Hellwig K, et al. Ovarian stimulation for IVF and endometrial receptivity—the missing link. Reprod Biomed Online. 2000;5(Suppl 1):36-43.
43. Wallach EE, Younis JS, Simon A, et al. Endometrial preparation: lessons from oocyte donation. Fertil Steril. 1996;66:873-84.
44. Weckstein LN, Jacobson A, Galen D, et al. Low-dose aspirin for oocyte donation recipients with a thin endometrium: prospective, randomized study. Fertil Steril. 1997;68(5): 927-30.
45. Xu B, Zhang Q, Hao J, et al. Two protocols to treat thin endometrium with granulocyte colony-stimulating factor during frozen embryo transfer cycles. Reprod Biomed Online. 2015;30(4):349-58.
46. Yarali H, Polat M, Mumusoglu S, et al. Preparation of endometrium for frozen embryo replacement cycles: a systematic review and meta-analysis. J Assist Reprod Genet. 2016;33:1287-304.
47. Young SL. Oestrogen and progesterone action on endometrium: a translational approach to understanding endometrial receptivity. Reprod Biomed Online. 2013; 27(5): 497-505.
48. Zadehmodarres S, Salehpour S, Saharkhiz N, et al. Treatment of thin endometrium with autologous platelet-rich plasma: a pilot study. JBRA Assist Reprod. 2017;21(1):54-6.
49. Zhao J, Zhang Q, Wang Y, et al. Rat bone marrow mesenchymal stem cells improve regeneration of thin endometrium in rat. Fertil Steril. 2014;101(2):587-94.

12

CHAPTER

Deciding on the Moment of Embryo Transfer: Discovering the Window of Implantation in ART

Mackens Shari, Racca Annalisa, Santos-Ribeiro Samuel, van de Vijver Arne, Christophe Blockeel

INTRODUCTION

A receptive endometrium is an endometrium that has developed the competence to let an embryo at blastocyst stage implant. The secretory changes that take place in the endometrial stromal compartment under the influence of progesterone, i.e. decidualization, are thought to be actively implicated in the selection of embryos seeking to implant. Hence, the timing of embryo transfer should ensure that a blastocyst encounters an optimal receptive, but also selective endometrium within the window of implantation (WOI).

In this chapter, we discuss how endometrial receptivity is altered following ovarian stimulation for *in vitro* fertilization (IVF)/intracytoplasmic sperm injection (ICSI), as well as the optimal frozen embryo transfer (FET) timing and the diagnostic possibilities to evaluate endometrial receptivity in daily clinical practice.

THE WINDOW OF IMPLANTATION IN ASSISTED REPRODUCTIVE TECHNOLOGY

Stimulated Cycles Followed by Fresh Embryo Transfer

Obtaining a receptive phenotype is a hormone driven process guided by the circulating serum concentrations of estrogen and progesterone (Young, 2013). It is, thus, easy to understand that ovarian stimulation (OS) for IVF/ICSI with its altered hormonal environment may strongly affect the endometrium (Bourgain and Devroey, 2003).

On the histological level, an endometrial advancement at the moment of oocyte retrieval has been described compared to natural cycles (Kolibianakis et al., 2002). Furthermore, distinct endometrial gene expression profiles in such biopsies have been detected in relation to the serum progesterone concentration (Van Vaerenbergh et al., 2011).

For endometrium harvested in the luteal phase during the WOI, limited differences have been put into evidence at the transcriptional level when appropriate luteal phase support (LPS) was used (Mirkin, et al., 2004) (Simón, et al., 2005). However, differences in gene expression were more pronounced when no LPS was provided (Horcajadas et al., 2005) (Humaidan et al., 2012), stressing its importance for the success rate of fresh embryo transfers. In contrast to the endometrial histological advancement seen at the moment of oocyte retrieval, research investigating the luteal phase endometrium not supplemented after OS suggests a functional delay in obtaining the receptive phenotype (Horcajadas et al., 2008). When comparing normal to high-responder patients, the level of the ovarian response also seems important for the subsequent endometrial transcriptome deregulation during the luteal phase (Liu et al., 2008). Furthermore, at this time-point, the impact of the serum progesterone level at the moment of triggering was confirmed (Labarta et al., 2011), although some describe an altered shift from prereceptive to receptive without the endometrial receptivity itself being affected (Haouzi et al., 2014).

It is evident that, during fresh embryo transfer cycles, one cannot ignore the impact of OS on the luteal phase endometrium, nor choose the day of embryo transfer. However, as cryopreservation strategies have improved (i.e. vitrification) (Loutradi et al., 2008) and as accumulating safety data are reassuring (Belva et al., 2016), the use of FET has increased vastly. This strategy method originally intended solely for surplus embryos has been extended to cases with late-follicular progesterone elevation (Healy et al., 2016) or embryo-endometrial asynchrony (Shapiro et al., 2008). Also, a freeze-all strategy following an agonist trigger with transfer of the embryo(s) in a subsequent FET cycle has been shown to be with high live birth rates (Blockeel et al., 2016) and may be associated with decreased maternal and neonatal morbidity (Ishihara et al., 2014) (Evans et al., 2014). Specifically, in repeated implantation failure (RIF) patients, a freeze all policy might be an option to improve treatment outcome (Magdi et al., 2017).

Frozen Embryo Transfer Cycles

Although the use of FET continues to increase [(European IVF-Monitoring Consortium (EIM) et al., 2016], the optimal endometrial preparation protocol remains to be elucidated and different strategies to prepare and to time the FET are used in current daily practice (Mackens et al., 2017). Preparation methods can typically be subdivided into two groups, namely in artificial and natural cycles. In the artificial or hormonal replacement therapy (HRT) cycles, the endometrial development is supported by exogenously administered estrogen and progesterone. In the natural cycle (NC), monitoring is performed by ultrasound and blood sampling evaluating serum hormone levels either to detect the timing of ovulation or to determine the best moment to trigger ovulation by human chorionic gonadotropin (hCG) (i.e. the difference between a true or a modified NC).

When deciding on the moment of embryo transfer, the differences in the above-mentioned protocols are of utmost importance to select the most appropriate time-point (Fig. 1). The WOI with its accompanying receptivity occurs once progesterone levels pass a critical threshold, initiating a tightly regulated endometrial transformation (Franasiak et al., 2016). Of course, a true NC, in which this process unfolds itself without any intervention, is the least prone to potential iatrogenic events. This issue has been raised when comparing the higher miscarriage rates of HRT FET compared to NC FET (Veleva et al., 2008), although others assign this observation to the fact that more polycystic ovary syndrome (PCOS) patients prepare FET with HRT because of irregular or absent natural cycles (Tomás et al., 2012). Moreover, in case of RIF, the analysis of the endometrial transcriptome favored NC over HRT (Altmäe et al., 2016). Nonetheless, retrospective clinical data comparing the outcome after NC or HRT FET have shown conflicting results (Ghobara and Vandekerckhove, 2008) (Givens et al., 2009) (Chang et al., 2011) (Groenewoud et al., 2013) (Guan et al., 2016) and a recent, large, multicenter, prospective trial failed to show a significant difference in terms of live birth rate after modified NC versus HRT FET (Groenewoud et al., 2016).

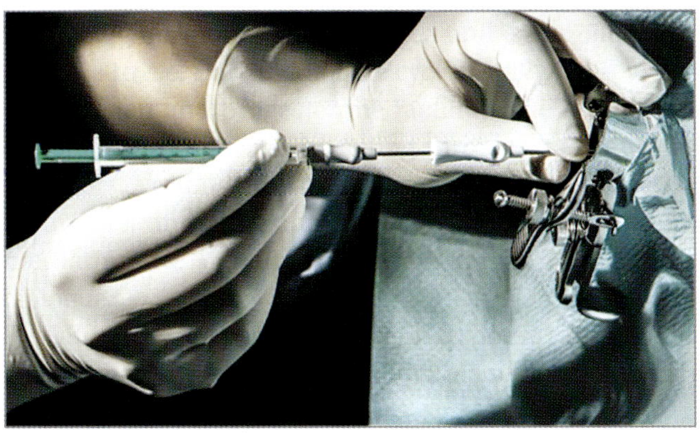

Fig. 1: Embryo transfer procedure.

In natural cycles, receptivity is achieved during a specific time interval called the WOI. This period in the menstrual cycle lasts about 3 to 4 days and is situated in the midluteal phase (Day 20–24) (Wilcox et al., 1999) (Norwitz et al., 2001). In NC FET, the luteinizing hormone (LH) surge is used to plan the moment of embryo transfer as normally the WOI opens 6 days after the progesterone elevation (Navot et al., 1991). However, one must be aware of the fact that an LH surge can occupy a period of 30 hours (Acosta et al., 2000) and that progesterone already rises slightly prior to ovulation, due to the peripheral granulosa cells producing LH (Hoff et al., 1983). Generally, we propose to perform true NC FET on LH +6 for the blastocyst stage with an adaptation respectively in case of cleavage stage embryo transfer (Fig. 2).

A difference in this timing could be considered for modified NC FET, as ovulation occurs probably later (i.e. 36–48 hr) after exogenous hCG administration (Kosmas et al., 2007). Therefore, we propose to perform modified NC FET on hCG +7 for the blastocyst stage, again with an adaptation respectively in case of cleavage stage embryo transfer (Fig. 2). Administering hCG while a spontaneous LH surge is already detected, has previously been linked to a detrimental outcome (Fatemi et al., 2010), although this was not confirmed in more recent research (Groenewoud et al., 2017). Nevertheless, the hypothesis needs to be studied further whether additional hCG, as well as additional early LPS in NC FET does not change the natural course of the endometrium toward receptivity with a different timing of the WOI and subsequent embryo-endometrial asynchrony.

The optimal exposure time to progesterone before transfer in HRT FET cycles has been the subject of many studies (Nawroth and Ludwig, 2005). Limited evidence

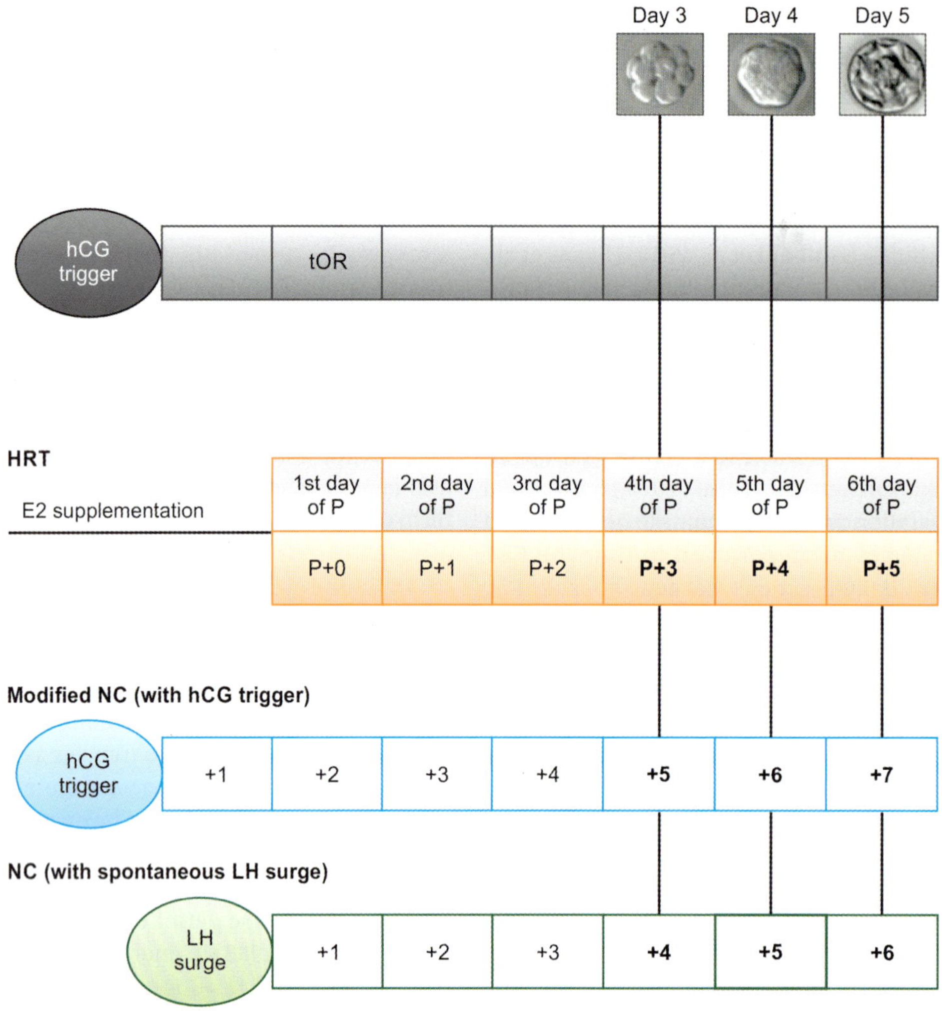

Fig. 2: Proposed embryo transfer timing according to the different preparation methods. (tOR: theoretical oocyte retrieval; E2: estradiol; P: progesterone; NC: natural cycle; hCG: human chorionic gonadotropin; HRT: hormonal replacement therapy; LH: luteinizing hormone)
Source: Reprinted from Mackens et al, 2017.

suggests that a short progesterone impregnation may be sufficient to reach endometrial receptivity (Imbar and Hurwitz, 2004) (Theodorou and Forman, 2012); however, a transfer of Day 4 embryos after three days of progesterone supplementation has been shown to be with a high risk of early pregnancy loss (van de Vijver et al., 2016). Conversely, an excessive exposure has been linked to a higher biochemical pregnancy rate (Escribá et al., 2006). It has indeed been suggested that the risk of early pregnancy loss increases when implantation takes place later in the WOI (Wilcox et al., 1999) and that a short supplementation may increase this risk due to delayed embryos having a higher chance of meeting a receptive endometrium when the WOI opens later (i.e. after more days of progesterone supplementation), allowing them to implant but afterward also being at increased risk for early pregnancy loss. Initiating progesterone one day earlier than the theoretical day of oocyte retrieval (Fig. 3), results in significantly lower pregnancy rates than starting on that day itself according to a Cochrane Database Review (Glujovsky et al., 2010). Furthermore, a recent randomized controlled trial (RCT) was in favor of the shortest protocol when comparing 5 versus 7 days of progesterone supplementation for blastocyst transfer, although not statistically significant in terms of clinical pregnancy rates (van de Vijver et al., 2017). Overall, the starting day of progesterone administration for HRT FET appears best when equal to the theoretical day of oocyte retrieval or one day later (Fig. 4). As the WOI is only present for a certain time, this detection of an optimal period is to be expected; implantation is probably possible

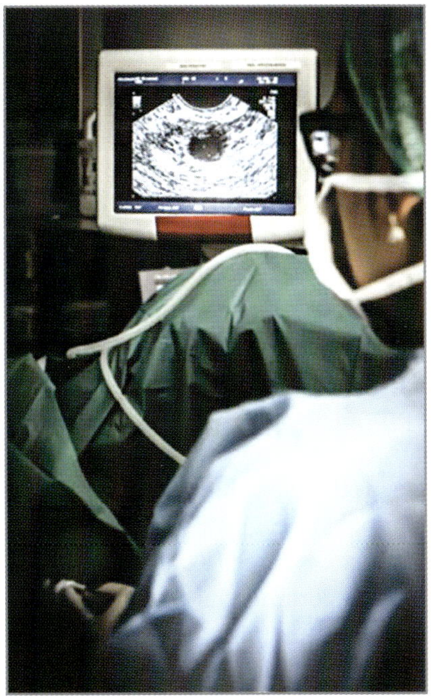

Fig. 3: Oocyte retrieval procedure under local anesthesia.

in a broader window, however optimal in a more narrow timeframe (Franasiak et al., 2016). The current proposed optimal timing for HRT FET is on the 6th day of progesterone administration, annotated as P+5, in case of blastocyst transfer, with an adaptation respectively in case of cleavage stage embryo transfer (Fig. 2).

This timing is in similarity with fresh embryo transfer timing following oocyte pick-up: the starting day of progesterone supplementation (P+0) mirrors the theoretical day of oocyte pick-up, which is from an embryonic point of view also Day 0.

Specific attention is needed when embryos are thawed and further developed *in vitro* preceding the embryo transfer. In this case, one should take into account the embryonic stage expected at the moment of transfer and not the stage of cryopreservation (Cercas et al., 2012) (Jin et al., 2013). So far, it is not known whether FET timing should differ following slow-freezing or vitrification. However, the method of freezing has been described to impact on post-thaw embryo development and metabolism (Balaban et al., 2008) (Cercas et al., 2012).

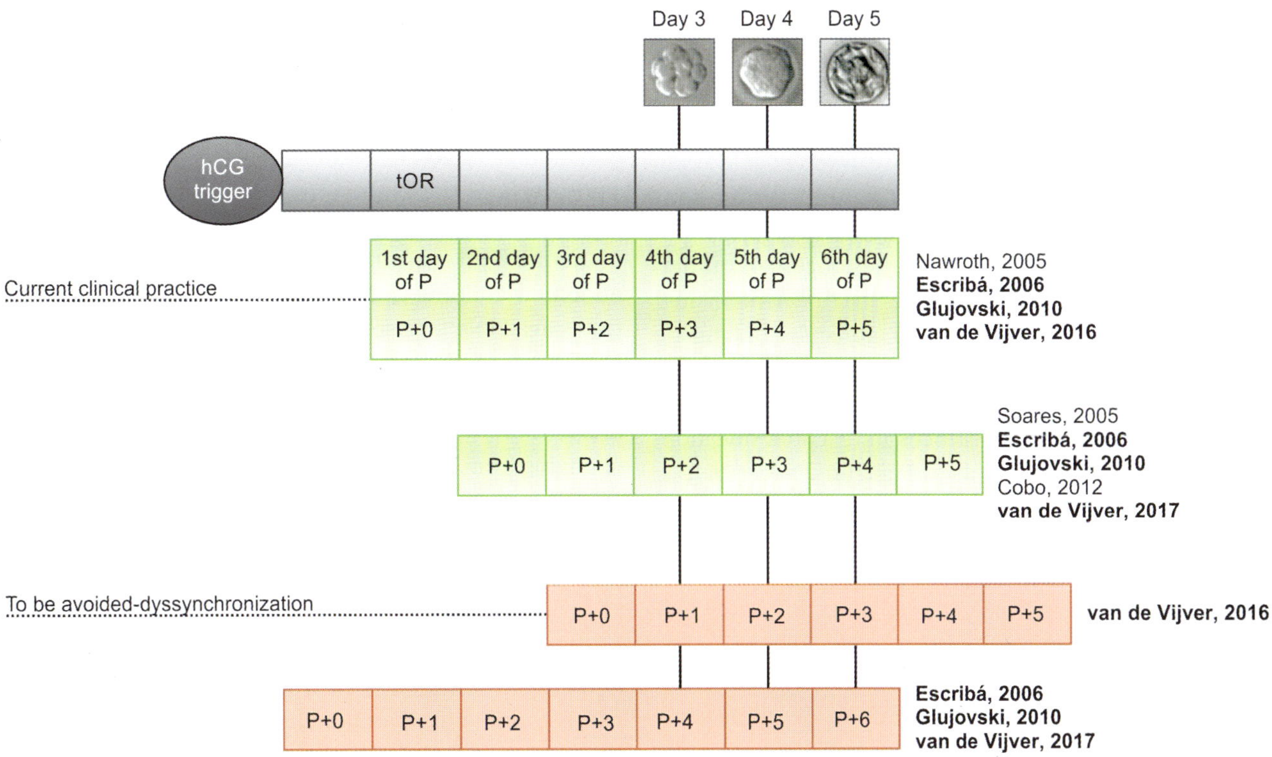

Fig. 4: Proposed embryo transfer timing in HRT cycles. (*In bold*: Studies with actual comparison of different embryo transfer days). (tOR: theoretical oocyte retrieval; P: progesterone; hCG: human chorionic gonadotropin)
Source: Reprinted from Mackens et al, 2017.

MOLECULAR ENDOMETRIAL RECEPTIVITY TESTING

Many researchers have attempted to develop a clinical test evaluating endometrial receptivity, but, at this time, no test is available that has been thoroughly validated by an RCT.

The optimal threshold for endometrial thickness measured by ultrasound remains unknown and although the often reported cut-off value of 7 mm has been linked to a lower pregnancy chance following meta-analysis, it is probably not justified to use it as a decision-making tool in clinic (Kasius et al., 2014). Furthermore, extrapolation of findings from fresh to FET cycles are not self-evident; the optimal endometrial thickness in HRT FET cycles has been reported to be between 9 mm and 14 mm (El-Toukhy et al., 2008), while no data for NC FET are present in current available literature.

Molecular analysis of endometrial biopsies offers possibilities to assess endometrial receptivity. At first, histological endometrial dating was proposed (Noyes et al., 1975), however, clinical efficacy was proven to be low (Murray et al., 2004) (Coutifaris et al., 2004), rendering it obsolete. In a next phase, single markers of endometrial receptivity (or limited combinations) have been researched (Lessey et al., 2000) (Guffanti et al., 2008), but also this approach raised scepticism as a one-by-one approach is not in line with the complexity of the process of implantation and the redundancy in pathways involved (Edgell et al., 2013). Since 2002 (Kao et al., 2002), high-throughput transcriptional data derived from endometrial biopsies are used to investigate receptivity and the process of human implantation. Currently, many studies have been published in the field, but, in clinical practice, molecular diagnostic evaluation of the endometrium remains limited, as the genes identified vary significantly between studies. This can largely be explained by differences in research question, experimental setting and statistical analysis. Nevertheless, commercially available tests analyzing the transcriptomic signature of freshly biopsied luteal phase endometria and discriminating between receptive and nonreceptive uteri have been developed (Díaz-Gimeno et al., 2013) (Koot et al., 2016).

The Endometrial Receptivity Array (ERA®, Igenomix, Spain) exists out of the quantification of the transcripts of 238 genes related to the receptivity state, subsequently analyzed by a trained predictor labeling the biopsy as pre-receptive, receptive or postreceptive (Díaz-Gimeno et al., 2013). The aim is to detect the most optimal moment for FET and in a subsequent cycle perform a personalized FET according to the test result. RCTs investigating the clinical usefulness of this test in various patient populations are awaited. Specifically in RIF patients, it has been proposed that the WOI might be too narrow and/or displaced (mostly delayed) (Ruiz-Alonso et al., 2013). However, also in the general population, in up to 25% a delayed endometrial development has been reported (Murray et al., 2004) and increased pregnancy rates have been associated with specific histological endometrial dating and corresponding adjustments in progesterone exposure (Gomaa et al., 2015).

Another promising luteal phase endometrial biopsy test is a specific transcriptomic signature linked to RIF with a 100% positive predictive value and the ability to subdivide RIF patients into distinct groups with different subsequent implantation success rates (Koot et al., 2016) (Macklon, 2017). Although a commercial test is not yet available for the clinic, this signature might become useful in the future in counseling and guiding further treatment in case of RIF.

Harvesting endometrial biopsies during the WOI, however, preclude embryo transfer in that same cycle. On the contrary, endometrial biopsies taken during the stimulation phase of IVF/ICSI treatment have previously been shown not to decrease the chances of implantation when performing fresh ET and differential gene expression profiles have been withheld between women that do achieve pregnancy versus women that do not (Zhou et al., 2008).

Another option to evaluate endometrial quality in the same cycle of the embryo transfer and even during the WOI, is the noninvasive approach in which a small amount of uterine fluid is aspirated without inducing injury to the endometrial lining (Edgell et al., 2013), however, no such test is available for use in clinic at this time. Nevertheless, continuous effort should be made to develop in-cycle endometrial functionality test as it has been shown that the uterus shows an enormous plasticity with the endometrium changing from cycle to cycle (Lucas et al., 2013).

KEYNOTE

Implantation failure after IVF/ICSI treatment can result from insufficient embryo quality, abnormal uterine receptivity or an improper dialogue between blastocyst and endometrium. It is clear that ovarian stimulation for IVF/ICSI influences endometrial receptivity in that cycle. Performing FET, preferably following vitrification, may offer a possibility to optimize endometrial receptivity on the day of embryo transfer (Fig. 5). However, whether transferring frozen embryos in a nonstimulated endometrium effectively

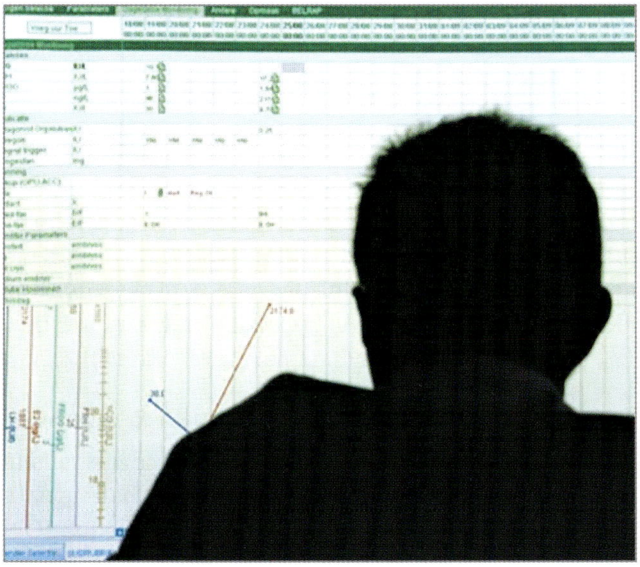

Fig. 5: Daily monitoring unit.

results in better reproductive outcome is still subject of debate and requires further investigation. Furthermore, no clinically randomized controlled trial validated test evaluating endometrial receptivity is available for daily practice so far.

KEY POINTS

- Following ovarian stimulation for IVF/ICSI, endometrial receptivity can be affected and the WOI shifted due to the hormonal impact of this stimulation on the endometrium. Furthermore, when performing fresh embryo transfer, there is no possibility to correct or optimize the moment of transfer.
- In frozen embryo transfer cycles, the optimal transfer timing is dependent on the used preparation protocol, which can be a HRT cycle or a natural cycle.
- If HRT is used for FET, progesterone intake can best be started at the theoretical day of oocyte retrieval (e.g. performing a blastocyst transfer on the 6th day of progesterone intake).
- If a natural cycle is used for FET, it is optimal to transfer the blastocyst stage embryo on LH+6 when a spontaneous ovulation is detected (true natural cycle) or on hCG+7 when ovulation is induced by exogenous hCG administration (modified natural cycle).
- Although endometrial receptivity tests are currently under development, further research to proof their efficacy in daily clinical practice is needed.

EDITORS' COMMENTS

1. Understanding the window of implantation is very important. The timing of embryo transfer should ensure that a blastocyst implantation meets the optimal receptive evaluation.
2. During a frozen embryo transfer on culturing the embryo after thawing, it is better to take in to account the resulting embryonic stage rather than stage at which it was frozen.
3. Implantation involves a complex cascade of molecular events. Luteal phase endometrial biopsy test might be a useful tool in the future for guiding RIF patients.

SUGGESTED READING

1. Acosta AA, Elberger L, Borghi M, et al. Endometrial dating and determination of the window of implantation in healthy fertile women. Fertil Steril. 2000;73(4):788-98.
2. Altmäe S, Tamm-Rosenstein K, Esteban FJ, et al. Endometrial transcriptome analysis indicates superiority of natural over artificial cycles in recurrent implantation failure patients undergoing frozen embryo transfer. Reprod Biomed Online. 2016;32(6):597-613.
3. Balaban B, Urman B, Ata B, et al. A randomized controlled study of human Day 3 embryo cryopreservation by slow freezing or vitrification: vitrification is associated with higher survival, metabolism and blastocyst formation. Hum Reprod. 2008;23(9):1976-82.
4. Belva F, Bonduelle M, Roelants M, et al. Neonatal health including congenital malformation risk of 1072 children born after vitrified embryo transfer. Hum Reprod. 2016;31(7):1610-20.
5. Blockeel C, Drakopoulos P, Santos-Ribeiro S, et al. A fresh look at the freeze-all protocol: a SWOT analysis. Hum Reprod. 2016;31(3):491-7.
6. Bourgain C, Devroey P. The endometrium in stimulated cycles for IVF. Hum Reprod Update. 2003;9(6):515-22.
7. Cercas R, Villas C, Pons I, et al. Vitrification can modify embryo cleavage stage after warming. Should we change endometrial preparation? J Assist Reprod Genet. 2012;29(12):1363-8.
8. Chang EM, Han JE, Kim YS, et al. Use of the natural cycle and vitrification thawed blastocyst transfer results in better in-vitro fertilization outcomes: cycle regimens of vitrification thawed blastocyst transfer. J Assist Reprod Genet. 2011;28(4):369-74.
9. Coutifaris C, Myers ER, Guzick DS, et al. Histological dating of timed endometrial biopsy tissue is not related to fertility status. Fertil Steril. 2004;82(5):1264-72.
10. Díaz-Gimeno P, Ruiz-Alonso M, Blesa D, et al. The accuracy and reproducibility of the endometrial receptivity array is superior to histology as a diagnostic method for endometrial receptivity. Fertil Steril. 2013;99(2):508-17.
11. Edgell TA, Rombauts LJF, Salamonsen LA. Assessing receptivity in the endometrium: the need for a rapid, noninvasive test. Reprod Biomed Online. 2013;27(5):486-96.

12. El-Toukhy T, Coomarasamy A, Khairy M, et al. The relationship between endometrial thickness and outcome of medicated frozen embryo replacement cycles. Fertil Steril. 2008;89(4):832-9.
13. Escribá M-J, Bellver J, Bosch E, et al. Delaying the initiation of progesterone supplementation until the day of fertilization does not compromise cycle outcome in patients receiving donated oocytes: a randomized study. Fertil Steril. 2006;86(1):92-7.
14. European IVF-Monitoring Consortium (EIM), European Society of Human Reproduction and Embryology (ESHRE), Kupka MS, et al. Assisted reproductive technology in Europe, 2011: results generated from European registers by ESHRE. Hum Reprod. 2016;31(2):233-48.
15. Evans J, Hannan NJ, Edgell TA, et al. Fresh versus frozen embryo transfer: backing clinical decisions with scientific and clinical evidence. Hum Reprod Update. 2014;20(6):808-21.
16. Fatemi HM, Kyrou D, Bourgain C, et al. Cryopreserved-thawed human embryo transfer: spontaneous natural cycle is superior to human chorionic gonadotropin-induced natural cycle. Fertil Steril. 2010;94(6):2054-8.
17. Franasiak JM, Ruiz-Alonso M, Scott RT, et al. Both slowly developing embryos and a variable pace of luteal endometrial progression may conspire to prevent normal birth in spite of a capable embryo. Fertil Steril. 2016;105(4):861-6.
18. Ghobara T, Gelbaya TA, Ayeleke RO. Cycle regimens for frozen-thawed embryo transfer. Cochrane Database Syst Rev. 2017:7.
19. Givens CR, Markun LC, Ryan IP, et al. Outcomes of natural cycles versus programmed cycles for 1677 frozen-thawed embryo transfers. Reprod Biomed Online. 2009;19(3):380-4.
20. Glujovsky D, Pesce R, Fiszbajn G, et al. Endometrial preparation for women undergoing embryo transfer with frozen embryos or embryos derived from donor oocytes. Cochrane Database Syst Rev. 2010;(1)CD006359
21. Gomaa H, Casper RF, Esfandiari N, et al. Nonsynchronized endometrium and its correction in nonovulatory cryopreserved embryo transfer cycles. Reprod Biomed Online. 2015;30(4):378-84.
22. Groenewoud ER, Cantineau AE, Kollen BJ, et al. What is the optimal means of preparing the endometrium in frozen-thawed embryo transfer cycles? A systematic review and meta-analysis. Hum Reprod Update. 2013;19(5):458-70.
23. Groenewoud ER, Cohlen BJ, Al-Oraiby A, et al. A randomized controlled, noninferiority trial of modified natural versus artificial cycle for cryo-thawed embryo transfer. Hum Reprod. 2016;31(7):1483-92.
24. Groenewoud ER, Macklon NS, Cohlen BJ, et al. The effect of elevated progesterone levels before HCG triggering in modified natural cycle frozen-thawed embryo transfer cycles. Reprod Biomed Online. 2017;34(5):546-54.
25. Guan Y, Fan H, Styer AK, et al. A modified natural cycle results in higher live birth rate in vitrified-thawed embryo transfer for women with regular menstruation. Syst Biol Reprod Med. 2016;62(5):335-42.
26. Guffanti E, Kittur N, Brodt ZN, et al. Nuclear pore complex proteins mark the implantation window in human endometrium. J Cell Sci. 2008;121(Pt12):2037-45.
27. Haouzi D, Bissonnette L, Gala A, et al. Endometrial receptivity profile in patients with premature progesterone elevation on the day of HCG administration. Biomed Res Int. 2014;2014:951937.
28. Healy MW, Patounakis G, Connell MT, et al. Does a frozen embryo transfer ameliorate the effect of elevated progesterone seen in fresh transfer cycles? Fertil Steril. 2016;105(1):93-9.
29. Hoff JD, Quigley ME, Yen SS. Hormonal dynamics at midcycle: a re-evaluation. J Clin Endocrinol Metab. 1983;57(4):792-6.
30. Horcajadas JA, Mínguez P, Dopazo J, et al. Controlled ovarian stimulation induces a functional genomic delay of the endometrium with potential clinical implications. J Clin Endocrinol Metab. 2008;93(11):4500-10.
31. Horcajadas JA, Riesewijk A, Polman J, et al. Effect of controlled ovarian hyperstimulation in IVF on endometrial gene expression profiles. Mol Hum Reprod. 2005;11(3):195-205.
32. Humaidan P, Van Vaerenbergh I, Bourgain C, et al. Endometrial gene expression in the early luteal phase is impacted by mode of triggering final oocyte maturation in recFSH stimulated and GnRH antagonist co-treated IVF cycles. Hum Reprod. 2012;27(11):3259-72.
33. Imbar T, Hurwitz A. Synchronization between endometrial and embryonic age is not absolutely crucial for implantation. Fertil Steril. 2004;82(2):472-4.
34. Ishihara O, Araki R, Kuwahara A, et al. Impact of frozen-thawed single-blastocyst transfer on maternal and neonatal outcome: an analysis of 277,042 single-embryo transfer cycles from 2008 to 2010 in Japan. Fertil Steril. 2014;101(1):128-33.
35. Jin R, Tong X, Wu L, et al. Extended culture of vitrified-warmed embryos in day-3 embryo transfer cycles: a randomized controlled pilot study. Reprod Biomed Online. 2013;26(4):384-92.
36. Kao LC, Tulac S, Lobo S, et al. Global gene profiling in human endometrium during the window of implantation. Endocrinology. 2002;143(6):2119-38.
37. Kasius A, Smit JG, Torrance HL, et al. Endometrial thickness and pregnancy rates after IVF: a systematic review and meta-analysis. Hum Reprod Update. 2014;20(4):530-41.
38. Kolibianakis E, Bourgain C, Albano C, et al. Effect of ovarian stimulation with recombinant follicle-stimulating hormone, gonadotropin releasing hormone antagonists, and human chorionic gonadotropin on endometrial maturation on the day of oocyte pick-up. Fertil Steril. 2002;78(5):1025-29.
39. Koot YEM, van Hooff SR, Boomsma CM, et al. An endometrial gene expression signature accurately predicts recurrent implantation failure after IVF. Sci Rep. 2016;6:19411.
40. Kosmas IP, Tatsioni A, Fatemi HM, et al. Human chorionic gonadotropin administration vs. luteinizing monitoring for intrauterine insemination timing, after administration of clomiphene citrate: a meta-analysis. Fertil Steril. 2007;87(3):607-12.
41. Labarta E, Martínez-Conejero JA, Alamá P, et al. Endometrial receptivity is affected in women with high circulating

progesterone levels at the end of the follicular phase: a functional genomics analysis. Hum Reprod. 2011;26(7): 1813-25.
42. Lessey BA, Castelbaum AJ, Wolf L, et al. Use of integrins to date the endometrium. Fertil Steril. 2000;73(4):779-87.
43. Liu Y, Lee K-F, Ng EHY, et al. Gene expression profiling of human peri-implantation endometria between natural and stimulated cycles. Fertil Steril. 2008;90(6):2152-64.
44. Loutradi KE, Kolibianakis EM, Venetis CA, et al. Cryopreservation of human embryos by vitrification or slow freezing: a systematic review and meta-analysis. Fertil Steril. 2008;90(1):186-93.
45. Lucas ES, Salker MS, Brosens JJ. Uterine plasticity and reproductive fitness. Reprod Biomed Online. 2013;27(5): 506-14.
46. Mackens S, Santos-Ribeiro S, van de Vijver A, et al. Frozen embryo transfer: a review on the optimal endometrial preparation and timing. Human Reprod. 2017;32(11): 2234-42.
47. Macklon N. Recurrent implantation failure is a pathology with a specific transcriptomic signature. Fertil Steril. 2017; 108(1):9-14.
48. Magdi Y, El-Damen A, Fathi AM, et al. Revisiting the management of recurrent implantation failure through freeze-all policy. Fertil Steril. 2017;108(1):72-7.
49. Mirkin S, Nikas G, Hsiu JG, et al. Gene expression profiles and structural/functional features of the peri-implantation endometrium in natural and gonadotropin-stimulated cycles. J Clin Endocrinol Metab. 2004;89(11):5742-52.
50. Murray MJ, Meyer WR, Zaino RJ, et al. A critical analysis of the accuracy, reproducibility, and clinical utility of histologic endometrial dating in fertile women. Fertil Steril. 2004;81(5):1333-43.
51. Navot D, Scott RT, Droesch K, et al. The window of embryo transfer and the efficiency of human conception in vitro. Fertil Steril. 1991;55(1):114-8.
52. Nawroth F, Ludwig M. What is the "ideal" duration of progesterone supplementation before the transfer of cryopreserved-thawed embryos in estrogen/progesterone replacement protocols. Human Reprod. 2005;20(5):1127-34.
53. Norwitz ER, Schust DJ, Fisher SJ. Implantation and the survival of early pregnancy. N Engl J Med. 2001;345(19):1400-8.
54. Noyes RW, Hertig AT, Rock J. Dating the endometrial biopsy. Am J Obstet Gynecol. 1975;122(2):262-3.
55. Ruiz-Alonso M, Blesa D, Díaz-Gimeno P, et al. The endometrial receptivity array for diagnosis and personalized embryo transfer as a treatment for patients with repeated implantation failure. Fertil Steril. 2013;100(3):818-24.
56. Shapiro BS, Daneshmand ST, Garner FC, et al. Contrasting patterns in vitro fertilization pregnancy rates among fresh autologous, fresh oocyte donor, and cryopreserved cycles with the use of day 5 or day 6 blastocysts may reflect differences in embryo-endometrium synchrony. Fertil Steril. 2008;89(1): 20-6.
57. Simón C, Oberyé J, Bellver J, et al. Similar endometrial development in oocyte donors treated with either high- or standard-dose GnRH antagonist compared to treatment with a GnRH agonist or in natural cycles. Human Reprod. 2005;20(12):3318-27.
58. Theodorou E, Forman R. Live birth after blastocyst transfer following only 2 days of progesterone administration in an agonadal oocyte recipient. Reprod Biomed Online. 2012;25(4):355-7.
59. Tomás C, Alsbjerg B, Martikainen H, et al. Pregnancy loss after frozen-embryo transfer—a comparison of three protocols. Fertil Steril. 2012;98(5):1165-9.
60. van de Vijver A, Drakopoulos P, Polyzos NP, et al. Vitrified-warmed blastocyst transfer on the 5th or 7th day of progesterone supplementation in an artificial cycle: a randomized controlled trial. Gynecol Endocrinol. 2017; 33(10):783-6.
61. van de Vijver A, Polyzos NP, Van Landuyt L, et al. What is the optimal duration of progesterone administration before transferring a vitrified-warmed cleavage stage embryo? A randomized controlled trial. Hum Reprod. 2016;31(5):1097-104.
62. Van Vaerenbergh I, Fatemi HM, Blockeel C, et al. Progesterone rise on HCG day in GnRH antagonist/rFSH stimulated cycles affects endometrial gene expression. Reprod Biomed Online. 2011;22(3):263-71.
63. Veleva Z, Tiitinen A, Vilska S, et al. High and low BMI increase the risk of miscarriage after IVF/ICSI and FET. Hum Reprod. 2008;23(4):878-84.
64. Wilcox AJ, Baird DD, Weinberg CR. Time of implantation of the conceptus and loss of pregnancy. N Engl J Med. 1999;340(23):1796-9.
65. Young SL. Estrogen and progesterone action on endometrium: a translational approach to understanding endometrial receptivity. Reprod Biomed Online. 2013;27(5):497-505.
66. Zhou L, Li R, Wang R, et al. Local injury to the endometrium in controlled ovarian hyperstimulation cycles improves implantation rates. Fertil Steril. 2008;89(5):1166-76.

13

CHAPTER

Freeze-all Strategy for All

Jatin P Shah

INTRODUCTION

In vitro fertilization (IVF) has been performed for more than 35 years, and it is estimated that in developed countries, more than 1% of all births are generated from assisted reproductive technology (ART). Rapid improvements made in cryopreservation techniques (vitrification) have led to few or no detrimental effects to the embryo and have resulted in no consequences to the offspring when compared to fresh embryos. This inspired the concept of the freeze-all policy (when all viable embryos are electively cryopreserved in the fresh cycle and transferred in a posterior cycle).

Controlled ovarian stimulation (COS) is considered an essential step during IVF treatment, its main objective being to induce the development of multiple follicles, more number of viable oocytes and embryos and maximize the chances of a positive outcome. Although fresh embryo transfer (ET) has been the norm, there are many concerns about the possible adverse effects of COS on endometrial receptivity and the uterine environment. COS may contribute to modifications in the endometrium (by way of the supraphysiologic levels of estradiol and progesterone), which might be related to poorer outcomes when fresh ET is performed. Despite rapid advances in laboratory technology, incubators, culture media and recombinant gonadotropins, live birth rates with fresh ET have remained in the range of 18–42% with an average of 32%. Also, in cycles with fresh ET, there is still a risk for the development of late onset and often severe ovarian hyperstimulation syndrome (OHSS), which is an iatrogenic, serious and potentially life threatening complication of COS. Furthermore, there is data to suggest that pregnancies from fresh ET are more prone (owing to COS and supraphysiologic hormonal levels) to early pregnancy losses, ectopic pregnancies, pregnancy-induced hypertension (PIH), low birth weight, abnormal placentation and accidental hemorrhage.

In the freeze-all strategy, the entire cohort of embryos is vitrified (not just the "surplus"), and the best embryos are transferred in a subsequent cycle with a more physiologic endometrium. In the past few years, the freeze-all strategy has emerged as a safer and more successful alternative to conventional fresh ET during IVF/intracytoplasmic sperm injection (ICSI) cycles. Data suggests that live birth rates are higher and obstetric and perinatal outcomes in pregnancies resulting from frozen embryo transfer (FET) are better than those from fresh ET. There is concern, however, about macrosomia and long-term implications of vitrification on the babies born.

At the same time, although the principle that COS may cause a less physiological milieu for embryos to implant, we must establish when and for whom this freeze-all approach is appropriate. How can we balance better implantation rates against the possible unnatural changes that we may be causing the embryo as a result of freezing? Is it time now to reconsider our freeze-all strategies and establish protocols for individualized segmented IVF and FET?

HOW DID THE "FREEZE-ALL" STRATEGY BEGIN?

Freeze-all strategy was first proposed for patients of polycystic ovary syndrome (PCOS) who are invariably prone to moderate or severe OHSS with COS protocols. Despite anticipation of OHSS [polycystic ovaries, high anti-Müllerian hormone (AMH) levels] and adjustment of the FSH dose (use of lower doses of FSH such as 100–112.5 IU), the incidence of moderate to severe OHSS requiring hospitalization is as high as 30–40%. Extremely elevated estradiol levels result in a nonreceptive endometrium and exaggerated uterine contractions with subsequent lower implantation rates. Studies have found that uterine contractility is much higher in stimulated cycles than in natural cycles. Fresh ET in patients with PCOS is also associated with higher risks of abnormal placentation (elevated E2 and VEGF) resulting in greater placental weight, placental previa, PIH and obstetric complications such as preterm delivery, low-birth weight LBW and higher lower segment cesarean section (LSCS) rate. Also, weaker implantation contributes to a higher rate of early pregnancy loss in these patients. Use of the antagonist instead of agonist helps reduce, but not eliminate the risk of OHSS in these patients. The antagonist brings with it the ability to use an agonist trigger (avoiding hCG eliminates the risk of OHSS) albeit with a deficient luteal phase and extremely low pregnancy rates. Efforts have been made to rescue the luteal phase with high doses of exogenous estradiol progesterone support often with add back low dose hCG but pregnancy rates remain disappointing. The "freeze-all" strategy with replacement of embryos in a subsequent estradiol-progesterone primed cycle gives extremely encouraging results. One of the initial reports by Atkinson showed a 50% cumulative pregnancy rate after two FET cycles employing the freeze all strategy in patients with PCOS.

In a trial by the author, 127 patients with elevated AMH levels and PCOS were subjected to a standard antagonist protocol using a starting dose of 150 IU of rFSH. Final oocyte maturation was triggered with 0.2 mg decapeptyl, oocytes were retrieved at 36 hour and embryos were vitrified at the 4-cell stage. FET was done with thawed 8-cell stage embryos in a subsequent down regulated E-P primed cycle. The clinical pregnancy rate in the first FET was 56.6% and after allowing for early pregnancy losses, the on-going pregnancy rate was 48.03%. Antagonist cycles with agonist trigger, "freeze-all" of all embryos and FET seems to be the most successful treatment for moderate to severe PCOS with a zero incidence of OHSS and excellent perinatal and obstetric outcomes on par with non-PCOS patients undergoing IVF. Elective cryopreservation and subsequent FET also reduces the odds of small for gestational-age (SGA) babies and PIH as compared to fresh ET in PCOS patients with elevated peak serum E2 levels (>3,450 pg/mL).

OTHER INDICATIONS FOR "FREEZE-ALL"

- *Patients with elevated serum progesterone levels (>1.5 ng/mL) on day of hCG*: It has been shown that patients with premature progesterone rise (PPR) are prone to endometrial advancement and lower pregnancy rates with fresh ET. Pregnancy rates are decreased from 31% to 19% in patients with PPR in both agonist and antagonist cycles. An endometrial advancement of >3 days is associated with a zero pregnancy rate. Also, it is interesting to note that it is only the endometrial receptivity and not oocyte quality that is affected by PPR as reflected in oocyte donation programs where elevated progesterone in the donor does not reduce pregnancy rates in the recipient. Freeze all and thaw transfer in a subsequent cycle is extremely successful for patients with PPR.
- *Patients with very low serum progesterone levels (<0.5 ng/mL) on day of hCG*: Very low levels of serum progesterone have been associated with significantly lower pregnancy rates (17% vs 30% as compared to patients with normal progesterone) with fresh ET. Freeze-all is preferred for these patients.
- *Patients of endometriosis*: It has always been proposed that patients of endometriosis do better with downregulation protocols. It is the author's experience that a majority of these patients have an already depleted ovarian reserve and low AMH levels especially after single/multiple laparoscopic surgeries. Studies have shown that it is better to avoid down regulation (for a better ovarian response in patients with reduced AMH levels) and use an antagonist protocol for the initial COHS cycle to get more oocytes and embryos and then down regulate the patient for the embryo transfer cycle. Freeze all and FET in a down regulated cycle, in patients with moderate to severe endometriosis, increases the pregnancy rates from 12% to 28%.
- *Patients with thin endometrium*: There are many patients who have a thin endometrium on the day of hCG (<8 mm) and would have lower pregnancy rates with fresh embryo transfer. Freeze-all is recommended for these patients as there would be ample time in a frozen-thaw transfer cycle to prepare the endometrium with GnRH agonist downregulation, high doses and prolonged administration of estradiol valerate, vaginal sildenafil, aspirin, LMW heparin and Intrauterine instillation of G-CSF. Measures to improve the endometrial thickness in a fresh cycle usually prove inadequate owing to a shortage of time in terms of days available for implementing these measures.

- *Patients of repeated implantation failures with fresh ET*: COHS results in supraphysiologic levels of estradiol and progesterone which impair endometrial receptivity and reduce pregnancy rates in fresh ET. Many of these failures are unexplained and occur in the presence of a normal looking endometrium and good quality embryos. A significant number of these patients achieve pregnancy with FET (owing to a more conducive uterine environment).
- *Endometrial polyp*: Often, endometrial polyps/septum/thin endometrium/adhesions are diagnosed during the course of ovarian stimulation creating a dilemma about ET. In these cases, it is advisable to freeze all the embryos, perform an operative hysteroscopy concurrent with the OPU procedure to correct the pathology and then do an FET in the next cycle. FET can be done as early as 35 days from the date of OPU with optimal pregnancy rates.
- *Low responders*: Patients with a poor ovarian response can benefit from accumulation of embryos over repeated COS cycles allowing them to achieve better pregnancy rates. FET is done once 3–4 good quality embryos have been obtained. Success rate of 20–30% have been reported with freeze all and embryo accumulation in poor responders.
- *Patients of advanced maternal age*: Freeze all is also attractive for patients of advanced maternal age who, in addition to being low responders, require pre-implantation genetic screening (PGS). Nowadays, there is a trend toward performing the PGS in the blastocyst stage with 24-chromosome screening. There is growing evidence showing higher implantation and delivery rates following the 24-chromosome screening when compared to fluorescence *in situ* hybridization (FISH)-PGS. The use of comprehensive chromosome screening (CCS) in blastocyst stage with elective single embryo transfer is as effective as double-embryo transfer of unscreened embryos and dramatically reduces the risk of twins. The embryos that undergo biopsy on Day 6 are not eligible for fresh transfer due to an asynchrony between the embryo and endometrium. In these cases, it is necessary to perform the cryopreservation of all embryos and a posterior frozen-thawed embryo transfer.
- Patient's with history of ectopic pregnancy/biochemical pregnancy/early pregnancy loss in a previous IVF cycle (with fresh embryo transfer). IVF with fresh embryo transfer is associated with a higher risk of ectopic pregnancy owing to increased uterine contractility and supraphysiologic hormonal levels during COS. There is a significant reduction in the incidence of ectopic pregnancies (by more than 50%) with freeze-all as compared to fresh embryo transfer.
- *Normal responders with normal progesterone levels*: The debate about whether freeze-all benefits normoresponders began with a recent meta-analysis which concluded that pregnancy rates and obstetric/perinatal outcomes are better with FET as compared to fresh ET even in normal responders with normal serum progesterone levels. However, this meta-analysis includes only three small studies and controversy still exists when it comes to normal responders. A recent study revealed no difference in terms of ongoing pregnancy and live birth rates between normal responders patients who underwent fresh and deferred embryo transfers. This was a retrospective study which included 882 patients, aged 20–44 who underwent their first or second IVF/ICSI cycle, in which a normal oocyte yield (4–20) was obtained. The raw analysis showed that ongoing pregnancy (36.2 vs 33.8%, $p = 0.51$) and live birth (33.2 vs 32.9%, $p = 0.94$) rates for freeze-all versus fresh cycles, respectively, were similar. Normal responders can face situations in which freeze-all may apply, such as those who undergo genetic screening, or present high progesterone levels, impaired endometrium, etc.
- *Social egg/embryo freezing*: Freeze-all allows women to preserve their fertility today, the so-called "social freezing" enabling them to have the same success rates as fresh embryo transfer at a later date in life.

A recent SWOT analysis (strengths, weaknesses, opportunities, and threats with freeze-all) by Christophe Blockeel summarized the strengths, weaknesses, opportunities, and threats of the freeze-all policy as described here.

Strengths

- *Establishing an OHSS free clinic*: Elimination of OHSS and enhanced maternal safety (Antagonist protocols, agonist trigger and freeze all).
- *Improved pregnancy rates as compared to fresh ET*: Reported by some but needs to be evaluated in more detail.
- *Better obstetric and perinatal outcomes*: FET pregnancies are significantly less likely to be complicated by perinatal mortality, SGA, LBW and APH as compared to fresh ET. The differences were even stronger when analyzing pregnancies within a single individual who conceived successive children with fresh and frozen ET. This proves that it is the "peri-implantation environment" created after COHS that is responsible for these changes.
- *Lower incidence of biochemical pregnancies*: Gonadotropins cause alterations in endometrial gene and

protein expression which might compromise the ability of embryos to develop once implanted, possible increasing the biochemical pregnancy rate with fresh ET.

- *Lower ectopic pregnancy rate*: Most centers report ectopic pregnancies in fresh ET cycles in the range of 3–7%. The risk factors are longer stimulation, elevated estradiol, and progesterone causing abnormal tubal and uterine contractions. FET cycles have a lower incidence of ectopic pregnancies (2.2% vs 5%), the incidence being lowest in blastocyst transfer cycles.

Weaknesses

- Increase in costs.
- Increased treatment duration time (2–3 months for one cycle).
- Patient disappointment for not having a fresh ET.
- Not enough randomized controlled trials (RCTs) comparing fresh and FET. Results of 5 major trials are awaited at the time of writing this chapter. Preliminary results from a Vuong (Vietnam) indicate no difference in pregnancy rate between fresh and FET (although PCOS was excluded from that study).
- Evidence of improved pregnancy rates in three RCTs only. Most studies limited to high responders and elimination of OHSS.

Opportunities

- Elimination of hormone monitoring and patient friendliness (can do away with cumbersome estimations of estradiol/progesterone).
- More oocytes with delayed triggering (no concern about the implantation window).
- Scheduling possibilities.

Threats

- Available evidence for superiority of freeze all is only for patients of PCOS.
- Extrapolation of these results to all IVF patients should be done with caution.
- There are reports of large for GA and macrosomic babies with FET (babies being heavier by 160 g) which warrants confirmation.
- Long-term implications of vitrification and FET on the babies are not known and need to be studied.

CONCLUSION

Freeze all seems to be promising for numerous reasons. There are confirmed reports of better obstetric and perinatal outcomes with significant reduction in incidence of early pregnancy losses, ectopic pregnancies, biochemical pregnancies, preterm labor, SGA, PIH, abnormal placentation, and LBW babies with the use of FET as compared to fresh ET. The author's own experience has been extremely fulfilling especially in high responders, poor responders (with embryo accumulation), endometriosis, PCOS, thin endometrium, inadvertent diagnosis of an endometrial polyp during the course of COS, repeated implantation failures and low/high serum progesterone levels on the day of hCG.

Whether "freeze-all" should be applied to all IVF patients (especially normoresponders without any complicating factors) is still under study. There is no concrete evidence to support this at the current moment. It is necessary to have the "best" laboratory and vitrification "technique" to successfully implement a freeze all program. Reports of macrosomic fetuses and long-term implications on the baby need to be studied in more detail.

AUTHOR'S RECOMMENDATIONS

Freeze-all (segmented IVF) seems to be ideal for patients with PCOS, poor responders, endometriosis, repeated implantation failures, thin endometrium and those having very low or elevated serum progesterone levels on the day of the hCG trigger.

Freeze-all is associated with a reduced risk of OHSS, improved endometrial receptivity and higher implantation rates. Also, the risk of ectopic pregnancy, biochemical pregnancy, early miscarriage, placenta previa, preterm birth, SGA and perinatal mortality is significantly reduced.

For a successful freeze-all program, it would be mandatory to have the "best" laboratory and vitrification technique to implement freeze all on a routine basis. The potential disadvantages of a freeze all policy are an increased (yet unconfirmed) risk of macrosomia, increased costs, not enough RCTs to prove its efficacy for all patients (especially normoresponders) and no data on poor responders. Although there are many potential advantages in performing FET over fresh ET, it seems that the freeze-all strategy is not designed for all IVF patients. There are a large number of patients that get pregnant and do not have any obstetric/perinatal complications even after fresh ET. A recent study by Roque et al. (presented at ESHRE, 2017) showed that there is no benefit with freeze-all in cycles where 4–9 oocytes are retrieved. Also, there is no benefit in poor responders (not undergoing embryo accumulation) where 1–3 oocytes are retrieved. However, the study showed that for patients with more than 10 oocytes, freeze-all strategy gives a higher live birth rate. The need of the hour is therefore, to individualize our clinical decisions (for normal responders) on the basis of number of oocytes retrieved and to develop a noninvasive test to evaluate the endometrial receptivity during a fresh cycle that will allow the selection of patients that would benefit from fresh embryo transfer or freeze-all.

EDITORS' COMMENTS

Freeze-all versus fresh embryo transfer is a topic of much debate. A number of recent randomized controlled trials compared the clinical and cost-effectiveness of a freeze-all policy followed by thawed frozen embryo transfer to the current practice of fresh embryo transfer. However, each trial is generally only powered for a primary outcome, thus making it difficult to identify, with precision, outcomes in key subgroups of couples (based on patient and treatment characteristics) who might benefit most from a freeze-all policy.

Recent literature has indicated that "freeze-all" is not for all, as the beneficial effect as seen in the early publications did not materialize when other patient subgroups were analyzed, including normal responders, poor responders, and suboptimal responders. Apparently, the main advantage of this strategy would be for patients at risk of OHSS and those who undergo preimplantation genetic testing for aneuploidy.[1,2]

Lastly, the term "freeze-all", although used extensively, is inaccurate because not all embryos are frozen; only good quality embryos are frozen. Even if the actual protocol of selective freezing is explained, the use of the term "freeze-all" carries the wrong message. A more adequate terminology would be one that refers to "cycles", not "embryos", such as "freeze-only IVF cycles".

SC Esteves, Campinas, Brazil

REFERENCES

1. Roque M, Haahr T, Esteves SC, et al. The "Big Freeze": freeze-all should not be used for everyone. Hum Reprod. 2018;33(8):1577-8.
2. Roque M, Nuto Nóbrega B, Valle M, et al. Freeze-all strategy in IVF/ICSI cycles: an update on clinical utility. Panminerva Med. 2019;61(1):52-7.

SUGGESTED READING

1. Aflatoonian A, Oskouian H, Ahmadi S, et al. Can fresh embryo transfers be replaced by cryopreserved-thawed embryo transfers in assisted reproductive cycles? A randomized controlled trial. J Assist Reprod Genet. 2010;27(7):357-63.
2. Blockeel C, Drakopoulos P, Santos-Ribeiro S, et al. A fresh look at the freeze-all protocol: a SWOT analysis. Human Reprod. 2016;31(3):491-7.
3. Celada P, Bosch E, De Los Santos MJ, et al. Elective frozen embryo transfer does not improve reproductive outcome in normoresponder patients. Hum Reprod. 2015;30(Suppl 1):i112.
4. Develioglu OH, Hsiu JG, Nikas G, et al. Endometrial estrogen and progesterone receptor and pinopode expression in stimulated cycles of oocyte doors. Fertil Steril. 1999;71(6): 1040-7.
5. Devroey P, Polyzos NP, Blockeel C. An OHSS-free clinic by segmentation of IVF treatment. Hum Reprod. 2011; 26(10):2593-7.
6. Fanchin R, Ayoubi JM, Oliviennes F, et al. Hormonal influence on the uterine contractility during ovarian stimulation. Hum Reprod. 2000;15(Suppl 1):90-100.
7. Fanchin R, Righini C, Olivennes F, et al. Uterine contractions at the time of embryo transfer alter pregnancy rates after IVF. Hum Reprod. 1998;13(7):1968-74.
8. Fang C, Huang R, Wei LN, et al. Frozen-thawed day 5 blastocyst transfer is associated with a lower risk of ectopic pregnancy than day 3 transfer and fresh transfer. Fertil Steril. 2015;103(3):655-61.
9. Fatemi HM, Popovic-Todrovic B, Humaidan P, et al. Severe ovarian hyperstimulation syndrome after gonadotropin-releasing hormone (GnRH) agonist trigger and "freeze-all" approach in GnRH antagonist protocol. Fertil Steril. 2014;101(4):1008-11.
10. Forman EJ, Hong KH, Ferry KM, et al. In vitro fertilizaion with single euploid blastocyst transfer: a randomized controlled trial. Fertil Steril. 2013;100(1):100-7.
11. Humaidan P, Bungum L, Bungum M, et al. Reproductive outcome using a GnRH antagonist for luteolysis and follicular synchronization in poor responder IVF/ICSI patients treated with a flexible GnRH antagonist protocol. Reprod Biomed Online. 2005;11(6):679-84.
12. Ishihara O, Araki R, Kuwahara A, et al. Impact of frozen-thawed single-blastocyst transfer on maternal and neonatal outcome: an analysis of 277,042 single-embryo transfer cycles from 2008–2010 in Japan. Fertil Steril. 2014;101(1):128-33.
13. Ishihara O, Kuwahara A, Saitoh H. Frozen-thawed blastocyst transfer reduces ectopic pregnancy risk: an analysis of single embryo transfer cycles in Japan. Fertil Steril. 2011;95(6): 1966-9.
14. Kol S, Humaidan P. GnRH agonist triggering: recent developments. Reprod Biomed Online. 2013;26(3):226-30.
15. Kolibianakis E, Bourgain C, Albano C, et al. Effect of ovarian stimulation with recombinant FSH, GnRH antagonists, and HCG on endometrial maturation on the day of oocyte pick-up. Fertil Steril. 2002;78(5):1025-9.
16. Li Z, Sullivan EA, Chapman M, et al. Risk of ectopic pregnancy lowest with transfer of single frozen blastocyst. Hum Reprod. 2015;30(9):2048-54.

17. Ling LP, Phoon JW, Lau MS, et al. GnRH agonist trigger and OHSS: relook at 'freeze-all' strategy. Reprod Biomed Online. 2014; 29(3):392-4.
18. Maheshwari A, Pandey S, Shetty A, et al. Obstetric and perinatal outcomes in singleton pregnancies resulting from the transfer of frozen thawed versus fresh embryos generated through IVF treatment: a systematic review and meta-analysis. Fertil Steril. 2012;98(2):368-77.
19. Mohamed AM, Chouliaras S, Jones CJ, et al. Live birth rate in fresh and frozen embryo transfer cycles in women with endometriosis. Eur J Obstet Gynecol Reprod Biol. 2011;156(2):177-80.
20. Nastri CO, Ferriani RA, Rocha IA, et al. Ovarian hyperstimulation syndrome: pathophysiology and prevention. J Assist Reprod Genet. 2010;27(2-3):121-8.
21. Ozgur K, Bulut H, Berkkanoglu M, et al. Concurrent oocyte retrieval and hysteroscopy: a novel approach in assisted reproduction freeze-all cycles. Reprod Biomed Online. 2016;33(2):206-13.
22. Pandey S, Shetty A, Hamilton M, et al. Obstetric and perinatal outcomes in singleton pregnancies resulting from IVF/ICSI: a systematic review and meta-analysis. Hum Reprod Update. 2012;18(5):485-503.
23. Petropanagos A, Cattapan A, Baylis F, et al. Social egg freezing: risk, benefits, and other considerations. CMAJ. 2015;187(9):666-9.
24. Pinborg A, Henningsen AA, Loft A, et al. Large baby syndrome in singletons born after frozen embryo transfer: is it due to maternal factors or the cryotechnique? Hum Reprod. 2014;29(3):618-27.
25. Pindborg A, Wennerholm UB, Romundstad LB, et al. Why do singletons conceived after ART have adverse perinatal outcomes? Systematic review and meta-analysis. Hum Reprod Update. 2013;19(2):87-104.
26. Roque M, Lattes K, Serra S, et al. Fresh embryo transfer versus frozen embryo transfer in IVF cycles: a systematic review and meta-analysis. Fertil Steril. 2013;99(1):156-62.
27. Roque M. Freeze-all policy: is it time for that? J Assist Reprod Genet. 2015;32(2):171-6.
28. Rubio C, Rodrigo L, Mir P, et al. Use of array comparative genomic hybridization (array-CGH) for embryo assessment: clinical results. Fertil Steril. 2013;99(4):1044-8.
29. Santos-Ribeiro S, Polyzos NP, Haentjens P, et al. Live birth rates are IVF are reduced by both low and high progesterone levels on the day of HCG administration. Hum Reprod. 2014;29(8):1698-705.
30. Scott Jr RT, Franasiak JM, Forman EJ. Comprehensive chromosome screening with synchronous blastocyst transfer: time for a paradigm shift. Fertil Steril. 2014;102(3):660-1.
31. Shapiro BS, Daneshmand ST, De Leon L, et al. Frozen-thawed embryo transfer is associated with a significantly reduced incidence of ectopic pregnancy. Fertil Steril. 2012;98(6): 1490-4.
32. Shapiro BS, Daneshmand ST, Garner FC, et al. Clinical rationale for cryopreservation of entire embryo cohorts in lieu of fresh transfer. Fertil Steril. 2014;102(1):3-9.
33. Shapiro BS, Daneshmand ST, Garner FC, et al. Evidence of impaired endometrial receptivity after ovarian stimulation for IVF: a prospective randomized trial comparing fresh and frozen-thawed embryo transfer in normal responders. Fertil Steril. 2011;96(2):344-8.
34. Shapiro BS, Daneshmand ST, Garner FC, et al. Evidence of impaired endometrial receptivity after ovarian stimulation for IVF: a prospective randomized trial comparing fresh and frozen-thawed embryo transfers in high responders. Fertil Steril. 2011;96(2):516-8.
35. Wennerholm UB, Henningsen AK, Romundstad LB, et al. Perinatal outcomes of children born after frozen-thawed embryo transfer: a Nordic cohort study from the CoNARTaS group. Hum Reprod. 2013;28(9):2545-53.
36. Youssef MA, van Wely M, Hassan MA, et al. Can dopamine agonists reduce the incidence and severity of OHSS in IVF/ICSI treatment cycles? A systematic review and meta-analysis. Hum Reprod Update. 2010;16(5):459-66.
37. Zhu L, Li Y, Xu A. Influence of controlled ovarian stimulation on uterine peristalsis in infertile women. Hum Reprod. 2012;27(9):2684-9.

14

CHAPTER

Procedure in Assisted Reproductive Technology

Kaberi Banerjee, Bhavana Singla

INTRODUCTION

Infertility is an inability to conceive after having regular unprotected sex for 1 year. The incidence of infertility has continued to rise over the last 20 years and it is estimated that it affects approximately 25% of couples of reproductive age. Worldwide, 186 million people are unable to have a child with male infertility contributing to over half of all cases of global childlessness.

Assisted reproductive technology is an interesting scientific branch after the birth of the world's first *in vitro* fertilization baby, Louise Brown, in the United Kingdom.

WHAT IS ASSISTED REPRODUCTIVE TECHNOLOGY?

Assisted reproductive technology (ART) is the term referring to techniques used to achieve pregnancy by artificial or partially artificial means. According to Centers for Disease Control and Prevention (CDC), ART includes all fertility treatments in which both eggs and sperm are handled.

ART Procedures

- Artificial insemination (AI) including intrauterine insemination (IUI)
- *In vitro* fertilization (IVF)
- Intracytoplasmic sperm injection (ICSI)
- Others [gamete intrafallopian transfer—(GIFT), zygote intrafallopian transfer (ZIFT)]
- Preimplantation genetic screening (PGS) or preimplantation genetic diagnosis (PGD)
- Assisted hatching (AH)
- Cryopreservation of sperms, oocytes and embryos
- Third party reproduction (donor eggs, donor sperms, and surrogacy).

Who Needs ART?

- Coital problems
- Ovulatory disorders
- Tubal pathology
- Endometriosis
- Thin endometrium
- Cervical factors
- Male factor infertility (problems related to sperms)
- Unexplained infertility
- Failure of other infertility treatments
- Familial genetic disorders.

ARTIFICIAL INSEMINATION

Artificial insemination is the procedure where sperms are placed into a woman's vagina, cervical canal or in the uterus. The types of AI are:

- Intravaginal insemination (IVI)
- Intrauterine insemination (IUI).

Intravaginal Insemination

It is a simple and painless procedure of artificial insemination by vaginal route. The basic idea of IVI treatment is to increase the sperm density near the site of fertilization in case of nonconsummation of marriage.

Who Needs IVI?

Nonconsummation of marriage due to:

- Vaginismus and dyspareunia in females
- Erectile dysfunction (ED) and premature ejaculation (PE) in males
- Combination of female and male factors.

How is it Performed?

The couples are consulted through history taking, physical examination and given questionnaire. After this initial assessment, the different treatment options are discussed with the couple. The process of IVI is demonstrated to the couple and they are doing the same at home on alternate day in fertile period of female in 3–6 cycles.

Artificial insemination kit is containing sterile semen container, a soft plastic IUI catheter, and a 5 cc syringe. The husband collects the semen sample by masturbation in a sterile plastic semen container. The sample is then processed and taken into an IUI catheter, and semen is injected slowly inside the cervical canal into the uterus and the patient is told to lie down for 20 min after the process.

What is the Success Rate and Risk of IVI?

Artificial vaginal insemination is an assisted conception method that can be used in selected couples. Intravaginal insemination is a simple, cheap, painless procedure for conception in nonconsummation of marriage without any risks.

The first study was done in our center to document the clinical pregnancy rates (CPR) using IVI in nonconsummation of marriage to the best of our knowledge. It was 69% in 20–30 years age group; 43% in 31–35 years age group and 25% in 36–40 years age group after 6 cycles of AI.

Intrauterine Insemination

It is a safe and easy treatment of artificial insemination where washed sperms are directly deposited in uterine cavity of wife. The basic idea of IUI treatment is to increase the pregnancy rate in the couple by increasing number of healthy sperm reaching to fertilization site.

Who Needs IUI?

- Cervical factor (abnormal mucus)
- Male infertility (Mild-to-moderate >10 million sperm)
- Failure to conceive after ovulation induction treatment
- Sexual dysfunction—ejaculatory disorder
- Retrograde ejaculation
- Unexplained infertility
- Use of donor sperms.

Intrauterine insemination is contraindicated in women with cervical stenosis, cervicitis, endometritis or bilateral tubal obstruction and in most cases of amenorrhea or severe oligospermia.

How is it Performed?

Intrauterine insemination can be done in a natural or stimulated cycle. In natural cycle, follicular monitoring starts from Day 9 or 10 of periods till follicle ruptures. IUI will be done on the day when follicle ruptures.

In a stimulated cycle (super ovulation), tablets or hormonal injections — clomiphene citrate (CC), letrozole (LE), human menopausal gonadotropin (hMG) or follicle stimulating hormone (FSH) starts from Day 2 of period and follicular monitoring starts from Day 8 or 9 of periods till follicle reaches 18 mm. Human chorionic gonadotropin (hCG) injection (5000–10,000 IU) is given to mature the eggs when the follicles reach an optimal size. IUI is performed 36 hours after the administration of the hCG injection.

Normal sperm stays in the female genital tract for 3–5 days, and an oocyte stays for 12–24 hours after ovulation.

The male partner is asked to collect the semen sample by masturbation in a sterile plastic semen container. The semen after liquefaction was examined according to the World Health Organization guidelines and processed using Sperm simple wash, swim-up or density gradient centrifugation. Insemination was carried out using an intrauterine catheter.

In case of donor sperms, it is thawed first, washed and then used for insemination.

Luteal phase support protocol is natural micronized progesterone or dydrogesterone which is to be started 3 days after ovulation and a serum or urine hCG assay is performed 16 days after IUI.

What is the Success Rate and Risk of IUI?

Intrauterine insemination is a simple and cost-effective therapy for cervical factor, anovulatory infertility, mild to moderate male factor, unexplained infertility and immunological infertility with clinical pregnancy rates from 7% to 12 %.

The pregnancy rate will be 7% per cycle with clomiphene citrate and IUI that is most common IUI protocol. It will be approximately 12% per cycle with ovarian stimulation with FSH and IUI treatment is 12% per cycle and 13% will be multiple pregnancy rate.

The average pregnancy rates with donor IUI are 4% higher than IUI with husband's sperm.

IN VITRO FERTILIZATION

It is a process that involves extraction of oocytes from ovaries after ovarian stimulation with hormonal injections followed by fertilization with the sperms in a laboratory and then the embryos were transferred to the uterus. The rationale of IVF is to bypass the fallopian tubes where the fertilization happens naturally.

Who Needs IVF?

- Ovulatory disorders
- Poor ovarian (egg) capacity
- Advanced maternal age
- Endometriosis
- Tubal damage or block
- Thin endometrium
- Absent or low sperm count (<5 million/mL)
- Failure of fertility treatment for more than 3 years
- Unexplained infertility
- Familial genetic disorders
- Recurrent abortions.

How is it Performed?

In vitro fertilization cycle involves the four steps — ovarian stimulation, egg collection, fertilization, embryo culture and embryo transfer. Ovarian stimulation involves daily injection of exogenous gonadotropins for 10–12 days to promote multifollicular development along with follicular monitoring. To prevent premature ovulation, gonadotropin-releasing hormone (GnRH) agonist or antagonist is added in IVF cycles that allow timed collection of mature oocytes also. hCG trigger or GnRH agonist is given to induce LH surge. Between 34 hour and 36 hour after hCG or GnRH agonist administration, oocyte pick up is performed via TVUS-guided needle aspiration under general anesthesia and rarely by abdominal route.

Oocyte pick-up is the removal of eggs from the ovary. A transvaginal ultrasound probe is used to visualize the follicles within the ovaries and a long needle is attached to the probe through guide which is connected to flexible tubing and connected through a test tube to a vacuum source. Vacuum source gives suction via test tube to needle to allow aspiration of oocyte from follicle with suction pressure of 100–120 mm Hg. The needle is inserted through vaginal wall into an ovarian follicle and follicular fluid containing cellular material including oocyte is aspirated which is delivered to IVF laboratory to identify and ova counting. The needle is withdrawn once all the ovarian follicles have been aspirated and the procedure is repeated on other ovary.

The eggs are fertilized with sperms in laboratory and the fertilized egg forms the embryo. It is performed shortly after oocyte retrieval either by conventional IVF or by ICSI. In conventional fertilization, each oocyte is incubated with approximately 50,000 sperms and fertilization happens naturally. For ICSI, one sperm is selected and directly injected into each oocyte. The indications for ICSI include: unexplained infertility, poor-quality oocytes, low oocyte yield, advanced maternal age, prior fertilization failure with IVF, routine use in all IVF cycles, preimplantation genetic screening (PGS), fertilization after *in vitro* maturation (IVM), and fertilization of cryopreserved oocytes. The ICSI is used to avoid fertilization failure in these cases. The oocyte is denuded from surrounding cumulus cells, stabilized by a micropipette, and injected with the sperm. Approximately 24 hour later, the oocytes are checked for fertilization. The embryos are examined by light microscopy for progression in development and cellular morphologic features at set time points following fertilization. The embryo is cultured in the laboratory for 2–5 days. Two-three best embryos are selected and transferred into the uterus on the second, third or fifth day. Day 5 transfer (blastocyst) is decided on case-to-case basis.

The embryo transfer is performed with transabdominal ultrasonography (USG) guidance for which full bladder is required (also straighten the cervico-uterine axis). After gentle insertion of speculum, cervical mucus plug is removed first, and then soft outer sheath followed by soft catheter containing embryos is introduced. The embryos are placed approximately 2 cm proximal to fundus under USG guidance and catheter is examined to check for retained embryos after embryo transfer.

Luteal phase support is given in the form of progesterone and estrogen and after 14 days, pregnancy test (β-hCG) is done.

What is the Success Rate and Risk of IVF?

The age of female partner is very important factor for pregnancy rates (PR) and live birth rates (LBR) in IVF. PR varies from 40% to 60% and LBR from 35% to 55% in age less than 35 years. The success rates go down with age. PR <10% and LBR ~5% per cycle will be in women more than 42 years of age.

The ICSI for all is not recommended to improve fertilization, implantation and chemical pregnancy rates. The fertilization rate per oocyte retrieved was higher with conventional insemination than with ICSI (58% vs 47%, $p < 0.0001$). In conventional IVF, fertilization failure occurred in 5% (11/206) and in ICSI group, 2% (4/209) was fertilization failure. In failed conventional IVFs, ICSI may improve fertilization rates (48%) in a subsequent cycle. ICSI may be of benefit for patients undergoing IVF with PGS, *in vitro* matured oocytes, and previously cryopreserved oocytes.

Maternal risks involved in IVF are ovarian hyperstimulation syndrome (OHSS), increased chances of multiple pregnancy, ectopic pregnancy, pre-eclampsia, placenta previa, placental abruption, gestational diabetes, and cesarean delivery. OHSS is a self-limiting condition but may be life-threatening condition and is characterized by ovarian enlargement, elevated sex steroids hormones, and vascular permeability resulting in fluid in third space leading to ascites and intravascular dehydration. Severe OHSS occurs in 0.5–5% of IVF cycles, and may result in multisystem organ failure and thromboembolism. The risk of multiple births associated with IVF is directly related to the number of embryos transferred in each cycle. There are 30% chances of multiple births after IVF.

Fetal risks in IVF are associated with multiple gestation, prematurity, LBW. ICSI may increase the risk of birth defects compared with those who conceived spontaneously (8.3% vs 5.8%).

Nowadays, GIFT and ZIFT offers little clinical advantage. The main disadvantages are general anesthesia and involvement of laparoscopy.

Gamete intrafallopian transfer is the procedure where unfertilized eggs and sperms are placed in the fallopian tubes and ZIFT is the procedure where eggs are fertilized with the sperms in the laboratory and the fertilized eggs (zygote) are placed in the fallopian tubes.

PREIMPLANTATION GENETIC SCREENING OR PREIMPLANTATION GENETIC DIAGNOSIS

Preimplantation genetic screening is the generalized screening of embryos whether they are genetically healthy or not.

Preimplantation genetic diagnosis is the screening of embryos for particular disorder (may be running in family).

Who Needs PGS/PGD?

- Recurrent miscarriages
- Repeated IVF failures
- Maternal age older than 38 years
- Severe male factor infertility
- One child already affected with a genetic disease
- Family history of inherited disease.

How is it Performed?

The PGS treatment involves the basic steps of IVF (hormonal injections to grow multiple eggs in the ovaries, extraction of all eggs through transvaginal aspiration and fertilization of eggs with sperms in IVF laboratory) followed by biopsy of embryos on Day 3 or day 5 (preferable).

Normally embryo biopsy is performed at the eighth cell stage of embryos on Day 3. In this one or two blastomeres of embryo are biopsied and healthy embryos can be transferred in the same cycle on Day 5. It is always better to give two blastomeres biopsy than single blastomere biopsy for accuracy but there is more risk of damage to the embryo development and implantation with 2 blastomere biopsies.

Another best method is Blastocyst stage biopsy. In this method, 5–10 trophectoderm cells are biopsied on Day 5. The blastocyst biopsy is preferred as we can collect more cells that provide better efficiency of result. The embryos are then cryopreserved in that cycle. The patient is then reprepared for the frozen embryo transfer, if the biopsied embryos are normal and then the embryos are thawed and transferred. Genetic analysis is done by fluorescence *in situ* hybridization (FISH), comparative genomic hybridization (CGH) or single nucleotide polymorphism (SNP) microarrays.

What is the Success Rate and Risk of PGS/PGD?

Preimplantation genetic screening or preimplantation genetic diagnosis in India is an uprising branch of ART that helps in improving the success rate of IVF.

For couples harboring a balanced chromosomal translocation, PGD using telomeric probes to identify and exclude embryos having an unbalanced genetic complement appears to decrease significantly the risk of spontaneous abortion (to <20%) and to increase significantly the likelihood of achieving a live birth. The clinical implantation rate per day-3 non-PGS embryos, PGS and non-PGS blastocysts range between 21.4% and 50%, 44% and 47.2%, and 39.3% and 65.5%, respectively.

Available evidence does not support the use of PGS as currently performed to improve live-birth rates in patients with advanced maternal age, recurrent implantation failure, and recurrent abortions.

There is a high incidence of mosaicism of human embryos associated with embryo biopsy at the cleavage stage may also contribute to the difficulties in assessing PGS outcomes. Technological improvements like the use of CGH and SNP microarrays can help meet some of these difficulties.

ASSISTED HATCHING

Assisted hatching is the manipulation of the zona pellucida (ZP) by laser, mechanical, or chemical means, with the aim of facilitating embryo implantation.

Who Needs AH?

Patients with a poor prognosis:
- ≥2 failed IVF cycles
- Poor embryo quality
- Older women (>38 years of age)

How is it Performed?

Assisted hatching involves the artificial thinning or breaching of the zona pellucida. The AH procedure is performed before to embryo transfer (ET) on Day 3 or 5 after fertilization by various methods. In this method, hole is created in the zona by drilling with acidified Tyrode's solution, partial zona dissection (PZD) with a glass microneedle, laser photoablation, or use of a piezo micromanipulator. The zona pellucida can also be thinned without breaching its integrity with proteolytic enzymes, acidified Tyrode's solution, or laser.

What is the Success Rate and Risk of AH?

Assisted hatching is associated with an increased chance of achieving clinical pregnancy and multiple pregnancies. There was a significant increase in clinical pregnancy (OR = 1.16, 95% CI = 1.00–1.36, $I^2 = 48.3\%$) and multiple pregnancy rates (OR = 1.50, 95% CI = 1.11–2.01, $I^2 = 44.0\%$) with AH.

The assisted hatching procedure may cause specific complications independent of the IVF procedure itself, including lethal damage to the embryo and damage to individual blastomeres with reduction of embryo viability. In addition, artificial manipulation of the ZP has been associated with an increased risk of monozygotic (MZ) twin pregnancy.

CRYOPRESERVATION

Cryopreservation of gametes and embryos is an essential aspect of ART.

Who Needs Sperm Cryopreservation?

- For sperm banks (donor sperms)
- Difficulty in sperm production (on OPU day)
- Malignancy (before RT or CT)
- Before vasectomy or surgical infertility treatments
- Azoospermia (TESA/PESA/Testicular biopsy sample).

Who Needs Oocyte Cryopreservation?

- Cancer patients —reproductive failure
- Desire to postpone childbearing
- Ethical opposition to embryo cryopreservation
- Partner unavailable
- Excess oocytes after superovulation therapy
- F/H of early menopause (wants fertility preservation)
- Oocyte donation programs.

Who Needs Embryo Cryopreservation?

- Spare embryos after a cycle of IVF
- For second pregnancy
- Embryo donation.

How is it Performed?

Freezing of gametes and embryos are done by vitrification (Better method) or slow freezing method. These are stored in liquid nitrogen (–196 °C).

What is the Success Rate and Risk of Cryopreservation?

In a randomized controlled trial of 3,000 fresh and 3,000 vitrified oocytes (92.5% survival) in an oocyte donation program, there was no detrimental effects of vitrification on subsequent fertilization, development, or implantation. Studies indicate that pregnancies and infants conceived after oocyte CP do not have increased risk of adverse obstetric outcomes or congenital anomalies.

Vitrification, as compared with slow freezing, looks to be better in terms of post-thawing survival rates both for cleavage-stage embryos [odds ratio (OR): 6.35, 95% confidence interval (CI): 1.14–35.26, random effects model] and for blastocysts (OR: 4.09, 95% CI: 2.45–6.84, random effects model). There was no significant difference in clinical pregnancy rates per transfer could be detected in two methods (OR: 1.66, 95% CI: 0.98–2.79).

THIRD-PARTY REPRODUCTION

Third-party reproduction is the process in which genetic material or gestation is provided by a third party or donor other than the one or two parents who will raise the resulting child.

Who Needs Third-party Reproduction?

Indications of Donor Sperms

- Severe male infertility - congenital or acquired
  - Obstructive (blockage of the ejaculatory ducts)
  - Nonobstructive (testicular failure) azoospermia
- Male partner carrying genetic disorder
- Option for single women or same sex female partners to conceive.

Indications of Donor Eggs

- Diminished ovarian function (Due to disease, chemotherapy, radiation therapy, or surgical removal of their ovaries)
- Absent ovaries
- Female carrying genetic diseases
- Infertility due to egg factor (multiple IVF failures, advanced reproductive age, and inadequate response to ovulation induction).

Indications of Donor Embryos

- Unexplained infertility involving both partners
- Unexplained infertility in a single woman
- Recurrent pregnancy loss due to factors related to embryos and genetic diseases affecting one or both partners.

Indications of Surrogacy

- After hysterectomy
  - For cancer
  - For postpartum hemorrhage
  - For menorrhagia
- Congenital absence of the uterus
- Repeated failure of IVF
- Recurrent abortion
- Severe medical conditions incompatible with pregnancy.

Third-party reproduction is complex process and requires regulations and guidelines. It has social, ethical, moral and legal issues but provides many couples opportunity to make their dream of parenthood a reality.

WHAT IS THE SUCCESS RATE FOR ART?

Various factors including age of female partner, sperm quality, the number of embryos transferred affects the success rate of ART. The success rate peaks with the transfer of three to four embryos. High degree of efficiency is required for the collection of eggs, fertilization, early embryo growth and embryo transfers.

The major problems to success are implantation after embryo transfer and early pregnancy loss. The rate of early pregnancy loss is slightly, but not significantly, higher with ART compared to spontaneous conception. The risk of early pregnancy loss increases with age of the female partner. After 40 years of age, ART success rates decline dramatically. Pregnancy complications tend to be higher with ART pregnancies, primarily because of the much higher rate of multiple pregnancies.

EDITORS' COMMENTS

1. In the last 5 years, the field of ART has evolved as the couple trying to conceive has become more aware and informed of the various options and the onus lies on the infertility specialist to guide them rightly to conceive as fast as possible.
2. With advancements in ART such as embryonic genetic testing, oocyte preservation, minimal stimulation protocols, optimizing techniques like IUI, etc. one must ensure that these resources are made available in a morally responsible and equitable manner.
3. Reproductive genetics in ART is gaining increasing importance in predicting possible outcomes of future pregnancies.

SUGGESTED READING

1. Abdelkader AM, Yeh J. The potential use of intrauterine insemination as a basic option for infertility: a review for technology-limited medical settings. Obstet Gynecol Int. 2009;2009:584837.
2. Banerjee K, Singla B. Pregnancy Outcome of home intravaginal insemination in couples with unconsummated marriage. J Hum Reprod Sci. 2017;10(4):293-6.
3. Bhattacharya S, Hamilton MP, Shaaban M, et al. Conventional in vitro fertilization versus intracytoplasmic sperm injection for the treatment of nonmale-factor infertility: a randomized controlled trial. Lancet. 2001;357(9274):2075-9.
4. Cobo A, Meseguer M, Remohi J, et al. Use of cryo-banked oocytes in an ovum donation program: a prospective, randomized, controlled, clinical trial. Human Reprod. 2010; 25(9):2239-46.
5. Coco R. Reprogenetics: preimplantational genetics diagnosis. Genet Mol Biol. 2014;37(Suppl 1):271-84.
6. Delvigne A, Rozenberg S. Epidemiology and prevention of ovarian hyperstimulation syndrome (OHSS): a review. Hum Reprod Update. 2002;8(6):559-77.
7. ESHRE Capri Workshop Group. Intrauterine insemination. Hum Reprod Update. 2009;15(3):265-77.
8. Goossens V, De Rycke M, De Vos A, et al. Diagnostic efficiency embryonic development and clinical outcome after the biopsy of one or two blastomeres for preimplantation genetic diagnosis. Hum Reprod. 2008;23(3):481-92.
9. Greenfeld DA. Effects and outcomes of third-party reproduction: parents. Fertil Steril. 2015;104(3):520-4.
10. Gunby J, Daya S. Assisted reproductive technologies (ART) in Canada: 2001 results from the Canadian ART Register. Fertil Steril. 2005;84(3):590-9.
11. Hershlag A, Paine T, Cooper GW, et al. Monozygotic twinning associated with mechanical assisted hatching. Fertil Steril. 1999;71(1):144-6.

12. Inhorn MC, Patrizio P. Infertility around the globe: new thinking on gender, reproductive technologies and global movements in the 21st century. Hum Reprod Update. 2015;21(4):411-26.
13. Kim HO, Sung N, Song IO. Predictors of live birth and pregnancy success after in vitro fertilization in infertile women aged 40 and over. Clin Exp Reprod Med. 2017;44(2):111-7.
14. Kokkali G, Vrettou C, Traeger-Synodinos J, et al. Birth of a healthy infant following trophectoderm biopsy from blastocytes for PGD of beta-thalasssemia major. Hum Reprod. 2005; 20(7):1855-9.
15. Kolibianakis EM, Venetis CA, Tarlatzis BC. Cryopreservation of human embryos by vitrification or slow freezing: which one is better? Curr Opin Obstet Gynecol. 2009;21(3):270-4.
16. Li D, Yang DL, An J, et al. Effect of assisted hatching on pregnancy outcomes: a systematic review and meta-analysis of randomized controlled trials. Sci Rep. 2016;6:31228.
17. Ly KD, Agarwal A, Nagy ZP. Preimplantation genetic screening: does it help or hinder IVF treatment and what is the role of the embryo? J Assist Reprod Genet. 2011;28(9):833-49.
18. Nejat EJ, Buyuk E. Reproductive technologies and the risk of birth defects. N Engl J Med. 2012; 367(9):875-6.
19. Noyes N, Porcu E, Borini A. Over 900 oocyte cryopreservation babies born with no apparent increase in congenital anomalies. Reprod Biomed Online. 2009;18(6):769-76.
20. Orvieto R. Preimplantation genetic screening the required RCT that has not yet been carried out. Reprod Biol Endocrinol. 2016;14:35.
21. Practice Committee of Society for Assisted Reproductive Technology; Practice Committee of American Society for Reproductive Medicine. Preimplantation genetic testing: a Practice Committee opinion. Fertil Steril. 2008;90(5 Suppl):S136-43.
22. Practice Committees of the American Society for Reproductive Medicine and Society for Assisted Reproductive Technology. Intracytoplasmic sperm injection (ICSI) for nonmale factor infertility: a committee opinion. Fertil Steril. 2012;98(6): 1395-9.
23. Rowell P, Braude P. Assisted conception. I—General principles. BMJ. 2003;327(7418):799-801.
24. Schieve LA, Meikle SF, Peterson HB, et al. Does assisted hatching pose a risk for monozygotic twinning in pregnancies conceived through in vitro fertilization? Fertil Steril. 2000; 74(2):288-94.
25. Shevell T, Malone FD, Vidaver J, et al. Assisted reproductive technology and pregnancy outcome. Obstet Gynecol. 2005;106(5 Pt 1):1039-45.
26. Stephens SM, Arnett DM, Meacham RB. The use of in vitro fertilization in the management of male infertility: what the urologist needs to know. Rev Urol. 2013;15(4):154-60.
27. Steptoe PC, Edwards RG. Birth after the reimplantation of a human embryo. Lancet. 1978;2(8085):366.
28. Van der Westerlaken L, Helmerhorst F, Dieben S, et al. Intracytoplasmic sperm injection as treatment for unexplained total fertilization failure or low fertilization after conventional in vitro fertilization. Fertil Steril. 2005;83(3): 612-7.
29. Verlinsky Y, Tur-Kaspa I, Cieslak J, et al. Preimplantation testing for chromosomal disorders improves reproductive outcome of poor-prognosis patients. Reprod Biomed Online. 2005;11(2):219-25.
30. World Health Organization. Temporal relationships between ovulation and defined changes in the concentration of plasma estradiol-17 beta, luteinizing hormone, follicle-stimulating hormone and progesterone. Am J Obstet Gynecol. 1980;138(4):383-90.

15

CHAPTER

Genetic Testing in Male Infertility

Rahul Gajbhiye

INTRODUCTION

Male infertility is reported in approximately 50% of the infertile couples. Several factors contribute to male infertility. Known genetic factors contribute approximately 20% of the male infertility. Recent advances in the field of genetics and genomics have contributed in better understanding of male infertility and also translated the knowledge into development of accurate genetic tests for diagnosis of male infertility. Karyotype analysis and Y-microdeletions testing are useful methods for men having nonobstructive azoospermia and severe oligozoospermia. Cystic fibrosis transmembrane conductance regulator (*CFTR*) gene mutation testing is useful in men having obstructive azoospermia due to vas aplasia. The genetic testing is not only useful for identification of genetic causes of male infertility but also useful for calculating the accurate genetic risk which is useful for providing genetic counseling to the infertile couples.

MALE INFERTILITY

As per the International Glossary on Infertility and Fertility Care, 2017, male infertility is defined as *infertility* due to male factors including altered semen parameters, anatomical, endocrine, genetic, functional or immunological abnormalities of the reproductive system, chronic disorders and sexual problems leading to difficulty in deposition of semen in the vagina. There is a limited information on burden of male infertility globally as well as India. It is estimated that men are responsible for 40–50% of infertility cases affecting approximately 7% of all men. Known genetic factors are responsible for approximately 20% of the male infertility. Majority of the azoospermia (30–60%) is still idiopathic and may need further investigations using genetic tests. There are different mechanisms responsible of genetics contributions of male infertility such as influencing physiological processes including hormonal homeostasis, spermatogenesis, and sperm quality.

Human Genome

The human genome is made up of two distinct parts: The nuclear and mitochondrial components. The nuclear genome consists of approximately 3,200,000,000 nucleotides of DNA, divided into 24 linear molecules, each contained in a different chromosome (Fig. 1). Out of 24 chromosomes, 22 are autosomes and X and Y are sex chromosomes. The mitochondrial genome is located in the mitochondria containing a circular DNA molecule of 16 569 nucleotides. Majority of the cells are diploid in nature containing two copies of each autosome along with two sex chromosomes, XX for females or XY for males (Total 46 chromosomes) and are therefore called as somatic cells. Whereas, the sex cells (gametes) are haploid in nature containing 23 chromosomes (one copy of each of 22 autosomes and one sex chromosome, either X or Y). The inheritance of genetic disorders can be broadly classified into: (1) chromosomal abnormalities, (2) Mendelian inheritance pattern, (3) mitochondrial, and (4) multifactorial or complex. Chromosomal abnormalities can be further divided into numerical abnormalities (polysomy and polyploidy) and structural abnormalities. Mendelian types of heritable disease are single-gene disorders inherited as autosomal dominant, autosomal recessive or X-linked. The mitochondrial genetic defects are maternally

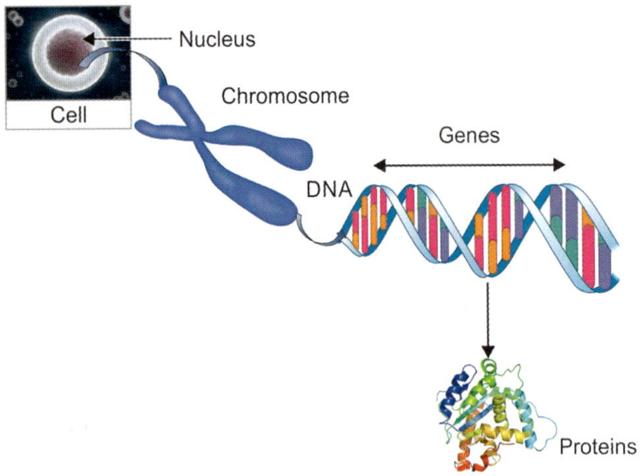

Fig. 1: Schematic representation of cell, nucleus, chromosome, genes, DNA, and proteins.

transmitted as sperm mitochondria do not survive in the oocytes. When multiple genes in combination with lifestyle and environmental factors contribute to a disease phenotype, it is referred as complex genetic inheritance.

Importance of Investigating the Genetic Factors

Recent advances in assisted reproductive technologies (ARTs) especially IVF-ICSI and sperm retrieval techniques such as percutaneous epididymal sperm aspiration (PESA), microsurgical epididymal sperm aspiration (MESA), testicular/epididymal sperm aspiration or extraction (TESA/TESE) and micro-TESE have significantly improved the male infertility management. However, these technological innovations were not followed up with long term research studies thereby lacking scientific evidence on safety of these technologies. For example, clinical application of ICSI was preceded without generating sufficient scientific evidence on the safety to the offspring and also its future genetic implications. Therefore, it is important to investigate the underlying genetic factors responsible for male factor infertility and identify abnormal phenotypes. Genetic defects transmitted due to IVF-ICSI technology can have serious implications on the developing zygote. Investigating the underlying genetic causes will help in early detection of genetic abnormalities, predicting prognosis, disease prevention, and treatment planning at or before onset of disease and most importantly predicting the health of the offspring.

Genetic Testing for Male Infertility

There are two main reasons for recommending genetic testing in male infertility. The first reason is to identify the possible genetic defects with risk transmission to the offspring through ARTs and secondly to detect the genetic disorders impacting the ability to obtain spermatozoa through sperm retrieval techniques such as micro-TESE, etc. There has been significant research on understanding the genetic factors contributing to male infertility. Genetics of male infertility is a complex and multifactorial in origin with broad spectrum of clinical manifestations. The genetic testing in male infertility includes karyotyping, *CFTR* gene mutation screening, Y chromosome microdeletions testing. When no underlying cause is detected, male infertility cases are termed as idiopathic (~40%). The Idiopathic male infertility cases might be due to genetic factors or/and associated with additional factors such as environment, endocrine disruptors, smoking, air pollution and epigenetics.

Screening of Nonobstructive Azoospermia/Severe Oligospermia

Karyotype

Karyotype analysis is recommended in all men having total motile sperm count <5 million and men with nonobstructive azoospermia. Although the frequency of karyotype abnormalities is low (0.6%) in general population, its frequency is relatively higher ranging from 2% to 14% in male infertility. The semen analysis of such males having chromosomal abnormalities suggests severe impairment of testicular function leading to azoospermia and severe oligozoospermia. Chromosomal abnormalities can be aneuploidy (e.g. trisomy) and/or structural (e.g. inversions or translocations). These numerical and structural chromosomal abnormalities are detected by following genetic techniques: (1) *karyotyping*—Giemsa/Trypsin staining on metaphases derived from peripheral blood lymphocytes and (2) *molecular cytogenetic methods*—fluorescence *in situ* hybridization (FISH), comparative genomic hybridization (CGH).

Klinefelter syndrome (KFS) having a 47, XXY karyotype, is reported as the most common chromosomal aneuploidy affecting 3–4% of infertile men and up to 12% men with azoospermia. Nonmosaic KFS contributes to 11% of men with azoospermia whereas mosaic KFS leads to oligozoospermia. KFS is characterized by gynecomastia, hypogonadism, ejaculatory azoospermia, seminiferous tubule dysgenesis, normal to moderately reduced Leydig cell function, scanty body hair, long arms, legs and elevated serum gonadotropin concentrations. Infertility in men having KFS is due to the defect in spermatogenesis leading to azoospermia or with occasionally severe oligozoospermia. Due to the variable symptoms severity, majority of patients remain undiagnosed leading to one-fourth of KFS patients to get detected for a very long period of time. Karyotype analysis is used to confirm a diagnosis of KFS. Around 80–90 % of the KFS patients show 47,XXY karyotype whereas 10–20% cases have 46,XY/47,XXY, 48,XXXY or 48,XXYY or structural abnormality of sex chromosome. Meiotic nondisjunction is the main genetic cause of KFS and intracytoplasmic sperm injection (ICSI) is the fertility treatment for KFS. Majority of the men with KFS are azoospermic requiring micro-TESE. Preimplantation genetic diagnosis (PGD) or amniocentesis is recommended due to risk of increase of sex chromosomal and autosomal abnormalities in the embryos of Klinefelter patients.

The most common structural chromosomal abnormalities detected on karyotyping are Robertsonian translocations, reciprocal translocations, inversions, complex rearrangements and marker chromosomes. Robertsonian translocations are caused due to fusion of two acrocentric chromosomes at the centromere. Reciprocal translocations occur when two nonhomologous chromosomes exchange segments. Breaking of a piece of chromosome at two points with reinsertion within the same chromosome leads to inversion. This can be of two types: pericentric and paracentric. Complex rearrangement is the structural rearrangement involving more than two breakpoints and more than two chromosomes. Supernumerary marker chromosomes are structurally abnormal chromosome fragments. These structural chromosomal abnormalities lead to risk of aneuploidy in embryos. Hence, such couples with structural abnormalities should undergo genetic counseling as well as PGD testing or amniocentesis.

Rarely, some of the men with azoospermia may have 46,XX disorder of sexual development. Couples in which male partner has defects in chromosome, there is an increased risk of miscarriages. Additionally, there is also a risk of chromosomal and congenital defects in the children. According to American Society for Reproductive Medicine (ASRM), men with nonobstructive azoospermia or severe oligozoospermia must be offered high-resolution karyotype before using their sperm for ICSI.

FISH analysis using chromosome specific DNA probes is now considered as faster, cheaper and alternative for detection of human sperm aneuploidy, sperm motility defects and other aspects of fertilization. FISH analysis for sperm aneuploidy could be useful in counseling and decision making before undergoing ICSI in following groups of patients:

- Klinefelter syndrome
- Men with structural defects in chromosomes
- Men with defective sperm morphology including macrocephalic, multinucleated and multiflagellate sperm
- Men with nonobstructive azoospermia with sperm retrieval from testicular biopsy.

Based on the FISH sperm analysis reports, the couples should be provided reassurance for low risk and option of ICSI combined with PDG in case of high risk.

Y Chromosome (AZF) Microdeletions

Y chromosome microdeletion is described as the absence of DNA segments or gene(s) from functionally active Y chromosome. It is the second most common genetic etiology of infertility in men after KFS with 10–15% prevalence in azoospermic men, 5–10% in oligozoospermic men. Microdeletions occur most frequently on the long arm of the Y chromosome, Yq. Y chromosome deleted regions are mapped to 3 azoospermia factor (AZF) regions namely, AZFa, AZFb, AZFc. These regions contain functionally active genes as well as transcription factors required for spermatogenesis. AZFa region contains 2 genes (*USP9Y* and *DBY*), AZFb region harbors 7 genes (*EIF1AY, RPS4Y2, SMCY, HSFY, XKRY, PRY, and RBMY*) whereas AZFc region contains 5 genes (*BPY2, CDY, DAZ, CSPG4LY,* and *GOLGAZLY*). Partial or complete deletion of AZF region leads to impaired spermatogenesis. Deletion of each of these regions leads to different phenotypic alterations. Sertoli-cell-only syndrome is caused by deletion of AZFa, spermatogenic arrest is caused by AZFb deletion and deletion of AZFc leading to phenotypes ranging from Sertoli-cell-only syndrome to oligozoospermia. AZFc deletions are the frequently detected (~80%) Y-microdeletions followed by AZFa (0.5–4%) and AZFb (1–5%) deletions. Apart from large deletions, it is also observed that partial deletions such as gr/gr (1.6 Mb), b1/b3 (1.6 Mb), b2/b3 (1.8 Mb), occur within the AZFc region. The AZFc region is very crucial as it contains genes that are required for normal spermatogenesis.

The *DAZ* gene has four copies on Y chromosome and is expressed in all the stages of germ cell development playing a crucial role in spermatogenesis. *DAZ* genes are essentially required for controlling process of meiosis and also required for primordial germ cell maintenance. Thus, deletions of *DAZ* gene can have deleterious effects ranging from oligozoospermia to azoospermia.

There is a genetic risk of transmitting these microdeletions to the sons of individuals having Y microdeletions. Therefore, ASRM has recommended that Y chromosome microdeletions testing should be carried out in infertile men having nonobstructive azoospermia and severe oligozoospermia before carrying out ICSI with their own sperm. Y-microdeletions are detected by polymerase chain reaction (PCR) techniques. It must be noted that failure to detect Y-microdeletion does not exclude a genetic defect, as there could be possibility of having unknown genetic defects on the Y or other chromosomes interfering the spermatogenesis.

CFTR Gene Defects and Obstructive Azoospermia

CFTR-related male infertility is subdivided into following phenotypes:

- Congenital bilateral absence of the vas deferens (CBAVD)
- CBAVD having unilateral renal anomalies (CBAVD-URA)
- Congenital unilateral absence of the vas deferens (CUAVD)
- Ejaculatory duct obstruction (EDO).

The incidence of CBAVD was reported to be 2–6% in infertile men and 25% in obstructive azoospermia. *CFTR* gene abnormalities are reported in CBAVD men and CBAVD is transmitted as autosomal recessive trait. The location of *CFTR* gene is on chromosome 7q31.2. *CFTR* gene contains 27 exons and there are >2500 mutations reported in *CFTR* gene leading to spectrum of *CFTR* disorders ranging from most lethal cystic fibrosis (CF) to mild phenotype CBAVD (Fig. 2). Our studies conducted in Indian population suggested that incidence of *CFTR*-related male infertility disorders could be same as that of Caucasians. However, the *CFTR* gene mutation spectrum is found to be different than the Caucasians. High frequency of F508del mutation is reported in Caucasian men with CBAVD than Asian men. In contrast, the IVS8-5T allele is detected in higher or of same frequency in non-Caucasian CBAVD men (Table 1). Renal anomalies are reported in 12–21% CBAVD men with higher incidence in unilateral absence of vas deference cases. The genetic association of *CFTR* gene mutations in CBAVD men having unilateral renal agenesis (CBAVD-URA) is yet to be established. We reported potential regulatory *CFTR* gene variants (c.1540A>G, c.2694T>G and c.4521G>A) along with IVS-9 c.1210-12[5] variant in three patients of CBAVD-URA indicating the need to conduct large scale studies. *CFTR* gene mutations were reported in 47% of men with idiopathic epididymal obstruction.

The current detection methods for *CFTR*-related infertility include the screening of common *CFTR* gene mutations including 5T by molecular methods. These mutation panels are mostly based on the mutation spectrum reported in Caucasian population. There are limitations of the currently available *CFTR* gene screening methods therefore negative *CFTR* testing results should be interpreted with caution. Using the approach of direct DNA sequencing of *CFTR* gene, *CFTR* gene mutations were detected in 66.3% of Indian CBAVD men and 33.7% Indian CBAVD men were reported no *CFTR* abnormalities (Gaikwad, et al., unpublished data) suggesting role of genetic factors other than *CFTR* gene.

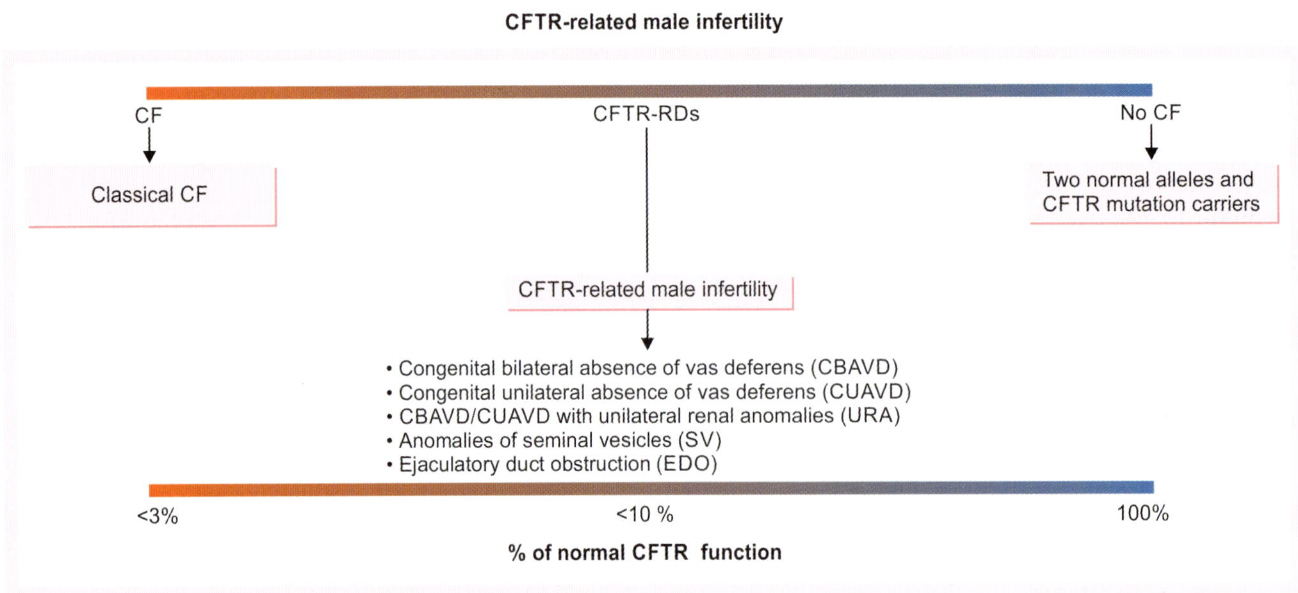

Fig. 2: Spectrum of CFTR-related disorders and male infertility.

TABLE 1 Population specific differences in CFTR mutation spectrum in CBAVD.

	F508del (%)	*5T (%)*	*R117H (%)*	*Others (%)*	*Reference*
Caucasian					
German (106)	26	13	11.3	30	Dork et al.,1997
Spanish (110)	18	23	4	38	Casals et al., 2000
French (800)	22	19	4.4	34	Claustress et al., 2000
Non-Caucasian					
Egyptian (20)	2.5	43.7	0	NA	Lissens et al.,1999
Turkish (51)	2.9	19.6	0	25	Dayangac et al., 2004
Taiwanese (27)	0	44.4	0	1	Wu et al., 2004
Japanese (19)	0	29	0	3	Anzai et al., 2003
Chinese (73)	0	46.5	0	NA	Li et al., 2012

Screening of the female partner for CF carrier is essential for calculating the accurate genetic risks and offering counseling and treatment options. Based on our experience and other studies conducted globally, it is observed that majority of the men with CBAVD harbor abnormal *CFTR* gene and therefore there is a risk of transmission of *CFTR* gene mutations to offspring if ICSI is performed. The *CFTR* gene mutations are also reported in increased frequency in men with azoospermia related to EDO, CUAVD therefore such men and their female partners should also undergo *CFTR* testing. It is likely that Cystic Fibrosis and CF related disorders like CBAVD are under diagnosed due to various reasons such as lack of diagnostic facilities, lack of knowledge and awareness about vas aplasia among general practitioners. In some of the countries such as UK, all men are screened for *CFTR* gene mutations before sperm donation. As per the recommendations of American Urological Association (AUA), *CFTR* gene testing must include a panel of common point mutations and the 5T allele. Preimplantation genetic screening is recommended when female partner of a CBAVD man has a *CFTR* mutation. AUA and ASRM recommended gene sequencing in couples with female partner CF carrier and CBAVD husband is *CFTR* negative.

X-linked Male Infertility and Autosomal Genetic Abnormalities

Men with nonobstructive azoospermia often have primary testicular failure but there is also a possibility of secondary testicular failure due to hypothalamic-pituitary axis deficiency. The most common cause of congenital hypogonadotropic hypogonadism (HH) is Kallmann syndrome. Kallmann syndrome is known to be associated with more than 20 genes including *ANOS1, CHD7, FGF8, FGFR1, PROK2* and *KAL1* (X-linked Kallmann syndrome). The genetic testing for *KAL1* gene and other autosomal genes should be carried out. Detection of mutations in *KAL1* gene or other autosomal or recessive genes will be useful for providing accurate genetic counseling and estimated risk to the offspring.

Androgen insensitivity syndrome (AIS) is a spectrum of variable phenotypes in 46,XY males. Individuals with karyotype analysis (46,XY) having under masculinization of external genitalia, spermatogenesis impairment with normal testes, absence or rudimentary mullerian structures should be investigated for detection of mutations in androgen receptor (AR) to establish the diagnosis of AIS. The algorithm for genetic investigations and diagnosis of male infertility is represented in Flowchart 1.

Other Genetic Disorders Leading to Male Infertility

Undescended testes (Cryptorchidism) is one of the most commonly seen congenital anomalies affecting 3–4% of newborn males with higher frequency up to 30% in premature infants associated with male infertility. *INSL3* gene and its receptor *LGR8* abnormalities were detected in some of the men with cryptorchidism. Mixed gonadal dysgenesis (MGD) have a karyotype XY, X consisting of 45,X/46,XY.

Majority of these MGD patients are infertile having azoospermia, rarely oligozoospermia.

Flowchart 1: Algorithm for genetic investigations of male infertility.

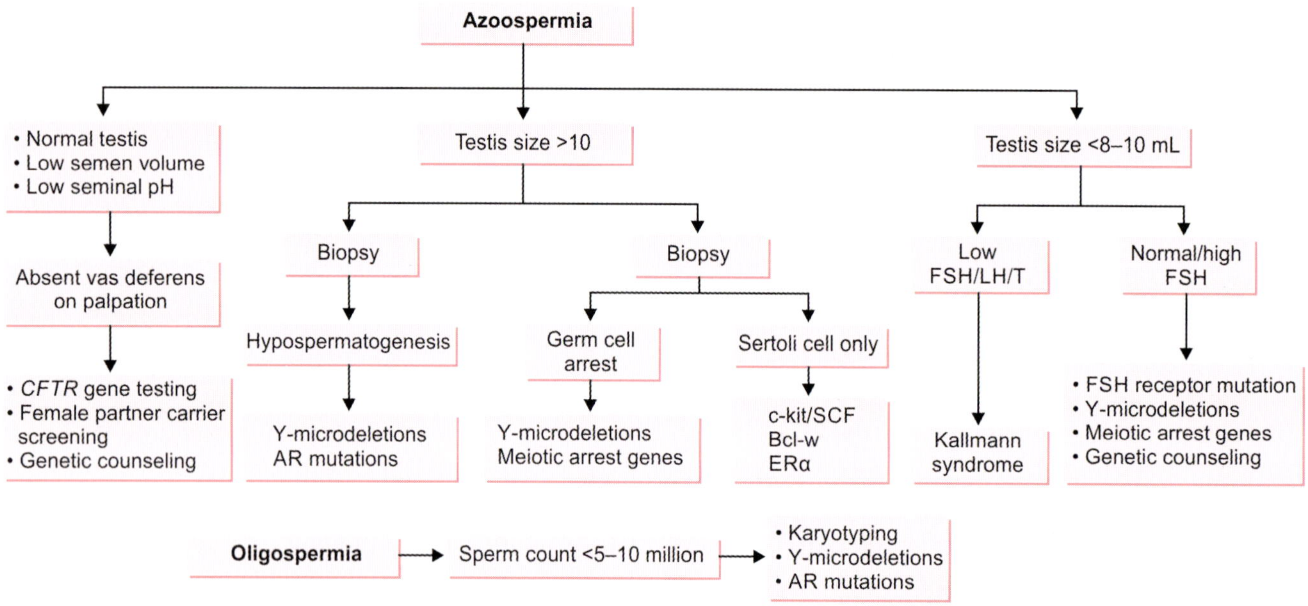

(AR: androgen receptor; FSH: follicle-stimulating hormone; LH: luteinizing hormone; T: testosterone)

GENETIC BASIS OF SPERM MOTILITY DEFECTS AND TESTING

Decreased sperm motility or asthenozoospermia (AZS) is one of the four sperm abnormalities reported in at least 50% of men having infertility. Primary ciliary dyskinesia (PCD) is autosomal recessive condition associated with AZS leading to male infertility. Kartagener's syndrome (KS) is associated with bronchiectasis and dextrocardia with sperm immotility or dysmotility. The sperm motility defect is due to axoneme abnormalities. *DNAI1* and *DNAH5* gene abnormalities are reported in infertile men having PCD.

RECENT ADVANCES IN GENETIC EVALUATION OF MALE INFERTILITY

Different factors involved in male infertility such as genetics, environmental, varicocele, systemic disorders, oxidative stress, and lifestyle contribute to sperm DNA fragmentation (SDF). High SDF was reported grades 2 and 3 varicocele. Varicocelectomy showed improvement of SDF in varicoceles of all grades. This is useful for selecting patients for surgery (varicocelectomy) especially those patients having varicocele and normal to below normal semen parameters. SDF can be measured by Comet, sperm chromatin dispersion, sperm chromatin structure assays, terminal deoxynucleotidyl transferase dUTP nick-end labeling and fluorescence flow cytometry. Recently published systematic review highlighted the merits and demerits of currently available SDF assays and suggested TUNEL as a reliable technique with high accuracy as an additional test in andrology laboratory. The genetic testing of infertile men has now become an integral part of clinical practice in reproductive medicine for providing correct diagnosis and management. There is a need of mandatory guidelines in India to screen for various genetic abnormalities leading to male infertility. There is a need to create awareness among the general practitioners, ART specialists on recommendation of genetic testing for male infertility.

KEY POINTS

- Genetic testing should be offered to men with severe oligozoospermia, nonobstructive azoospermia and obstructive azoospermia.
- Most commonly used genetic tests are karyotyping for chromosomal abnormalities, PCR to detect Y-microdeletions or *CFTR* gene mutations.
- KFS is the most common X chromosome abnormality leading to male infertility.
- AZFc Y-chromosome microdeletions contribute to around 60% of the Y-microdeletions.
- ΔF508 and IVS8-5T variant are the most common *CFTR* gene mutations in Caucasians CBAVD men. For Indian CBAVD, extensive *CFTR* gene screening is required along with female partner CF carrier screening.

- ART centers in India need to be equipped with genetic screening facilities and provide appropriate genetic counseling to the couple.

EDITOR'S COMMENTS

In recent years, the management of male factor infertility has undergone important changes with the introduction of novel concepts, advanced testing, and therapeutic interventions. This chapter on *Genetic Testing in Male Infertility* by Dr Gajbhiye provides readers a practical overview of the genetic conditions associated with male infertility, the recommendations for testing, as well as the current existing methods for male infertility genetic evaluation. Importantly, the author also discusses his clinical experience with genetic mutations affecting Indian men with obstructive azoospermia due to congenital absence of vas deferens.

Apparently, men with either severe oligozoospermia or azoospermia are the most affected by genetic conditions.[1,2] However, recent knowledge shows that men with conventional semen parameters within normal levels may also harbor genetic and or epigenetic sperm deficiencies.[2-4] It is therefore crucial that reproductive specialists have an understanding of the most common genetic conditions affecting the infertile male. Equally important is to provide eligible patients the appropriate testing and adequate counseling and treatment.

As discussed by Dr Gajbhiye, molecular technology has allowed the recognition of three AZF subregions in the Y chromosome, namely AZFa, AZFb, and AZFc, each one including a major candidate gene involved in spermatogenesis. Deletions differentially affecting these AZF subregions cause a distinct disruption of germ cell development. AZFa deletions affecting the entire AZFa are invariably associated with complete absence of spermatogenesis.[1] AZFb and AZFbc deletions are similar to AZFa deletions, thus meaning that sperm retrieval (SR) success is virtually nil. In contrast, AZFc deletions are often associated with residual spermatogenesis and the SR success varies from 50% to 70%.[1]

Notwithstanding, the male offspring originated from fathers with AZFc microdeletions will inherit the Y chromosome microdeletion and as a result infertility. However, there is a potential risk for the 45,X0 karyotype and to the mosaic 45,X0/46,XY in the offspring, which may lead to spontaneous abortion and genital ambiguity. Genetic testing is, therefore, essential in men with severe oligozoospermia and nonobstructive azoospermia (NOA), who are at risk of harboring AZF microdeletions. In face of AZF microdeletions, counseling is aimed at giving information about the chances of success in harvesting sperm from the seminiferous tubules among men with NOA, and informing the affected patient about the risks of conceiving a son with infertility and other genetic abnormalities.[1,3,5,6] To sum up, NOA candidates for SR and ICSI should be screened for Y chromosome microdeletions since diagnosing a deletion has prognostic value and influence the therapeutic options. Sperm retrieval is not recommended to men with complete deletions involving the AZFa and/or AZFb regions. Lastly, genetic counseling should be offered to the patients with AZFc deletions because such deletions will be invariably transmitted from father to son.

SC Esteves, Campinas, Brazil

REFERENCES

1. Esteves SC. Clinical management of infertile men with nonobstructive azoospermia. Asian J Androl. 2015;17(3):459-70.
2. Esteves SC. Novel concepts in male factor infertility: clinical and laboratory perspectives. J Assist Reprod Genet. 2016;33(10):1319-35.
3. Esteves SC. A clinical appraisal of the genetic basis in unexplained male infertility. J Hum Reprod Sci. 2013;6(3):176-82.
4. Esteves SC, Hamada A, Kondray V, et al. What every gynecologist should know about male infertility: an update. Arch Gynecol Obstet. 2012;286(1):217-29.
5. Esteves SC, Roque M, Bedoschi G, et al. Intracytoplasmic sperm injection for male infertility and consequences for offspring. Nat Rev Urol. 2018;15(9):535-62.
6. Agarwal A, Hamada A, Esteves SC. Engaging practicing gynecologists in the management of infertile men. J Obstet Gynaecol India. 2015;65(2):75-87.

SUGGESTED READING

1. Agarwal A, Majzoub A, Esteves SC, et al. Clinical utility of sperm DNA fragmentation testing: practice recommendations based on clinical scenarios. Transl Androl Urol. 2016;5(6):935-50.
2. Anguiano A, Oates RD, Amos JA, et al. Congenital bilateral absence of the vas deferens: a primarily genital form of cystic fibrosis. JAMA. 1992;267(13):1794-7.
3. Bansal SK, Jaiswal D, Gupta N, et al. Gr/gr deletions on Y-chromosome correlate with male infertility: an original study, meta-analyses, and trial sequential analyses. Sci Rep. 2016;6:19798.
4. Bojesen A, Juul S, Gravholt CH. Prenatal and postnatal prevalence of Klinefelter syndrome: a national registry study. J Clin Endocrinol Metab. 2003;88(2):622-6.

5. Bombieri C, Claustres M, De Boeck K, et al. Recommendations for the classification of diseases as *CFTR*-related disorders. J Cyst Fibros. 2011;10(Suppl 2):S86-102.
6. Flannigan R, Schlegel PN. Genetic diagnostics of male infertility in clinical practice. Best Pract Res Clin Obstet Gynaecol. 2017;44:26-37.
7. Gaikwad A, Khan S, Kadam S, et al. The *CFTR* gene mild variants poly-T, TG repeats and M470V detection in Indian men with congenital bilateral absence of vas deferens. Andrologia. 2018;50(2).
8. Gajbhiye R, Gaikwad A. Cystic fibrosis, *CFTR* gene, and male infertility. In: Singh R, Singh K (Eds). Male Infertility: Understanding, Causes and Treatment. Singapore: Springer; 2017.
9. Gajbhiye R, Kadam K, Khole A, et al. Cystic fibrosis transmembrane conductance regulator (*CFTR*) gene abnormalities in Indian males with congenital bilateral absence of vas deferens and renal anomalies. Indian J Med Res. 2016;143(5):616-23.
10. Hamada AJ, Esteves SC, Agarwal A. A comprehensive review of genetics and genetic testing in azoospermia. Clinics (Sao Paulo). 2013;68(Suppl 1):39-60.
11. Harper JC, Aittomäki K, Borry P, et al. Recent developments in genetics and medically assisted reproduction: from research to clinical applications. Eur J Hum Genet. 2018;26(1):12-33.
12. Harton GL, Tempest HG. Chromosomal disorders and male infertility. Asian J Androl. 2012;14(1):32-9.
13. Hotaling J, Carrell DT. Clinical genetic testing for male factor infertility: current applications and future directions. Andrology. 2014;2(3):339-50.
14. Jarvi K, Zielenski J, Wilschanski M, et al. Cystic fibrosis transmembrane conductance regulator and obstructive azoospermia. Lancet. 1995;345(8964):1578.
15. Kim SY, Lee BY, Oh AR, et al. Clinical, hormonal, and genetic evaluation of idiopathic nonobstructive azoospermia and Klinefelter syndrome patients. Cytogenet Genome Res. 2017;153(4):190-7.
16. Kumar N, Singh AK. Trends of male factor infertility, an important cause of infertility: A review of literature. J Hum Reprod Sci. 2015;8(4):191-6.
17. Lewis-Jones DI, Gazvani MR, Mountford R. Cystic fibrosis in infertility: screening before assisted reproduction: Opinion. Hum Reprod. 2000;15(11):2415-7.
18. Male Infertility Best Practice Policy Committee of the American Urological Association, Practice Committee of the American Society for Reproductive Medicine. Report on evaluation of the azoospermic male. Fertil Steril. 2006;86(5 Suppl 1):S210-5.
19. O'Flynn O'Brien KL, Varghese AC, Agarwal A. The genetic causes of male factor infertility: a review. Fertil Steril. 2010;93(1):1-12.
20. Panner Selvam MK, Agarwal A. A systematic review on sperm DNA fragmentation in male factor infertility: laboratory assessment. Arab J Urol. 2018;16(1):65-76.
21. Practice Committee of American Society for Reproductive Medicine. The clinical utility of sperm DNA integrity testing. Fertil Steril. 2008;90(5 Suppl):S178-80.
22. Practice Committee of the American Society for Reproductive Medicine. Diagnostic evaluation of the infertile male: a committee opinion. Fertil Steril. 2015;103(3):e18-25.
23. Thonneau PF, Candia P, Mieusset R. Cryptorchidism: Incidence, risk factors, and potential role of environment; An Update. J Androl. 2003;24(2):155-62.
24. Zhang Y-S, Li LL, Xue LT, et al. Complete azoospermia factor b deletion of Y chromosome in an infertile male with severe Oligoasthenozoospermia: Case report and literature review. Urology. 2017;102:111-5.

16

CHAPTER

Medical Management of Male Infertility

Niket Patel, Yuvraj Jadeja

INTRODUCTION

Male reproductive health has become an important issue in the current medical scenario of assisted reproduction. It is astonishing to know that males are responsible for up to 50% of the total infertility cases and surprisingly amongst them 30% cases are solely related to male factor issues.

Despite the enormity of these numbers, the medical treatment of male infertility is continually proving to be challenging, in light of the numerous etiologies but only a handful of them can be effectively managed by medical management. With most male infertility attributable to idiopathic oligospermia and other sperm anomalies, empirical interventions have failed to resolve this condition. However, with the advent of techniques like intrauterine insemination (IUI), *in vitro* fertilization (IVF), intracytoplasmic sperm injection (ICSI), intracytoplasmic morphologically selected sperm injection (IMSI) and nonsurgical as well as surgical methods of sperm retrieval, there are now immense newer options that have revolutionized the treatment of male infertility. In this chapter, we have tried to review and evaluate the diagnostic work up of various etiologies of male infertility and put into perspective the relevant medical treatment.

Out of the multiple known causes of male infertility, only a handful can be managed medically with a good success rate. Empirical therapy is typically given in cases of idiopathic or genetic causes. The art of use of medical therapy in male infertility requires a proper understanding of the physiology of the hypothalamus-pituitary-gonadal (HPG) axis.

The use of medical therapy has been aimed at optimizing testosterone (T) production from the Leydig cells to normalize the testosterone/estrogen (T/E) ratio, increasing the follicle-stimulating hormone (FSH) levels to inturn stimulate Sertoli cells and hence spermatogenesis.

Luteinizing hormone (LH) and FSH both bind to the Leydig cells and promote the synthesis of testosterone—LH directly and FSH by enhancing the production of LH receptors. Increased levels of testosterone then create a negative feedback loop at the level of hypothalamus and pituitary, thereby decreasing the LH and gonadotropin-releasing hormone (GnRH) secretion.

FSH acts at the level of the seminiferous tubules to stimulate spermatogenesis. It appears that FSH, together with testosterone, acts directly on the Sertoli cells, and that they influence the germ cells only indirectly. However, it has been determined that the Sertoli cells, in response to FSH, produce various proteins that affect the germ cell or its immediate environment. One of these is androgen-binding protein, which is secreted into the lumen of the seminiferous tubule. When testosterone and dihydrotestosterone diffuse from the Leydig cells into the tubules, they are bound by androgen-binding protein, greatly increasing the local intraluminal concentration of androgen. This high local androgen concentration (relative to the plasma) is necessary for effective spermatogenesis and maturation. FSH is also under negative feedback control, but not primarily by testosterone or other steroid hormones; rather, the Sertoli cells, in response to FSH, secrete a glycoprotein (inhibin) that suppresses FSH secretion in the pituitary (Fig. 1).

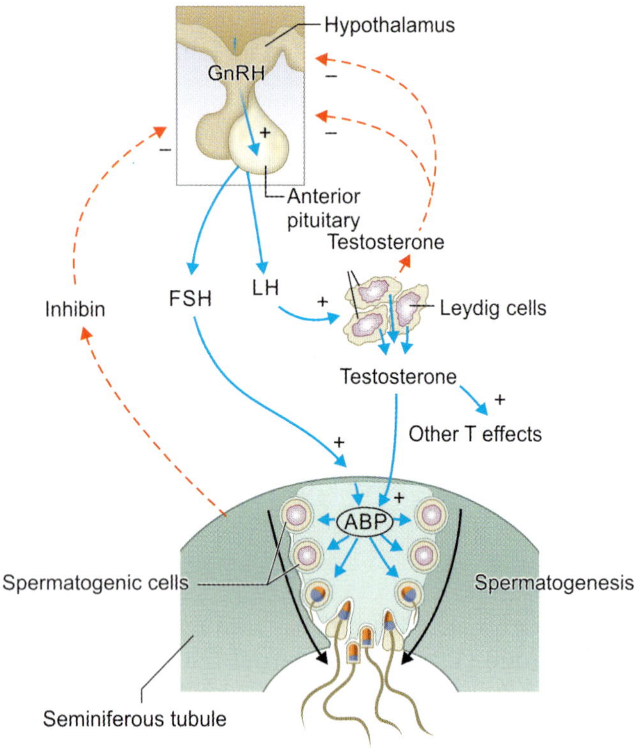

Fig. 1: Hormonal regulation of male reproductive system. (GnRH: gonadotropin-releasing hormone; FSH: follicle-stimulating hormone; LH: luteinizing hormone; ABP: androgen-binding protein)

PRETREATMENT INVESTIGATIONS

A thorough medical history which apart from the routine questions must include:

- Sexual history
- Childhood and developmental history
- Personal history/social history
- Medication history and previous surgical history
- Gonadotoxin exposure
- Family history
- Current health status.

Physical Examination (Mandatory)

- Evaluate appropriate sexual development, body habitus, pattern of hair distribution, gynecomastia.
- *Thorough genital examination*:
  - Urinary meatus
  - Curvature of phallus
  - For STD.

A thorough physical examination to rule out causes of suboptimal spermatogenesis such as varicoceles, ectopic testis should be done.

We usually perform endocrine evaluation when:

- Sperm concentration is less than10 million/mL
- Erectile dysfunction
- Hypospermia (volume <1 mL)
- Signs and symptoms of endocrinopathies or hypogonadism.

Tests: Sr. FSH, Sr. LH, total testosterone, Sr. TSH, Estradiol (if required).

Complementary workup includes:

- Genetic evaluation (viz. karyotyping, Y-chromosome microdeletion and CTFR gene mutation)
- Transrectal, scrotal and renal ultrasonography
- Sperm function laboratory tests
- Postejaculatory urine examination
- Vasography
- Testis BIOPSY.

MEDICATIONS

GnRH analogs

Gonadotropin-releasing hormone administered in a pulsatile manner is an effective modality of treatment for infertile men with hypogonadotropic hypogonadism due to lack of secretion from hypothalamus (viz. Kallmann syndrome, idiopathic hypogonadotropic hypogonadism). Fertility in these men is usually restored by re-establishing high intratesticular testosterone and FSH stimulation of Sertoli cells.

Dose: Subcutaneous infusion pump 25–200 ng/kg/pulse every 2 hour (5–20 mcg/2 hour pulse).

Pulsatile GnRH therapy induces spermatogenesis in about 85% of patients and on an average 60% of couples will conceive by 12 months. Pulsatile GnRH therapy can maximum be taken up to 2 years.

We need to first understand the various parameters related to the two types of azoospermia viz.

1. Nonobstructive azoospermia

	FSH	*LH*	*Testosterone*	*Testicular volume*
Primary testicular failure	High	High	Low	Low/Normal
Hypogonado-tropic hypogonadism	Low	Low	Low	Low

2. Obstructive azoospermia has all of the above parameters in the normal range and hence can be treated with a potentially curable surgery rather than any form of hormonal therapy.

Azoospermia does not necessarily warrant the use of a gonadotropin. If the sperm concentration is nil, semen volume is low, and the hormones are normal, then a postejaculatory urinalysis and transrectal ultrasound should be performed to look for evidence of retrograde ejaculation or ejaculatory tract obstruction. Also, analysis for mutations of the cystic fibrosis transmembrane conductance regulator should be performed in all men with unilateral or bilateral absence of the vasa deferentia.

Hence, we need to be very careful with the use of gonadotropins in different scenarios.

GnRH has been administered in doses of 4–20 µm in a pulsatile therapy every 2 hours subcutaneously and doses are adjusted until midnormal levels of serum testosterone are achieved. Also, for men who have had cryptorchidism, GnRH analogs tend to improve spermatogenesis when used as an adjunct to orchidopexy.

However, GnRH should not be used as therapy in idiopathic male infertility.

Gonadotropins

Treatment of men with pituitary insufficiency (viz. pituitary adenoma, systematic diseases such as hemochromatosis and sarcoidosis) is based on the use of gonadotropins as spontaneous production of testosterone cannot be induced by pulsatile GnRH. Human chorionic gonadotropin (hCG) is an LH analog that stimulates intratesticular testosterone production by acting on the Leydig cells. Among various available drugs, there have been no differences in the purity, safety profile, and clinical efficacy between recombinant and highly purified gonadotropins.

For hypogonadotropic hypogonadism, we at our center usually prescribe 1,000–2,500 IU of hCG IM or SC twice a week and check testosterone levels after 3 months. We also perform a semen analysis every 3 months while the patient is on hCG therapy. If the patient does not respond to hCG alone for 6–9 months even after increasing the dosage up to 2,500 IU IM thrice weekly and the FSH level is low or normal, then, we add highly purified hMG or recombinant human FSH in a dose of 75–225 IU subcutaneously three times a week. Gonadotropins not only increase intratesticular testosterone but also increase the testicular volume. The treatment continues until the ejaculate shows the presence of sperm which sometimes might take up to 1–2 years to appear. Low BMI (<30 kg/m^2) and testicular volume of 8 mL or more are more likely to respond than vice versa. The cost of these injections is pretty high which restricts their use and acts as a major drawback of gonadotropin therapy.

Majority of patients with idiopathic infertility may have a raised FSH level where adding rFSH or LH has no role. FSH monotherapy has yet not been proved to be used in treating idiopathic male infertility.

Androgen/Testosterone Therapy

Various studies have shown that there is no role of androgen therapy in idiopathic male infertility owing to the fact that it causes a negative feedback on hypothalamic pituitary axis and thereby leading to inhibition of LH and FSH and hence spermatogenesis.

Rebound effect: There is a transient increase in the gonadotropin levels and sperm concentration upon sudden stopping of testosterone which is termed as rebound effect.

Testosterone undecanoate can be used in a dose of 120–240 mg/day. However, testosterone monotherapy has no role in idiopathic male infertility. However, testosterone when used in combination with tamoxifen has been shown to improve parameters leading to a higher pregnancy rates in couples where infertility is related to idiopathic oligozoospermia. This can be attributed to the inferior androgenic environment in the reproductive tract of oligozoospermic men which may compromise epididymal maturation of spermatozoa which can be overcome by this combination of tamoxifen with testosterone.

Dopamine Agonist

Hyperprolactinemia is often a missed cause of male infertility. Optimum prolactin levels help maintain the fertility as well as the normal sexual drive in the male. Normal prolactin levels in men are usually less than 15 mg/mL. High prolactin levels inhibit the pulsatile secretion of the gonadotropin releasing hormone, which causes decreased pulsatile release of FSH, LH, and T, which in turn causes spermatogenic arrest, impaired sperm motility, and altered sperm quality. Prolactin receptors are also present on Sertoli and Leydig cells in testis and as a result of which hyperprolactinemia directly acts on these receptors and produces primary infertility and hypogonadism. Although, this is a correctible cause, one needs to be mindful and should not miss this investigation. It can be managed by simple medications like cabergoline or bromocriptine. Cabergoline can be given in a dose of 0.125–0.5 mg weekly until stabilization of prolactin levels.

Aromatase Inhibitors

Synonymous with its name, these compounds block the enzyme aromatase, which is responsible for the conversion of testosterone to estradiol, the main source of estrogen in men.

There are steroidal as well as non-steroidal aromatase inhibitors, but as of now the non-steroidal ones have taken over the market in terms of treating infertility. They can cause reversible enzyme inhibition and can increase endogenous testosterone production and serum testosterone levels in men. They can do this without the associated increase in estrogen seen with estrogen receptor modulators such as clomiphene. Letrozole (2.5 mg daily) and anastrazole (1 mg daily) are the most commonly used nonsteroidal aromatase inhibitors.

Aromatase inhibitors are best used in patients with low testosterone and high estradiol levels or in other words in patients with low T/E ratios as their action is exactly opposite viz. AI's will increase testosterone, decrease estrogen and inhibit the peripheral metabolism of testosterone.

Men with low testosterone levels or T/E <10:1 are most likely to benefit from this therapy especially who have a stamped diagnosis of NOA or idiopathic oligo-asthenozoospermia.

Growth Hormone Therapy

It acts on gonads directly or through insulin like growth factor (IGF-1). Recombinant GH, when given for a period of 8–12 weeks in males with oligoasthenozoospermia may lead to sexual growth and differentiation, gonadal steroidogenesis and gametogenesis. The use of growth hormone in men still needs to be studied further to be used extensively.

Selective Estrogen Receptor Modulators

Clomiphene citrate has now been prescribed by medical practitioners over 30 years for idiopathic male infertility as well as male hypogonadism. Selective estrogen receptor modulators (SERMs) block negative feedback at the level of the hypothalamus and the pituitary and as a result of this blockade, it indirectly enhances LH and FSH excretion from the anterior pituitary, increasing both testosterone and spermatogenesis.

Tamoxifen on the other hand is an oral antiestrogen compound but with absolutely no estrogenic activity. It is usually prescribed in a dose of 20 mg once daily for 3–6 months. Tamoxifen has been used in combination with testosterone as mentioned above and also in combination with kallikrein. Tamoxifen 20 mg/day along with kallikrein 600 IU/day daily for three months has been shown to improve both sperm count and motility.

Among the recent data available, a meta-analysis was performed by Chua et al. in 2013 analyzed 11 randomized controlled trials that evaluated SERMs (clomiphene or tamoxifen) for idiopathic male infertility. They found that the use of SERMs was associated with a statistically significant increase in sperm concentration of 5.24 million sperm/mL and 4.55% increase in sperm motility. Most importantly, although, the meta-analysis revealed an increase in pregnancy rates which was not seen in the prior Cochrane review.

At our center, we generally prescribe clomiphene citrate for idiopathic male infertility when the sperm count is below 10 million sperm/mL. We then do a repeat semen analysis at 3 months and again at 6 months. We usually do not keep a patient on continuous therapy for more than 9 months. Clomiphene is usually given in oral daily doses of 25–50 mg for a 6–9 month period. We usually do the blood tests and recommend clomiphene in patients with low testosterone and normal or low FSH as clomiphene will not work in patients with pretreatment elevated FSH.

Next generation clomiphene that is enclomiphene is under research and development. We believe that isomerically pure enclomiphene is more favorable than clomiphene as a progonadotropin for the treatment of male hypogonadism.

Antioxidants

Two factors protect the sperm DNA from an oxidative insult: (1) the characteristic tight packaging of the DNA and (2) the antioxidants present in the seminal plasma. Oxidative stress can cause DNA fracture.

Measures to reduce or negate the harmful effects of oxidative stress:

- Lifestyle characteristics such as smoking, alcohol, sheesha, drugs, unhealthy diet, obesity, and psychological stress have been implicated in increasing ROS. It is therefore wise to reduce/refrain from any sort of substance abuse.
- Avoiding activities that may impart heat to the scrotum such as steam baths, prolonged hot water baths, and saunas.
- Use of protective equipment at workplace involving hot vapors and chemicals.
- Antioxidants as discussed above also play a key role in reducing the harmful effects of free radicals. Antioxidants can be preventive or scavenging. Dietary antioxidants mainly obtained from fruits, vegetables and dry fruits form an essential part of the human antioxidant defense system.
  - Vitamin C and E are chain breaking antioxidants present in the extracellular fluid and cell membrane respectively. In clinical trials, vitamin A was shown to improve semen parameters, most significantly by improving the oxidant stress levels of the semen.
  - Beta-carotene protects the plasma membrane against lipid peroxidation.
  - Lycopene also appears to be highly concentrated in the testes, where sperms are produced. Therefore, lycopene and lycopene-rich foods, such as tomatoes, are expected to improve male infertility by enhancing the antioxidant capacity of sperm.

Ideally, the patient should be put on antioxidants after initial evaluation in addition to any other medications required to treat their overlying conditions, such as antibiotics, SERMS, etc. According to urologists, the antioxidants are to be taken for at least 3–6 months. This typically includes 500 mg of vitamin C, 400 IU of vitamin E, 50 mg of zinc, 100 mg of selenium and 5 mg of folate.

Newer Antioxidants:

- *Coenzyme Q10*: It is a component of the mitochondrial respiratory chain. It is well known that reactive oxygen species (ROS) are responsible for sperm dysfunction and male infertility. Ubiquinol is the reduced state of reduced CoQ10 (CoQ10H2-reduced) (Fig. 2). Ubiquinol is a strong lipophilic antioxidant that can regenerate other antioxidants. Studies have revealed that ubiquinol-10 inhibits organic peroxide formation in both the seminal fluid and seminal plasma, which reduces the oxidative stress on the sperm cells. In addition, coenzyme Q10 has also been shown to reduce serum FSH and LH and increase inhibin B and hence associated with better spermatogenesis and sperm parameters. Also, there is a positive correlation between coenzyme Q10 (ubiquinol) levels, sperm count and motility. Although, there is no evidence showing that coenzyme Q10 increases pregnancy rates and live birth rates but it does seem to improve the global sperm parameters and intragenital milieu. We usually prescribe a dose of 100–200 mg/day for 3 months.
- *Zinc*: Zinc increases spermatogenesis by actively participating in spermatozoa maturation and preservation of germinal epithelium. It also plays a key role in production and secretion of testosterone from Leydig cells, which, along with follicle-stimulating hormone (FSH) regulates

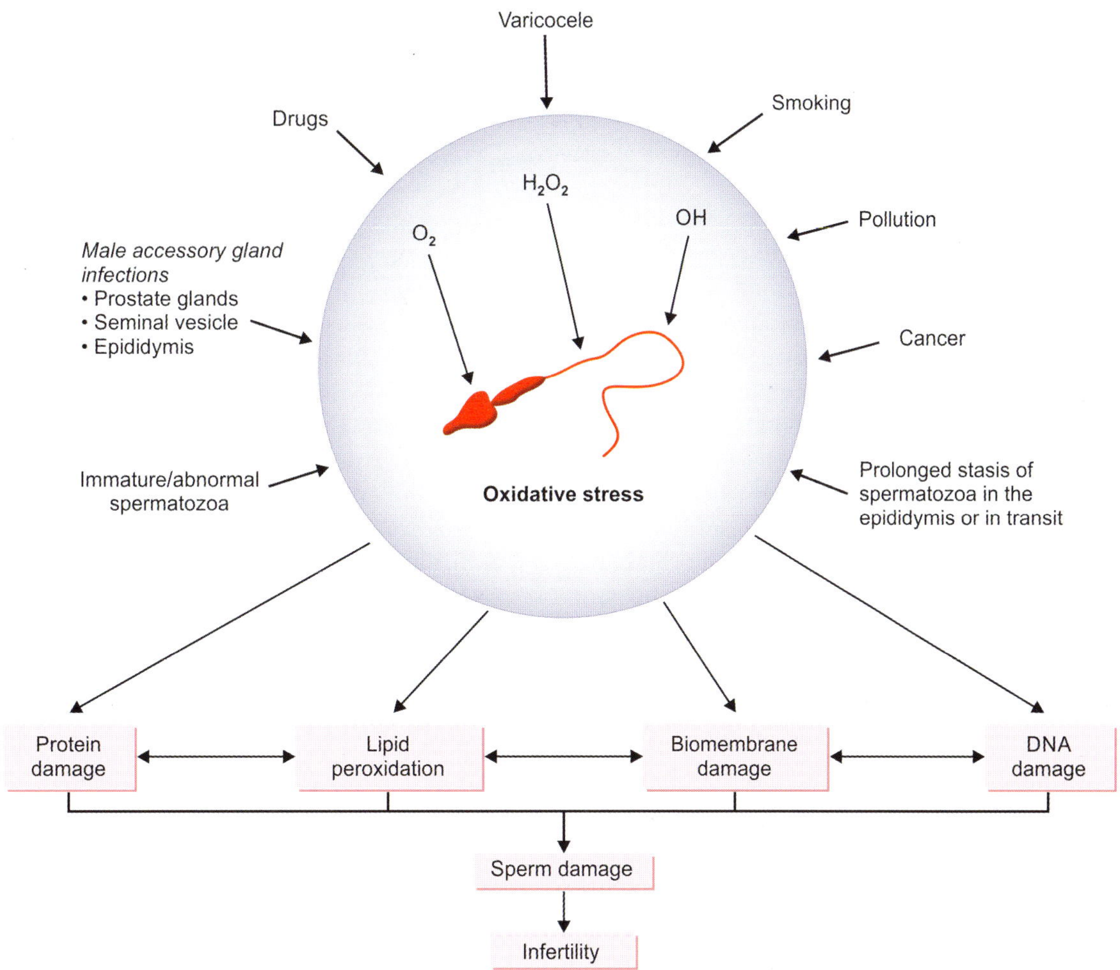

Fig. 2: Association of reactive oxygen species production with infertility.

spermatogenesis. Zinc deficiency leads to gonadal dysfunction, decrease in testicular weight and shrinkage of seminiferous tubules. Zinc also has its well-known antibacterial property which makes its presence all the more important.

Specific Medical Therapy

1. *Hypogonadotropic hypogonadism*: FSH and LH or GnRH Pulse therapy
2. *Chronic filarial epididymo-orchitis*: Antifilarial and anti-inflammatory drugs
3. *Accessory gland infection*: Antibiotics
4. *ASA*: IUI or steroids
5. *Chronic scrotal fungal dermatitis*: Antifungal topical cream

Emission failure and retrograde ejaculation (2 week trial):
- *Imipramine*: 50 mg once a day
- *Pseudoephedrine*: 60 mg QID 7
- *Ephedrine*: 30 mg QID
- *Phenylpropanolamine*: 75 mg QID

Oxytocin, when given as intravenous injections or intranasal just before ejaculation seems to promote sperm progression by increasing the epididymal contractility but there is a lack of evidence warranting its use in male infertility.

Psychological support is of great help in males who face depression and anxiety due to infertility or subnormal performance. Often, it is noticed that in males in our part of the world face a sense of isolation and reduced self-esteem. Therefore, an intervention in the form of time to time counseling and positive reappraisal coping interventions need to be made when a vulnerable mental state is noticed.

Newer forms of therapy like conveyer of modulating radiance (that is short sessions of light therapy with radioelectric conveyer apparatus) have also been found to be useful in improving spermatogenesis and neuropsychomotor functions. Naturopathy, kinesiology reflexology and acupuncture have also been tried not necessarily to just improve sperm quality but also to improve the mental state of the person. There have been circulars designed for cognitive coping strategies with limited success.

OPTIMIZING SURGICAL SPERM EXTRACTION

High levels of intratesticular testosterone and FSH stimulation of Sertoli cells can prove to be beneficial in males with nonobstructive azoospermia and focal testicular failure. Gonadotropins, clomiphene citrate, and aromatase inhibitors can be used to increase the intratesticular testosterone and normalize estradiol levels and enhance the chances of retrieving sperms by invasive technique but the results are still controversial.

CONCLUSION

It must be noted that despite wide use of medical therapy in idiopathic male infertility guidelines issued by several urological societies such as AUA and EUA do not recommend empirical therapy. Pharmacologic therapy is only effective in a handful of known causes of male infertility where the causes are relatively well-defined and understood. Recent several hormonal studies have shown promise in management of male idiopathic infertility but further trials are needed to warrant its use in routine clinical practice. Psychological support provided to the infertile male will not only help him cope with his current condition but also enhance his relationship with spouse and the surrounding community which will definitely improve his quality of life.

EDITORS' COMMENTS

1. Pharmacological therapy for male infertility is still an area which requires a lot of research owing to the fact that the current medical approach is effective in only a handful of patients.
2. Optimizing the sperm retrieval procedure by the use of gonadotropins is controversial.
3. Understanding the HPG axis and the effect of estrogen excess is critical for the assessment and treatment of male infertility. Optimizing LH levels, stimulating testosterone secretion from the Leydig cells and eliminating estrogen excess is the key to induce spermatogenesis.

SUGGESTED READING

1. Alleva R, Scararmucci A, Mantero F, et al. The protective role of ubiquinol-10 against formation of lipid hydroperoxides in human seminal fluid. Mol Aspects Med. 1997;18(Suppl): S221-8.
2. Cheah Y, Yang W. Functions of essential nutrition for high quality spermatogenesis. Adv Biosci Biotechnol. 2011; 2(4):182-97.

17

CHAPTER

Advances in Sperm Retrieval Techniques in Azoospermic Men

Rupin Shah

INTRODUCTION

In the past, with the exception of a few men who benefited from reconstructive surgery, the only option for men with azoospermia was donor insemination or adoption.

This has changed dramatically with the advent of intracytoplasmic sperm injection (ICSI) which has made it possible to achieve a pregnancy with sperm recovered from the testis or epididymis. There are a variety of operative techniques to retrieve these sperms and it is important to be well versed in the various procedures so that one can offer the best procedure suited to a given patient.

INDICATIONS FOR OPERATIVE SPERM RETRIEVAL

- *Obstructive azoospermia (OA)*: This can often be treated by reconstructive surgery to bypass the obstruction. However, sometimes reconstruction is not possible (vas aplasia, multiple obstructions, complete fibrosis of epididymis or ejaculatory duct), or the procedure may have failed. In these cases, sperm can be retrieved from the epididymis or testis and used for ICSI.
- *Nonobstructive azoospermia (NOA)*: These men are azoospermic because of testicular failure. However, some of them still have a few sperm in the testes but are azoospermic, despite no obstruction, because sperm appear in the ejaculate only after a minimal threshold of sperm production is reached. In such men, these scanty sperm can be surgically recovered from the testes and used for ICSI.

These few sperm may be scattered throughout the testis (homogeneously distributed), or may be present at a few locations only (heterogeneous pattern). In the former, a single conventional biopsy may be sufficient to retrieve sperm, while in the latter case the entire testis may have to be explored to find a few sperm.

Accordingly a number of techniques, including specialized microsurgical procedures, have evolved to optimize sperm retrieval (SR) in men with NOA.

- *Necrozoospermia*: When all the ejaculated sperms are dead, and therefore immotile, then testicular sperms can be aspirated and used for ICSI since testicular sperms are usually viable even when nonmotile.
- *Ejaculatory failure*: If a man cannot ejaculate naturally, then the next step is use of vibratory stimulation or electro-ejaculation. If these are unsuccessful, or unavailable, then testicular sperms can be used for ICSI.

SPERM RETRIEVAL TECHNIQUES

The methods of sperm retrieval are listed in Table 1.

Percutaneous Sperm Aspiration

The caput epididymis is held between forefinger and thumb and punctured with a fine needle while suction is applied with a syringe to aspirate epididymal fluid. The needle is passed in and out in several directions. We use a tuberculin syringe with a 26G needle, containing 0.1 mL of sperm washing medium. The use of a 22G scalp vein needle has also been described. The procedure may have to be repeated at different locations since sperm quality will differ in

TABLE 1 Techniques for operative sperm retrieval.

	Epididymal	*Testicular*
Percutaneous	PESA	TEFNA/TESA nTESE/NAB
Open	OFNA MESA	cTESE Mapping TESE (SST) micro-TESE

(cTESE: conventional testicular sperm extraction; mapping TESE: mapping testicular sperm extraction; MESA: microsurgical epididymal sperm aspiration; micro-TESE: microdissection testicular sperm extraction; NAB: needle aspiration biopsy; nTESE: needle testicular sperm extraction; OFNA: open fine needle aspiration; PESA: percutaneous epididymal sperm aspiration; SST: single seminiferous tubule technique; TEFNA: testicular fine needle aspiration; TESA: testicular sperm aspiration)

different lobules of the epididymal caput ranging from no sperm to dead sperm to many active sperm.

Comment: This is a quick and simple method for retrieving sperm from the epididymis. It is successful in most cases and can retrieve enough sperm for ICSI and freezing for future cycles.

Open Fine Needle Aspiration

The epididymis is exposed through a small scrotal incision. A dilated tubule in the caput is punctured with a tuberculin syringe and fluid is aspirated. When the needle is withdrawn, fluid leaks out on to the surface of the epididymis. This is aspirated with the tuberculin syringe, keeping the bevel of the needle facing the epididymis. The aspirate is flushed with sperm washing medium and checked for sperm. The procedure is repeated on other tubules till enough motile sperms are retrieved.

Comment: This technique is useful if open epididymal sperm aspiration is indicated. It is simple, quick, and does not require microsurgery.

Microsurgical Epididymal Sperm Aspiration

Through a scrotal incision, the epididymis is exposed and examined under a surgical microscope. An enlarged tubule is identified and exposed by incising the tunica. The tubule is opened and the effluxing fluid is aspirated and checked for sperm. The procedure is repeated over additional tubules till sufficient sperms are obtained.

Comment: This was one of the early techniques used to collect epididymal sperm. It is an unnecessarily complicated procedure compared to simple epididymal aspiration.

Testicular Fine Needle Aspiration/Testicular Sperm Aspiration

This is like a cytology examination. A fine needle is inserted into the testis. Multiple passes are made in different directions while applying suction with a 10 mL or 20 mL syringe. The aspirate, consisting of fluid and tiny pieces of testicular tissue, is inspected for sperm.

Comment: This is not a good procedure for sperm retrieval, or diagnosis, for two reasons:

1. It is not an efficient way of retrieving sperm; sperm retrieval rates are significantly lower than open testicular sperm extraction (TESE).
2. The repeated passage of the needle in various directions macerates testicular tissue and can damage intratesticular vessels creating intratesticular hematomas. Thus, while it looks innocuous, this procedure is actually quite damaging to the testis. As a result, sperm may be found in the first testicular sperm aspiration (TESA), but not during the second attempt, especially if the procedure is repeated within a short interval.

Needle Testicular Sperm Extraction/Needle Aspiration Biopsy

The scrotal skin is stretched tightly over the testis. A scalp vein needle (18G or 20G), connected to a 10 mL syringe, is inserted into the testis and moved in and out in *one direction only*. After a few passes, the tubing is clamped near the syringe. This maintains suction while preventing the aspirated tubules from being sucked into the syringe. The needle is slowly withdrawn. As the needle emerges, it pulls out a strand of seminiferous tubule. This is held using nonserrated fine-tipped forceps and more tissue is pulled out from the testis. The tubules are pulled out of the needle and transferred into medium. The needle is then flushed with air (using the syringe) to recover additional tissue from the tubing and needle.

Some centers use an angiocath to aspirate the tissue but this does not allow multiple passes to aspirate more tissue. A Tru-cut® biopsy needle can also be used for the same purpose but is more traumatic since it cuts through the parenchyma instead of pulling tubules out.

Comment: Superficially, this may seem the same as testicular fine needle aspiration (TEFNA), and often the term TESA is used loosely to refer to either procedure, but, in fact, needle testicular sperm extraction/needle aspiration biopsy (nTESE/NAB) differs significantly from TESA, both in technique and sperm retrieval rates. Unlike TEFNA, which mainly aspirates only fluid, NAB recovers intact seminiferous tubules and a much larger sample, equivalent to an open biopsy. Usually, large pieces can be obtained, adequate for both sperm retrieval and histology. At the same time, NAB causes less damage than TEFNA, though a larger bore needle is used, since it is passed only in one direction, thus minimizing parenchymal damage.

NAB technique will fail to recover tissue if the testis is fibrotic or very small.

Single Seminiferous Tubule Mapping TESE

This is an open procedure. The exposed testis is examined under magnification and an avascular spot is punctured using a 21G needle. Seminiferous tubules will extrude through the puncture hole, which can be gently enlarged with a microforceps if needed. The tubule is grasped with microforceps and is gently extracted from the testis. If inspection under magnification reveals it to be thin and gelatinous, then no more is pulled out. If the tubule looks healthy, then extraction is continued till a good length of tubule is obtained. The tubule is dissected and checked for sperm. If sperms are found, then more tissue is recovered from the same site. Otherwise, the procedure is continued at other locations till the entire testicular surface has been checked with 20–30 microbiopsies. Thus, adequate tissue can be obtained from all over the testis, mapping it comprehensively, without an incision or suture on the tunica.

Comment: This is the least traumatic method for extensively sampling the testis. Since the tunica is punctured and not cut, and the tubule is recovered from the surface, there is minimal risk of damaging any blood vessel.

Also, the technique can be performed with minimal magnification (loupes) and without special training in microsurgery, providing an alternative to micro-TESE for centers that lack that facility.

The single seminiferous tubule (SST) method will fail to extract tubules when the testis is small and fibrotic. Also, it does not take tissue from the interior of the testis and hence may miss sperm-containing tubules when there is a very focal area of sperm production.

Microdissection TESE

The testis is exposed and the tunica is incised along the transverse axis. The protruding parenchyma is inspected and favorable tubules are biopsied. The edges of the tunica are then pulled apart with hemostats to split the testis. The internal parenchyma is examined and biopsied. The two hemispheres are then explored from the hilum toward the outer surface, separating the testicular lobules between the radially oriented blood vessels. As the parenchyma is dissected, it is spread open and everted. The tubules are inspected, looking for tubules that are larger than the surrounding thin, atretic tubules. Favorable tubules are biopsied. If the parenchyma has a uniform pattern, then random microbiopsies are taken from multiple locations. The biopsies are processed and checked for sperm. After hemostasis with microbipolar cautery, the tunica is sutured with 5-0 Prolene®. The opposite side is explored if there are no sperms in the first side (in the author's experience sperms are found only on one side in 10% of cases).

Comment: Microdissection TESE enables the most extensive search for a sperm-producing focus in the testis and hence is the final step in sperm retrieval in NOA. However, it is a misconception that it is not traumatic because only a small amount of testicular tissue is extracted. The procedure involves a long incision through the tunica and occasionally an arterial branch will be cut in the process; since these are end-arteries, this will cause devascularization of some part of the testis. The process involves extensive dissection of the parenchyma, and also coagulation of multiple small vessels during this dissection; this will cause fibrosis during the healing phase and many patients seen a year after surgery show a measureable reduction in testicular size. This is also reflected in the significant fall in testosterone levels that may be seen in some patients after the procedure.

CHOICE OF SPERM RETRIEVAL METHOD

The ideal technique is one that retrieves maximum sperm with least trauma to the testes. In some men, sperm will be found by a simple procedure while others may need an aggressive search. Hence, procedure should be customized to each patient.

Sperm Retrieval in Obstructive Azoospermia

In these men, large numbers of active, mature sperm can be aspirated from the epididymis. The aspirate is convenient for the embryologist to handle, with easy recovery of sperm in adequate numbers for ICSI and cryopreservation in multiple vials. While many centers still use the older technique of microsurgical epididymal sperm aspiration (MESA), in most cases percutaneous sperm aspiration (PESA) is sufficient to retrieve good numbers of sperm and is much quicker and simpler. PESA being a blind procedure, multiple aspirations from different areas of the head may be needed to get a good sample. If open retrieval is preferred, then the open fine needle aspiration (OFNA) technique is quicker and simpler than MESA and does not need a surgical microscope.

Percutaneous sperm aspiration may not retrieve sperm if the entire epididymis is fibrosed (tuberculosis or filariasis), if there is a block at the rete testis, or if the epididymis is atretic (as in some cases of vas aplasia). In such cases, sperm can be easily retrieved from the testis by the NAB technique. In OA, the testicular sperms are numerous and of good quality, and pregnancy rates are the same with epididymal or testicular sperm. Some authors recommend routine use of testicular sperm, in all OA cases, because testicular sperms have lower DNA fragmentation, but this recommendation is not supported by the clinical experience of high pregnancy rates with epididymal sperm.

Sperm Retrieval in Nonobstructive Azoospermia

In these men, there are no sperm in the epididymis; sperm retrieval has to be done from the testis. Some centers (without advanced andrological facilities) limit themselves to needle aspiration or open biopsies. If they fail to find sperm, then either they do not proceed further, or may subsequently refer the man for micro-TESE. Other centers subject all patients of NOA to micro-TESE. Neither approach can be considered ideal.

Many studies have reported that in NOA even simple TESE (needle or open) will retrieve sperm in about 35% of cases, while micro-TESE will retrieve sperm in about 50% of cases. Thus, if only simple TESE is performed then sperm will be missed in 15% of men. If, instead, micro-TESE is offered to all patients then 35% men would have an unnecessarily invasive and expensive procedure, when a simpler nTESE would have sufficed.

There is an additional problem with the approach of doing only TESE first, and then referring the patient for a micro-TESE later on if no sperms are found. This is because the testicular aspiration can traumatize the testis and compromise spermatogenesis, thus reducing the chances of success during the later micro-TESE. Evidence for this comes from cases where there were sperms in the first NAB but no sperms were found during a repeat procedure a few months later.

A similar problem arises with diagnostic testicular mapping. Turek reported that in men with very poor sperm production, in whom only three or less aspirated sites showed sperms during the diagnostic mapping, sperms were subsequently retrieved in only 81% of men. Thus, in one of five men with very poor sperm production, the needle aspiration compromised subsequent micro-TESE. This is why we do not recommend diagnostic testicular mapping prior to definitive sperm retrieval.

Thus, some men with NOA will need only a NAB, while others will have sperm retrieved only on micro-TESE. Also, the first attempt should be the best attempt. Hence, we have integrated all the techniques into a staged approach performed at a single sperm retrieval surgery—single session staged sperm retrieval.

The preparation is as for micro-TESE. First, three NABs are taken from one testis. If adequate sperms are found the procedure is over.

If no sperms are found, then three NABs are repeated on the opposite testis.

If both sides are negative, then the scrotum is incised to expose one testis, and testicular mapping is done by taking 20–30 biopsies by the SST technique. This is real-time mapping with the tissue being simultaneously examined by the in vitro fertilization (IVF) laboratory for sperm. If no sperms are found, then SST mapping is done on the opposite testis.

If bilateral mapping is negative, or the SST technique does not yield tubules (small, fibrotic testis) then we proceed with micro-TESE. If the first side is negative, then the opposite side is explored. This approach ensures the best chance of sperm retrieval while minimizing testicular damage.

Sperm Retrieval in Ejaculatory Failure

It is best to retrieve testicular sperm by NAB. PESA may fail to retrieve sperm, since the epididymis is not obstructed and distended. Also, an epididymal puncture may create an iatrogenic block.

Sperm Retrieval in Necrozoospermia

When all ejaculated sperms are immotile, they have to be checked for viability. If most are nonviable, then testicular sperm should be retrieved by NAB and used for ICSI since these sperms will be viable and may even be motile!

COMPLICATIONS OF OPERATIVE SPERM RETRIEVAL

Percutaneous procedures seem simple and safe but can lead to a large hematocele if the puncture point is not compressed for 5–10 minutes after a needle biopsy of the testis.

Single seminiferous tubule procedure is generally free of complications but the puncture points can occasionally bleed and must be coagulated with a microbipolar forceps if bleeding is persistent.

Microdissection TESE is an extensive and invasive procedure. Major complications include vascular damage to testicular blood supply leading to partial atrophy later on, postoperative hematocele, testicular infection, and persistent postoperative pain. Late complications include reduction in testis size and fall in testosterone levels that may take up to a year to recover. Some men, especially those with small testes, or low testosterone to start with, may need lifelong testosterone replacement after a bilateral micro-TESE.

HORMONAL STIMULATION BEFORE SPERM RETRIEVAL

Men with OA do not need hormonal therapy prior to sperm retrieval.

Hormonal stimulation of men with NOA would also seem unnecessary since most of them already have high levels of follicle-stimulating hormone (FSH) and luteinizing hormone (LH). However, there is some evidence that stimulation of a failing testis may still induce improved function.

Following stimulation with clomiphene or human chorionic gonadotropin (hCG), to elevate testosterone and FSH, Alayman et al. reported improvement in sperm retrieval rates by 15%. Shiraishi et al. treated men who had no sperm retrieved by micro-TESE with high doses of gonadotropins and were able to find sperm in 20% during repeat micro-TESE.

The evidence supporting the use of hormone therapy in men with NOA is limited and indiscriminate use of gonadotropins should be avoided. Possible candidates for hormone therapy are men with low or low-normal testosterone and normal gonadotropin levels. If testosterone is already above 400 ng/dL, then hormone stimulation seems unwarranted.

PREDICTORS OF SPERM RETRIEVAL

Before starting IVF, couples often ask about the chances of finding sperm. However, there are no predictors that are 100% sensitive or specific for predicting sperm retrieval. Some authors have reported a reducing probability of finding sperm as FSH rises, inhibin falls, and testis size reduces; others have not found such a correlation. In either case, one cannot predict positive or negative outcomes absolutely, for sperm may be present in a small testis with high FSH and low testosterone, or may be absent despite normal FSH and good testicular volume.

Sperm can be found in men with Klinefelter's syndrome, and even in men with azoospermia due to late orchiopexy, mumps orchitis, or chemotherapy.

When there is a microdeletion in the azoospermia factor a (AZFa) or AZFb regions of the Y chromosome, then sperm will not be found. But in men with AZFc deletions, sperm can be found in 30–50% of cases.

CONCLUSION

There are many different ways of retrieving sperm from the testes of men with NOA. A simple aspiration may suffice for some, while others may need an extensive dissection and search. Subjecting all patients to one standard procedure will result in either unnecessary trauma for some or an inadequate search for others. A staged approach, as discussed previously, starting with the least invasive method and progressing further if required, all in the same session, will ensure that the first attempt is the best, and will avoid unnecessary procedures in many men.

KEYNOTE

Sperm can be surgically retrieved in all men with obstructive azoospermia and in some men with nonobstructive azoospermia (primary testicular failure). A variety of percutaneous and open surgical procedures are available. They have varying degrees of invasiveness, success, and complications. The ideal technique is one that gives the best possibility of sperm retrieval with the least invasiveness and complications. There is no one single ideal technique. The procedure used for a given case should be selected as per the specific clinical considerations—etiology, prior attempts, local findings, etc. of that individual.

KEY POINTS

- Methods of sperm retrieval from epididymis and testis
- Selection of optimal technique
- Complications of surgical procedures
- Predictors of successful sperm retrieval
- Role of medical therapy before sperm retrieval.

EDITORS' COMMENTS

While retrieval method has no apparent impact on outcomes in men with obstructive azoospermia,[1] the use of microsurgical methods has been shown to be superior in men with nonobstructive azoospermia. In this scenario, retrieval rates are approximately 1.5 higher with microdissection testicular sperm extraction than conventional testicular sperm extraction.[2] Importantly, among men with NOA, sperm retrieval methods should be compared not only concerning sperm retrieval rates but also other potential benefits. Microsurgical approaches offer the benefit of extracting less testicular parenchyma, thus making the process more efficient as embryologists will take less time to search the whole specimen.[3] Moreover, less tissue extraction is advantageous as many men with NOA are already hypogonadal, a condition that might get worse with large tissue extraction.[4] For the reasons above, micro-TESE is our preferable SR method for men with NOA due to spermatogenic failure. A short movie depicts the key steps of microdissection testicular sperm extraction (http://www.brazjurol.com.br/videos/may_june_2013/Esteves_440_441video.htm).[5] Our results indicate that retrieval rates are higher by micro-TESE than conventional TESE, and favorable results might be obtained even in the worst-case scenarios such those of Sertoli cell-only syndrome and Klinefelter syndrome.[4-6]

In his chapter, Dr Shah rightly points out that it is important to individualize the SR method according to factors like previous history of successful retrieval, availability of andrological armamentarium, etc. Along these lines, MESA might be the optimal approach for retrieving sperm in men with OA concerning cost-effectiveness. Despite the fact that percutaneous methods are highly successful in this scenario,[7] MESA allows the surgeon to harvest lots of sperm, which can be cryopreserved in multiple vials, thus precluding the need of repeat attempts in case of ICSI failure.[1]

As for clinical results, live birth rates are lower in NOA than in OA,[8,9] thus suggesting that severity of infertility has a role on the likelihood of parenthood. Nevertheless, the health of resulting offspring from azoospermic fathers seems not be affected overall.[9,10]

SC Esteves, Campinas, Brazil

REFERENCES

1. Miyaoka R, Esteves SC. Predictive factors for sperm retrieval and sperm injection outcomes in obstructive azoospermia: do etiology, retrieval techniques and gamete source play a role? Clinics (Sao Paulo). 2013;68 Suppl 1:111-9.
2. Bernie AM, Mata DA, Ramasamy R, et al. Comparison of microdissection testicular sperm extraction, conventional testicular sperm extraction, and testicular sperm aspiration for nonobstructive azoospermia: a systematic review and meta-analysis. Fertil Steril. 2015;104(5):1099-103.e1-3.
3. Esteves SC, Varghese AC. Laboratory handling of epididymal and testicular spermatozoa: What can be done to improve sperm injections outcome. J Hum Reprod Sci. 2012;5(3): 233-43.
4. Esteves SC. Clinical management of infertile men with nonobstructive azoospermia. Asian J Androl. 2015;17(3): 459-70.
5. Esteves SC. Microdissection testicular sperm extraction (micro-TESE) as a sperm acquisition method for men with nonobstructive azoospermia seeking fertility: operative and laboratory aspects. Int Braz J Urol. 2013;39(3):440; discussion 441.
6. Ashraf MC, Singh S, Raj D, et al. Micro-dissection testicular sperm extraction as an alternative for sperm acquisition in the most difficult cases of Azoospermia: Technique and preliminary results in India. J Hum Reprod Sci. 2013;6(2): 111-23.
7. Esteves SC, Lee W, Benjamin DJ, et al. Reproductive potential of men with obstructive azoospermia undergoing percutaneous sperm retrieval and intracytoplasmic sperm injection according to the cause of obstruction. J Urol. 2013; 189(1):232-7.
8. Esteves SC, Prudencio C, Seol B, et al. Comparison of sperm retrieval and reproductive outcome in azoospermic men with testicular failure and obstructive azoospermia treated for infertility. Asian J Androl. 2014;16(4):602-6.
9. Esteves SC, Agarwal A. Reproductive outcomes, including neonatal data, following sperm injection in men with obstructive and nonobstructive azoospermia: case series and systematic review. Clinics (Sao Paulo). 2013;68 Suppl 1:141-50.
10. Esteves SC, Roque M, Bedoschi G, et al. Intracytoplasmic sperm injection for male infertility and consequences for offspring. Nat Rev Urol. 2018;15(9):535-62.

SUGGESTED READING

1. Amer M, Ateyah A, Hany R, et al. Prospective comparative study between microsurgical and conventional testicular sperm extraction in non-obstructive azoospermia: follow-up by serial ultrasound examinations. Hum Reprod. 2000;15: 653-6.
2. Bernie AM, Mata DA, Ramasamy R, et al. Comparison of microdissection testicular sperm extraction, conventional testicular sperm extraction, and testicular sperm aspiration for nonobstructive azoospermia: a systematic review and meta-analysis. Fertil Steril. 2015;104:1099-103. e1-3.
3. Colpi GM, Colpi EM, Piediferro G, et al. Microsurgical TESE versus conventional TESE for ICSI in non-obstructive azoospermia: a randomized controlled study. Reprod BioMed Online. 2009;18:315-9.
4. Craft I, Tsirigotis M. Simplified recovery, preparation and cryopreservation of testicular sperm. Hum Reprod. 1995;10:1623-7.
5. Deruyver Y, Vanderschueren D, Van der Aa F. Outcome of microdissection TESE compared with conventional TESE in non-obstructive azoospermia: a systematic review. Andrology. 2014;2:20-4.
6. Esteves SC. Clinical management of infertile men with nonobstructive azoospermia. Asian J Androl. 2015;17:459-70.
7. Everaert K, De Croo I, Kerckhaert W, et al. Long term effects of micro-surgical testicular sperm extraction on androgen status in patients with non obstructive azoospermia. BMC Urol. 2006;20:6-9.

8. Ghalayini IF, Al-Ghazo MA, Hani OB, et al. Clinical comparison of conventional testicular sperm extraction and microdissection techniques for non-obstructive azoospermia. J Clin Med Res. 2011;3:124-31.
9. Girardi SK, Schlegel P. MESA: review of techniques, preoperative considerations and results. J Androl. 1996;17:5-9.
10. Hussein A, Ozgok Y, Ross L, et al. Optimization of spermatogenesis-regulating hormones in patients with non-obstructive azoospermia and its impact on sperm retrieval: a multicentre study. BJU Int. 2013;111:E110-4.
11. Jensen CF, Ohl DA, Hiner MR, et al. Multiple needle-pass percutaneous testicular sperm aspiration as first-line treatment in azoospermic men. Andrology. 2016;4:257-62.
12. Kovac JR, Lehmann KJ, Fischer MA. A single-center study examining the outcomes of percutaneous epididymal sperm aspiration in the treatment of obstructive azoospermia. Urol Ann. 2014;6:41-5.
13. Plotton I, Brosse A, Cuzin B, et al. Klinefelter syndrome and TESE-ICSI. Ann Endocrinol (Paris). 2014;75:118-25.
14. Schlegel PN. Testicular sperm extraction: microdissection improves sperm yield with minimal tissue excision. Hum Reprod. 1999;14:131-5.
15. Shah R, Gupta C. Advances in sperm retrieval techniques in azoospermic men: A systematic review. Arab J Urol. 2018;16:125-31.
16. Shah RS. Surgical and non-surgical methods of sperm retrieval. In: Hansotia M, Desai S, Parihar M (Eds). Advanced Infertility Management. New Delhi: Jaypee Brothers; 2002. pp. 253-8.
17. Shah RS. Surgical sperm retrieval: techniques and their indications. Ind J Urol. 2011;27:102-9.
18. Shin DH, Turek PJ. Sperm retrieval techniques. Nat Rev Urol. 2013;10:723-30.
19. Shiraishi K, Ohmi C, Shimabukuro T, et al. Human chorionic gonadotropin treatment prior to microdissection testicular sperm extraction in non-obstructive azoospermia. Hum Reprod. 2012;27:331-9.
20. Stahl PJ, Masson P, Mielnik A, et al. A decade of experience emphasizes that testing for Y microdeletions is essential in American men with azoospermia and severe oligozoospermia. Fertil Steril. 2010;94:1753-6.
21. Vernaeve V, Tournaye H, Schiettecatte J, et al. Serum inhibin B cannot predict testicular sperm retrieval in patients with non-obstructive azoospermia. Hum Reprod. 2002;17:971-6.

18

CHAPTER

Ultrasound in Infertility

Asha Rao, Padmashri, C Rathi Lavanya, Vedapriya

INTRODUCTION

Ultrasound (US) forms an integral part of diagnosing and treating infertility problems. With the advent of transvaginal ultrasound (TVS) and three-dimensional (3D) imaging, there has been a major breakthrough in the field of infertility. The ultimate goal is to assist the clinician in timely diagnosis of underlying cause and provide a safe effective treatment that leads to high probability of conception.

This chapter deals with the role of US in infertility under two major headings:

1. Evaluation of uterine, ovarian, and other adnexal pathology
2. Monitoring ovarian stimulation, oocyte retrieval (OCR), and embryo transfer (ET) in assisted reproductive technology (ART).

EVALUATION OF UTERINE, OVARIAN, AND ADNEXAL PATHOLOGY

All patients with infertility should have a baseline scan best done during early follicular phase and should be done by TVS with empty bladder. It includes:

Evaluation of the uterus: Uterus is screened in sagittal and transverse planes. Position, size, mobility, texture of myometrium in terms of thickness, homogenecity, presence of mass, uniformity of the endometrium, endomyometrial junction (EMJ) cervix and cervical canal assessment is done. Transabdominal scan is necessary in case of large pelvic mass.

Evaluation of ovaries: Confirm the presence of ovaries, ovarian volume, antral follicle count (AFC), stromal echogenicity, and detection of abnormalities.

Evaluation of pelvic peritoneum and tubes: Detection of hydrosalpinges, peritoneal cysts, and pelvic adhesions.

EVALUATION OF THE UTERUS

Any irregularity in the outer contour of the uterus denotes the presence of an abnormality in the uterus. The absence of "sliding sign" and a retroverted uterus suggests pelvic adhesions are more common in endometriosis.

Müllerian Anomalies

Congenital abnormalities in uterine cavity contribute to infertility and have an impact on its treatment course (Figs. 1A to F). They may be diagnosed by TVS but 3D US is recommended as the first diagnostic tool due to the high positive predictive value (PPV) (96.3%) and negative predictive value (NPV) (100%). 3D US criteria for classification of congenital uterine anomalies are seen in the Table 1. The recent European Society of Human Reproduction and Embryology—European Society of Gastrointestinal Endoscopy (ESHRE-ESGE) consensus on the diagnosis of uterine anomalies recommends performing 3D US in midcycle or luteal phase to achieve a clearer outline of uterine cavity (Figs. 2A and B). Septate and subseptate uteri are associated with subfertility.

The use of color Doppler to determine vascularity of septum is important as the vascular septae contributes to higher prevalence of early pregnancy failure and late pregnancy complications than those with nonvascularized septae. No consensus exists on removal of septae versus nonremoval prior to an *in vitro* fertilization (IVF) cycle. However, reports have been published showing increased pregnancy rate (PR) after hysteroscopic metroplasty.

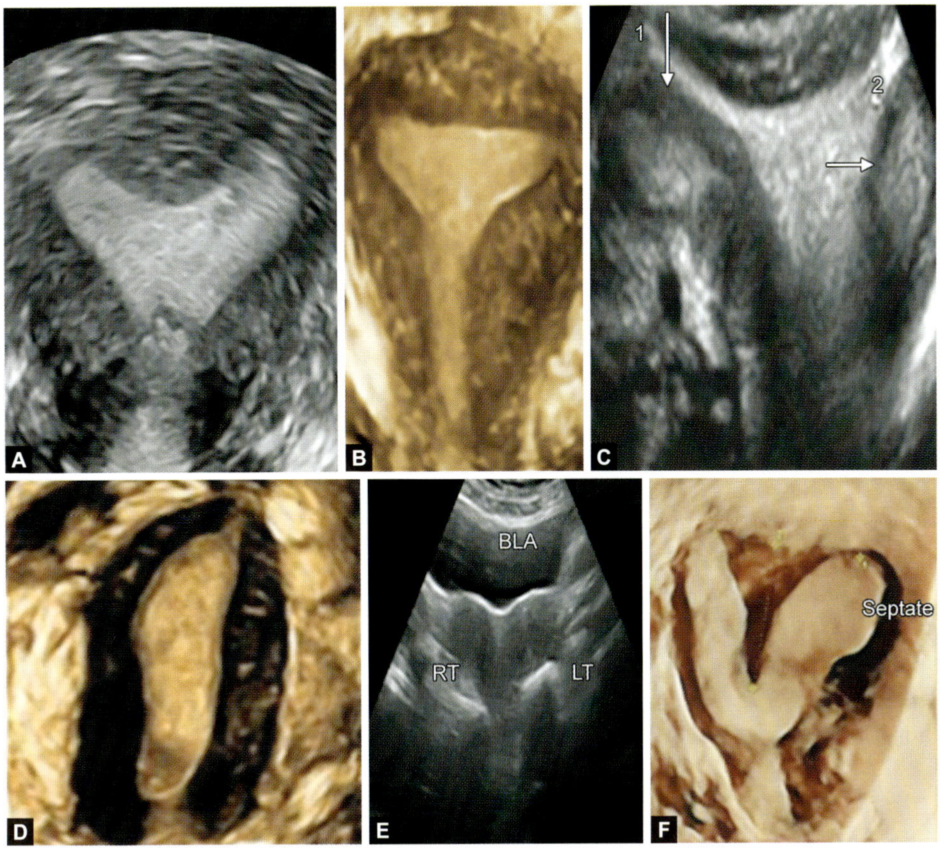

Figs. 1A to F: Sonographic appearance of Müllerian anomalies. (A) Arcuate uterus; (B) T-shaped uterus; (C) Uterus didelphys; (D) Unicornuate uterus; (E) Bicornuate uterus; (F) Septate uterus.

TABLE 1 Three-dimensional ultrasound criteria for classification of congenital uterine anomalies.

Uterine morphology	*Fundal contour*	*External contour*
Normal	Straight or convex	Uniformly convex or with indentation <10 mm
Arcuate	Concave fundal indentation with central point of indentation at obtuse angle (>90°)	Uniformly convex or with indentation <10 mm
Partial septate	Presence of septum (does not extend to cervix) with central point of septum at an acute angle (<90°)	Uniformly convex or with indentation <10 mm
Complete septate	Presence of septum that completely divides cavity from fundus to cervix	Uniformly convex or with indentation <10 mm
Bicornuate	Two well-formed uterine cornua	Fundal indentation >10 mm dividing the two cornua
Unicornuate uterus	Single well-formed uterine cavity with a single interstitial portion of Fallopian tube and concave fundal contour	Fundal indentation >10 mm dividing the two cornua if a rudimentary horn is present

Source: Bazot M, Daraï E. Role of transvaginal sonography and magnetic resonance imaging in the diagnosis of uterine adenomyosis. Fertil Steril. 2018;109(3):389-97.

Due to significant intracycle variation of uterine cavity indentation on 3D US in both natural and stimulated cycles, it is advisable to make comparison of post-operative 3D US at the same time of cycle as preoperative 3D US.

Myometrium

Fibroids

Fibroids appear as hypoechoic areas arising from within the myometrium causing attenuation of US beam and

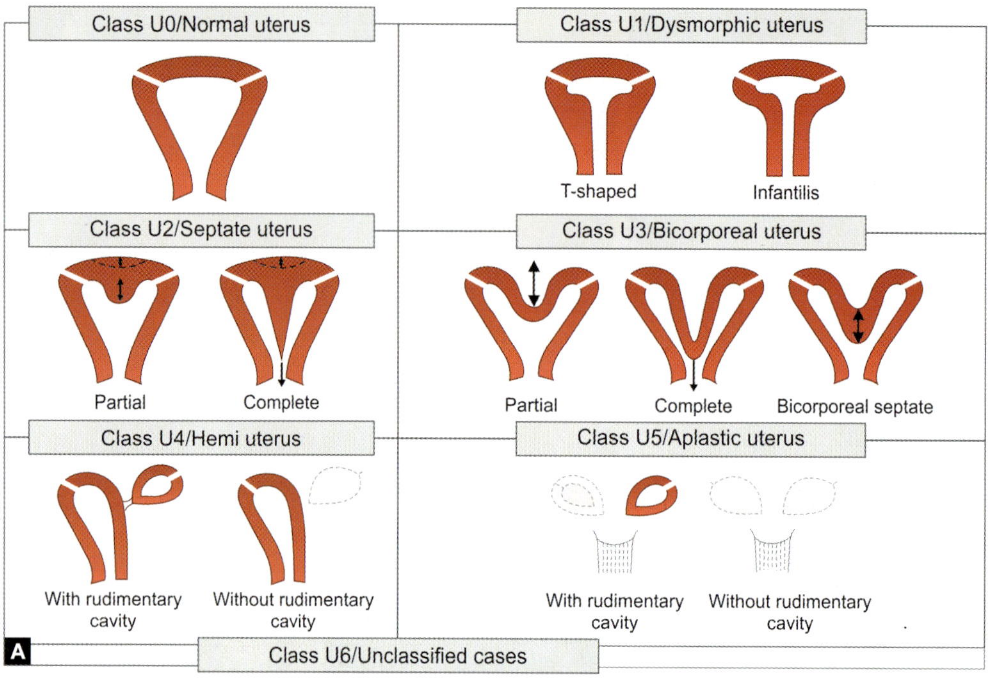

Subclass	C0	Normal cervix
	C1	Septate cervix
	C2	Double "normal" cervix
	C3	Unilateral cervical aplasia
	C4	Cervical aplasia

Subclass	V0	Normal vagina
	V1	Longitudinal non-obstructing vaginal septum
	V2	Longitudinal obstructing vaginal septum
	V3	Transverse vaginal septum and/or imperforate hymen
	V4	Vaginal aplasia

B

Figs. 2A and B: ESHRE/ESGE classification of uterine anomalies—main classes and subclasses.
(ESHRE/ESGE: European Society of Human Reproduction and Embryology—European Society of Gastrointestinal Endoscopy)

distal shadowing with a well-defined outline. Peripheral vascularity is typical of fibroid. Degeneration in fibroid results in heterogeneous echogenicity. Calcification can be identified. The size and location of each fibroid and its relation to endometrial cavity are an important consideration in infertility management.

Volume ultrasonography (USG) can play an important role in assessing the invasion or distortion of cavity as the coronal plane can bring out the relationship of fibroid to the endometrium (Figs. 3A to C) and is useful in follow-up of patients with gonadotropin-releasing hormone agonist (GnRHa) therapy. US plays a significant role in medical management for size reduction of fibroids prior to surgical removal. Approximately 50% of symptomatic women conceived after myomectomy and IVF outcomes may improve.

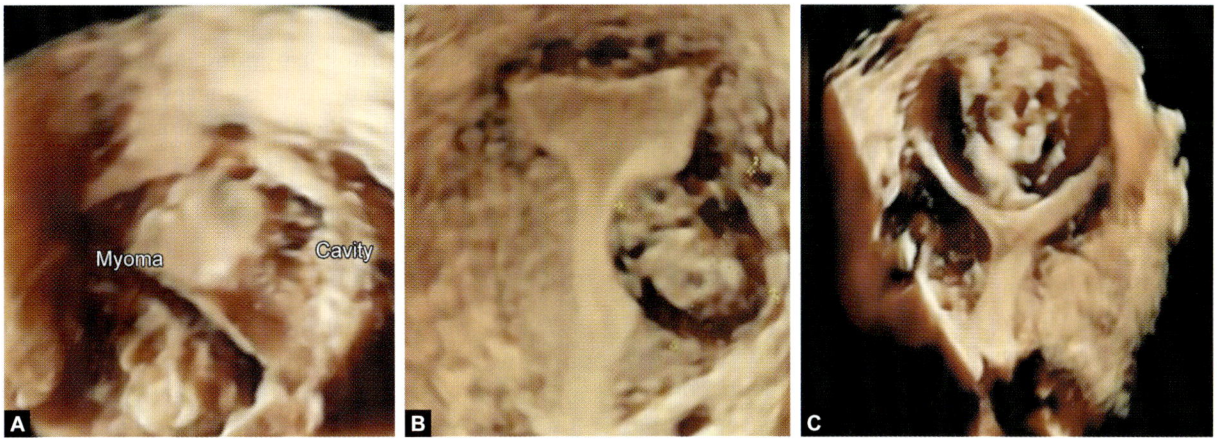

Figs. 3A to C: 3D Ultrasound coronal plan in HD live render mode. (A) Saline infusion sonography showing Grade 0 submucous myoma; (B) Submucous myoma indenting the cavity; (C) Grade 2 submucous myoma.

Classification of submucous fibroid:

- *Type 0*: If they are pedunculated and 100% in the cavity
- *Type 1*: If fibroid is >50% in cavity
- *Type 2*: If fibroid is less than 50% protruding in the cavity.

Type 0 and type 1 submucous fibroids can be removed hysteroscopically; whereas type 2 fibroid needs laparoscopy. 3D US is useful to counsel the patient regarding treatment options.

Adenomyosis

The visualization of a big, regular, heterogeneous uterus containing tiny cystic lesions of 2–9 mm in TVS is suggestive of adenomyosis. Adenomyosis may be generalized or localized. Asymmetrical thickening of myometrium with ill-defined EMJ is characteristic of adenomyosis. In the presence of features mimicking fibroids, power Doppler US showing vessels perpendicular to the endometrial surface reveals the presence of adenomyosis. Magnetic resonance imaging (MRI) is more useful than TVS in the diagnosis of adenomyosis. Both fibroids and adenomyosis pose difficulties during monitoring of ovulation due to acoustic shadowing.

Volume US in adenomyosis: Endomyometrial junctional zone (JZ) can be seen as subendometrial halo below the endometrial layer. Adenomyosis leads to focal or diffuse thickening of EMJ (Figs. 4A and B). 3D US with volume contrast imaging (VCI) and volume rendering can assess the JZ as it acquires uterine volume and hence coronal plane. JZ alteration occurs due to distortion and infiltration of hypoechoic inner myometrium by hyperechoic endometrial tissue. 3D US findings of JZ of greater than 8 mm, JZ difference of greater than or equal to 4 mm, and JZ alteration show greater sensitivity in the diagnosis of adenomyosis.

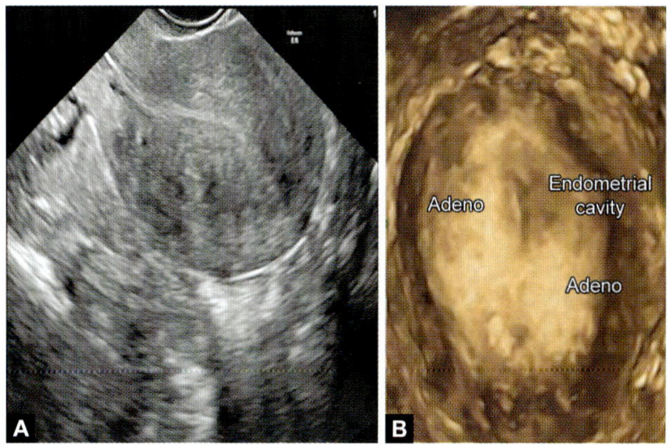

Figs. 4A and B: (A) Two-dimensional adnenomyosis; (B) Three-dimensional adnenomyosis with increased junctional zone thickness.

Cervix

In IVF cycles, measurement of cervical length and assessment of uterocervical angle aid in facilitating clinical touch ET. Cervical polyps and fibroids can be clearly identified by USG. The presence of nabothian cysts is a normal finding and does not interfere with IVF cycles.

Endometrium

The endometrium undergoes morphological changes in concordance with the changes in ovarian follicular development and luteal function in the ovaries during normal menstrual cycles. The endometrium appears as a thin, simple hyperechoic stripe of 1-4 mm thickness following menses. A triple-lined echotextural pattern of up to 11 mm thickness is seen in the periovulatory period mirroring the rising estradiol (E2) levels. Following ovulation, the endometrium becomes homogeneous hyperechoic under the progesterone effect in luteal phase.

The endometrial measurement should be taken in the sagittal plane, using a line drawn from endometrial-myometrial interface, on the superior to inferior aspects of endometrial cavity within 5–10 mm of the fundal aspect of the endometrium. 3D imaging provides a better coronal view of the endometrial cavity, with the site of tubal insertion and fundal myometrium in the same view.

Endometrial Polyps

- Appear as solid echogenic lesion within the cavity arising from endometrial wall
- Periovulatory period is the best time to visualize polyp
- Feeding vessel helps to identify polyp
- Polyps can be differentiated from submucosal fibroids which are generally hypoechoic.
- 3D USG helps for localization of polyps (Fig. 5).

They account for recurrent implantation failure in up to 50% of infertile women despite normal screening with TVS and hysterosalpingography (HSG). There are few studies to support hysteroscopic polypectomy before oocyte retrieval (OCR) without cancellation of IVF cycles. The interval between polyp resection and ET was about 2–16 days according to the reported studies.

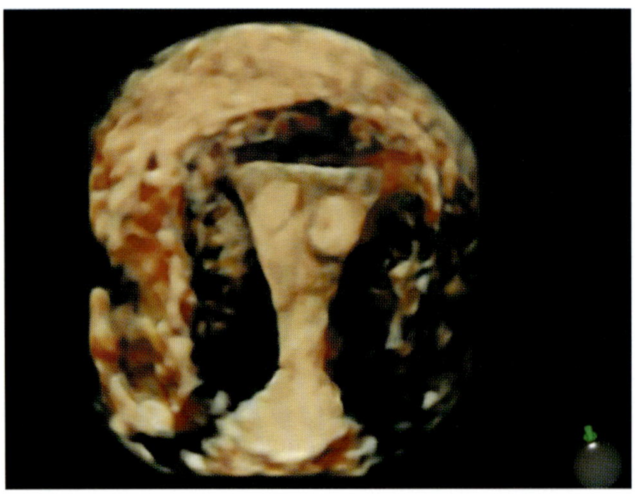

Fig. 5: Three-dimensional ultrasound with multiple endometrial polyps.

Intrauterine Adhesions

Failure to visualize a uniform endometrial lining and a thin and echogenic endometrium is suggestive of intrauterine adhesion (IUA), which develops as fibrous strands between the endometrial walls due to infection or surgical insult.

Sonohysterography: It can visualize the failure of distension of cavity with saline. Clear fluid being anechoic provides excellent contrast. Endometrial lesions can be clearly seen.

3D Ultrasound: It can help in exact assessment of restriction of cavity, whereas hysteroscopy offers a "see and treat" approach for patients with IUA. Selective hysteroscopic resection of residual trophoblastic tissue after miscarriage even on term delivery reduces the incidence of IUA and increases PRs when compared to US-guided evacuation of a curette.

EVALUATION OF OVARIES

It is always essential to confirm the presence of ovaries. The assessment of ovaries is an integral part of baseline scan. The scan is done to predict ovarian reserve and to classify the ovaries in one of the three categories: polycystic ovaries, normal ovaries, and low-reserve ovaries. The site and mobility of ovaries prior to start of cycle treatment is assessed.

Two-dimensional US assessment of the ovaries consists of measurement of ovarian diameter, ovarian volume, and AFC.

Antral Follicular Count

- It is the number of antral follicles measuring 2–10 mm in both ovaries on Day 2 or 3 of the cycle.
- Antral follicular count is strongly associated with anti-Müllerian hormone (AMH). It is helpful in counseling the patient and determining the stimulation protocol.
- Antral follicular count of 10–22 is considered optimum cutoff levels for prediction of poor and exaggerated ovarian response, respectively.
- Antral follicular count is considered the test of choice for the assessment of diminished ovarian reserve.
- Antral follicular count and AMH have shown to be the best predictor for ovarian hyperstimulation syndrome (OHSS).

Addition of color and power Doppler aids to measure the vascular indices. A normal-reserve ovary has a diameter of 2–3.5 cm, volume of 3–6.6 cc, stromal resistance index (RI) of 0.6–0.7, stromal peak systolic volume (PSV) of 5–10 cm/sec, and follicle number per ovary of 5–12.

Three-dimensional US is more accurate in determining the ovarian volume using virtual organ computer aided analysis (VOCAL, GE Kretz) technique. This technique employs a rotational method which involves manual delineation of the ovarian volumc in various planes until a calculated volume is generated. Similarly, 3D US techniques are now available for sonography-based automated volume count (Sono AVC), which color codes each follicle and shows x, y, z diameters, mean diameter r, and volume of each follicle. Advantages are that it is faster, precise, and more efficient with better reproducibility.

Polycystic Ovaries

Sonographic criteria for polycystic ovaries from 2003 Rotterdam's conference include ≥12 follicles of 2–9 mm in diameter or an increased ovarian volume (>10 mL) or both. Only one ovary with these findings is sufficient to define polycystic ovary syndrome (PCOS). This criterion does not apply to women on contraceptive pills.

Apart from these findings, stromal volume is increased in PCOS and stromal hypertrophy is a common and specific indicator of ovarian hyperandrogenism. The ratio of stromal area to ovarian area (S/A) is defined by the periphery of the hyperechoic stroma divided by the perimeter of the ovary in maximum plane and this could be the most efficient US parameter for hyperandrogenism with a cutoff value of 0.32.

Stromal vascularity is more in PCOS than in normal ovarics, but may bc higher in PCOS with hyperandrogenemia.

When the number of follicles is more as in PCOS, counting by 2D can be inaccurate. Sono AVC (Figs. 6A and B) by 3D US can give accurate follicle count because of automated volume where recounting is avoided. Inter- and intraobserver variability is less. Total ovarian volume and stromal volume were significantly higher in PCOS. This can be assessed by threshold volume in 3D US using VOCAL software. Stromal abundance is a feature of PCOS.

Functional Cysts

They appear as unilocular cysts with a uniform, nonvascular wall, and hypoechoic clear content of size less than 5 cm. Some cysts appear after stimulation with GnRH analogs due to flare effect that may result in downregulation and failure of the E2 levels to drop. According to Kumbak et al., basal ovarian cysts should not be considered a contraindication to gonadotropin initiation in normal response ART patients, provided E2 levels show downregulation as there is no difference in implantation rates, PR, and live birth rate in conservatively managed and cyst aspiration group.

Endometriotic Cyst

Endometrioma appears as unilocular cyst with a ground-glass appearance due to the presence of low echogenic content. It appears as thick, shaggy-walled with or without septae. Probe tenderness can be exhibited. The US sensitivity and specificity for diagnosis of endometriomas is 77% and around 94–100%, respectively. Studies show that an endometrioma is associated with lower response to ovarian stimulation, but surgical removal of endometrioma can also affect the ovarian response and decrease the reserve.

Hemorrhagic Cysts

They also appear as unilocular, basically clear but have echogenic thread-like strands giving a cobweb-like

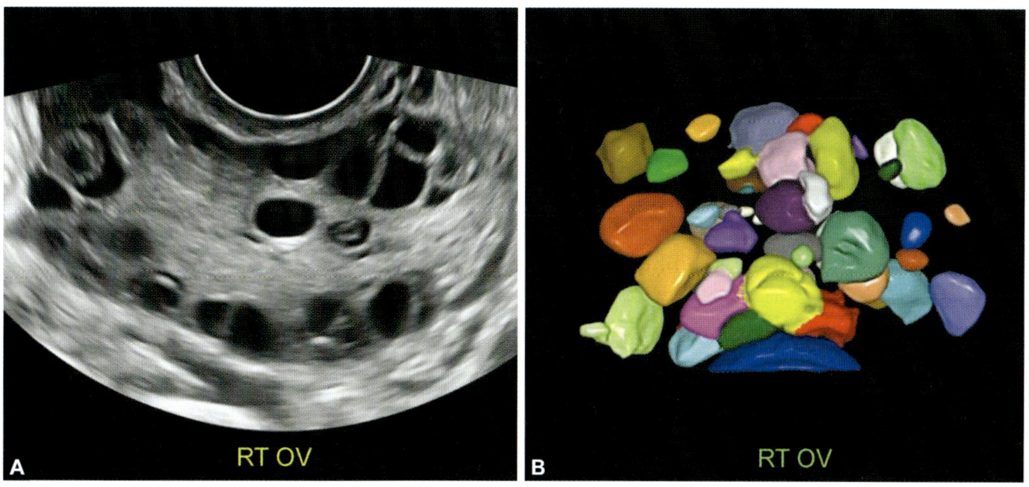

Figs. 6A and B: Two-dimensional PCOS and Sono AVC.
(PCOS: polycystic ovary syndrome; Sono AVC: sonography-based automated volume count)

appearance. They are normally avascular by color Doppler except for corpus luteal cyst, which shows vascularity all around the cyst.

Dermoid Cysts

They present as solid, hyperechoic, heterogeneous masses with a mixed pattern of solid and cystic areas. They may contain calcification, fat, and hair. The hair particles can float in the sebum giving a "tip of the iceberg" sign. They should be removed prior to IVF if they are causing pain or if there is a question of malignancy. During OCR, care should be taken to avoid puncture due to high risk of peritonitis.

EVALUATION OF OTHER ADNEXAL PATHOLOGIES

- Paraovarian cysts are hypoechoic clear avascular cysts seen outside and separate from normal ovarian tissue. They have no effect on induction of ovulation and ovarian response.
- Hydrosalpinges appear as tubular cystic structure separate from ovary with incomplete septations or internal projections giving a cog wheel (or) beads-on-a-string appearance. Any visible hydrosalpinx by US should be removed by laparoscopic salpingectomy or tubal disconnection. Patients with hydrosalpinx show a decreased endometrial and subendometrial flow.
- Presence of peritoneal or pseudoperitoneal cysts should be ruled out in patients with previous pelvic surgeries and pelvic adhesions.

ROLE OF ULTRASOUND IN ART

Monitoring the Course of Ovarian Stimulation

Ultrasonography is used to assess the direct effects of stimulatory drugs on the ovaries in ovarian stimulation protocols. It is necessary to individualize the stimulation protocol to the number of oocytes desired and balance it against the risk of OHSS.

Baseline scan is done to assess uterocervical length (UCL) in midsagittal section of uterus from fundus of endometrial cavity to internal os and external os. It serves as a roadmap for intrauterine insemination/embryo transfer (IUI/ET).

Ovarian stimulation is monitored by manual counting of the follicles. Optimum pressure is applied on TV probe to avoid compression of follicle. Follicular diameter is measured by taking mean of two perpendicular diameters. The rate of growth of individual follicles is useful in predicting ovulation and the risk of ovarian hyperstimulation than follicle diameter alone. The usual growth rate is 1.5 mm/day irrespective of whether they develop during natural or stimulated cycle. With the advent of 3D US, using Sono AVC technique, it has become easy to measure mean diameter and volume of hypoechoic areas within the ovary representing the follicle in shorter period of time with great accuracy.

Features of Mature Follicle

A mature follicle of 16–18 mm size will have thin wall, regular outline without echogenicity and cumulus which appears 36 hours before rupture.

Doppler features of mature pre-human chorionic gonadotropin (pre-hCG) follicle are—(1) perifollicular blood flow covering three-fourths of follicular circumference (Grade 3–4 vascularity). Chu I et al. graded the follicular flow as Grade 1–4 when the flow covered <25%, 25–50%, 50–75%, and >75% of follicular circumference, and (2) PSV of >10 cm/sec. Lower PSV indicates ovum hypoxia and have higher chance of chromosomal abnormalities.

Human chorionic gonadotropin is usually administered when there is minimum one follicle of 16–18 mm in size. Number should be three or more of this size in IVF cycles.

Ultrasound features of secondary risk factors are >14 follicles with a diameter of 11 mm on the day of trigger. This could be useful in deciding the type of trigger.

Signs of Ovulation

- Irregular or disappearance of pre-existing follicle
- Presence of corpus luteum with vascular ring
- Free fluid in pouch of Douglas (POD)
- Corresponding hyperechogenic endometrium.

Endometrial Assessment and Doppler Study

A good blood supply toward the endometrium is essential for normal implantation. The receptivity of endometrium depends on the endometrial thickness, pattern, volume, and vascularity.

Optimum endometrial thickness is 8 mm with multi-layered endometrial pattern. Morphologically, endometrium is graded as:

- *Grade A*: Triple line with intervening area as hypoechoic as myometrium
- *Grade B*: Multilayered with hypoechoic intervening area
- *Grade C*: Homogeneous isoechoic endometrium.

The changes in the endometrial vascularity on color Doppler examination may correlate with its histologic changes. The endometrial and periendometrial areas are divided into the following four zones by Applebaum:

- *Zone 1*: 2 mm thick area surrounding the hyperechoic outer layer of the endometrium

- *Zone 2*: Hyperechoic outer layer of the endometrium
- *Zone 3*: Hypoechoic inner layer of the endometrium
- *Zone 4*: Endometrial cavity.

The variations in the depth of vascular penetration are noted before, during, and after the midcycle and in many patients the vascularity reaches Zone 3 by the midcycle. It is important to know that inadequate vascular penetration of endometrial blood flow (not within Zone 3) prior to ET has been associated with an unfavorable outcome. Another parameter that has been used in prediction is Doppler USG of uterine artery. Usually, a pulsatility index (PI) more than 3 and a RI more than 0.95 before ET were associated with a low probability of conception.

3D US IN ENDOMETRIAL RECEPTIVITY

Prediction of failure in pretransfer stage could prevent embryo wastage by freezing and a more favorable outcome in subsequent cycle. 3D Volume analysis and volume histogram will automatically give the endometrial volume and endometrial perfusion status with vascular indices: vascular index (VI), flow index (FI), and vascular flow index (VFI) (Figs. 7A to C). Compared to 2D color Doppler, 3D power Doppler shows the global vascularity. 3D US is reliable and reproducible. 3D endometrial volume is a better parameter than endometrial thickness since the thickness may not be uniform throughout.

Pregnancy and implantation rate were significantly lower when endometrial volume is 1–2 mL (Kupesic et al.). Hence, the endometrial volume and 3D power Doppler indices are important in predicting cycle outcome when single ET policy is adopted.

ULTRASOUND-GUIDED PROCEDURES

Oocyte Retrieval

Before the advent of US, OCR was done laparoscopically. But now, it is routinely done under TVS guidance. An aspiration needle of 18G with echogenic tip is introduced through a guide attached to a transvaginal probe and is inserted into ovary through the fornices. The follicular fluid is aspirated by gentle suction with a negative pressure of 110–120 mm Hg once the needle enters the follicle. Vessel can be identified by moving the probe in sagittal and transverse plane and by Doppler. There are two types of aspiration needle: single-lumen and double-lumen needle. Use of double-lumen catheter increases the chances of OCR. Flushing is recommended only if there are very few follicles.

Complications like pelvic infection, injury to iliac vessels, and puncture of endometrioma or hydrosalpinx should be avoided.

Embryo Transfer

Patients are placed in lithotomy position and a speculum is used to visualize the cervix. After removing mucus and secretions, it is cleansed with culture media and tip of the transfer catheter is introduced into the cervix. A 3–4 MHz large aperture transabdominal transducer is used and the uterus and cervix are visualized in sagittal plane under full bladder window. The catheter tip is carefully guided through uterine lumen under real time imaging and ejection of transfer media containing embryos and air bubbles can be visualized. The placement of embryos is usually at a distance of 1.5 cm from the fundus in the thickest portion of endometrium to decrease uterine contractions, to facilitate the easy atraumatic transfers.

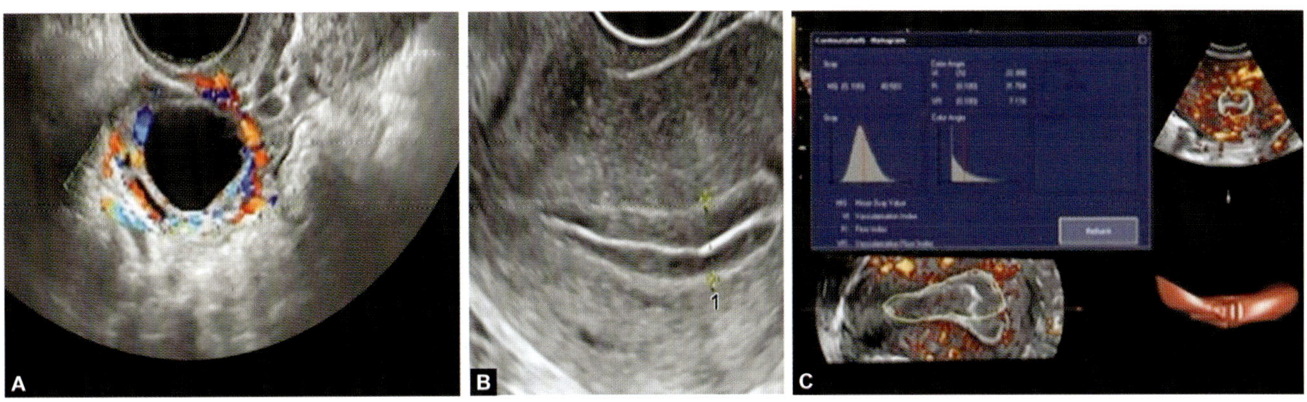

Figs. 7A to C: Follicle with peripheral vascularity, endometrium showing triple line and VOCAL with volume histogram. (VOCAL: virtual organ computer aided analysis)

KEY POINTS

- Accuracy and ease of use of US in monitoring of ovulation induction is unchallenged.
- It provides information needed to permit the safe use of medications and to avoid acute risks of hyperstimulation syndrome and long-term sequelae associated with multiple pregnancies.
- Sono AVC provides automated measures of follicle size and may have implications in IVF centers. Sono AVC can help for calculation of antral follicles or calculation of follicular diameter or volume or multiple pre-hCG follicles of controlled ovarian hyperstimulation.
- Antral follicle count is a reliable marker of ovarian reserve.
- Estimation of ovarian response by US is simple and noninvasive.
- Three-dimensional US is more reliable and reproducible. Coronal plane is unique to 3D US for diagnosing congenital uterine abnormalities, and myometrial and endometrial pathologies. Volume US has made volume calculations more accurate. 3D power Doppler gives global vascularity.
- Three-dimensional US may improve the sonographic diagnosis of adenomyosis.
- Ultrasound helps in diagnosing and assessing the number, size, and type of fibroids and polyps which is important in counseling women about their chances of treatment success.
- Saline infusion sonography with 3D can be used to evaluate uterine cavity in particular assessing sub-mucosal fibroids before hysteroscopy.
- Ultrasound is an indispensable tool for OCR and ET. Effective egg retrieval relies on USG. US can monitor, guide, and verify proper embryo deposition in the uterus.

EDITORS' COMMENTS

Accurate and skilled ultrasound finding plays a vital role in diagnosis, treatment, and prognostication of treatment in infertility.

- All forms of USG 2D/3D/4D/Sono AVC/SIS have their own diagnostic value in obstetrics and gynecology.

Fine diagnosis through USG in terms of follicular Doppler studies, endometrial blood flow, and diagnosis of polyps and adhesions, and timely treatment can go a long way in improving treatment outcome in ART.

SUGGESTED READING

1. Bazot M, Daraï E. Role of transvaginal sonography and magnetic resonance imaging in the diagnosis of uterine adenomyosis. Fertil Steril. 2018;109(3):389-97.
2. Belosi C, Selvaggi L, Apa R, et al. Is the PCOS diagnosis solved by ESHRE/ASRM 2003 consensus or could it include ultrasound examination of the ovarian stroma? Hum Reprod. 2006;21(12):3108-15.
3. Coroleu B, Barri PN, Carreras O, et al. The influence of the depth of embryo replacement into the uterine cavity on implantation rates after IVF: a controlled, ultrasound-guided study. Hum Reprod. 2002;17(2):341-6.
4. Heinonen PK, Kuismanen K, Ashorn R. Assisted reproduction in women with uterine anomalies. European J Obstet Gynecol Reprod Biol. 2000;89(2):181-4.
5. Kumbak B, Kahraman S. Management of prestimulation ovarian cysts during assisted reproductive treatments: impact of aspiration on the outcome. Arch Gynecol Obstet. 2009;279(6):875-80.
6. Kupesic S, Bekavac I, Bjelos D, Kurjak A. Assessment of endometrial receptivity by transvaginal color Doppler and three-dimensional power Doppler ultrasonography in patients undergoing in vitro fertilization procedures. J Ultrasound Med. 1994;20:125-34.
7. Lam PM, Jhonson IR, Rainne-Fenning NJ. 3D US features of PCOS and the effect of different phenotype expressions on these parameters. Hum Reprod. 2007;22:3116-223.
8. Madani T, Ghaffari F, Kiani K, et al. Hysteroscopic polypectomy without cycle cancellation in IVF cycles. Reprod BioMed Online. 2009;18(3):412-5.
9. Malzoni M, Tinelli R, Cosentino F, et al. Laparoscopy versus minilaparotomy in women with symptomatic uterine myomas: short-term and fertility results. Fertil Steril. 2010; 93(7):2368-73.
10. Mercé LT, Barco MJ, Bau S, et al. Are endometrial parameters by three-dimensional ultrasound and power Doppler angiography related to in vitro fertilization/embryo transfer outcome? Fertil Steril. 2008;89(1):111-7.
11. Nargund G, Bourne TH, Doyle PE, et al. Association between ultrasound indices of follicular blood flow, oocyte recovery and preimplantation embryo quality. Hum Reprod. 1996;11:109-13.
12. Rein DT, Schmidt T, Hess AP, et al. Hysteroscopic management of residual trophoblastic tissue is superior to ultrasound-guided curettage. J Minim Invas Gynecol. 2011;18(6):774-8.
13. Salim R, Woelfer B, Backos M, et al. Reproducibility of three-dimensional ultrasound diagnosis of congenital uterine anomalies. Ultrasound Obstet Gynecol. 2003;21(6):578-82.
14. Saravelos SH, Li TC. Intra-cycle variation of the uterine cavity indentation assessed with three-dimensional ultrasound in natural and stimulated cycles. Reprod BioMed Online. 2016;32(5):545-50.
15. Somigliana E, Vercellini P, Viganó P, et al. Should endometriomas be treated before IVF-ICSI cycles? Hum Reprod Update. 2006;12(1):57-64.

19

CHAPTER

Color Doppler in Infertility

Sonal Panchal

INTRODUCTION

Ultrasound has been long considered now to be the modality of choice for monitoring of the patients on treatment for infertility, may it be intrauterine insemination (IUI) cycles or *in vitro* fertilization (IVF) cycles. The reason for this is that it is patient friendly, easy to use repeatedly, and is financially also viable. Moreover, when used with Doppler, it also gives idea about the hormonal changes occurring during the entire cycle. This is so because the hormonal changes reflect as vascular changes followed by morphological changes.

The discussion about the role of ultrasound during the entire treatment cycle will be divided into three sections:

1. Baseline scan and deciding the stimulation protocol
2. Preovulatory scan and decision on trigger
3. Luteal phase scan.

BASELINE SCAN AND DECIDING THE STIMULATION PROTOCOL

This scan is done when estrogen and progesterone levels are at baseline on day 2–3 of the menstrual cycle. The ovaries are silent, and have no active follicle or corpus luteum at this stage. Route of scan has to be transvaginal always to allow better resolution and more anatomical details of ovary and endometrium. All the scans are done using B-mode ultrasound with color Doppler, pulse Doppler, three-dimensional (3D) ultrasound, and 3D power Doppler.

Technique

Ovary is located by following the transverse section of the uterus, laterally along the adnexal soft tissue. Once ovary is located, the probe is rotated to find out the long plane of the ovary, and then the probe is spanned across this plane to find out the longest section. This image is stored as one frame on a dual screen. Then probe is rotated 90°, with no other movements of the probe to get a true transverse section of the ovary. Measure the largest longitudinal and anteroposterior (AP) diameter of the ovary in centimeters (cm) on long section and transverse diameter on transverse section. Ovarian volume can be calculated by the ($x \times y \times z \times 0.523$). Antral follicles can be counted by eyeballing, when spanning across the ovary in any one plane, without rotation of the probe. For color Doppler assessment, machine is set for pulse repetition frequency (PRF) of 0.3–0.4 and wall filter is set at the lowest for both color and the power Doppler. After B-mode assessment, the color is switched on and the vessels in the middle of the stroma are the stromal vessels on the baseline scan. For the preovulatory scan, perifollicular blood vessels are the vessels that overlap the follicular margin. Uterus is assessed in its midsagittal plane and the endometrial thickness is measured from outer margin of hyperechoic line to outer margin of hyperechoic line, perpendicular to the central line. The Doppler assessment of the endometrium is done in this plane only.

Baseline Scan

In 2002, Kupesic et al. used 3D ultrasound for assessment of ovarian response in IVF cycles. The antral follicle count (AFC) and ovarian stromal flow parameters on the baseline scan were shown to be most predictive of the ovarian response after pituitary downregulation in this study, followed by total ovarian volume, ovarian stromal area, and age. Popovic-Todorovic et al., in 2003, combined age, body

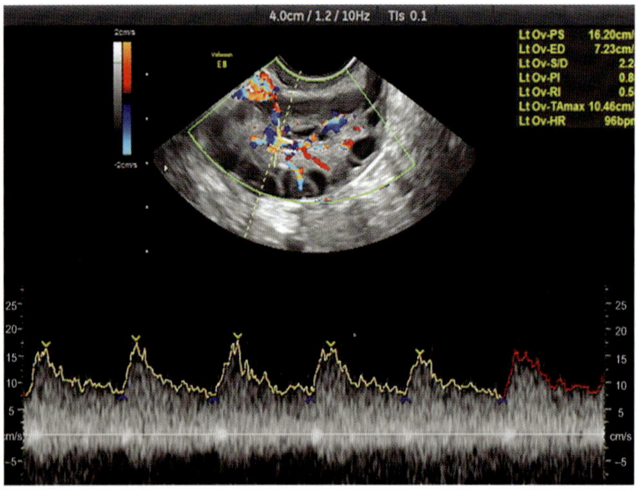

Fig. 1: Ovarian stromal flow as seen on color Doppler and pulse Doppler.

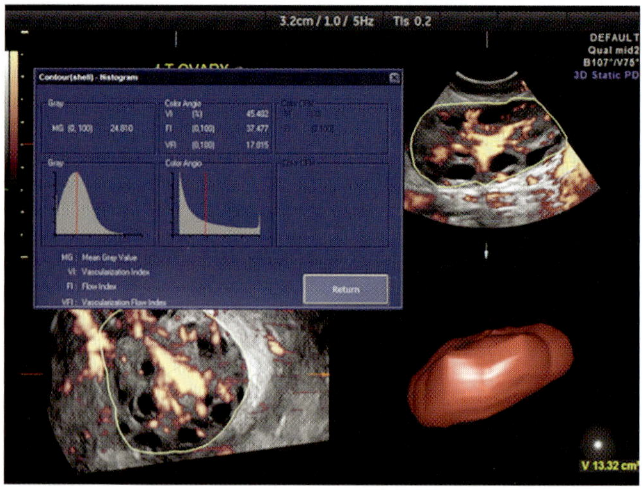

Fig. 2: Three-dimensional power Doppler ultrasound image with VOCAL calculated volume with volume histogram (blue box) showing VI, FI, and VFI parameters.
(VI: vascularization index; FI: flow index; VFI: vascularization flow index; VOCAL: virtual organ computer-aided analysis)

mass index (BMI), cycle length, and smoking status and ultrasound features of the ovaries also to design a dosage nomogram of recombinant follicle-stimulating hormone (rFSH) for *in vitro* fertilization/intracytoplasmic sperm injection (IVF/ICSI) patients. According to this study, total number of antral follicles and ovarian stromal blood flow were the two most significant predictors of ovarian response and ovarian volume was highly significant predictor of number of follicles and oocytes retrieved. Nomogram for dose calculation was evaluated by the same group in another study. The results of this study were in absolute favor of individualizing dose according to the dosage nomogram proving the reliability of ultrasound parameters and age and BMI for decision on stimulation doses.

An ultrasound-based study on prediction of ovarian response in 2007 by Merce et al. evaluated ovarian volume, AFC, and 3D power Doppler indices—vascularization index (VI), flow index (FI), and vascularization flow index (VFI) for their reliability to calculate the number of follicles grown, oocyte retrieved, and embryos transferred.

The parameters that we have used to calculate the dose for gonadotropin-stimulation protocol for IUI cycles in our study are age, BMI, AFC, ovarian volume, stromal RI, and peak systolic velocity (PSV). Inclusion of stromal blood flows (Fig. 1) as one of the decision-making parameters is also considered. It has been shown that measurement of ovarian stromal flow in early follicular phase is related to subsequent ovarian response in IVF treatment.

Ovarian stromal PSV after pituitary suppression is predictive of ovarian responsiveness and outcome of IVF treatment. Kupesic has shown correlation between the ovarian stromal flow index and the number of mature oocytes retrieved in IVF cycles and pregnancy rates (Fig. 2). Stromal FI <11, low responder; 11–14, good reponder; >15, risk of ovarian hyperstimulation syndrome (OHSS).

The ovarian stromal blood flow was found to be negatively correlated with age. Ovarian blood flow predicts ovarian responsiveness and hence provides a noninvasive and cost-effective prognostic factor of IVF outcome. The flow in the ovarian stroma is less in obese patients as compared to controls.

Based on all these facts and findings, it is understood that ovaries that have high resistance, low-velocity flow, require higher doses of gonadotropins for stimulation. Whereas, those with low resistance, high-velocity flow requires lower doses of gonadotropins for stimulation.

The final dose calculation can be based on following factors and we would prefer to simplify it as shown in Table 1.

This study we believe may prove to be an important guide for safe use of gonadotropins for ovulation induction in assisted reproductive technology (ART) cycles.

A follicle that is >10 mm in diameter grows at a rate of 2–3 mm per day, has no internal echogenicity, and has thin (pencil-line like) walls, is not only more likely to become the leading follicle but will also give mature healthy ovum.

B-mode Features of a Mature Follicle

The follicular diameter is measured when the follicle is seen as a rounded structure, or at least three orthogonal measurements and take a mean measurement as follicular

TABLE 1 Factors affecting gonadotropin dose for ovulation induction.

	Increase the dose when	*Decrease the dose when*
Age	> 35 years	< 25 years
BMI	> 28 kg/m^2	< 20 kg/m^2
AFC	< 3 (FNPO)	> 12 (FNPO)
Stromal RI	> 0.7	< 0.5
Stromal PSV	< 5 cm/sec	> 10 cm/sec
Stromal FI	< 11	> 15
Ovarian volume	< 3 cc	> 10 cc

(AFC: antral follicle count; BMI: body mass index; FI: flow index; FNPO: follicle number per ovary; PSV: peak systolic velocity; RI: resistance index)

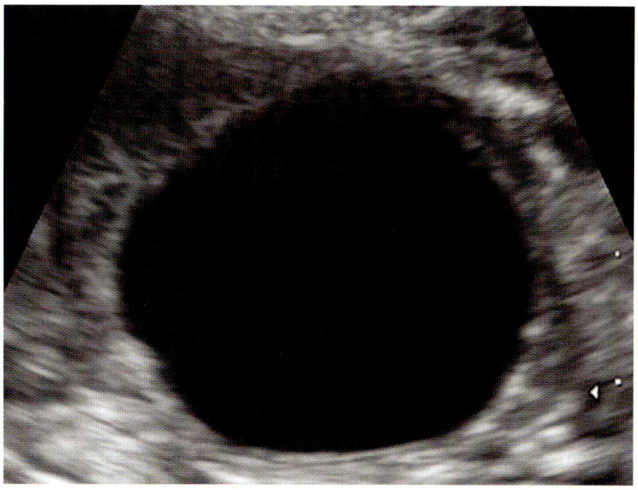

Fig. 3: B-mode ultrasound image of a mature follicle.

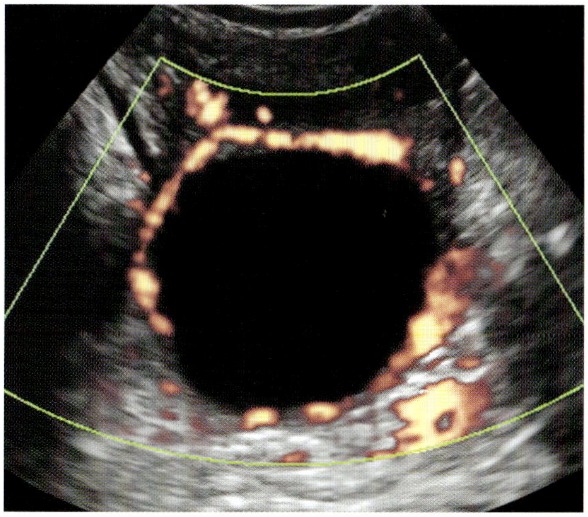

Fig. 4: Perifollicular vascularity seen on color Doppler.

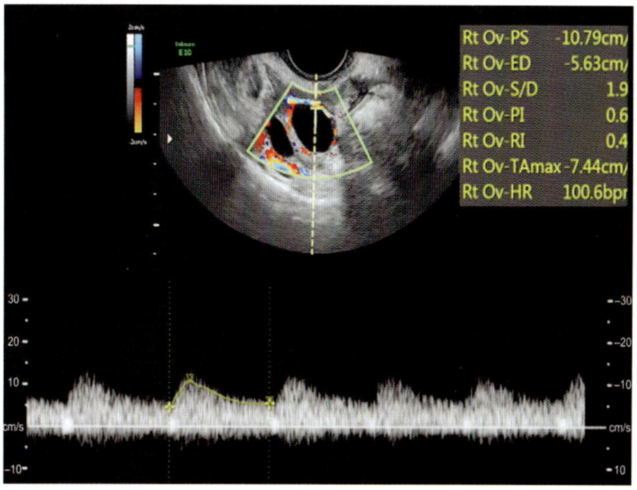

Fig. 5: Pulse Doppler image of the low resistance perifollicular flow.

diameter. A mature follicle is 16–18 mm (Fig. 3), has thin walls, regular round shape, and no echogenicity in the lumen and shows a thin hypoechoic rim surrounding the follicle. This thin hypoechoic rim develops approximately 36 hours before rupture.

Doppler Features of a Good Pre-human Chorionic Gonadotropin Follicle

Increase in perifollicular vascularity of dominant follicle in theca layer starts developing as early as 8th day of the cycle. Fall in perifollicular RI starts 2 days before ovulation, reaches nadir at ovulation, remains low for 4 days, and then with gradual rise reaches 0.5 in mid-luteal phase.

When functionally mature, on color Doppler, the follicle shows blood vessels covering at least three-fourths of the follicular circumference (Fig. 4). Chui et al. graded the follicular flow on the day of oocyte collection as grade 1–4 when in a single cross area slice the flow covered less than 25%, 25–50%, 50–75%, and > 75% of follicular circumference. The conception was related to grade 3–4 vascularity.

On pulse Doppler, these blood vessels show RI of 0.4–0.48 and PSV of >10 cm/sec (Fig. 5).

The PRF settings for color Doppler are set at 0.3 and wall filter at the lowest. The perifollicular vessels are only those that obliterate the follicular wall with color. If the follicular wall is seen and the vessel is seen just besides it, it is not a perifollicular vessel. Ovarian flow correlates well with oocyte recovery rates and hence may be useful in determining the most appropriate time to administer human chorionic gonadotropin (hCG) to optimize recovery rate. It has been quoted in a study by Nargund et al. that embryos produced by fertilization of the ova obtained from the follicles which had a perifollicular PSV of <10 cm/sec, are less likely to be grade 1 embryos and also have higher chance of chromosomal malformations. In the same study, it has been shown that the probability of developing a grade 1 or 2 embryo is 75% if PSV was >10 cm/sec, 40% if PSV was <10 cm/sec, and 24% if there was no perifollicular flow. There is yet another study that supports this finding. Oocytes from severely hypoxic follicles are associated with high frequency of abnormalities of organization of chromosomes on metaphase spindle and may lead to segregation disorders and catastrophic mosaics in embryo.

It has been shown that follicular fluid concentrations of leptin, a follicular angiogenesis-related factor, are inversely related to the stromal blood FI. It has also been suggested that the follicles containing oocytes capable to produce a pregnancy have a perifollicular vascular network more uniform and distinctive. This can be best assessed by 3D power Doppler. In our study, we have found perifollicular VI of between 6 and 20 and perifollicular FI >35 as most optimum for best conception rates.

According to this study, 68.4% of patients conceived when the VI was between 6 and 18 and 50% when it was between 18 and 20. However, the pregnancy rates were <25% when VI was <6 and only 7.4% when VI was >20. This can be explained by the fact that the vascularity of the follicle is very low or absent around the ovulation site. The differences in perifollicular blood flow may be of crucial importance for normal release of the mature oocyte.

It was only 7.4% of patients with FI <27 who conceived whereas beyond 27, the conception rates rose consistently. Conception rate was 50% with FI between 27 and 35, 70% when FI was between 35 and 43, and almost all patients had conceived when FI was >43. Although it is possible to assess the follicular flow as expressed by the PSV and perifollicular color map, it is the 3D power Doppler that gives the most precise information about the vascularization and follicular blood flow. hCG plays a major role in inducing influx of blood within follicles. At the luteinizing hormone (LH) surge, the perifollicular PSV is 10 cm/sec. This means that if the follicle is said to be functionally mature when PSV is 10 cm/sec, that is the time when the LH surge starts and under the effect of that LH, the perifollicular PSV keeps on rising constantly. This derives that a rising PSV with steady low RI suggests that the follicle is close to rupture.

Implantation has been the weakest link in the success of infertility treatment. Endometrium is a receptor organ for majority of the hormones involved in fertility and therefore study of its morphology and vascularity is thought to explain the mysteries of implantation failure. Therefore, like follicle, endometrium is also assessed by transvaginal 2D US and color Doppler before planning for hCG during any ARTs.

B-mode Features of Endometrium with Good Receptivity

On transvaginal sonography (TVS), an endometrial thickness of minimum 6 mm is required on the day of hCG, but 8–10 mm is optimum. Endometrial thickness has more negative predictive value for implantation. But it is also important to remember that endometrium also has a definite growth rate and the healthy one is 1–2 mm a day. The dynamicity of the endometrium is an important feature to be documented while evaluating the endometrium for its receptivity. Morphology of the endometrium is as important as thickness of the endometrium. In all the healthy endometria, the endometrio-myometrial interface is always seen as a clear hypoechoic halo surrounding the whole endometrium. Breach or irregularity of endometrio-myometrial junction is an indication of unhealthy endometrium and therefore poor receptivity.

Popularly multilayered endometrium is considered as a desired endometrial pattern (Fig. 6). Morphologically, the endometrium is graded as the best grade A, when it is a triple line endometrium with the intervening area as hypoechoic as the anterior myometrium. This is because of secretions in endometrial glands and scarce stromal edema. The endometrium is graded as intermediate or grade B when it is multilayered or triple line with hypoechoic intervening area. In grade C or the most unfavorable endometrium would

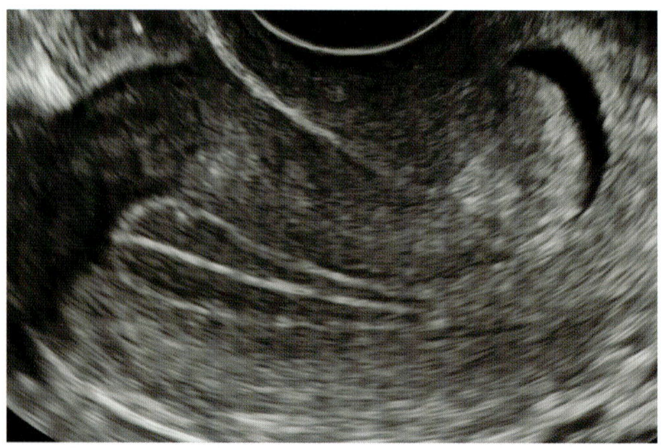

Fig. 6: B-mode ultrasound image of multilayered endometrium.

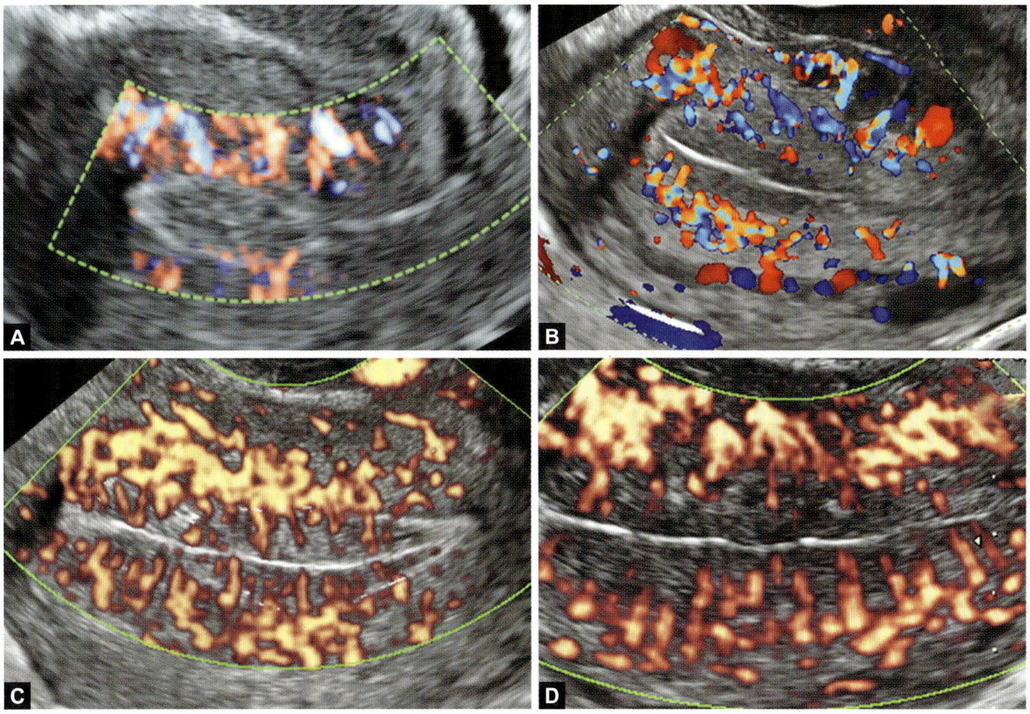

Figs. 7A to D: Doppler images of the zones 1–4 endometrial vascularity clockwise starting from left upper image.

be a homogeneous isoechoic endometrium. Though some studies have shown no significant difference in pregnancy rates amongst different morphological patterns.

There are several reports by different groups that agree on the fact that implantation rates can be more correlated to the vascularity of the endometrium rather than the thickness and morphology of the endometrium.

Doppler Features of Endometrium with Good Receptivity

Segmental uterine artery perfusion demonstrates significant correlation with hormonal and histological markers of uterine receptivity, reaching the highest sensitivity for subendometrial blood flow. On color Doppler, the endometrium that has good receptivity should show vascularity in zones 3 and 4 or may be called subendometrial and endometrial layers (Figs. 7A to D).

The zones of vascularity are defined according to Applebaum as zone 1 when the vascularity on power Doppler is seen only up to endometrio-myometrial junction, zone 2 when vessels penetrate through the hyperechogenic endometrial edge, zone 3 when blood vessels reach intervening hypoechogenic zone, and zone 4 when vessels reach the endometrial cavity. The pregnancy rates related to the zones of vascular penetration are 26.7% for zone 1, 36.4% for zone 2, and 37.9% for zone 3.

TABLE 2 Correlation of endometrial vascularity zone and conception rates.

Vascularity	*Conception rate study 1*	*Conception rate study 2*
Zone 1	3.5–7.5%	5.2%
Zone 2	15.8–29.7%	28.7%
Zone 3	24.2–47.8%	52%
Zone 4	67.3%	74%

TABLE 3 Endometrial vascularity zone and conception and abortion rates.

Vascularity	*Zone 1*	*Zone 2*	*Zone 3*	*Zone 4*
% of patients	6.69%	20.73%	58%	14.47%
+ β-hCG	19%	21.87%	39.77%	70.14%
Gestational sac	9.6%	14.58%	36.8%	68.65%
Abortions	50%	23.8%	5.6%	1.5%

(β-hCG: beta human chorionic gonadotropin)

One more comparative study has also shown similar results (Table 2).

Another study has shown not only higher conception rates but significantly low abortion rates when the vascularity was present in zones 3 and 4 (Table 3).

Zaidi et al. reported that absence of flow in the endometrial and subendometrial zones on day of hCG indicates total failure of implantation. The vessels that reach

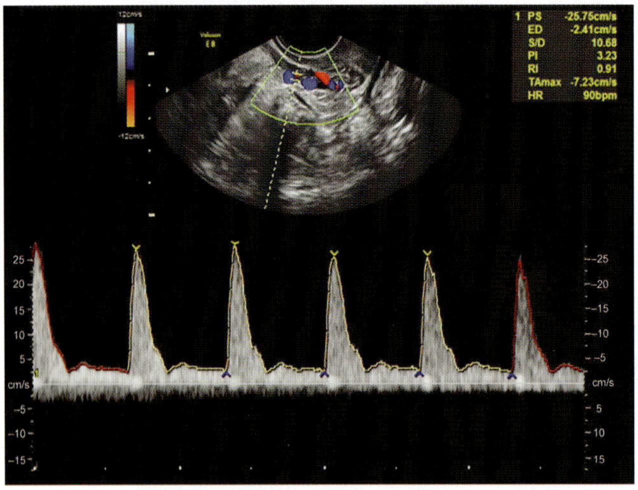

Fig. 8: Pulse Doppler image showing high resistance uterine artery flow waveform.

TABLE 4 Parameters indicating pretrigger follicular maturity and endometrial receptivity.

	Follicle	*Endometrium*
Size/thickness	16–18 mm	8–10 mm
Morphology	Thin wall, no internal echoes, halo	Grade A/B
Vascularity	3/4th circumference	Zone 3–4
RI	0.4–0.48	< 0.5
PSV	>10 cm/sec	–
Uterine artery PI	–	< 3.2
Volume	3–7 cc	3–7 cc
3D morphology	Cumulus	Intact endo-myo junction
3D PD	More symmetrical the better	Higher the better

(PD: power Doppler; PSV: peak systolic velocity; RI: resistance index; PI: pulsatility index)

the endometrium are the spiral arteries. The pulse Doppler of these arteries should have an RI of between 0.6 and 0.8 or PI of between 1.1 and 2.3 for the endometrium to be called receptive for implantation.

Moreover, the pulse Doppler analysis of the uterine artery waveform is done and its PI should be <3.2 (Fig. 8). Several authors have shown that the optimum uterine receptivity was obtained when average PI of the uterine artery was between 2 and 3 on the day of transfer or on the day of hCG. Coulam et al. have also shown that no pregnancy was achieved after embryo transfer when uterine artery PI was above 3.3 in an IVF program. Cacciatore et al. reported that implantation is unlikely when PI is >3.3 and RI >0.95 or when no velocities are seen at the end of the diastole. In such cases therefore in IUI cycles, hCG is withhold or postponed till satisfactory Doppler parameters are achieved and in IVF cycles, embryos are frozen for transfer in subsequent cycles when optimum Doppler parameters are achieved.

Three-dimensional power Doppler assessment of the endometrium gives idea about the global vascularity of the endometrium. This can be assessed subjectively, but the 3D power Doppler parameters—vascularization index (VI), FI, and VFI give more precise information about the vascularity of the endometrium. Endometrial volume by 3D US volume calculation of the endometrium may help to correlate the cycle outcome with quantitative parameter rather than endometrial thickness. Study by Kupesic et al. also shows no pregnancy when endometrial volume was <2 mL, or when exceeded 8 mL. According to a study by Merce et al., no pregnancy was achieved when endometrial volume was <3 mL and VI was <10, whereas exceptionally better pregnancy rates are achieved with endometrial volume >7 mL and subendometrial VI between 10% and 35%.

A study by Kupesic et al. shows lower resistance index of 0.49–0.57 in subendometrial vessels and FI of 11.0–15.4 as compared to 9.5–13.3 otherwise in the conception cycles.

In spite of so much of evidence that clearly shows better conception rates when the endometrium shows better vascularity, a clear correlation between the endometrial vascularity and the pregnancy rates has not been proved. This is because implantation is not a function of endometrium alone; the embryo also needs to be of a good quality to achieve pregnancy. Correlation between the endometrial Doppler indices and conception rates has been demonstrated when non-grade 1 embryos are transfered.

To summarize, the ultrasound features of follicular maturity and good endometrial receptivity are shown in Table 4.

Secretory Phase Assessment

Rupture of the follicle leads to formation of corpus luteum. Corpus luteum is responsible for progesterone production. The functional efficacy of the corpus luteum can be assessed by Doppler by assessing the pericorpus luteal vascularity.

A clear correlation between RI of corpus luteum and plasma progesterone levels has been seen in natural cycle. RI of the corpus luteum can therefore be used as an adjunct to plasma progesterone assay as an index of luteal function. A corpus luteum that is functionally normal and produces adequate amount of progesterone shows corpus luteal flow: RI 0.35–0.50 (Figs. 9A and B).

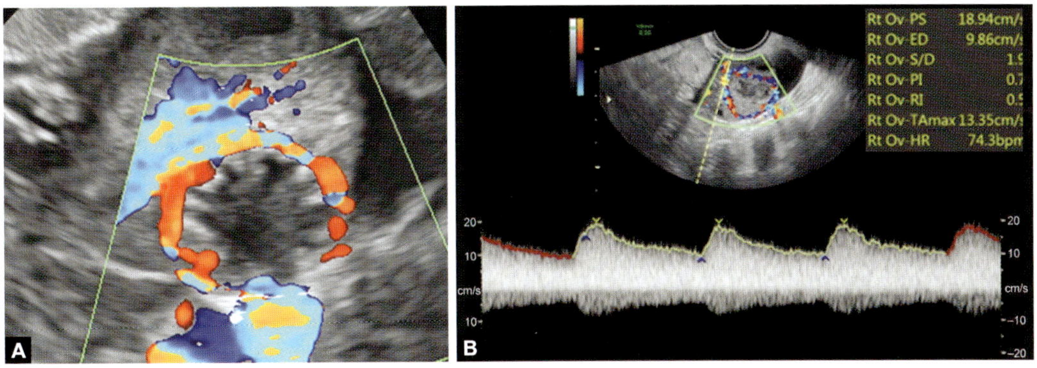

Figs. 9A and B: Normal corpus luteal flow seen on (A) color Doppler and (B) pulse Doppler.

TABLE 5 Follicular and corpus luteal RI in normal cycle and in patient with luteal phase defect.

Phase	*Normal RI*	*LPD RI*
Perifollicular	0.56 ± 0.06	0.58 ± 0.04
LH peak day	0.44 ± 0.04	0.58 ± 0.04
Midluteal phase	0.42 ± 0.06	0.58 ± 0.04
Late luteal phase	0.50 ± 0.04	0.58 ± 0.04

(LPD: luteal phase defect; RI: resistance index).

TABLE 6 Endometrial RI in normal cycle and in patient with luteal phase defect.

Phase	*Control RI*	*LPD RI*
Periovulatory	0.53 ± 0.04	0.70 ± 0.06
Midluteal	0.50 ± 0.02	0.72 ± 0.06
Late luteal	0.51 ± 0.04	0.72 ± 0.04

(LPD: luteal phase defect; RI: resistance index).

The receptor organ for progesterone also (like estrogen) is endometrium and its vascular studies can be a reliable clue to adequate progesterone production. Soon after rupture of the follicle, the outer margin of the endometrium starts becoming fluffy and blurred. It is after this that the endometrial outer margin starts becoming hyperechoic and the hyperechogenicity progresses toward the central line of the endometrium, to make the entire endometrium hyperechoic in the mid-luteal phase. With adequate progesterone levels, in the mid-luteal phase, the spiral arteries show RI 0.48–0.52 (low resistance flow) and uterine artery shows PI of 2.0–2.5. The flow is assessed in the uterine artery of the dominant side (on the side of ovulation). This PI is lower than observed in the preovulatory phase because of smooth muscle relaxing effect of progesterone. Inadequate progesterone production due to corpus luteal inadequacy is suggested by high resistance flow in corpus luteal vessels. Whereas high spiral artery resistance would suggest inadequate response of endometrium to progesterone. This is because of inadequate progesterone receptors in the endometrium or because of local endometrial cause, like endometrial injury or chronic endometritis.

In luteal phase defect because of low progesterone levels, the resistance in the peri-corpus luteal vessels is high. Because of low progesterone levels, there is inadequate relaxation of the muscularis of the uterine artery and therefore the uterine artery resistance is high along with higher resistance in its branches—the spiral vessels.

Comparative values of corpus luteal RI and spiral artery RI in normal cycle and luteal phase defect are shown in the Tables 5 and 6.

CONCLUSION

Ultrasound is an excellent tool for assessment of the menstrual cycle. Hormonal changes occurring day to day during the menstrual cycle reflect as morphological and vascular changes in the ovary and the uterus. Assessing these changes by transvaginal ultrasound and Doppler and correctly interpreting can explain the hormonal basis of these changes. Ultrasound with Doppler can thus be used as the only modality for cycle assessment in patients undergoing assisted reproduction technology and may be of help to reduce the cost of the cycle by avoiding certain hormonal assessments and still maintaining close and accurate watch on the hormonal changes occurring during treatment cycle.

EDITORS' COMMENTS

1. Color Doppler in infertility can prove to be a very informative technique when used with expertise in medicated situation.
2. Color Doppler evaluation of endometrium and uterine artery parameters can help to give additional information and could have prognostic value in ART outcome.
3. Doppler evaluation of dominant follicles, ovaries, and uterine flow can help to some extent in optimizing ART outcome.

SUGGESTED READING

1. Applebaum M. The 'steel' or 'teflon' endometrium—ultrasound visualization of endometrial vascularity in IVF patients and outcome. Presented at The third World Congress of Ultrasound in Obstetrics and Gynecology. Ultrasound Obstet Gynecol. 1993;3(Suppl 2):10.
2. Arora A, Gainder S, Dhaliwal L, et al. Clinical significance of ovarian stromal blood flow in assessment of ovarian response in stimulated cycle for in vitro fertilization. Int J Reprod Contracept Obstet Gynecol. 2015;4(5):1380-3.
3. Bourne TH, Jurkovic D, Waterstone J, et al. Intrafollicular blood flow during human ovulation. Ultrasound Obstet Gynecol. 1991;1:53-9.
4. Brannstrorm M, Zackrisson U, Hangstroom HG, et al. Preovulatory changes of blood flow in different regions of the human follicle. Fertil Steril. 1998;69:435-42.
5. Cacciatore B, Simberg N, Fusaro P, et al. Transvaginal Doppler study of uterine artery blood flow in in vitro fertilization embryo transfer cycles. Fertil Steril. 1996;66:130-4.
6. Chui DK, Pugh ND, Walker SM, et al. Follicular vascularity—the predictive value of transvaginal power doppler ultrasonography in an in-vitro fertilization programme: a preliminary study. Hum Reprod. 1997;12(1):191-6.
7. Coulam CB, Stern JJ, Soenksen DM, et al. Comparison of pulsatility indexes on the day of oocyte retrieval and embryo transfer. Hum Reprod. 1995;10:82-4.
8. Engmann L, Saldkevicius P, Agrawal R, et al. Value of ovarian stromal blood flow velocity measurement after pituitary suppression in the prediction of ovarian responsiveness and outcome of in vitro fertilization treatment. Fertil Steril. 1999;71(1):22-9.
9. Fleischer AC, Keppe DM. Benign conditions of the uterus, cervix and endometrium. In: Nyberg A, Hill LM, Bohm-Velez M, Mendelson EB (Eds). Transvaginal Ultrasound. St Louis: Mosby Year Book; 1992. pp. 21-43.
10. Glock JL, Brumsted JR. Colour flow pulsed Doppler ultrasound in diagnosing luteal phase defect. Fertil Steril. 1995;64:500-4.
11. Jokubkeine L, Sladkevicius P, Rovas L, et al. Assessment of changes in volume and vascularity of ovaries during the normal menstrual cycle using three dimensional power Doppler ultrasound. Hum Reprod. 2006;21(10):2661-8.
12. Kupesic S, Bekavac I, Bjelos D, et al. Assessment of endometrial receptivity by transvaginal colour Doppler and three dimensional power Doppler ultrasonography in patients undergoing in vitro fertilization procedures. J Ultrasound Med. 2001;20:125-34.
13. Kupesić S, Kurjak A, Vujisić S, et al. Luteal phase defect: Comparison between Doppler velocimetry, histological and hormonal markers. Ultrasound Obstet Gynecol. 1997; 9(2):105-12.
14. Kupesic S, Kurjak A. Predictors of IVF outcome by three-dimensional ultrasound. Hum Reprod. 2002;17(4):950-5.
15. Lam PM, Johnson IR, Rainne-Fenning NJ. Three dimensional ultrasound features of the polycystic ovary and the effect of different phenotypic expressions on these parameters. Hum Reprod. 2007;22(12):3116-23.
16. Merce LT, Barco MJ, Bau S, et al. Are endometrial parameters by three-dimensional ultrasound and power Doppler angiography related to in vitro fertilization/embryo transfer outcome? Fertil Steril. 2008;89(1):111-7.
17. Merce LT, Barco MJ, Bau S, et al. Prediction of ovarian response and IVF/ICSI outcome by three dimensional ultrasonography and power Doppler angiography. Eur J Obstet Gynecol Reprod Biol. 2007;132(1):93-100.
18. Merce LT, Barco MJ, Kupesic S, et al. 2D and 3D power Doppler ultrasound from ovulation to implantation. In: Kurjak A, Chervenak F (Eds). Textbook of Perinatal Medicine. London: Parthenon Publishing; 2005.
19. Merce LT. 2D and 3D power Doppler ultrasound study of endometrium as implantation marker. Text book of Transvaginal Sonography. New Delhi: Jaypee Brothers Medical Publishers; 2006. pp. 241-2.
20. Merce LT. Ultrasound markers of implantation. Ultrasound Rev Obstet Gynecol. 2002;2:110-23.
21. Nagori C, Panchal S. Endometrial vascularity: Its relation to implantation rates. Int J Infertil Fetal Med. 2012;3(2):48-50.
22. Nargund G, Bourne TH, Doyle PE, et al. Association between ultrasound indices of follicular blood flow, oocyte recovery and preimplantation embryo quality. Hum Reprod. 1996;11:109-13.
23. Nargund G, Doyle PE, Bourne TH, et al. Ultrasound-deviced indices of follicular blood flow before hCG administration and prediction of oocyte recovery and preimplantation embryo quality. Hum Reprod. 1996;11:2512-7.
24. Panchal S, Nagori C. Baseline scan and ultrasound diagnosis of PCOS. DSJUOG. 2012;6(3):290-9.
25. Panchal S, Nagori CB. Ultrasound based decision making on stimulation protocol for superovulated IUI cycles. IJIFM. 2016;1:7-13.
26. Panchal S, Nagori CB. Ultrasound Based decision making on stimulation protocol in IVF. DSJUOG. 2016;10(3):330-7.
27. Panchal SY, Nagori CB. Can 3D PD be a better tool for assessing the pre hCG follicle and endometrium? A randomized study of 500 cases. Presented at 16th World Congress on Ultrasound in Obstetrics and Gynecology, 2006, London. J Ultrasound Obstet Gynecol. 2006;28(4):504.

28. Popovic-Todorovic B, Loft A, Lindhard A, et al. A prospective study of predictive factors of ovarian response in 'standard' IVF/ICSI patients treated with recombinant FSH. A suggestion for recombinant FSH dosage normogram. Hum Reprod. 2003;18(4):781-7.
29. Smith B, Porter R, Ahuja K, et al. Ultrasonic assessment of endometrial changes in stimulated cycles in an in vitro fertilization and embryo transfer program. J In Vitro Fertil Embryo Transf. 1984;1:233-8.
30. Steer CV, Campbell S, Tan SL, et al. The use of transvaginal colour flow imaging after in vitro fertilization to identify optimum uterine conditions before embryo transfer. Fertil Steril. 1992;57:372-6.
31. Van Blerkom, Antezak M, Schrader R. The developmental potential of human oocyte is related to the dissolved oxygen content of follicular fluid: association with vascular endothelial growth factor levels and perifollicular blood flow characteristics. Hum Reprod. 1997;12(5):1047-55.
32. Vlaisavljevic V, Reljic M, Gavric LV, et al. Measurement of perifollicular blood flow of the dominant preovulatory follicle using three dimensional power Doppler. Ultrasound Obstet Gynecol. 2003;22:520-6.
33. Wittmack FM, Kreger DO, Blasco L, et al. Effect of follicular size on oocyte retrieval, fertilization, cleavage and embryo quality in in vitro fertilization cycles: a 6 year data collection. Fertil Steril. 1994;62:1205-10.
34. Wu MH, Tsai SJ, Pan HA, et al. Three dimensional power Doppler imaging of ovarian stromal blood flow in women with endometriosis undergoing in vitro fertilization. Ultrasound Obstet Gynecol. 2003;21:480-5.
35. Zaidi J, Barber J, Kyei-Mensah A, et al. Relationship of ovarian stromal blood flow at baseline ultrasound to subsequent follicular response in an in vitro fertilization program. Obstet Gynecol. 1996;88:779-84.
36. Zaidi J, Campbell S, Pittrof R, et al. Endometrial thickness, morphology, vascular penetration and velocimetry in predicting implantation in an in vitro fertilization program. Ultrasound Obstet Gynecol. 1995;6:191-8.
37. Zaidi J, Pittrof R, Shaker A, et al. Assessment of uterine artery blood flow on the day of human chorionic gonadotropin administration by transvaginal colour Doppler ultrasound in an in vitro fertilization program. Fertil Steril. 1996;65: 377-81.

20

CHAPTER

Hysteroscopy in ART

Divyesh V Shukla, Shilpi Shukla

"When a yam doesn't grow well, we don't blame it; it is because of the soil".

—*Emily Davila*

INTRODUCTION

Despite of increasing advances in *in vitro* fertilization/intracytoplasmic sperm injection (IVF/ICSI) technology, the implantation rate per embryo remains 30%. Precautions must be taken to nullify the uterine causes for implantation failure as success of IVF treatment also depends upon normal the uterine cavity and endometrial receptivity.

For assessing uterine cavity and intrauterine pathology, transvaginal 3D ultrasound with color Doppler examination and hysteroscopy are considered standard. Hysteroscopy is generally used for the assessment of the uterine cavity, endometrium, diagnosis, and complete treatment of intrauterine pathology. Use of three-dimensional (3D) color Doppler ultrasound is to identify the precise type of uterine malformation, intrauterine pathology, examination of the myometrium, junctional zone (JZ) abnormalities, blood flow in myometrium and endometrium, blood flow in pathology identified, and associated adnexal pathologies.

INVESTIGATIONS FOR EVALUATION OF UTERINE CAVITY

To evaluate uterine cavity in case of infertility, 3D transvaginal sonography (TVS), saline infusion hysterography, hysterosalpingography (HSG), magnetic resonance imaging (MRI), and/or hysteroscopy are performed in cases of infertility.

Three-dimensional Transvaginal Sonography with Color Doppler

This is the first investigation after clinical examination. It has high sensitivity and specificity for detecting polyps, fibroids, endometrial hyperplasia, fibroids, uterine malformations, JZ abnormality, myometrial vascularity, including intrauterine adhesions and fibrosis, foreign body, and intrauterine presence of fluid. If fibroids are seen, their size and location as per International Federation of Gynecology and Obstetrics (FIGO) type is defined and their closeness to JZ should also be seen and reported. Color Doppler flow imaging of fibroids helps raising suspicion of sarcoma depending upon the vascular pattern. In many cases fibroids and adenomyomas are coexistent.

Saline Infusion Hysterography

Injecting saline in uterine cavity while performing TVS improves endometrial pathology detection rates. While performing sonosalpingography at the end, when cannula is withdrawn, infusing saline in uterine cavity helps in additional evaluation of uterine cavity. However, a separate procedure as sonohysterography can also be done. Sonohysterography along with 3D imaging increases chance to detect intrauterine polyps and intrauterine adhesions.

Hysterosalpingography

It is more painful and invasive procedure more commonly used as tubal patency test procedure along with uterine cavity evaluation. The patient is required to be shifted to radiology unit. Factors which may modify the reports of HSG are day of menstrual cycle when the procedure is scheduled, air bubbles, and intrauterine debris consisting of mucus and menstrual blood. They lead to false interpretations. Generally, water soluble contrast media is used for the procedure. The sensitivity of HSG in detecting uterine problems is reported ranging from 60% to 80% in comparison to hysteroscopy. Primarily the procedure is performed to assess tubal patency.

However, use of oil contrast media results in significantly higher pregnancy rates as compared to patients where this procedure is not performed, as it may cause tubal flushing of debris and mucous plugs. The oil contrast might also influence peritoneal macrophage activity and so on endometrial receptivity, thereby enhancing fertility.

Magnetic Resonance Imaging

T2-weighed images of the uterus help to diagnose JZ interruptions and pathologies. It is also used for diagnosis of adenomyoma, adenomyosis and fibroids, their number, location, and their closeness to JZ. It has also role in diagnosis of various congenital Müllerian dysgenesis when the diagnosis is in doubt. MRI is also performed when suspicion of uterine sarcoma is raised. They appear as infiltrating myometrial mass of heterogeneous hypointensity on T1-weighted images, with irregular and ill-defined margins. On T2-weighted images, they usually show intermediate-to-high signal intensity with central hyperintensity indicative of extensive necrosis.

WHY HYSTEROSCOPY?

Role of hysteroscopic examination before all scheduled IVF procedure was suggested especially in repeated implantation failure as there was additional 30–60% rate of pathology detected even with normal HSG findings reported. Hysteroscopic surgery performed in the same setting further helps to treat the pathology and was treated in the same setting. Preoperative HSG, saline infusion sonohysterography or TVS failed to detect intrauterine pathologies in many reported studies.

Overall, comparative studies of HSG or ultrasound in the evaluation of uterine cavity abnormalities showed high false negative rates, low positive predictive values, and poor diagnostic accuracy values. Such undetected pathologies may reduce implantation rate after IVF/ICSI. Hysteroscopy along with treatment of these undetected abnormalities improved reproductive outcome in these patients. From our unpublished hospital records we have found <10% failure of preoperative ultrasound diagnosis of intrauterine pathology in our group of infertile patients. The difference could be because of difference in the study design or the type of ultrasound machines used for ultrasonography.

Newer smaller diameter telescopes (2.9 mm and 1.9 mm diameter) with diagnostic and operative sheath help even performing operative hysteroscopy procedure without use of anesthesia as office procedure. Availability of 18 Fr and 22 Fr resectoscopes also eases cervical entry without dilation and can treat all size of pathology without increase in operative timing with the same results.

In majority of institutions, diagnostic and operative hysteroscopy procedures now are being carried out by using normal saline and bipolar electrosurgery reducing the complications related to glycine intravasation with comparable or better results.

The success of IVF depends on many factors and there is a chance, couple may require multiple cycles of treatment hence it becomes mandatory to diagnose and treat intrauterine pathologies before the procedure.

A systemic review and meta-analysis were performed to assess the efficacy of diagnostic and operative hysteroscopy in improving the live birth rate of infertile women, with and without intrauterine abnormalities, at any stage of the infertility workup. The meta-analysis suggested robust and high-quality randomized controlled trials (RCTs) are still needed before hysteroscopy can be regarded as a first-line procedure in all infertile women, especially during the basal clinical assessment of the couple, when assisted reproductive treatment is not indicated yet.

Low-to-moderate evidence is present for practice of performing hysteroscopy prior to each IVF/ICSI cycle or in patient with one or more implantation failures after IVF/ICSI.

Hysteroscopy procedure itself has been said to be of beneficial as irrigation of the uterine cavity mechanically removes glycodelin which is derived from endometrium (antiadhesive glycoprotein molecules on the endometrial surface involved in endometrial receptivity). Elevated levels are washed away and implantation rates improve. Glycodelin actions are in dose-dependent manner, higher levels inhibit binding of human sperm to the zona pellucida. Around ovulation the levels are low. It facilitates implantation by its elevated levels at the time of implantation by suppressing natural killer cell activity and protects embryo immunosuppressive action by suppressing natural killer cell activity.

Hysteroscopic mechanical endometrial injury or endometrial scratching in the cycle preceding IVF or during the same cycle along with ovarian stimulation improves pregnancy rate. Endometrial gene expressions in natural and stimulated cycles are different. Genes that were upregulated in the endometrial samples of the scratching or biopsy-treated patients are mucin 1 transmembrane

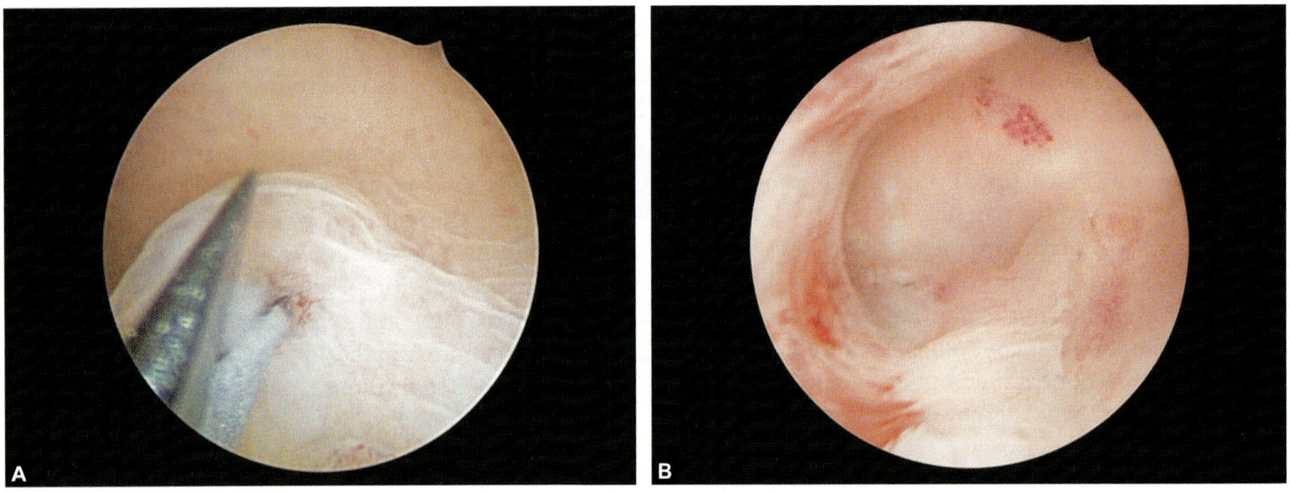

Figs. 1A and B: Hysteroscopic-guided endometrial scratching.

(MUC1), crystalline alpha B, apolipoprotein D (APOD), phospholipase A2 (PLA2), and uroplakin Ib (UPIb). They are required for endometrial preparation. Endometrial scratching also delays endometrial maturation and this is attained by modulating expression of glycodelin A. However, this can be done in outpatient department (OPD) under ultrasonography (USG) guidance using intrauterine insemination (IUI) cannula (Figs. 1A and B).

The procedure of hysteroscopy itself may ease embryo transfer procedure as because of this procedure correct assessment of direction of endocervical canal can be made, intracervical adhesions can be cut, cervical stenosis can be corrected, and dilation of internal cervical orifice (OS) can be done in case required. All these are possible explanation for the improved IVF outcome after hysteroscopy scheduled in these patients (Figs. 2A to C)

Intrauterine polyps single or multiple of size 15 mm or more located in upper part of body of the uterus can interfere with fertility. Hysteroscopic polypectomy by atraumatic graspers, scissors, hysteroscopic mechanical morcellators or use of resectoscope is very effective method to treat polyps. Several authors including from our unpublished records of hysteroscopy suggest that it can effectively treat intrauterine polyps by atraumatic graspers, resectoscope, scissors or mechanical morcellators even in an ongoing IVF cycle. In fact, the procedure increases the success of IVF in the same cycle. Hysteroscopic polypectomy improves implantation failure and pregnancy loss after previous IVF failures. Conception resulting in the same cycle of hysteroscopy procedure suggests tissue healing and remodeling after hysteroscopy does not negatively affect endometrial receptivity (Figs. 3A to E).

Submucous fibroids interfere with implantation by altering character of endometrium over it and altering myometrial contractility. Submucous fibroids should be removed in infertile patients, regardless of the size or the presence of symptoms. With increasing experience of the procedure even FIGO type 2 fibroids can be removed in single setting. There is strong evidence favoring hysteroscopic myomectomy in women before undergoing ART. Multiple published studies have shown hysteroscopic resection of fibroids is a safe, minimally invasive, and very effective procedure. For smaller intracavitary lesions, hysteroscopic morcellators may be used while for large lesions and lesions with intramyometrial location resectoscopes are preferred (Figs. 4A to E).

History of 1st and/or 2nd trimester abortions and infertility has higher prevalence of congenital uterine anomalies when compared with the unselected population. Septate uterus is the most common structural uterine anomaly associated with the highest incidence of reproductive failure. Hysteroscopic metroplasty improves reproductive outcome. Arcuate cavity does not require correction. High rate of abortions reported in patients with arcuate uterus by some indicated causal relationship. After septal metroplasty abortions, preterm delivery and full-term delivery rates improved (Figs. 5A to E).

Hysteroscopy surgery using scissors only or use of mono- or bipolar needle is used to treat intrauterine adhesions. Surgery involves cutting intracervical adhesions to lyse intrauterine fibrotic or muscular adhesions. In case of complete obliteration of cavity more extensive adhesiolysis is required. This is followed by sequential hormonal therapy, with or without use of platelet-rich plasma or endometrial

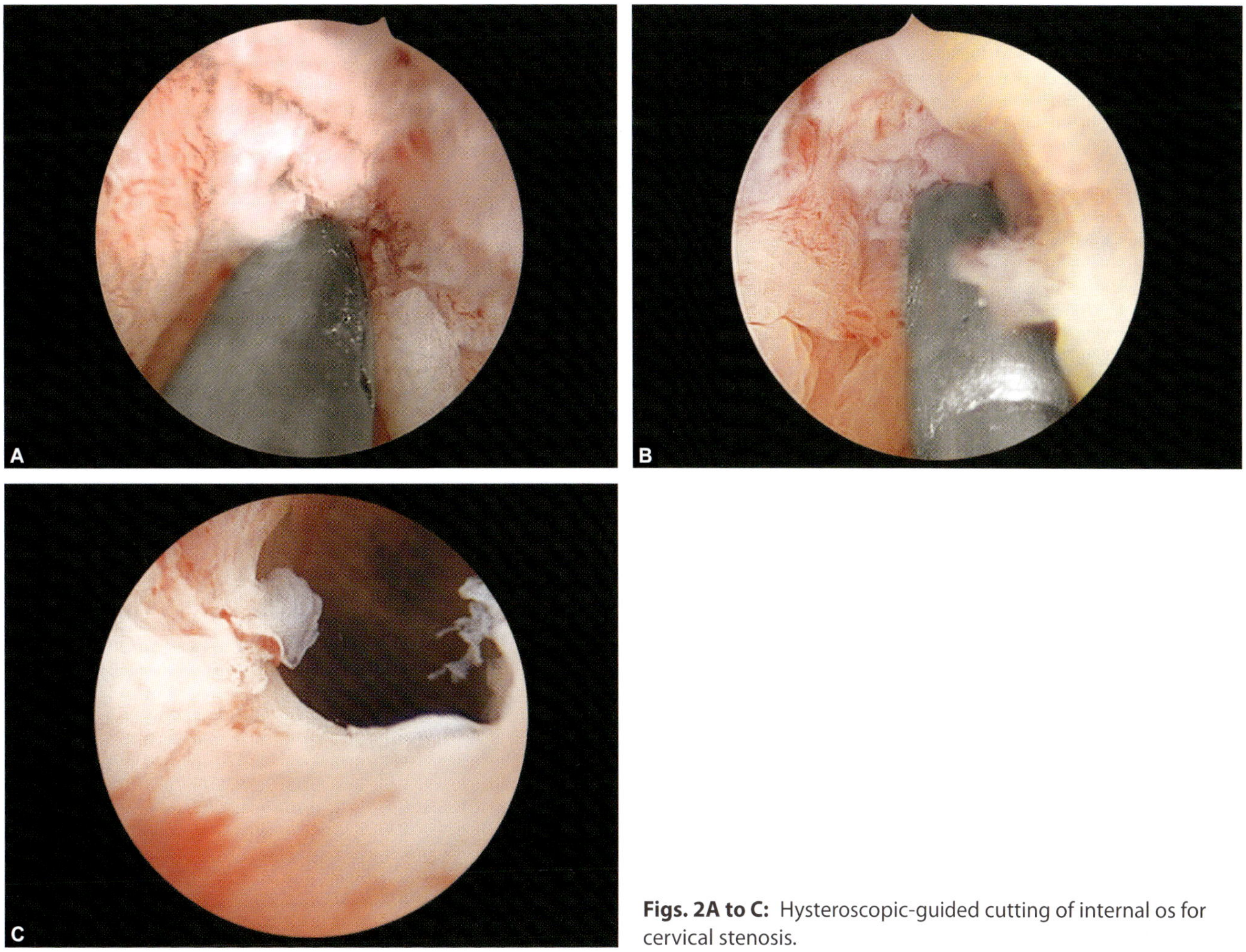

Figs. 2A to C: Hysteroscopic-guided cutting of internal os for cervical stenosis.

or mesenchymal cells, this practice is under research. Hysteroscopic adhesiolysis has very encouraging results in patients with infertility. However, these patients will require one or multiple repeat hysteroscopic procedures and use of antiadhesives for normalizing cavity and to evaluate the endometrium after surgery (effect of hormones and other drugs) depending upon the grade of Asherman's before subjecting them for IVF (Figs. 6A to H).

Hysteroscopic metroplasty for asymmetric cavities and abnormal shape cavity or unicornuate cavity to increase the size of cavity are usually performed only after prior pregnancy losses. The procedure if performed by scissors or bipolar resectoscope using Colin's knife, aim of surgery is to make the cavity triangular and symmetric. Preoperative 3D TVS USG is performed to assess cornual width and lateral wall indentations in case of T- and Y-shaped cavity (Figs. 7A to F).

Evidence of chronic endometritis and tuberculosis endometritis can be only obtained by visual appearance, vascularity, cornual vascularity, endometrial characteristic, and endometrial or fibrous adhesions on hysteroscopic examination. Multiple micropolyps and/or associated fragile endometrium, surface vascularity of endometrium appearing as broken capillary may be indicative of endometritis. Cavity may be pale looking with intrauterine adhesions. Endometrial biopsy is taken and polymerase chain reaction (PCR) for tuberculosis is performed. PCR assays can detect <10 bacilli/mL including dead bacilli and has a testing time of 8–12 hours. Sensitivity of PCR is higher than culture and histopathology and specificity may be as high as 100% in detecting female genital tuberculosis (FGTB). However, the false positive rates are high so other findings on laparoscopy can be taken in consideration before starting treatment (Figs. 8A to E).

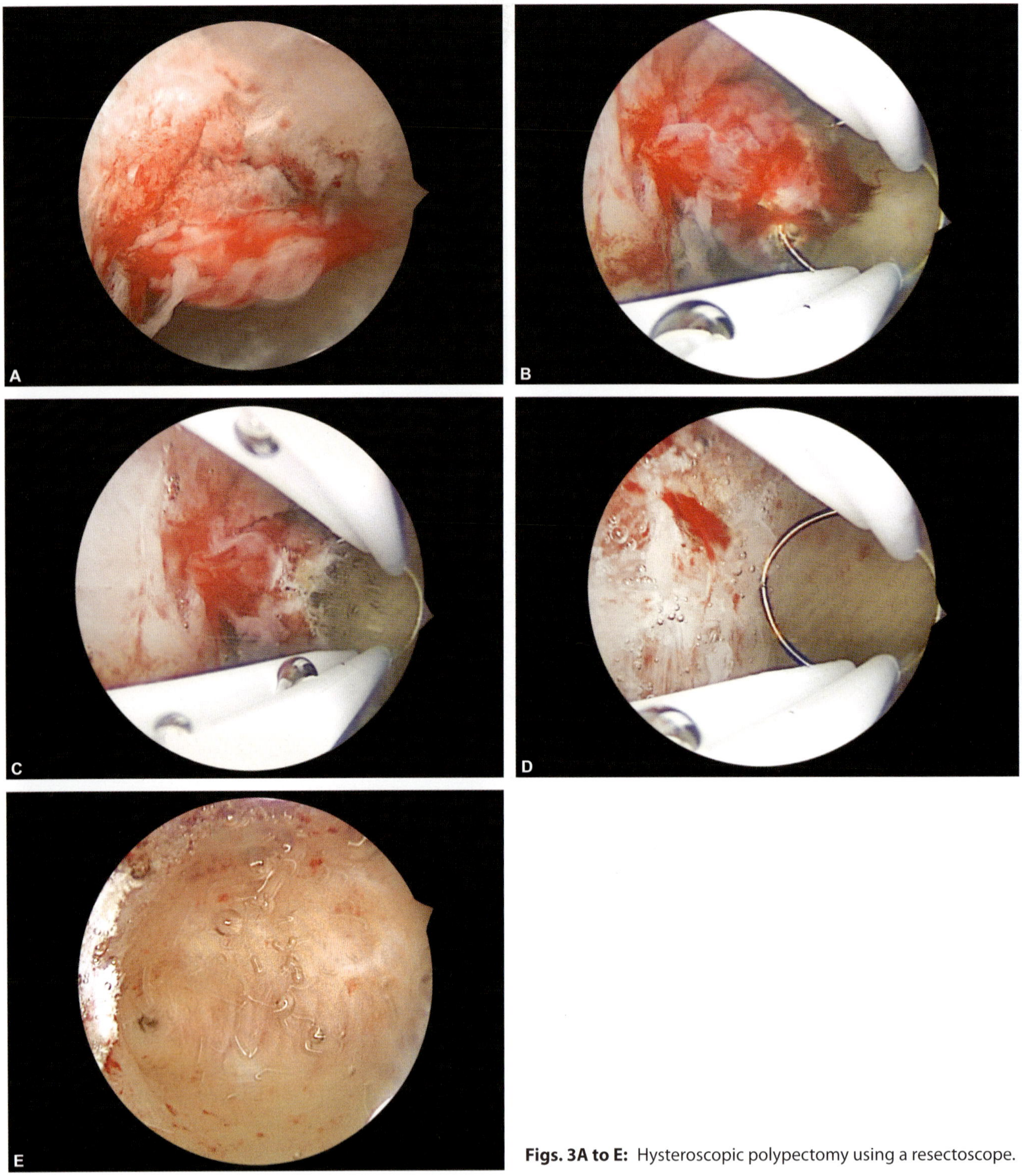

Figs. 3A to E: Hysteroscopic polypectomy using a resectoscope.

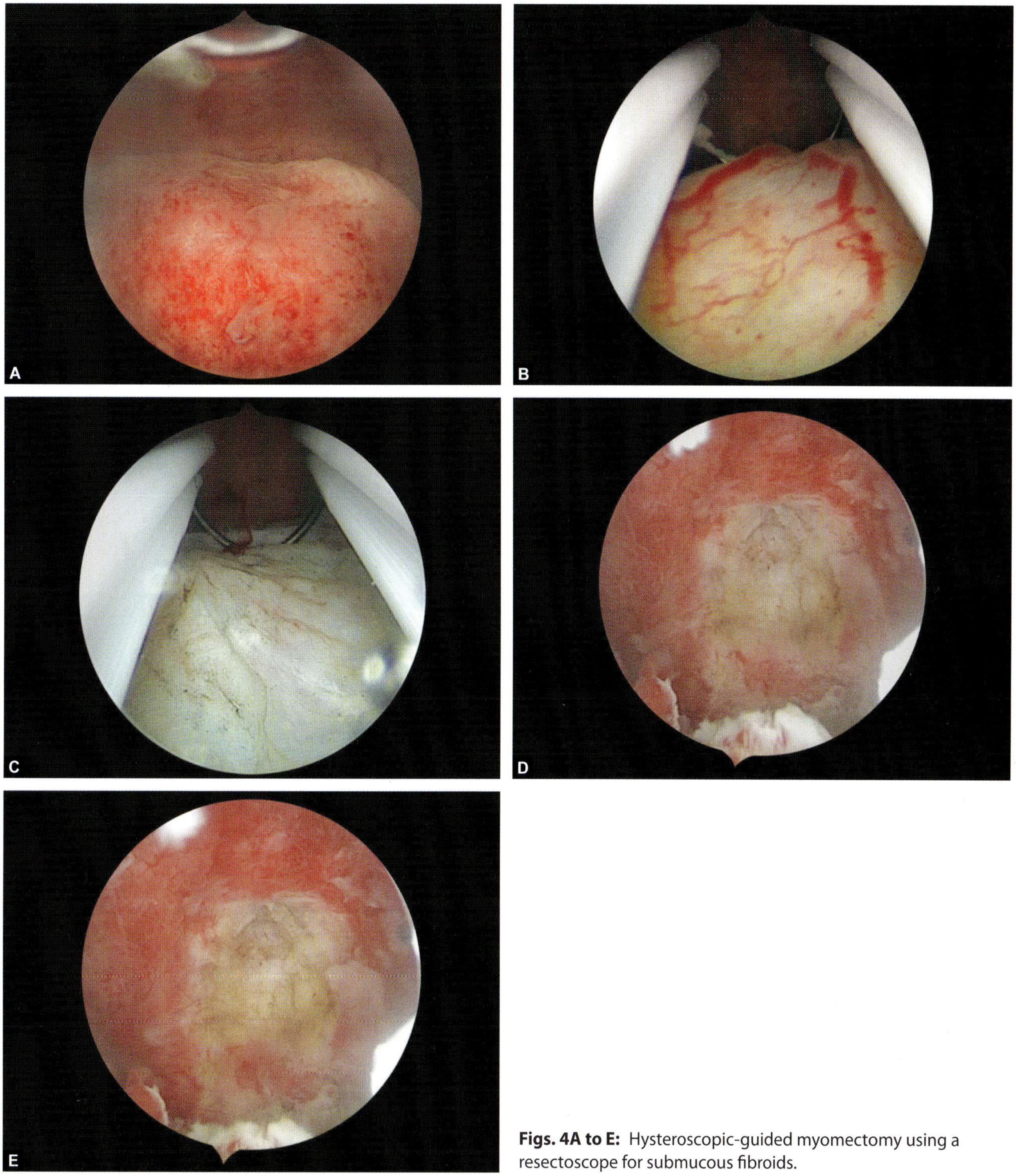

Figs. 4A to E: Hysteroscopic-guided myomectomy using a resectoscope for submucous fibroids.

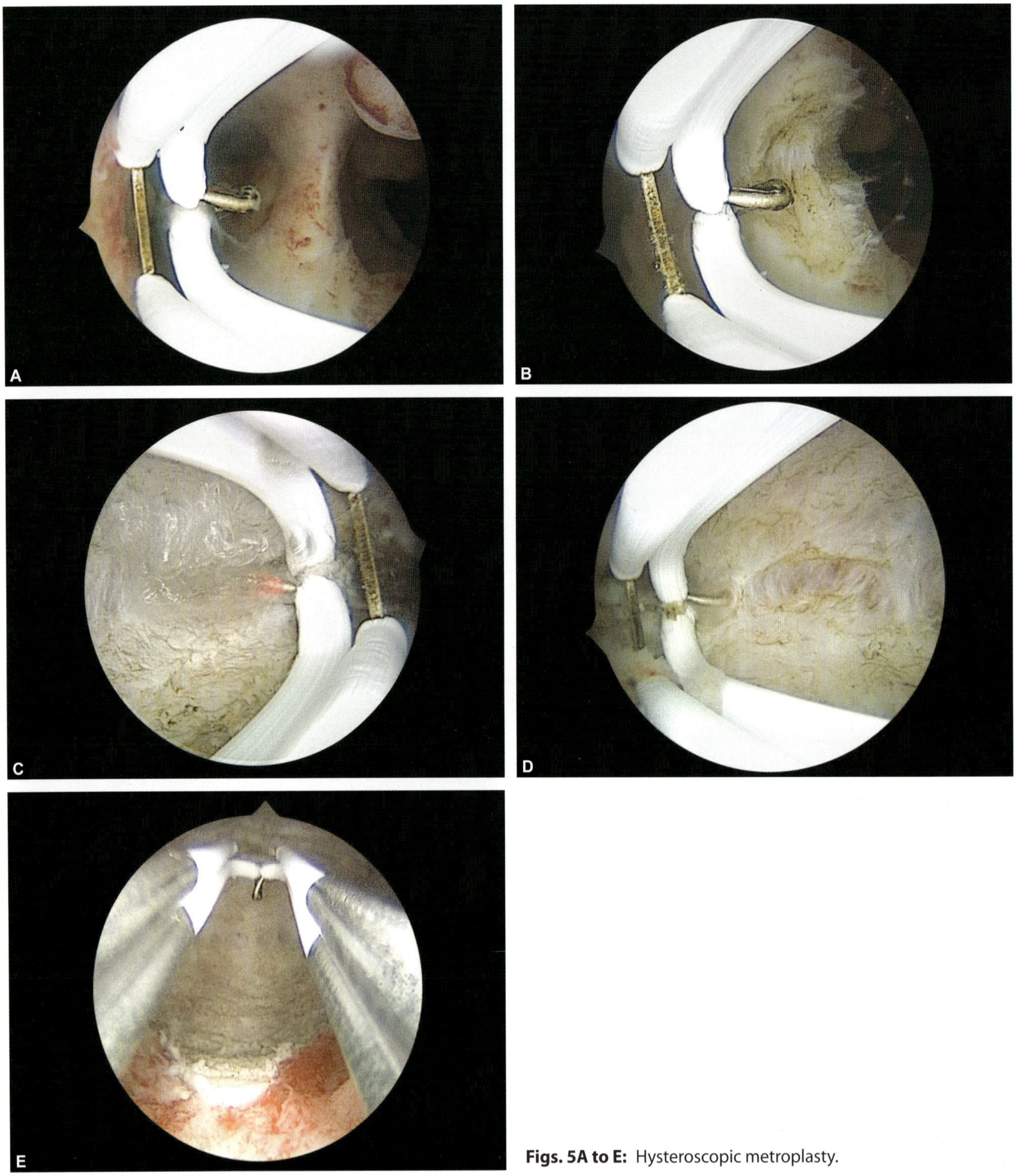

Figs. 5A to E: Hysteroscopic metroplasty.

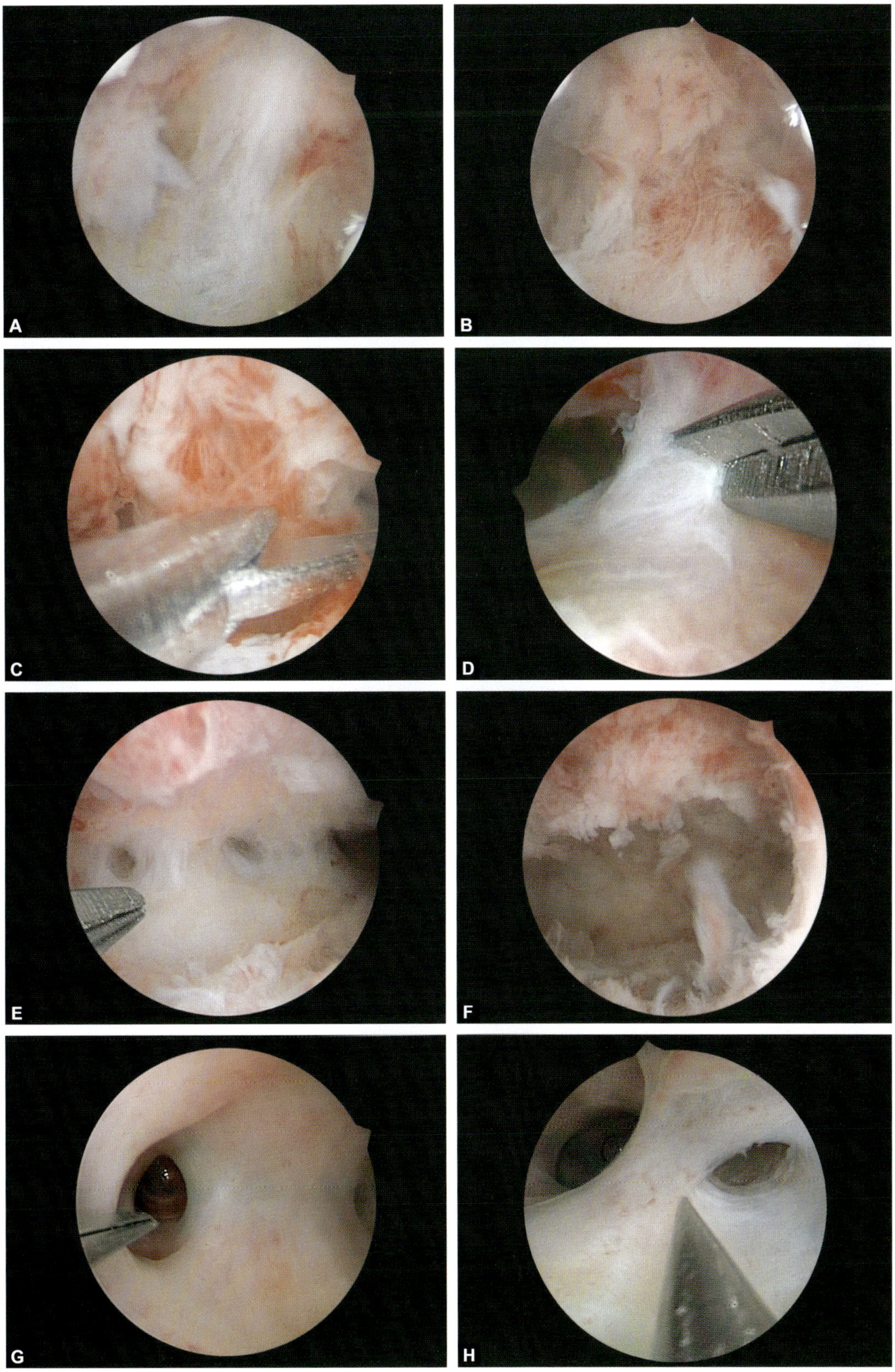

Figs. 6A to H: Treatment of Asherman's fibrosis by hysteroscopic scissors.

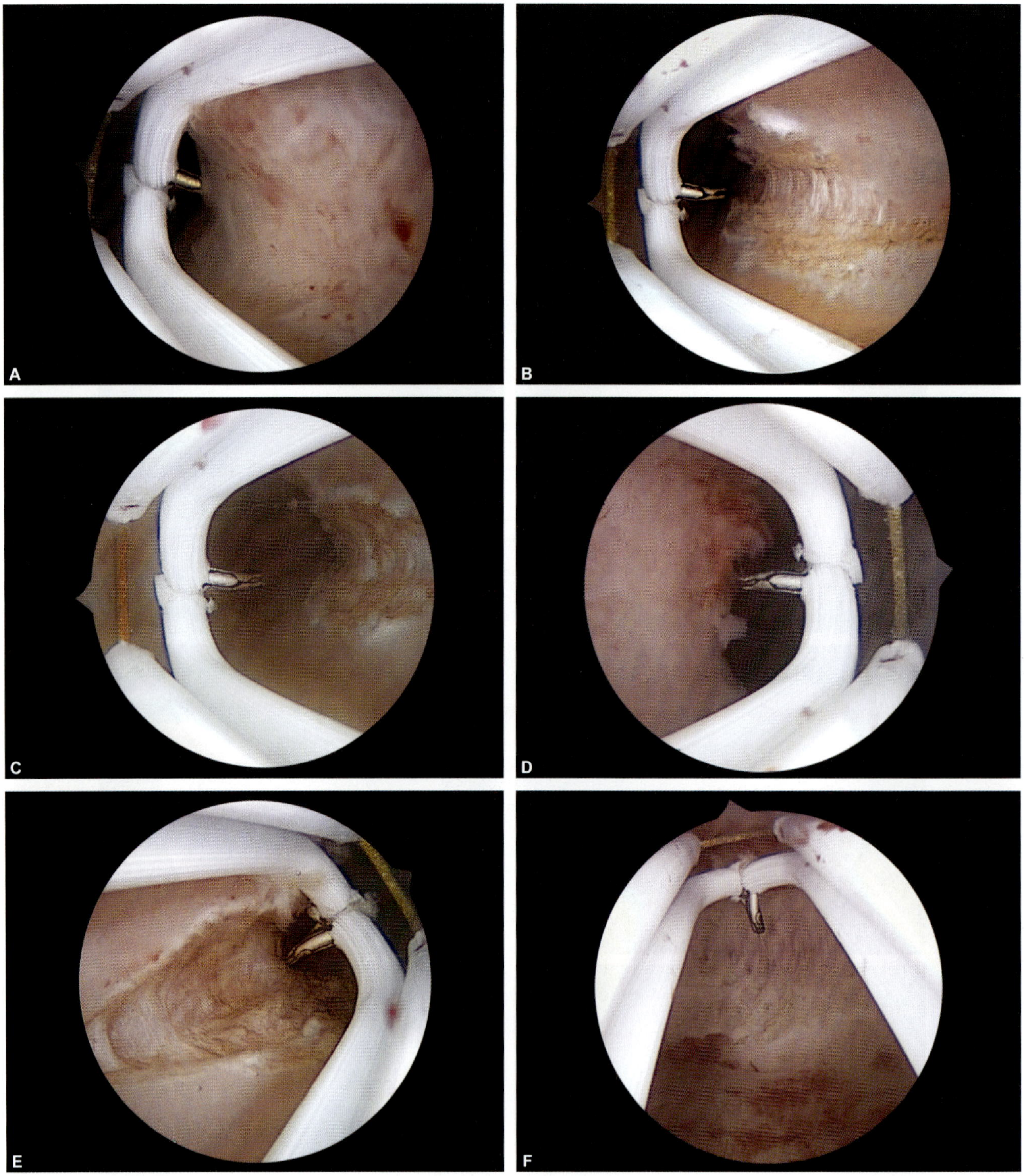

Figs. 7A to F: Lateral metroplasty.

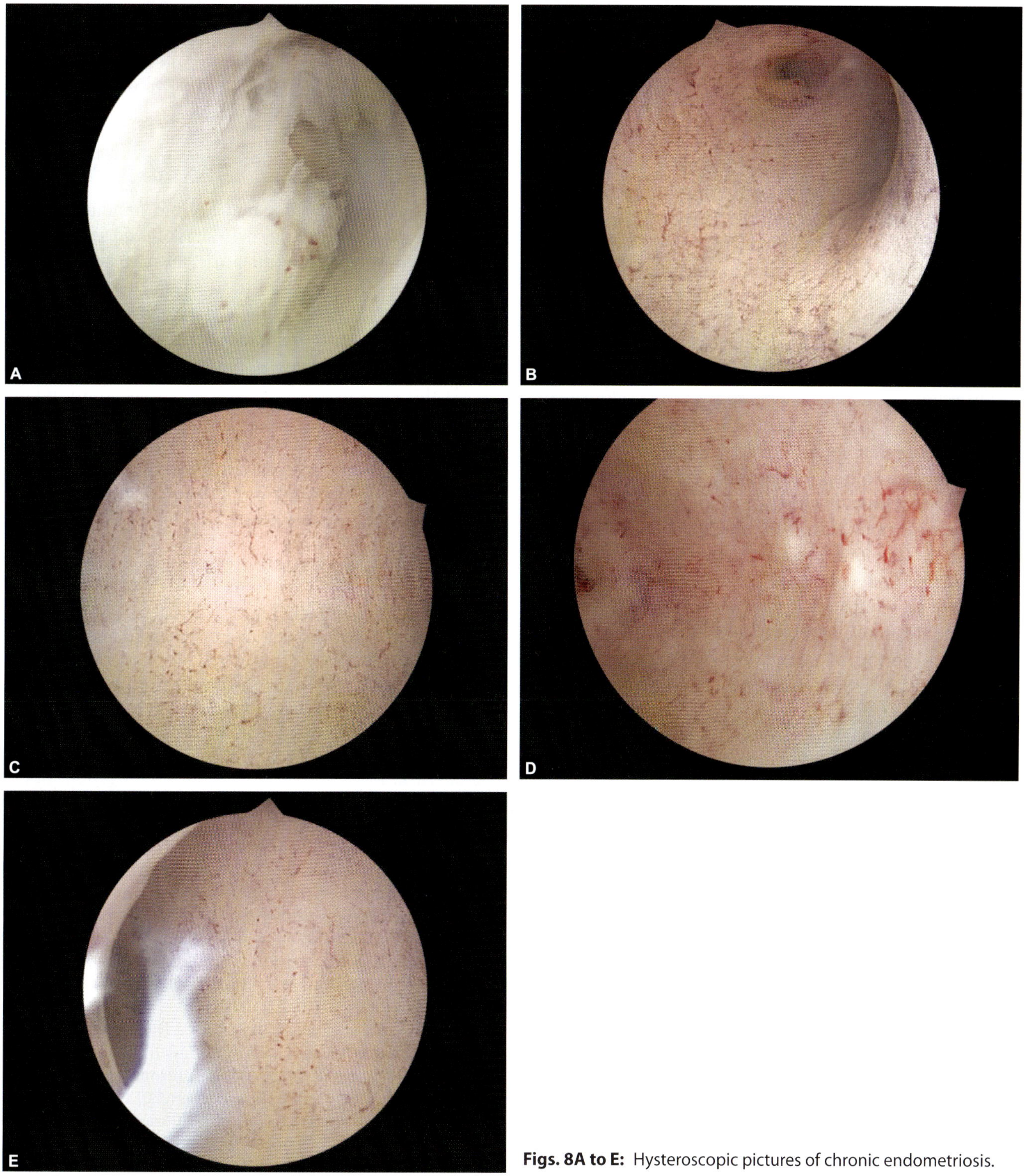

Figs. 8A to E: Hysteroscopic pictures of chronic endometriosis.

Negative effect of hydrosalpinx on success of IVF is well known, hysteroscopic occlusion of interstitial portion of Fallopian tube by Essure device has been reported in many studies. This precludes requirement of laparoscopy in this condition.

Hysteroscopic-guided embryo transfer (ET) also has been reported in case of difficult transfers. This is a visual procedure and placement or implantation of a single embryo, the hysteroscopic embryo delivery procedures will help optimize the results and decrease major side effects. These include: multiple pregnancies, ectopic or heterotopic pregnancies, and placenta previa from IVF. Abbreviations as HEED (hysteroscopic endometrial embryo transfer) and SEED (subendometrial embryo delivery) are used for these procedures.

In group of patients undergoing IVF with no abnormality reported on TVS prevalence of minor intrauterine abnormalities were reported as high as 20–50% on hysteroscopy. But the recent published data indicate this figure to be less (11% versus 20–45%).

Contrary to the above-mentioned published reports, the TROPHY trial in 2016 reports opposite. The TROPHY trial was a single-blind multicenter RCT conducted in 8 hospitals in 4 European countries. This study reports when patients had normal ultrasound reports even with history with prior IVF failure, performing outpatient hysteroscopy does not improve live birth rates, conception rate, and implantation or abortions.

Contrary to TROPHY multicentric data, another study published reports performing hysteroscopy in cases with recurrent IVF failure detects abnormalities in 39% of patients even when USG reveals normal findings.

SUMMARY

Role of hysteroscopy in infertile female before ART remains under debate despite of its safety and possibility of it being performed as outpatient procedure.

In routine clinical practice, TVS or 3D TVS and HSG are the first-line investigations offered as an infertility investigation. Hysteroscopy is usually indicated only if there is an abnormality reported on above investigations or there are recurrent IVF failures.

Routine practice of hysteroscopy before IVF when TVS is normal does not improve the live birth rate following IVF.

Hysteroscopic septal resection improves IVF results but other procedures performed for correction of uterine cavity need more evaluation. More RCTs are necessary to study effectiveness of hysteroscopic polypectomy and submucous fibroid resection.

Finally, the role of hysteroscopy cannot be denied in success of IVF as various observational and retrospective studies have documented definite role of hysteroscopic surgeries to diagnose and treat intrauterine pathologies and subsequent improvement of IVF success rates.

EDITORS' COMMENTS

1. In spite of hysteroscopy being a gold standard investigation to assess uterine cavity, it is offered as a second-line therapy mainly because of its invasiveness and cost.
2. Apart from being a tool to be visualized and correct uterine structural defects, hysteroscopy benefits implantation and pregnancy rates as saline irrigation mechanically removes harmful antiadhesive molecules on the endometrial surface affecting endometrial receptivity.
3. In difficult embryo transfer, hysteroscopy can be used as HEED/SEED procedure for visual placement and implantation of a single embryo but, this technique has not shown promising results.

SUGGESTED READING

1. Almog B, Shalom-Paz E, Dufort D, et al. Promoting implantation by local injury to the endometrium. Fertil Steril. 2010;94(6):2026-9.
2. Alobaidy EJ. Comparison the diagnostic accuracy of hysterosalpingography and hysteroscopy in the detection of intrauterine abnormality in recurrent pregnancy loss. J Pharm Sci Res. 2018;10(4):900-2.
3. Al-Turki HA. Hysteroscopy as an investigation tool in recurrent implantation failure in vitro fertilization. Saudi Med J. 2018;39(3):243-6.
4. Apirakviriya C, Rungruxsirivorn T, Phupong V, et al. Diagnostic accuracy of 3D-transvaginal ultrasound in detecting uterine cavity abnormalities in infertile patients as compared with hysteroscopy. Eur J Obstet Gynecol Reprod Biol. 2016;200:24-8.
5. Carneiro MM. What is the role of hysteroscopic surgery in the management of female infertility? A review of the literature. Surg Res Pract. 2014;2014:105412.
6. Cenksoy P, Ficicioglu C, Yıldırım G, et al. Hysteroscopic findings in women with recurrent IVF failures and the effect of correction of hysteroscopic findings on subsequent pregnancy rates. Arch Gynecol Obstet. 2013;287(2):357-60.
7. Di Spiezio Sardo A, Di Carlo C, Minozzi S, et al. Efficacy of hysteroscopy in improving reproductive outcomes of infertile couples: A systematic review and meta-analysis. Hum Reprod Update. 2016;22(4):479-96.
8. El-Toukhy T, Campo R, Khalaf Y, et al. Hysteroscopy in recurrent in-vitro fertilisation failure (TROPHY): A multicentre, randomised controlled trial. Lancet. 2016;387(10038): 2614-21.

9. Fatemi HM, Kasius JC, Timmermans A, et al. Prevalence of unsuspected uterine cavity abnormalities diagnosed by office hysteroscopy prior to in vitro fertilization. Hum Reprod. 2010;25(8):1959-65.
10. Ganglion R, Valentini A, Pistilli E. A comparison of hysterosalpingography and hysteroscopy. Int J Gynecol Obstet. 1996;52:151-3.
11. Grace GA, Devaleenal DB, Natrajan M. Genital tuberculosis in females. Indian J Med Res. 2017;145(4):425-36.
12. Javadian M, Esmaeilzadeh S, Farzadmanesh M, et al. Is hysteroscopy a routine investigation before assisted reproductive techniques? Caspian J Reprod Med. 2015;1(1): 31-4.
13. Johnson JV, Montoya IA, Olive DL. Ethiodol oil contrast medium inhibits macrophage phagocytosis and adherence by altering membrane electronegativity and microviscosity. Fertil Steril. 1992;58:511-7.
14. Johnson NP, Farquhar CM, Hadden WE, et al. The FLUSH trial, flushing with lipiodol for unexplained (and endometriosis-related) subfertility by hysterosalpingography: A randomized trial. Hum Reprod. 2004;19:2043-51.
15. Johnson NP. Review of lipiodol treatment for infertility—an innovative treatment for endometriosis-related infertility? Aust N Z J Obstet Gynaecol. 2014;54:9-12.
16. Kalma Y, Granot I, Gnainsky Y, et al. Endometrial biopsy-induced gene modulation: First evidence for the expression of bladder-transmembranal uroplakin Ib in human endometrium. Fertil Steril. 2009;91:1042-9.
17. Kamra M. Hysteroscopic embryo transfer: HEED and SEED. Hysteroscopy. 2017;193-9.
18. Kumar SC, Awasthi RT, Gokale N. Assessment of uterine factor in infertile women: Hysterosalpingography vs hysteroscopy. MIJAFI. 2003;60:39-41.
19. Pereira N, Amrane S, Estes JL, et al. Does the time interval between hysteroscopic polypectomy and start of in vitro fertilization affect outcomes? Fertil Steril. 2016;105(2):539-44.
20. Richlin SS, Ramachandran S, Shanti A, et al. Glycodelin levels in uterine flushings and in plasma of patients with leiomyomas and polyps: Implications for implantation. Hum Reprod. 2002;17(10):2742-7.
21. Roma Dalfó A, Ubeda B, Ubeda A, et al. Diagnostic value of hysterosalpingography in the detection of intrauterine abnormality: A comparison hysteroscopy. Am J Roentgenol. 2004;183(5):1405-9.
22. Sharma JB. Current diagnosis and management of female genital tuberculosis. J Obstet Gynaecol India. 2015;65(6): 362-71.
23. Stamatellos I, Apostolides A, Stamatopoulos P, et al. Pregnancy rates after hysteroscopic polypectomy depending on the size or number of the polyps. Arch Gynecol Obstet. 2008;277(5):395-9.
24. Takahashi K, Mukaida T, Tomiyam T, et al. High pregnancy rate after hysteroscopy with irrigation in uterine cavity prior to blastocyst transfer in patients who have failed to conceive after blastocyst transfer. Fertil Steril. 2000;74:206.
25. Vitner D, Filmer S, Goldstein I, et al. A comparison between ultrasonography and hysteroscopy in the diagnosis of uterine pathology. Eur J Obstet Gynecol Reprod Biol. 2013;171(1): 143-5.
26. Xu W, Zhang Y, Yang Y, et al. Effect of early second-look hysteroscopy on reproductive outcomes after hysteroscopic adhesiolysis in patients with intrauterine adhesion: A retrospective study in China. Int J Surg. 2018;50:49-54.

CHAPTER 21

Fertility-enhancing Surgeries in ART

Sanjay Patel

INTRODUCTION

Laparoscopy nowadays is routinely performed for evaluating and treating infertility. In this era of assisted reproductive technique (ART) and *in vitro* fertilization (IVF), laparoscopy has an advantage due to its minimal invasive nature and direct visualization of the pelvic reproductive anatomy.

Laparoscopy is helpful in following conditions interfering with fertility:
- Endometriosis
- Adhesions
- Adenomyosis
- Ovarian cysts
- Fallopian tube damage
- Congenital abnormalities
- Fibroids
- Polycystic ovaries.

Benefits of endoscopy:
- Definitive
- Minimal invasive
- Treatment benefits
- Shorter hospital stay
- Less postoperative morbidity
- Cosmetic benefits.

Assessment of internal female pelvic anatomy particularly tubal patency (chromopertubation) and uterine cavity is important for evaluation of infertility.

Tubal infertility: Seen in 40% of female with infertility.

Types of tubal surgery:
- Hysteroscopic tubal cannulation
- Laparoscopic tubal microsurgery
- Laparoscopic salpingo-ovariolysis and fimbrioplasty.

HYSTEROSCOPIC TUBAL CANNULATION

Patients having proximal tubal occlusion (PTO) are candidates for hysteroscopic tubal cannulation.

Proximal tubal occlusion accounts for 10–25% of tubal disease as found on hysterosalpingograms.

Causes of PTO are shown in Table 1.

These infections may damage other areas of the tube, which will affect the prognosis of the treatment.

Contraindications to hysteroscopic tubal cannulation include active infection, heavy uterine bleeding, potential pregnancy, and uterine malignancy.

Adverse effects of hysteroscopic tubal cannulation include damage to normal tube which may be either dissection or perforation and other is ectopic pregnancy.

LAPAROSCOPIC TUBAL MICROSURGERY

Laparoscopic tuboplasty has an advantage of both microsurgery and laparoscopy.

TABLE 1 Causes of proximal tubal occlusion.

Noninfectious causes	*Infectious causes*
Obstruction due to tubal spasm	Salpingitis isthmica nodosa
Plugging by mucus and amorphous material	Pelvic inflammatory disease
Occlusion from fibrosis or endometriosis	Tuberculosis

Benefits of laparoscopic tuboplasty:

- Follow microsurgical principles (tissue handling, magnification, homeostasis, and lavage).
- Less tissue handling and trauma
- Less adhesions
- Cosmetic benefit
- Fast recovery
- Single-step procedure contrast to IVF.

Indications

- Tubal sterilization reversal
- Midtubal block
- Salpingitis isthmica nodosa (SIN).

Contraindications

- Age ≥40 years
- Low anti-Müllerian hormone (AMH) and ovarian failure
- Major tubal damage (salpingoscopy ≥3)
- Hydrosalpinx tubal diameter >3 cm
- Small proximal/distal tubal stump for tuboplasty
- Post-tuboplasty tubal length <3 cm
- Frozen pelvis with tubal involvement
- Distorted uterine cavity
- Contraindication of pregnancy/surgery
- Advanced male infertility/sterility.

Intraoperative Evaluation

Before proceeding for the tubal reconstruction one must evaluate the inside of the tube, so as to be confirmed that the anastomosis is going to be fruitful or not at all worthwhile. This involves salpingoscopy and falloposcopy.

- Salpingoscopy allows direct inspection of tubal mucosa in the ampullary part.
- The degree of tubal mucosal damage is probably the major factor in establishing the prognosis for tubal surgery.
- Brosen's classification is useful for evaluation according to degree of mucosal atrophy and mucosal adhesions.

Salpingoscopy Grade 1 (Fig. 1): Normal intraluminal findings with healthy major (primary) and minor (secondary) folds.

Salpingoscopy Grade 2 (Fig. 2): Mucosal nuclear staining with methylene blue dye.

Salpingoscopy Grade 3 (Fig. 3): Minimal flattening and minimal adhesion (→) of endosalpinx.

Salpingoscopy Grade 4 (Fig. 4): Moderate flattening of endosalpinx with intraluminal adhesion.

Salpingoscopy Grade 5 (Fig. 5): Severe flattening of mucosa with severe intraluminal adhesions.

Types of anastomosis (Fig. 6):

- Isthmo-isthmic anastomosis
- *Isthmo-ampullary anastomosis*: Difficulty of luminal disparity is managed by cutting the isthmic end
- *Ampullo-ampullary anastomosis*: Thin muscularis and mucosal folds prolapse can cause difficulty
- *Tubo-cornual anastomosis*: Cornual wedge excision and mobilization of interstitial portion.

Our Experience

Pregnancy rates were comparable with open tubal recanalization. Average surgical duration was 2 hours and 30 minutes. The average hospital stay was 2 days.

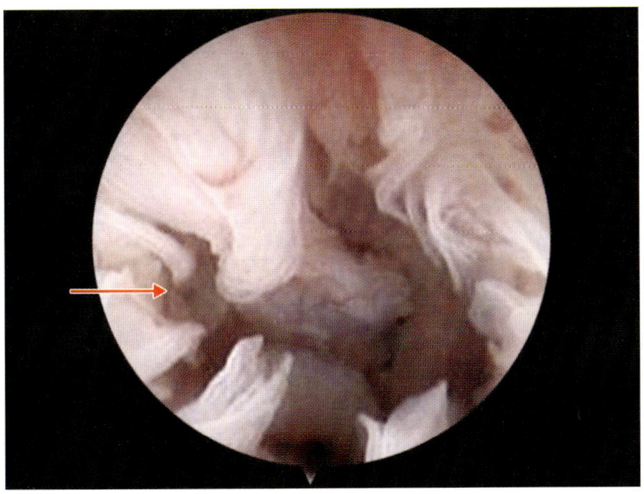

Fig. 1: Salpingoscopy Grade 1.

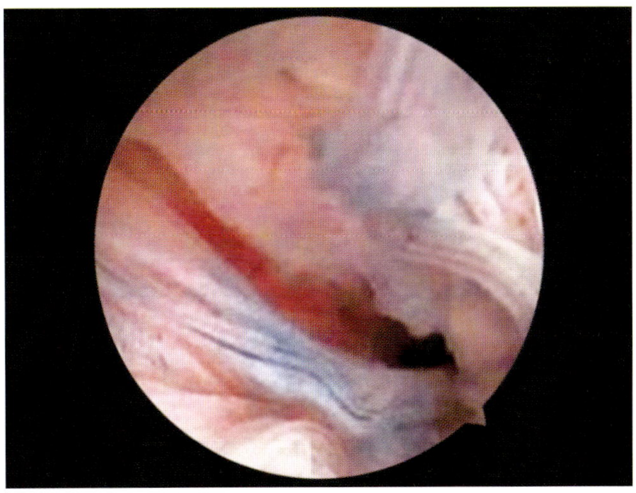

Fig. 2: Salpingoscopy Grade 2.

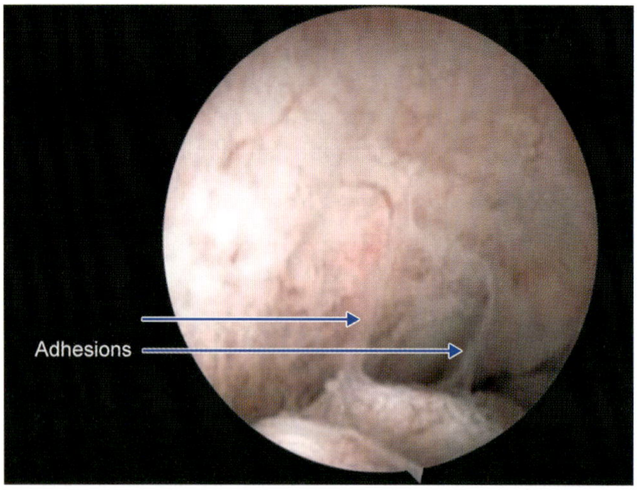

Fig. 3: Salpingoscopy Grade 3.

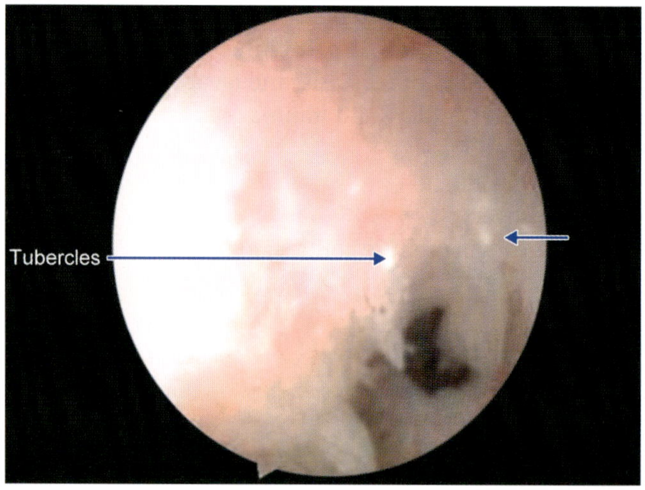

Fig. 4: Salpingoscopy Grade 4.

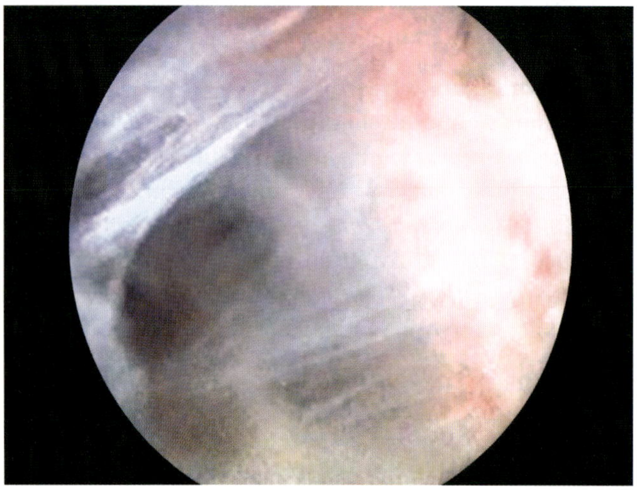

Fig. 5: Salpingoscopy Grade 5.

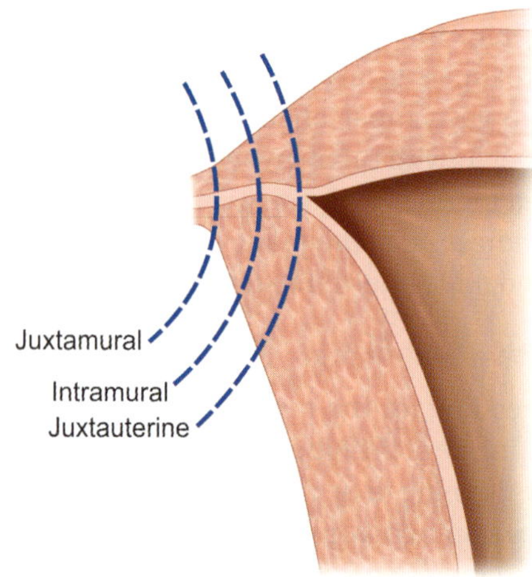

Fig. 6: Types of anastomosis.

Study between 1996 and 2006

TL reversal	*Tubal block due to PID*	*Tubal block secondary to ectopic pregnancy*	*Failed tubal cannulation for proximal block*	*Total*
299 (68.57%)	90 (20.64%)	16 (3.66%)	31 (7.11%)	436 cases

Types of anastomosis

Bilateral	*Unilateral*	*Incomplete (due to multiple blocks)*	*Total*
324 (74.31%)	92 (21.1%)	20 (4.58%)	436 cases

Types of anastomosis and its result

Types of anastomosis	*Isthmo-isthmic*	*Isthmo-ampullary*	*Ampullo-ampullary*	*Juxtamural-isthmic*	*Juxtauterine-isthmic*	*Intramural-isthmic*	*Total*
Total no.	186 (42.66%)	137 (31.42%)	57 (13.0%)	26 (5.96%)	12 (2.75%)	18 (4.13%)	436
Cases conceived	165 (88.7%)	119 (86.86%)	26 (45.61%)	13 (50%)	03 (25%)	5 (27.77%)	331 (75.92%)

Case type versus results

Type of cases	*Tl reversal (n = 299)*	*Pathological tubes (n = 137)*	*Total (n = 436)*
Cases conceived	266 (88.96%)	65 (47.45%)	331 (75.92%)

Total 436 successful surgeries, 331 (75.92%) get pregnancy [14 had an ectopic (4.2%)].

LAPAROSCOPIC SALPINGO-OVARIOLYSIS, FIMBRIOPLASTY, AND ADHESIOLYSIS

Microsurgical principals are used to treat pelvic adhesions and restore pelvic anatomy and tubo-ovarian relationship. There is a correlation of fertility results after adhesiolysis with the type and extent of the adhesions.

Risk Factors

- Previous surgery
- Previous ruptured appendix
- Endometriosis pelvic inflammatory disease (PID)
- Inflammatory bowel diseases
- Bacterial peritonitis
- Chemical peritonitis and peritoneal dialysis
- Tuberculosis (TB)
- Foreign body reaction.

Cause of Infertility

- Mechanical blockage to the fallopian tubes-preventing oocyte retrieval
- Follicular growth may be suppressed by ovarian entrapment from adhesions around the tubes and ovaries
- Motility of tube and transportation can be affected by adhesion around and in the tubes
- Slow embryo movement.

Technique

Prerequisite

- Possible benefit of adhesiolysis
- Requirement of sharp or blunt dissection
- Risk of injury to vital organs.

Adhesions should cut and excised fibrotic portion, coagulation of vascular adhesions by fine bipolar, avascular flimsy adhesions are stretched and cut with sharp dissection, vascular pedicle like adhesions coagulated and cut.

To avoid trauma adhesions band or the ovarian ligaments are held instead of the ovarian cortex and mobilized from pouch of Douglas (POD) and tubo-ovarian relationship is established.

After homeostasis and adhesiolysis, saline is filled in POD, any flimsy avascular adhesions over ovary and fimbria that floats in the saline, are excised with sharp dissection without coagulation.

Tips to Tackle Adhesion

- Fimbriae may be buried, dye test is helpful.
- Blunt dissection
- Sharp dissection
- Fimbrial adhesions in endometriosis
- Do not use energy near bowel, ureter, and urinary bladder.

Conclusions

- Establishment of tubal patency is the most important task in fertility enhancement.
- Ectopic pregnancy with <2 cm sac, segmental excision as discussed.
- Salpingoscopy in pathological block has a prognostic and predictive role.
- Significant rise in pregnancy rate in infertile women after laparoscopic adhesiolysis.
- Aim is to restore near normal anatomy.
- Follow microsurgical principles.
- Hydrosalpinx, TB, and endometriosis have poor prognosis.
- Salpingectomy for hydrosalpinx doubles the chances of pregnancy in IVF.
- In extensive adhesions, may opt for proximal ligation with distal fenestration.
- Single-step treatment and cost effective when compared to IVF.
- *In vitro* fertilization is a better option in poor prognosis after tuboplasty.

ROLE OF SALPINGECTOMY BEFORE IVF

Fluid of hydrosalpinx causes reduction by almost half in the success rate of ART by reducing the endometrial receptivity. Laparoscopic salpingectomy in hydrosalpinges as a pre-IVF treatment improves pregnancy and live birth rate.

ROLE OF LAPAROSCOPY IN ENDOMETRIOSIS

Affected population is reproductive-aged women due to its estrogen dependency with prevalence rate of 20–50% in infertile women which increases to 71–87% in chronic

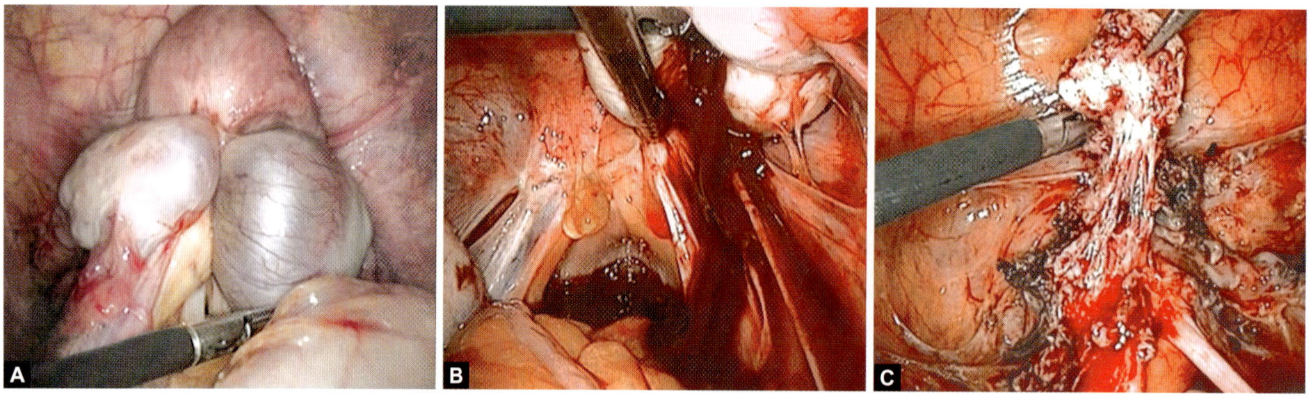

Figs. 7A to C: Role of laparoscopy in the treatment of endometriosis.

pelvic pain. The laparoscopic route is ideal for conservative treatment of endometriosis (Figs. 7A to C).

Pathophysiology

- High level of prostaglandins
- Reduced sperm motility and binding
- Decreased implantation of embryo
- Abnormal immunological factors
- High vascular endothelial growth factor
- High tumor necrosis factor alpha
- Irregular follicular development.

Grade 1/2 endometriosis or normal pelvic anatomy can cause infertility.

Surgical Techniques

- Excision/ablation of implants
- Cystectomy/resection of ovarian endometriomas
- Excision of adhesions, endometrial growths, and fibrotic tissue
- Establishing normal anatomy.

Laser or electrodiathermy ablation has a recurrence rate of 19% and is same for all methods.

Management of Endometrioma

The gold standard is laparoscopic cystectomy in endometrioma with good pain relief and fertility rates compared to drainage. Gonadotropin-releasing hormone agonists only decrease the size of the cyst but have no effect on pain relief.

Fenestration, ablation or drainage is less effective with high recurrences than excision.

Complications

- Surgical injuries to adjacent structures (e.g. nerves, blood vessels, ureters, bowels) at the time of excision or ablation, wound infection, and adhesion formation.

ROLE OF LAPAROSCOPY IN FIBROID OF UTERUS

Prevalence is 20–40% in reproductive-aged women.

Based on location:
- Subserous
- Intramural
- Submucous.

Assisted reproductive technique in fibroid has low success rates.

Causes of infertility due to myomas:
- Mechanical obstruction in sperm and embryo transport and implantation
- Endometrial blood flow and biochemical imbalance
- Inflammation
- Irregular contraction of uterus.

The American College of Obstetricians and Gynecologists (ACOG) and American Society for Reproductive Medicine (ASRM) criteria for myomectomy:
- Menorrhagia and anemia
- Severe acute pain
- Infertility with cavity distortion
- Large size producing compression symptoms.

Nowadays laparoscopic approach for myoma removal is justified, safe with pregnancy, and has the same cumulative pregnancy and live birth rates, less pain, shorter hospitalization compared to laparotomy with no difference in complication and recurrence.

Complications of Myomectomy

- Secondary hemorrhage
- Gastrointestinal (GI) injuries
- Adhesion
- Inflammation
- Rupture of uterus in pregnancy and delivery.

LAPAROSCOPY FOR POLYCYSTIC OVARY SYNDROME AND INFERTILITY

The incidence of polycystic ovary syndrome (PCOS) varies between 3% and 15% with some of them are infertile, irregular ovulation, and high miscarriage.

Ovarian Drilling

Ovarian drilling way have a role in clomiphene-resistant PCOS with accompanied indication for laparoscopy [Society of Obstetricians and Gynecologists of Canada (SOGC)]. A small French study also suggested that surgical management via ovarian drilling with hydrolaparoscopy may be beneficial in cases of PCOS that are resistant to clomiphene citrate to induce the ovulation.

Advantages:

- Minimal invasive
- Safe
- Improves gonadotropins sensitivity
- Reduce multiple pregnancy and ovarian hyper-stimulation with concerns about the long-term effects of ovarian drilling on ovarian function.
- Cost-effective.

Adenomyosis

In Indian women, when medical line of therapy is not available or effective or effective, adenomyoma resection is done to relive the symptoms. It improved the success rate of infertility treatment. Many studies have reported various adenomyomectomy methods that preserve the uterus as conservative surgical techniques (Figs. 8A and B).

Aim of Adenoma Resection

The aim of resection is to reduce tension in myometrium [similar to debulking surgery of benign space-occupying lesion (SOL) of brain without injuring vital areas of brain], which can be achieved by debulking the affected myometrium, which is sometimes up to 50%, leading to hemihysterectomy.

Classification: As per its morphological occurrence (1) localized adenomyoma and (2) diffused adenomyosis.

Our Classification of Adenomyosis (Figs. 9A and B)

Three techniques of adenoma resection (Figs. 10A and B):

1. Elliptical strip excision technique
2. Hood technique
3. Slice technique.

Elliptical strip excision technique for Grade-I and Grade-II A with involvement of serosal layer of uterus by adenomyosis: Elliptical strip excision would be better for adenoma resection rather than attempting enucleation as in fibroid.

Hood technique for Grade-I and Grade-II A without involvement of serosal layer of uterus by adenomyosis (intramural adenomyoma): Posterior wall adenoma with normal serosa, incision is made using monopolar needle, Hood is made by coring below the normal uterine serosa, suturing is done by slip knot technique.

Slice technique for large Grade-II B and some of the Grade-III with involvement of serosal layer of uterus by adenomyosis: Posterior wall adenoma with serosal involvement by the disease, injection Pitressin (1:200 mL dilution) is injected

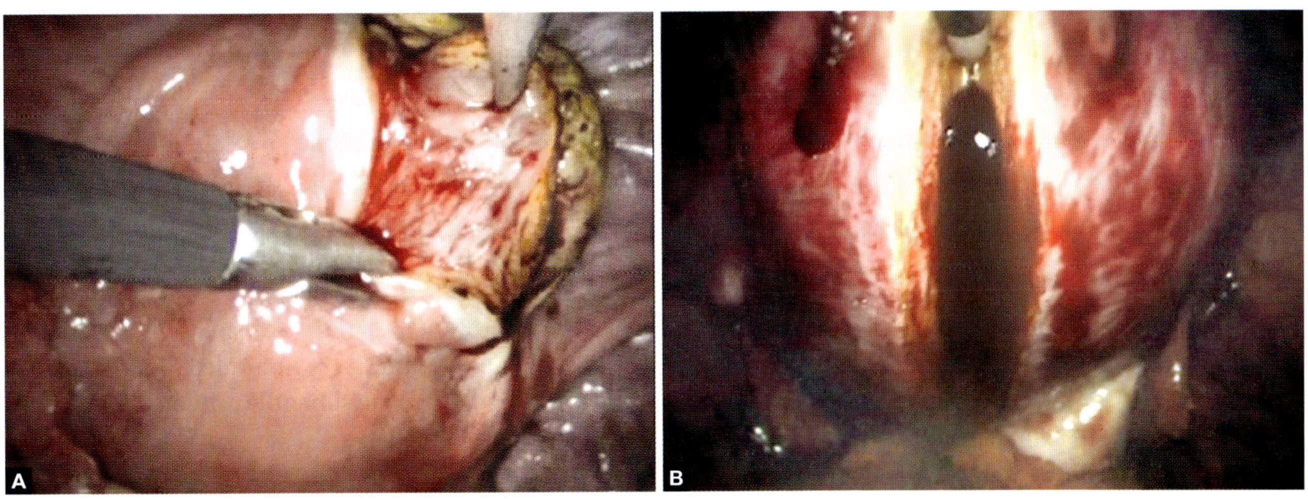

Figs. 8A and B: Adenomyoma resection.

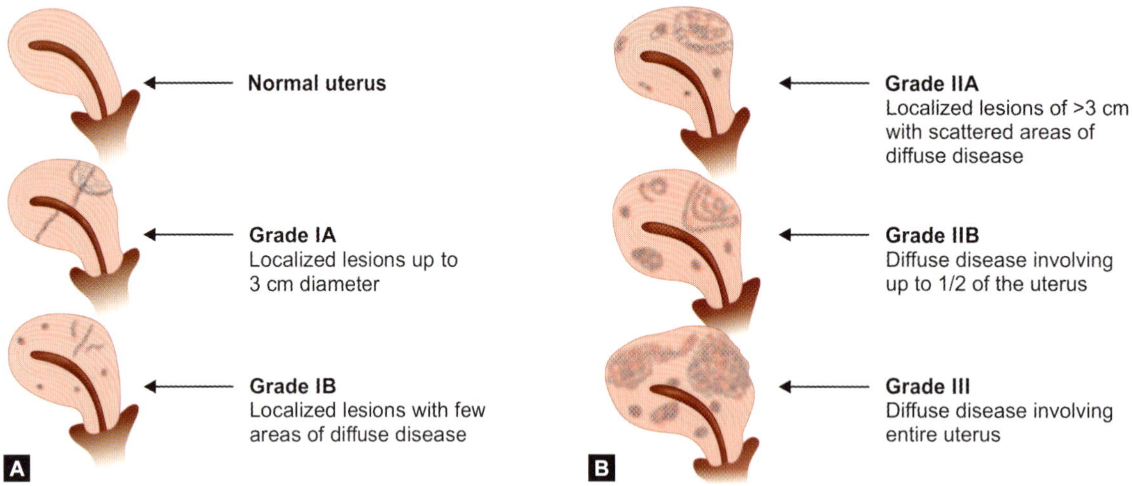

Figs. 9A and B: Pregnancy outcome in different grades of adenomyosis.

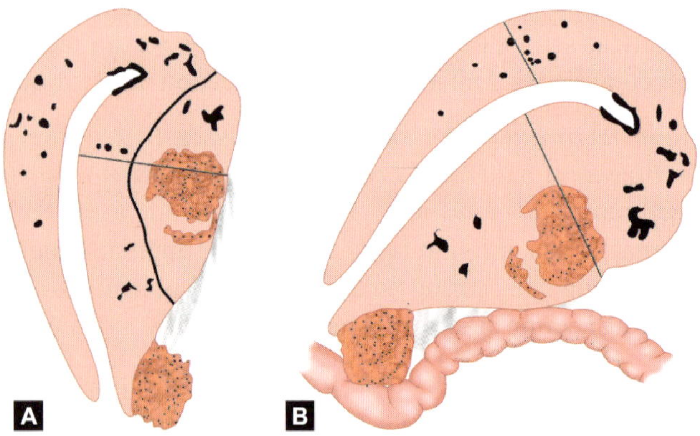

Figs. 10A and B: Techniques of adenoma resection.

in adenoma with lateral mobilization of the ureter, uterine artery is ligated at the origin, slice of adenoma excised, half of the adenomyotic tissue of posterior wall is removed, surgical (j&j) is placed over the raw area for homeostasis.

Conclusion

Adenoma resection is technically more difficult but quite a rewarding surgery in early stage of the disease in terms of fertility and improvement in symptomatology in which hysterectomy cannot be advised.

Laparoscopy Complications (1–2% by ASRM Usually Minor)

Complications:

- Bowel, bladder, and ureteric injury
- Vascular injury and hemorrhage
- Neuronal injury
- Infection
- Anesthesia complication
- Urinary tract infection and urinary retention
- Wound infection
- Re-adhesion
- Hematomas
- Hypersensitivity
- Weeping peritoneum.

Contraindication or caution for laparoscopy:

- Congestive heart failure (CHF), cardiac disease
- Severe pulmonary problem/chronic obstructive pulmonary disease
- Distended bowel
- Previous laparotomy incisions.

It requires experience for surgeons to get best possible outcome of laparoscopic surgery and its complications.

EDITORS' COMMENTS

1. Advances in endoscopic surgery have revolutionized our approaches to gynecological surgeries and now most of the fertility spanning surgeries can be done with laparoscopically requisite skill.
2. Diagnostic hysteroscopy and laparoscopy is one of the most basic and commonly performed surgeries in ART; it can be performed in subfertile patients without other factors.
3. Robotics is a new developing field in ART to reckon in future.

4. Clinical research in the field of reproductive surgery should ideally be guided by high-quality randomized trials (current gold standard), whenever there is uncertainty about effectiveness of a specific surgical intervention.

SUGGESTED READING

1. Alborzi S, Momtahan M, Parsanezhad ME, et al. A prospective, randomized study comparing laparoscopic ovarian cystectomy versus fenestration and coagulation in patients with endometriomas. Fertil Steril. 2004;82(6):1633-7.
2. American College of Obstetricians and Gynecologists. ACOG technical bulletin. Sterilization. Number 222—April 1996 (replaces no. 113, February 1998). Int J Gynaecol Obstet. 1996;53(3):281-8.
3. Bateman BG, Nunley WC, Kitchin III JD. Surgical management of distal tubal obstruction—are we making progress? Fertil Steril. 1988;48:523-42.
4. Beretta P, Franchi M, Ghezzi F, et al. Randomized clinical trial of two laparoscopic treatments of endometriomas: Cystectomy versus drainage and coagulation. Fertil Steril. 1998;70(6):1176-80.
5. Carter JE. Combined hysteroscopic and laparoscopic findings in patients with chronic pelvic pain. J Am Assoc Gynecol Laparosc. 1994;2(1):43-7.
6. Cook AS, Rock JA. The role of laparoscopy in the treatment of endometriosis. Fertil Steril. 1991;55(4):663-80.
7. Darai E, Dechaud H, Benifla JL, et al. Fertility after laparoscopic myomectomy: Preliminary results. Hum Reprod. 1997;12(9):1931-4.
8. Demir SC, Cetin MT, Kadayifçi O. The effect of tubal ligation scoring and sterilization counseling on the request for tubal reanastomosis. Eur J Contracept Reprod Health Care. 2006;11(3):215-9.
9. Donnez J, Nisolle M, Clerckx F. Evaluation of preoperative use of danazol, gestrinone, lynestrol, buserelin spray and buserelin implant in the treatment of endometriosis-related infertility. In: Chadha DR, Buttram VC Jr (Eds). Current Concepts in Endometriosis. New York, NY: Alan R. Liss; 1990. pp. 427-42.
10. Dubuisson JB, Chaperon C, Nos C, et al. Sterilization reversal: Fertility results. Hum Reprod. 1995;10(5):1145-51.
11. Dubuisson JB, Chapron C, Fauconnier A, et al. Laparoscopic myomectomy and myolysis. Curr Opin Obstet Gynecol. 1997;9(4):233-8.
12. Eldar-Geva T, Meagher S, Healy DL, et al. Effect of intramural, subserosal, and submucosal uterine fibroids on the outcome of assisted reproductive technology treatment. Fertil Steril. 1998;70(4):687-91.
13. Farquhar C, Lilford RJ, Marjoribanks J, et al. Laparoscopic 'drilling' by diathermy or laser for ovulation induction in anovulatory polycystic ovary syndrome. Cochrane Database Syst Rev. 2007;CD001122.
14. Gomel V. Microsurgical reversal of female sterilization: A reappraisal. Fertil Steril. 1980;33(6):587-97.
15. Hasson HM, Rotman C, Rana N, et al. Laparoscopic myomectomy. Obstet Gynecol. 1992;80(5):884-8.
16. Hurst BS, Matthews ML, Marshburn PB. Laparoscopic myomectomy for symptomatic uterine myomas. Fertil Steril. 2005;83(1):1-23.
17. Hyams LL. Adenomyosis: its conservative surgical treatment (hysteroplasty) in young women. N Y State J Med. 1952;52:2778-84.
18. Levgur M. Therapeutic options for adenomyosis: A review. Arch Gynecol Obstet. 2007;276:1-15.
19. Mage G, Pouly JL, Bouquet de Jolinière J, et al. A preoperative classification to predict the intrauterine and ectopic pregnancy rates after distal microsurgery. Fertil Steril. 1986;46:807-10.
20. Nezhat F, Yadav J. In: Nezhat C, Nezhat F, Nezhat CH (Eds). Nezhat's Operative Gynecologic Laparoscopy and Hysteroscopy, 3rd ed. Cambridge: Cambridge University Press; 2008.
21. Osada H. Uterine adenomyosis and adenomyoma: The surgical approach. Fertil Steril. 2018;109(3):406-17.
22. Palomba S, Zupi E, Falbo, A, et al. A multicenter randomized, controlled study comparing laparoscopic versus minilaparotomic myomectomy: Reproductive outcomes. Fertil Steril. 2007;88:933-41.
23. Parker W. Uterine myomas: Management. Fertil Steril. 2007;88:255-71.
24. Peacock K, Hurst BS. Laparoscopic myomectomy. Surg Technol Int. 2006;15:141-5.
25. Poujade O, Gervaise A, Faivre E, et al. Surgical management of infertility due to polycystic ovarian syndrome after failure of medical management. Eur J Obstet Gynecol Reprod Biol. 2011;158(2):242-7.
26. Practice bulletin no. 114: Management of endometriosis. Obstet Gynecol. 2010;116(1):223-36.
27. Rawson JM. Prevalence of endometriosis in asymptomatic women. J Reprod Med. 1991;36(7):513-5.
28. Reich H, McGlynn F, Parente C, et al. Laparoscopic tubal anastomosis. J Am Assoc Gynecol Laparosc. 1993;(1):16-9.
29. Reich H. Laparoscopic treatment of extensive pelvic adhesions, including hydrosalpinx. J Reprod Med. 1987;32:736-42.
30. Revelli A, Modotti M, Ansaldi C, et al. Recurrent endometriosis: A review of biological and clinical aspects. Obstet Gynecol Surv. 1995;50(10):747-54.
31. Revised American Fertility Society classification of endometriosis: 1985. Fertil Steril. 1985;43:351-2.
32. Saidi MH, Vancaillie TG, White AJ, et al. Complications of major operative laparoscopy. A review of 452 cases. J Reprod Med. 1996;41(7):471-6.
33. Sauer MV. In: Mishell DR, Davajan V, Lobo RA (Eds). Infertility, Contraception and Reproductive Endocrinology, 3rd edition. Boston: Blackwell Scientific Publications; 1991. pp. 682-707.
34. Seinera P, Arisio R, Decko A, et al. Laparoscopic myomectomy: Indications, surgical technique, and complications. Hum Reprod. 1997;12(9):1927-30.

35. Seracchioli R, Manuzzi L, Vianello F, et al. Obstetric and delivery outcome of pregnancies achieved after laparoscopic myomectomy. Fertil Steril. 2006;86:159-65.
36. Stovall DW, Parrish SB, Van Voorhis BJ, et al. Uterine leiomyomas reduce the efficacy of assisted reproduction cycles: Results of a matched follow-up study. Hum Reprod. 1998;13(1):192-7.
37. Strathy JH, Molgaard CA, Coulam CB, et al. Endometriosis and infertility: A laparoscopic study of endometriosis among fertile and infertile women. Fertil Steril. 1982;38(6):667-72.
38. Swolin K. [50 fertility operations. I. Literature and methods]. Acta Obstet Gynecol Scand. 1967;46(2):234-50.
39. Taylor E, Gomel V. The uterus and fertility. Fertil Steril. 2008;89:1-16.
40. Van Voorhis B. Comparison of tubal ligation reversal procedures. Clin Obstet Gynecol. 2000;43(3):641-9.
41. Vause TD, Cheung AP, Sierra S, et al. Ovulation induction in polycystic ovary syndrome. J Obstet Gynaecol Can. 2010;32(5):495-502.
42. Verkauf BS. Incidence, symptoms, and signs of endometriosis in fertile and infertile women. J Fla Med Assoc. 1987;74(9):671-5.
43. Wada S, Kudo M, Minakami H. Spontaneous uterine rupture of a twin pregnancy after a laparoscopic adenomyomectomy: A case report. J Minim Invasive Gynecol. 2006;13:166-8.
44. Wallach EE, Vlahos NF. Uterine myomas: An overview of development, clinical features, and management. Obstet Gynecol. 2004;104(2):393-406.

22

CHAPTER

Newer Concepts in the Management of PCOS

Duru Shah, Sabahat Rasool

INTRODUCTION

Polycystic ovary syndrome (PCOS) is a complex endocrine spectrum disorder ranging from anovulation to metabolic syndrome. Insulin resistance (IR) and consequent hyperinsulinemia is central to the pathophysiology of PCOS. PCOS is the major cause of anovulatory infertility, accounting for >80% of World Health Organization (WHO) Group II of anovulatory infertility. If lifestyle measures like weight restriction, regular exercise and hypocaloric diet, and ovulation induction with clomiphene citrate (CC) and letrozole fail, low-dose gonadotropins (Gns) or ovarian drilling may be tried. For those who still remain anovulatory, assisted reproductive techniques (ARTs) are reasonable options.

DIAGNOSTIC CRITERIA

The Rotterdam definition of 2003 is the most widely accepted and used definition of PCOS. Two of the following criteria are required to diagnose PCOS:

1. Oligo- and anovulation
2. Clinical hyperandrogenism or biochemical hyperandrogenemia
3. Polycystic ovary morphology on ultrasound with 12 or more follicles measuring between 2 mm and 9 mm and/or ovarian volume >10 mL in at least one ovary.

It has been observed that there is a significant increase in follicles measuring between 2 mm and 5 mm, and no change in follicle numbers measuring between 6 mm and 9 mm. After initial recruitment, it is possible that there is a follicular arrest consequent to hyperandrogenic milieu.

PCOS AND SUBFERTILITY

Anovulation is the leading cause of subfertility in women with PCOS but there may be other contributing factors like IR obesity, hormonal imbalances, and inflammation worsening the oocyte quality. The oocyte competence is compromised leading to reduced fertilization, abnormal meiosis, and embryo formation. IR and hyperinsulinemia lead to impaired glucose metabolism in the follicles with detrimental effect on oocyte energy production. This is followed by an altered expression of key genes for chromosomal alignment and segregation, further worsened by hyperandrogenic microenvironment.

Ovulation Induction

Clomiphene citrate was introduced as an ovarian stimulant in 1961. It is a selective estrogen receptor modulator (SERM) exerting weak agonist effect on some tissue and moderate antiestrogenic effects on others. CC causes prolonged depletion of hypothalamic-pituitary estrogen receptors, thus blocking the negative feedback, leading to a rise in release of pituitary Gn. CC achieves an ovulation rate of 70–92% but a pregnancy rate (PR) only ranging between 20% and 40%. Low PRs are explained by the antiestrogenic effect of CC on cervix, endometrium and tubal motility, decreased uterine blood flow, and endometrium-embryo asynchrony.

Letrozole is a nonsteroidal competitive inhibitor of aromatase. It blocks estrogen synthesis temporarily, releasing hypothalamic-pituitary block, and thus normalizing the pulsatile release of follicle-stimulating hormone (FSH). There is no antiestrogenic effect on endometrium, cervix, and tubes.

Clomiphene Citrate versus Letrozole

In a systematic review and meta-analysis including 1,833 PCOS patients, live birth rates (LBRs), and PRs were found to be statistically significantly higher with letrozole compared to CC. Another meta-analysis of 26 randomized controlled trials (RCTs) with 5,560 PCOS women found letrozole to improve PR and LBR compared to CC. A double-blind RCT of letrozole vs. CC in PCOS women by Amer SA et al. concluded the superiority of letrozole over CC as a primary ovulation induction agent, with 40% increase in PR and with a shorter time-to-pregnancy interval. A recent meta-analysis of 57 RCTs with nearly 8,000 participants concluded that compared to CC alone, both letrozole and combination of CC and metformin showed higher ovulation and PR. Letrozole was the only treatment with significantly higher LBR.

Superovulation Strategies

As far as different Gn preparations are concerned, there is no difference in the outcome between human menopausal gonadotropin (hMG) and recombinant-FSH. The number of oocytes retrieved, LBR, miscarriage, multiple pregnancy, and ovarian hyperstimulation rates are not significantly different among various Gn preparations.

Gonadotropin-releasing Hormone Antagonist

With no gonadotropin-releasing hormone (GnRH) receptor activation and a rapid suppression in secretion within hours of administration, GnRH antagonist (GnRH-ant) regimens offer shorter treatments compared to GnRH agonist regimens. A Cochrane review showed significantly lower incidence of ovarian hyperstimulation syndrome (OHSS) in antagonist regimens with no difference in LBRs in PCOS patients. Lainas TG et al. found an earlier follicular growth and higher estradiol levels during GnRH-ant protocols compared to GnRH agonist long protocol. The oocyte yield, fertilization, and clinical PRs were similar but the OHSS rates were significantly lower in the antagonist group. GnRH-ant regimens are the standard treatment of choice for all PCOS patients in view of marked reduction in incidence of OHSS.

Oocyte Maturation Triggers

GnRH Agonist Trigger

With the use of GnRH-ant protocol, there is an advantage of using GnRH agonist trigger for ovulation. GnRH agonist displaces GnRH-ant from GnRH receptors and induces final oocyte maturation and development. This trigger has a shorter half-life compared to human chorionic gonadotropin (hCG) (60 minutes vs. 32–34 hours) and a lower risk of OHSS. The various agonist triggers used are buserelin intranasal or subcutaneous, triptorelin, and leuprolide subcutaneous. Agonist triggers produce comparable oocyte yield, embryo quality, and implantation and PRs. However, a Cochrane review demonstrated an inferior LBR but reduced rates of OHSS with the use of agonist trigger. The low LBR was attributed to dramatically deficient luteal phase consequent to agonist trigger. Short t1/2 of luteinizing hormone (LH), while being beneficial in reducing OHSS, is not able to sustain and support the corpus luteum for pregnancy.

The various strategies proposed and used for modifying and augmenting luteal phase support following an agonist trigger include a combination of low dose of hCG, and estradiol and progesterone supplementation. Various studies have reported equal LBR after modifying the luteal phase support.

Recombinant LH Trigger

Recombinant LH (r-LH) has a longer half-life compared to native LH and can be used to mimic the mid-cycle LH surge. r-LH is safer than hCG as far as OHSS is concerned. Compared to r-hCG, r-LH demonstrated lower rates of moderate-to-severe OHSS.

Kisspeptin Trigger

A novel agent for oocyte maturation trigger in high risk of OHSS is kisspeptin. Kisspeptins are hypothalamic peptides encoded by *KISS1* gene and are potent stimulants of hypothalamic-pituitary-ovary axis. Kisspeptin 54 has been studied as an ovulation trigger in high responders and was found to be effective as well as safe.

Insulin Resistance and Insulin Sensitizers

Hyperinsulinemia consequent to IR causes hyperandrogenemia besides being a harbinger of metabolic and cardiovascular diseases in women with PCOS. IR is best screened by 75 g oral glucose tolerance test. Insulin sensitizers include metformin, pioglitazone, and inositols.

Metformin: The evidence of metformin in improving LBR in PCOS women undergoing *in vitro* fertilization (IVF) is conflicting. A Cochrane review of five RCTs comparing Gn plus metformin vs. Gn alone concluded that metformin may increase the LBR among women undergoing ovulation induction with Gn. Abu Hashim summarized and critically appraised RCTs and concluded that metformin with CC should be considered as an effective option for CC-resistant PCOS. With Gn ovulation induction, metformin significantly increases LBR and PR with reduced risk of cycle cancellation. In women undergoing ART, metformin confers a beneficial effect on clinical PR and reduces the risk of OHSS. There was no risk of major anomalies with the use of metformin. A Cochrane review of insulin-sensitizing drugs in 4,451 PCOs women with subfertility suggested that metformin alone may be beneficial over placebo for LBR. Metformin plus CC showed a higher clinical PR and ovulation rate compared to CC alone.

Metformin treatment before and during IVF reduces the risk of OHSS.

Inositols: Inositols are being studied extensively for their use in PCOS. Treatment with the two isomers, myo-inositol (MI) and d-chiro-inositol (DCI), in the physiological ration of 40:1 has shown promise in improving hyperandrogenism and metabolic syndrome, thus improving the cardiovascular risk. While MI improves metabolic profile, DCI reduces hyperandrogenism better. DCI at higher doses, however, is detrimental to the oocyte quality. Till there is conclusive evidence about the positive effect of inositols on reproductive outcomes in PCOS women, their use remains largely experimental, and is not recommended as of now.

In Vitro Maturation

Polycystic ovary syndrome patients have hypersensitive ovaries which lead to an overexaggerated response to supraphysiological doses of Gn used for controlled ovarian hyperstimulation. This results in development of a large cohort of follicles being recruited, retrieval of immature oocytes, and increased odds of OHSS. In vitro maturation (IVM) is a potentially effective alternative for women with PCOS, whereby early retrieval of immature oocytes at germinal vesicle stage is done either from unstimulated or minimally stimulated ovaries. These oocytes are isolated by washing the follicular aspirate, then matured *in vitro* in specially formulated IVM medium with melatonin at 37°C and 5% CO_2 for 24–48 hours. The oocytes are then fertilized with intracytoplasmic sperm injection (ICSI) and assessed for fertilization 16–18 hours later. Due to prolonged culture, there is a hardening of zona pellucida, because of which ICSI is preferred even in the absence of male factor. More number of oocytes are retrieved from the polycystic ovary compared to the normal ovary. The maturation and fertilization rates are comparable but pregnancy and LBR are significantly higher in PCOS patients compared to those with normal and polycystic ovaries. The oocyte yield and implantation rates are significantly lower from an IVM cycle compared to the conventional IVF. The PRs per transfer vary between 4% and 27% and implantation rates between 2% and 14%. This is attributed to reduced oocyte development potential, higher odds of abnormal meiotic spindles and chromosomal alignment, nuclear-cytoplasmic asynchrony, imperfect culture conditions, and reduced endometrial receptivity. In a Cochrane review to compare outcomes of IVM followed by either IVF or ICSI, it was concluded that there is still no evidence from RCTs upon which to base any practice recommendations regarding IVM. A meta-analysis of 11 trials with 268 PCOS, 100 PCO, and 440 women with other causes of infertility concluded that IVM appears to be a more efficient treatment option in women with PCOS in terms of clinical pregnancy, implantation, and cycle cancellation rates. In view of poorer pregnancy outcomes with IVM compared to conventional IVF, it becomes a difficult decision for clinicians as well as patients to choose IVM over IVF.

Natural cycle IVM includes a baseline sonography on 2nd or 3rd day of periods followed by another sonography on 6th or 8th day of periods to assess follicular growth and endometrial thickness. Human chorionic gonadotropin trigger is given when the dominant follicle reaches a size of more than 12 and less than 14 mm and endometrium needs to be between 5 mm and 6 mm. Some studies suggested that oocytes obtained after Gn and hCG priming have better developmental competence and maturation rate. Other studies were not able to prove this beneficial effect of Gn priming. Mild ovarian stimulation involves administration of 75 IU of Gn till follicles reach a size of 12 mm. Human chorionic gonadotropin trigger of 10,000 IU is given at follicle size of 12 mm and oocytes retrieved 35–36 hours later. Since the follicular phase length is reduced, endometrial preparation with 6–12 mg of estradiol valerate is started on the day of oocyte retrieval. Progesterone support is begun from the day of oocyte retrieval. The obstetric outcome of babies born through IVM is comparable.

OVARIAN HYPERSTIMULATION SYNDROME

Ovarian hyperstimulation syndrome is a serious iatrogenic complication of ovarian stimulation ranging from mild ovarian enlargement to severe life-threatening complications like pleural/pericardial effusion, adult respiratory distress syndrome, thromboembolic events, and even death. PCOS is the strongest risk factor for the development of OHSS (Fig. 1).

Etiopathogenesis of OHSS

Ovarian hyperstimulation syndrome is an utterly hCG-dependent condition, and consists of ovarian enlargement

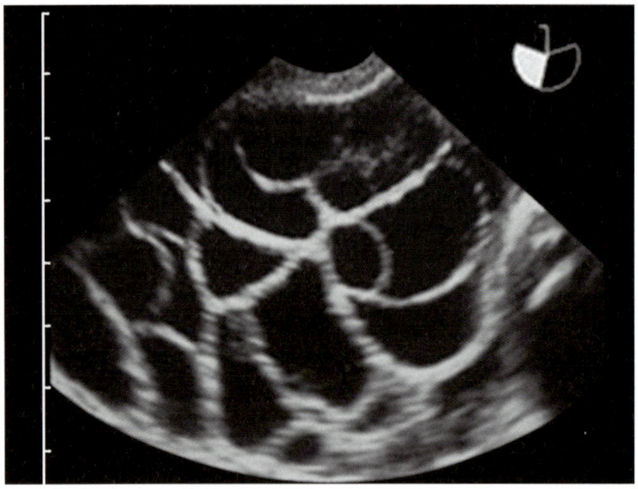

Fig. 1: Hyperstimulated ovary.

and massive production of ovarian hormones and vasoactive substances like rennin, prostaglandins, angiotensin II, vascular endothelial growth factor (VEGF), tumor necrosis factor, and interleukins which promote neoangiogenesis and hyperpermeability state. VEGF levels correlate the best with disease severity.

Classification

The syndrome is classified as early and late. Early OHSS occurs within 3–7 days of hCG triggering, and late OHSS occurs more than 10 days after hCG trigger. Late OHSS only occurs in case of a pregnancy and accounts for 70% of all severe OHSS cases.

Based on severity, OHSS is classified as mild, moderate, severe, and critical (Table 1).

Prevention of OHSS

- Definition of at-risk population is essential for following preventive strategies. The most important risk factor for OHSS is PCO on transvaginal ultrasound having a high antral follicle count with "necklace sign" or "string of pearls" appearance (Table 2).
- Chronic low-dose step-up and step-down methods of ovarian stimulation have been used. Chronic low-dose regimen is more likely to significantly reduce OHSS. Step-down protocol also allows more follicular atresia.
- Coasting/withholding Gn works by altering the VEGF production by granulosa cells. There is conflicting evidence of coasting on oocyte yield and PRs.

TABLE 1 Ovarian hyperstimulation syndrome (OHSS) classification.

Mild	*Moderate*	*Severe*	*Critical*
Bloating	Vomiting	Massive ascites	Tense ascites
Nausea	Abdominal pain	Hydrothorax	Hypoxemia, pericardial effusion
Abdominal distension	Ultrasound evidence of ascites		
	Hematocrit >41%	Hematocrit >45%	Hematocrit >55%
Ovaries ≤5 cm	Ovaries >5 cm	Ovaries enlarged variably	Ovaries enlarged variably
	Leucocyte (WBC) count >10,000/mm^3	WBC count >15,000/mm^3	WBC count >25,000/mm^3
		Oliguria	Oliguria/anuria
		Serum creatinine 1–1.5 mg/dL	Creatinine >1.5 mg/dL
		Hepatic dysfunction	Renal failure, adult respiratory distress syndrome
		Anasarca	Thrombo-embolism

TABLE 2 Risk factors for OHSS.

High risk	*Low risk*
Young <35 years	Older than 35 years
Polycystic ovaries	Hypogonadotropic
Lean built	Heavy built
E2 >4,000 pg/mL in ART >1,700 pg/mL in ovulation induction (OI)	Low E2
Follicles >20 in ART >6 in OI	Poor response to Gn
Necklace sign	Fewer antral follicles
Pregnancy	High basal FSH
hCG luteal support	Progesterone or no luteal support
GnRH agonist cycle	CC/hMG protocol
High AMH	

(AMH: anti-Müllerian hormone; ART: assisted reproductive technology; CC: clomiphene citrate; E2: estradiol; FSH: follicle-stimulating hormone; Gn: gonadotropin; GnRH: gonadotropin-releasing hormone; hCG: human chorionic gonadotropin; hMG: human menopausal gonadotropin; OHSS: ovarian hyperstimulation syndrome)

- Gonadotropin-releasing hormone antagonist cycles with agonist trigger and modified luteal phase support with best toward the preventive of OHSS (as discussed earlier in detail).

- *Blastocyst transfer*: To assess the degree of OHSS before embryo transfer, it is advisable to do a blastocyst transfer. This is because a blastocyst transfer takes place on the 7th day of hCG injection and we can safely assess OHSS before transfer. Elective single blastocyst transfer is being widely advocated in women prone to develop OHSS to minimize the odds of multiple pregnancies.
- *Embryo cryopreservation*: For prevention of severe OHSS in patients showing early signs of hyperstimulation, freeze-all strategy may be employed.

Miscellaneous Preventive Strategies

Human albumin and hydroxyethyl starch (HES) administration at the time of oocyte retrieval has been used extensively. Albumin administration has a significant role in treatment of fully developed OHSS. However, albumin administered may lead to allergic reactions and there is a possibility of prion and virus transmission.

Among other modalities for prevention of OHSS are laparoscopic ovarian drilling prior to controlled ovarian stimulation (COS), use of metformin, calcium infusion, kisspeptin trigger, dopamine agonists, and VEGF-antagonist. Cabergoline, a dopamine agonist, blocks VEGF receptor 2. With a daily dose of 0.5 mg, there is a 50% reduction in the incidence of moderate OHSS.

The American Society of Reproductive Medicine endorses the use of low-dose aspirin in prevention of OHSS.

Treatment of OHSS

Vascular endothelial growth factor and cytokine antagonist therapies are still experimental. Treatment must be individualized. Mild cases need reassurance and follow-up and usually resolve spontaneously. Moderate cases need best rest, plenty of fluid intake especially oral isotonic electrolyte drinks. Patients should be educated to watch out for worsening of symptoms, decreased urine output, and significant weight gain and abdominal distension.

Hemoconcentration is the best marker of severity of OHSS. Leucocytosis is yet another marker to assess severity of the condition. If oral intake is poor or the patient does not tolerate orally, intravenous fluids become mandatory. Crystalloids with NaCl remain the mainstay of treatment, despite hyperpermeable vascular system.

A strict input-output balance should be maintained along with the assessment of body weight, abdominal growth, hematocrit, creatinine, leucocyte count, electrolytes, coagulation profile, and liver enzymes.

About 25% albumin in doses of 50–100 g should be given intravenously every 2–12 hours till hematocrit falls below 45% and urine output increases.

Paracentesis is only indicated for symptomatic relief, tense ascites with venacaval compression, oliguria not corrected by volume expansion, and hemoconcentration unresponsive to medical treatment. Up to 4 L of ascitic fluid can be drained slowly to gravity under aseptic precautions. There is a risk of hemorrhage, infection, and leakage with paracentesis. Women with OHSS must be given prophylactic anticoagulation therapy with either unfractionated or low-molecular weight heparin. Severe and critical forms of OHSS need multidisciplinary intensive care.

EDITORS' COMMENTS

1. Polycystic ovary syndrome is one of the most common endocrinological disorders seen in infertile females. Understanding of complex pathophysiology is required to treat its endocrinological, gynecological, and reproductive issues.
2. Recently released CRE-PCOS guidelines are an extensive compilation of various societies around the world for diagnosis and management of PCOS.
3. Various super ovulation strategies have been developed in PCOS for treatment of infertility.
4. Adjuvants like melatonin, N-acetyl cysteine, myo-inositols, chromium, L-methyl folate have documented beneficial effect on metabolic profile and ovarian function. However, their use has to be customized and discussed
5. Allelic variants of (YPIKa), (have a role in etiology of hyperandrogenemia and/or PCOS), (YP-21 mutation), (YP-17 expression dysregulation and SNP polymorphism etc. have been identified as genetic advancements in the understanding of PCOS.
6. Apart from the infertility point of view one must not neglect the endocrinology metabolic psychological and other long-term complications of PCOS.

SUGGESTED READING

1. Abbara A, Jayasena CN, Christopoulos C, et al. Efficacy of kisspeptin-54 to trigger oocyte maturation in women at high risk of ovarian hyperstimulation during IVF therapy. J Clin Endocrinol Metab. 2015;100:3322-31.
2. Abdalla H, Nicopoullos JDM. The effect of duration of coasting and estradiol drop on the outcome of assisted reproduction: 13 years of experience in 1068 coasted cycles to prevent OHSS. Fertil Steril. 2010;94:1757-63.
3. Aboulghar M, Evers JH, Al-Inany H. Intravenous albumin for preventing severe OHSS: A Cochrane review. Hum Reprod. 2002;17:3027-32.

4. Abu Hashim H. Twenty years of ovulation induction with metformin in PCOS: What is the best available evidence? Reprod Biomed Online. 2016;32(1):44-53.
5. Al-Inany HG, Youssef MAFM, Aboulghar M. GnRH antagonists are safer than agonists: An update of a Cochrane review. Hum Reprod Update. 2011;17(4):435.
6. Alvarez C, Marti-Bonmati L, Novella-Maestre E, et al. Dopamine agonist cabergoline reduces hemoconcentration and ascites in hyperstimulated women undergoing assisted reproduction. J Clin Endocrinol Metab. 2007;92:2931-7.
7. Amer SA, Smith J, Maharan A, et al. Double-blind randomized controlled trial of letrozole versus clomiphene citrate in subfertile women with polycystic ovary syndrome. Hum Reprod. 2017;32(8):1631-38.
8. Anderson AN, Devroey P, Arce JC. Clinical outcome following stimulation with highly purified hMG or recombinant FSH in patients undergoing IVF: A randomized assessor-blind controlled trial. Hum Reprod. 2006;21(12):3217-27.
9. Babayof R, Margalioth EJ, Huleihel M, et al. Serum inhibin A, VEGF and TNF alpha levels after triggering oocyte maturation with hCG in women with PCOS undergoing IVF treatment: A prospective randomized trial. Hum Reprod. 2006;21(5): 1260-5.
10. Balen AH, Laven JSE, Tan SL, et al. Ultrasound assessment of polycystic ovary: International Consensus definitions. Hum Reprod Update. 2003;9(6):505-14.
11. Bergh PA, Navot D. OHSS – A review of pathophysiology. J Assist Reprod Genet. 1992;9:429-38.
12. Bordewijk EM, Nahius M, Costello MF, et al. Metformin during ovulation induction with Gn followed by timed intercourse or intrauterine insemination for subfertility associated with PCOS. Cochrane Database Syst Rev. 2017:1:CD009090.
13. Buckett WM, Chian RC, Barrington K, et al. Obstetric, neonatal and infant outcome in babies conceived by IVM: Initial five-year result 1998-2003. Fertil Steril. 2004;82:S133.
14. Buckett WM, Chian RC, Holzer H, et al. Congenital abnormalities and perinatal outcome in pregnancies following IVM, IVF, and ICSI delivered in a single center. Fertil Steril. 2006;85:11-12.
15. Cha KY, Chian RC. Maturation in in vitro of immature human oocytes for clinical use. Hum Reprod Update. 1998;4(2): 103-20.
16. Chian RC. In vitro maturation of immature oocytes for infertile women with PCOS. Reprod Biomed Online. 2004;8(5):547-52.
17. Child TJ, Abdul Jalil AK, Gulekli B, et al. In vitro maturation and fertilization of oocytes from unstimulated ovaries, polycystic ovaries and women with PCOS. Fertil Steril. 2001;76(5):936-42.
18. Clark JH, Peck EJ, Andersen JN. Estrogen receptors and antagonism of steroid hormone action. Nature. 1974;251: 446-8.
19. De Neuborg D, Mangelschots K, van Royen E, et al. Singleton pregnancies are as affected by OHSS as twin pregnancies. Fertil Steril. 2004;2:1691-3.
20. Delvigne A, Rozenberg S. Review of clinical course and treatment of ovarian hyperstimulation. Hum Reprod Update. 2003;9(1):77-96.
21. Dinicola S, Chiu TT, Unfer V, et al. The rationale of the myo- and d-chiro inositols combined treatment for PCOS. J Clin Pharmacol. 2014;54(10):1079-92.
22. Du A, Kadoch IJ, Bourcigaux N, et al. In vitro maturation for the infertility associated with PCOS: The French experience. Hum Reprod. 2005;20(2):420-4.
23. Dumesic DA, Padmanabhan V, Abbott DH. PCOS and oocyte developmental competence. Obstet Gynecol Surv. 2008;63(1):39-48.
24. European recombinant LH Study Group. Human recombinant LH is as effective as but safer than urinary hCG in inducing final follicular maturation and ovulation in IVF procedures: Results of a multi-center double-blind study. J clin Endocrinol Metab. 2001;86:2607-18.
25. Fauser BC, de Jong D, Olivenness F, et al. Endocrine profiles after triggering of final oocyte maturation with GnRH agonist after co-treatment with GnRH antagonist Ganirelix during ovarian hyperstimulation for IVF. J Clin Endocrinol Metab. 2002;87(2):709-15.
26. Formosa C, Stracquadanio M, Crotta L. Myoinositol vs. d-chiro inositols in PCOS treatment. Minerva Ginecol. 2015;67(4):321-5.
27. Franik S, Kremer JA, Nelen WL, et al. Aromatase inhibitors for subfertile women with PCOS. Cochrane Database Syst Rev. 2014;2(2):CD010287.
28. Gardener DK, Weissman A, Howles CM, et al. Severe ovarian hyperstimulation syndrome. Textbook of Assisted Reproductive Techniques, 5th edition. CRC Press; 2018.
29. Garlisi G, Navot D. Cryopreservation of semen, oocytes, and embryos. Curr Opin Obstet Gynecol. 1992;4:726-31.
30. Humaidan P, Engmann L, Benadiva C. Luteal phase supplementation after GnRH agonist trigger in fresh embryo transfer: The American and European approaches. Fertil Steril. 2015;103(4):879-85.
31. Iliodromoti S, Blockeel C, Tremellen KP, et al. Consistent high clinical pregnancy rates and low ovarian OHSS rates in high-risk patients after GnRH agonist triggering and modified luteal support: A retrospective multi-center study. Hum Reprod. 2013;28(9):2529-36.
32. Isaza V, Garcia-Velasco JA, Aragones M, et al. Oocyte and embryo quality after coasting. The experience from egg donation. Human Reprod. 2002;17:1777-82.
33. Jonard S, Robert Y, Corlet-Rudelli C, et al. Ultrasound examination of polycystic ovaries: Is it with counting the follicles? Hum Reprod. 2003;18(3):598-603.
34. Kinget K, Nijs M, Cox AM, et al. A novel approach for patients at a risk of OHSS: Elective transfer of a single zona-free blastocyst on day 5. Reprod Biomed Online. 2002;4:51-5.
35. Lainas TG, Petsas GK, Zorzovlis IZ, et al. Initiation of GnRH antagonist on day 1 of stimulation as compared to the long agonist protocol in PCOS patients. A randomized controlled trial: Effect on hormonal levels and follicular development. Hum Reprod Update. 2007;22(6):1540-6.
36. Lee C, Tummon L, Martin J, et al. Does with holding gonadotropin administration prevent severe OHSS? Human Reprod. 1998;13:1151-8.

37. Li Y, Feng HL, Cao YJ, et al. Confocal microscopic analysis of the spindle and chromosome configurations of human oocytes matured in vitro. Fertil Steril. 2006;85(4):827-32.
38. Loumaye E, Piazzi A, Engrand P. Results of a phase III, dose finding, clinical study, comparing r-LH with hCG to induce final follicular maturation prior to IVF. Sixteenth World Congress Fertility & Sterility. San Francisco, CA, October 4-9, 1988 (Abst. O-236).
39. Mikkelsen AL, Smith S, Lindenberg S. Possible factors affecting development of oocytes in in vitro maturation. Hum Reprod. 2000;15(Suppl 5):11-7.
40. Mikkelson AL, Indenberg S. Benefit of FSH priming of women with PCOS to the in vitro maturation procedure and the outcome: A randomized prospective study. Reproduction. 2001;122(4):587-92.
41. Moran LJ, Misso ML, Wild RA, et al. Impaired glucose tolerance, type 2 diabetes and metabolic syndrome in PCOS: A systematic review and meta-analysis. Hum Reprod Update. 2010;16(4):347-63.
42. Morley LC, Tang T, Yasmin E, et al. Insulin-sensitizing drugs for women with PCOS, oligomenorrhea and subfertility. Cochrane Database Syst Rev. 2017;11:CD003053.
43. Navot D, Beigh PA, Laufer N. OHSS in novel reproductive technologies: Prevention and treatment. Fertil Steril. 1992; 58:249-61.
44. Out JH, Coelingh Bennick HJ. Clomiphene citrate or gonadotropins for ovulation induction? Hum Reprod. 1998; 13(9):2358-61.
45. Polson DW, Adams J, Wadsworth J, et al. Polycystic ovaries: A common finding in normal women. Lancet. 1988;1(8590): 870-2.
46. Practice Committee of the American Society of Reproductive Medicine. Prevention and treatment of moderate and severe ovarian hyperstimulation syndrome: A guideline. Fertil Steril. 2016;106:1634-47.
47. Roque M, Tostes AC, Valle M, et al. Letrozole versus CC in PCOS: Systematic review and meta-analysis. Gynecol Endocrinol. 2015;31(12):917-21.
48. Rotterdam ESHRE/ASRM-sponsored PCOS Consensus Workshop Group. Revised 2003 Consensus on diagnostic criteria and long-term health risks related to polycystic ovary syndrome. Fertil Steril. 2004;81:19-25.
49. Russell JB, Knezevich KM, Fabian KF, et al. Unstimulated immature oocyte retrieval: Early versus midfollicular endometrial priming. Fertil Steril. 1997;67(4):616-20.
50. Siristatidis C, Sergentanis TN, Vogiatzi P, et al. In vitro maturation in women with vs. without PCOS: A systematic review and meta-analysis. PLoS One. 2015;10(8):e0134696.
51. Skov V, Glintborg D, Knudsen S, et al. Reduced expression of nuclear-encoded genes involved in mitochondrial oxidative metabolism in skeletal muscle of insulin-resistant women with polycystic ovary syndrome. Diabetes. 2007;56(9): 2349-55.
52. Thaler I, Yoffe M, Kaftory JK, et al. Treatment of OHSS: The physiologic basis for a modified approach. Fertil Steril. 1981;26:110-3.
53. Tsilchorozidou T, Overton C, Conway GS. The pathophysiology of polycystic ovary syndrome. Clin Endocrinol. 2004;60(1): 1-17.
54. Tso LO, Costello MF, Albuquerque LE, et al. Metformin treatment before and during IVF or ICSI in women with PCOS. Cochrane Database Syst Rev. 2014;11:CD006105.
55. Van Wely M, Kwan I, Burt AL, et al. Recombinant versus urinary gonadotropins for ovarian stimulation in ART cycles. Cochrane Database Syst Rev. 2011;2:CD005354.
56. Wang R, Kim BV, van Wely M, et al. Treatment strategies for women with WHO group II anovulation: Systematic review and network meta-analysis. BMJ. 2017;356:j138.
57. Wheetan LG III, Vlahos NF. The ovarian hyperstimulation syndrome. Fertil Steril. 2000;73:883-96.
58. Wood JR, Dumesic DA, Abbott H, et al. Molecular abnormalities in oocytes from women with polycystic ovary syndrome revealed by microarray analysis. J Clin Endocrinol Metab. 2007;92(2):705-13.
59. Wynn P, Picton HM, Krapez JA, et al. Pretreatment with follicle stimulating hormone promotes the numbers of human oocytes reaching metaphase II by in vitro maturation. Hum Reprod. 1998;13(11):3132-8.

23

CHAPTER

Recent Advances in Endometriosis in ART

Kanthi Bansal, Sugandha Goel

INTRODUCTION

Endometriosis is a gynecologic pathology that is frequently considered enigmatic. It is a chronic inflammatory disease, disabling 15–20% reproductive group women. Endometriosis presents a diagnostic and clinical challenge and is the second most common gynecological condition after fibroids. It is defined as the growth of endometrial-like tissue outside the uterus. Although its exact cause is unknown, it is hormone mediated and is associated with menstruation.

EPIDEMIOLOGY

Endometriosis is a very common debilitating disease affecting 5–10% women by leading to pain and infertility. In 25–40% infertile women, the etiology is due to endometriosis. The fecundity rate per month of women suffering from this disease is 0.02–0.10 in comparison to fertile women which is around 0.15–0.20.

ENDOMETRIOSIS AND INFERTILITY

Mild endometriosis is common in women with infertility, however, the grade of endometriosis is the reason for infertility and effect depends upon the severity of endometriosis. Around 40% of patients with mild grade conceive by giving expectant management only, whereas quarter patients suffering from moderate disease and very few patients with severe endometriosis are successful.

The mechanisms for endometriosis-related infertility are not fully understood and seem to be different in different stages of endometriosis as follows:

- *Distorted pelvic anatomy*: Impairment of oocyte release owing to pelvic adhesions and endometrioma, impaired tubal transport, and blockage of sperm migration.
- *Altered peritoneal function*: Peritoneal fluid volume raised, concentration of peritoneal fluid increased of the following activated macrophages, prostaglandins, interleukin-1, tumor necrosis factor and proteases, ovum capture inhibitor present in peritoneal fluid which prevents normal cumulus-fimbria interaction, alterations in peritoneal fluid impact sperm, oocyte, embryo or fallopian tube function.
- *Hormonal change and cell-mediated function*: IgA and IgG autoantibodies and lymphocytes alter implantation and receptivity of endometrium. Autoantibodies to endometrial antigens can increase endocrine and ovulatory abnormalities.
- Endometriosis patients may have risk of the following:
  - Abnormal follicle growth
  - Luteinized unruptured follicle syndrome
  - Luteal phase defect
  - Impaired implantation
  - Premature luteinizing hormone (LH) surges.

MEDICAL VERSUS SURGICAL TREATMENT: WHAT IS THE BEST CHOICE AND WHAT COMES FIRST?

The current debate is about whether it is necessary to medically treat, operate, and/or combine both treatments in infertile women. In recent time, a study regarding the combination treatment of gonadotropin-releasing hormone (GnRH) agonists with laparoscopic surgery whether the most suitable treatment or not was published. The optimal treatment protocol is difficult to define for patients with endometriosis. The result shows that in minimal or mild disease, there is no role of medical therapy in patients with minimal or mild endometriosis. Surgical correction with sandwich therapy followed immediately by assisted reproductive technique (ART) should be the standard of care for moderate and severe endometriosis.

Medical Treatment

Whether hormonal treatment [oral contraceptive pill (OCP), GnRH agonists, medroxyprogesterone acetate, danazol] has a role in the treatment of infertility due to endometriosis has been evaluated by meta-analysis done by Hughes et al. Suppression of ovarian function (by means of danazol, GnRH analogues, OCP) to improve fertility in minimal-to-mild endometriosis is not effective and should not be offered for this indication alone.

Cochrane review found no difference between different drugs and their effects on spontaneous pregnancy or live births rates when compared to placebo or no treatment.

Recommendation: Good Clinical Practice Recommendations (GCPR) on endometriosis—The Federation of Obstetric and Gynecological Societies of India (FOGSI)

- Medical management in the form of ovulation suppression is ineffective in improving the pregnancy rates [Evidence level A].
- Guideline development group (GDG) recommends no benefits of adjunctive hormonal therapy before surgery to improve spontaneous pregnancy rates [Evidence level (good practice point) GPP].
- Clinicians should not prescribe adjunctive hormonal therapy after surgery to improve spontaneous pregnancy rates [Evidence level A].
- Guideline development group does not recommend nutritional supplement, complementary or alternate medicine in the treatment of endometriosis-associated infertility [Evidence level GPP].

GnRH Agonist as a Treatment for Endometriosis

Gonadotropin-releasing hormone agonists are synthetic hormones similar to the natural GnRH, causes increase in the follicle-stimulating hormone (FSH) and LH production rapidly. Pituitary gland prevents the production of FSH and LH after their elevated levels, and thus avoids ovulation. Hypothesis says that GnRH agonist acts by regulating the mechanisms of apoptosis and angiogenesis on cells of endometrium and thus inhibiting their growth and proliferation.

There are some latest studies which show that GnRH agonist decreases vascular endothelial growth factor A (VEGF-A) and interleukin 1β (IL-1β) production in endometrium cells and inhibiting the increase in endometriosis.

Dose and Administration

Gonadotropin-releasing hormone agonist is given for 3–6 months, however, the authors of the Cochrane review stressed that the recommendation is based on only one properly randomized study and called for further research, particularly on the mechanism of action.

A 3-month course of treatment may relieve pain symptoms as effectively as a 6-month course but treatment for 6 months appears to lead to a longer delay before the return of symptoms. Based on the drug, the mode of administration and dosage varies.

Recommendation: GCPR on endometriosis—FOGSI

- Ultra-long protocol of GnRH agonists for a period of 3–6 months before ART improves the clinical pregnancy rates [Evidence level A].

Effect of GnRH Agonist in Recurrent Ovarian Endometriomas after Conservative Laparoscopic Management

After surgery, the cumulative rate of ultrasonographic recurrence has been reported to be 11.7% at 4 years and 18.9% at 5 years. The rate of recurrence is directly proportional to duration and follow-up. After surgery, GnRH agonist for 6 months may decrease the pain for 12–24 months when compared to expectant management or placebo. Recently an updated online version of the European Society of Human Reproduction and Embryology (ESHRE) guidelines mentioned that treatment for 3 months with GnRH agonist may be as effective as 6 months in terms of pain relief. Treatment with GnRH agonists for 6 months had a beneficial impact on ultrasonographic recurrence rate after conservative laparoscopic surgery for ovarian endometriosis (Endometriosis Stage III/IV) at 24/36 months follow-up.

Surgical Treatment for Endometriosis-associated Infertility

Surgical Management

Surgery is preferably performed by laparoscopy as it leads to reduced adhesions and requires shorter hospital stay compared to laparotomy. There is insufficient evidence and data available to recommend whether surgical excision in moderate-severe endometriosis enhances pregnancy rates.

The issue of whether surgery improves the chances of a women conceiving spontaneously (naturally) is complex.

But both the Cochrane reviews and the Royal College of Obstetricians and Gynaecologists (RCOG) guidelines are in agreement that there is definite improvement in fertility associated with endometriosis following laparoscopic surgery. Surgical treatment is more efficient by ablating the lesions for the improvement of fertility in the type of minimal-to-mild endometriosis. In addition, pain relief is an added advantage. For ovarian endometriomas, the green top guidelines clearly state that compared to drainage and coagulation the laparoscopic cystectomy is superior. There is good data that excision of endometrioma provides a more favorable outcome than drainage and ablation with regard to the recurrence of the endometrioma, recurrence of pain symptoms, and in women who were previously subfertile, subsequent spontaneous pregnancy.

Excision cystectomy is the ideal method for endometrial cysts in pain and fertility and can be aided by the use of mesna and initial circular excision. An absorbable adhesion barrier, 4% icodextrin solution, and a viscoelastic gel are safe and beneficial products for reducing the adhesion formation in laparoscopic surgery.

The Cochrane review suggests that cystectomy is associated with lesser recurrences of endometriomas as well as recurrence of pain than drainage and coagulation. Excision surgeries also provide the benefit of providing tissue for histology but there is a risk of loss of ovarian tissue and decrease in ovarian reserve. Excision technique is related to increase in rate of pregnancy and a decrease in the rate of recurrence, and can lead to severe damage to the ovarian reserve as per randomized controlled trials. Combined excision-vaporization technique or replacement of diathermy coagulation by suture may improve the latter aspect. There are studies which show positive evidence with Interceed, Oxiplex/AP gel and Adept solution but are based on second look laparoscopies performed few weeks after the intervention and data on fertility is missing.

Clinical Tips

- Adherence to principles of microsurgery such as diligent hemostasis, reduced fulguration, and limited use of sutures may improve fertility.
- Excision is preferred over fenestration, drainage, or ablation of the cyst lining for the treatment of an ovarian endometrioma.
- Use of adhesion-prevention adjuncts may help reduce adhesion formation but improvement in fertility is unknown.

Recommendation: GCPR on endometriosis—FOGSI

- Laparoscopic ablation or excision and adhesiolysis improve pregnancy rate in stage I and II endometriosis when compared to diagnostic laparoscopy alone. [Evidence level A].
- Operative laparoscopy is the treatment for stage III and IV endometriosis to increase spontaneous pregnancy rate [Evidence level B].
- Excision of endometrioma, i.e. cystectomy is better than drainage or coagulation and is recommended as treatment of choice [Evidence level A].
- The GDG recommends clinicians to counsel women with endometrioma regarding the reduction of ovarian reserve following surgery. In the event of previous surgery, the decisions for repeat surgery should be done carefully [Evidence level GPP].
- Excision of endometrioma is strongly recommended in infertile women, when there is suspicion of malignancy or when there is rupture or torsion of the cyst [Evidence level A].

MANAGEMENT OF OVARIAN ENDOMETRIOMA

There is still controversy in understanding the role of endometrioma in leading to infertility but a study showed that patients with infertility due to endometriosis present 17–44% ovarian endometrioma. A large endometrioma may replace most of the normal ovarian tissue. Presence of peritubal and periovarian adhesions may distort the pelvic anatomy. Follicular defects like abnormal follicular growth, decreased follicular size, and shortened follicular phase are observed in women with mild endometriosis. Impaired ovarian function, pituitary ovarian dysfunction, granulosa cell impairment, and uterine function impact on oocyte quality and embryo quality, resulting in ovulatory, fertilization, and implantation disorders.

In endometrioma, the follicular development is compromised, quality of oocyte and embryos is poor which leads to decrease in fertility outcomes. Surgical removal of endometrioma leads to decline in ovarian reserve and the response to stimulation. Expectant management, aspiration with ultrasonography (USG), endometriotic cyst drainage and vaporization of the cyst wall, ovarian fenestration with bipolar electrocoagulation, and laparoscopic cystectomy are advised for endometrioma with infertility. Regarding spontaneous pregnancies and recurrence of the cysts and symptoms, a recent systemic review shows that laparoscopic cystectomy is the best treatment compared to drainage or coagulation.

Alborzi et al. prospectively evaluated 52 patients submitted to laparoscopic cystectomy and observed spontaneous pregnancy rates of nearly 60% in the first year after surgery, which were statistically significant when compared with the 23.3% obtained after endometrioma fenestration and coagulation.

After surgery, for patients under 35 years of age, expectant therapy can be a good choice for spontaneous pregnancy, but over 35 years or patients with ovarian functional impairment should not go for expectant treatment as they have low ovarian reserve and low ovarian response. For such patient ART has to be considered as first line of treatment.

For ovarian endometrioma, ≥4 cm in diameter laparoscopic ovarian cystectomy is suggested. Surgical approach confirms the diagnosis histologically, reduces the risk of recurrence, better access to follicles, increased ovarian response, and prevents endometriosis progression. There is risk of reduced ovarian function postsurgery for which woman needs to be counseled and the decision should be reconsidered if she has had previous ovarian surgery (RCOG GTG 24).

Garcia-Velasco et al. have done a retrospective study, 189 women who had undergone in vitro fertilization (IVF) treatment were evaluated following laparoscopic approach to excise lesions and observed no differences between the groups, whatever variety analyzed. Among operated women, pregnancy occurred in 25.4% patients and among patients with intact cysts, pregnancy occurred in 22.7% patients; showed no statistical significance concluding no additional benefits were provided by cystectomy.

Normal ovarian tissue removal might have a negative effect on controlled ovarian hyperstimulation (COH) due to cystectomy. Accidental removal of ovarian tissue during cystectomy and the damage inflicted by both surgery-related local inflammation and electrosurgical coagulation of ovarian stroma and vascularization may add to the problem but do not affect the mean number of dominant follicles and pregnancy rate.

Treatment of Endometrioma before Starting IVF

Commonly in clinical practice it is found that many patients who are planning for ART have endometrioma. Ovarian reserve is reduced due to surgical excision and there is reduction in healthy tissue of ovaries. But nonremoval of endometriomas might have certain drawbacks such as increasing the risk of infection, rupture, and follicular fluid contamination during oocyte retrieval. Both the ESHRE and RCOG have recommended surgical excision when an endometrioma has a diameter more than 3 cm as probably size more than this may cause difficulties during oocyte pick-up. According to the American Society for Reproductive Medicine (ASRM), there is doubt about any benefit of the excision procedure. Surgery before IVF is also needed if there is hydrosalpinx.

If salpingectomy is surgically challenging due to the extent of endometriotic disease, then proximal resection, clipping or even aspiration at time of IVF can be the options.

For these women undergoing IVF, pretreatment includes surgery, expectant management, and medical treatment. According to a study, there is no significant effect on the rate of pregnancy and on the stimulation response of ovary when compared with no treatment.

However, some author observe that laparoscopic removal of endometriomas before IVF does not compromise the number or quality of oocytes obtained with COH, but at the same time it does not improve fertility outcomes. Hence, cystectomy may be an option when patient has pelvic pain as an associated symptom with infertility.

An ESHRE-sponsored survey to learn the strategies employed for the management of endometrioma (>3 cm) prior to IVF found that surgical management was the most common treatment (82.2%), with cyst wall excision and drainage being the preferred surgical treatment (78.5%). The situation was different for women with previous ovarian surgery or recurrent endometrioma where surgical treatment was less commonly offered. Expectant management of endometrioma remains a major approach in these patients.

Women with normal ovarian reserve can be down-regulated for prolong period based on the study which shows that it may improve the rate of pregnancy compare to women with poor ovarian reserve.

With regard to women who had previous ovarian surgery for endometrioma, implantation and clinical pregnancy rates were higher with the GnRH-agonist protocol than with the GnRH-antagonist protocol (22.6% and 39% vs 15.9% and 27.5%, respectively). There was insufficient data to recommend surgical approach for treatment of endometrioma in asymptomatic subfertile women. According to ESHRE guidelines, for less than 4 cm endometrioma and recurrence, expectant management can be offered. Women should be reassured that IVF does not influence the likelihood of endometriosis recurrence.

Recommendation: GCPR on endometriosis—FOGSI

- In stage I and II endometriosis patients undergoing laparoscopy before ART, consider the complete surgical removal of endometriosis to improve live birth rate, although the benefit is not well-established [Evidence level C].

- In infertile women with endometrioma smaller than 3 cm cystectomy prior to ART does not improve pregnancy rates [Evidence level A].
- In women with endometrioma larger than 3 cm, cystectomy is indicated prior to ART when it is associated with pain or inaccessibility of follicles [Evidence level GPP].

ASSISTED REPRODUCTION AND ENDOMETRIOSIS

Intrauterine Insemination

There is evidence from several randomized controlled trial (RCT) that controlled ovarian stimulation combined with intrauterine insemination (IUI) may be effective in improving fertility in patients with stage I and II endometriosis.

Recommendation: GCPR on Endometriosis—FOGSI

- In stage I and II endometriosis, treatment with super ovulation and IUI improve fertility compared to expectant management. Clinicians should take into consideration, age, duration of infertility, ovarian reserve and male factor [Evidence level A].
- Previous ovarian surgery results in longer stimulation, higher FSH requirement, decreased oocyte number but no difference in fertilization, pregnancy outcome in subsequent ART cycles.

In Vitro Fertilization

Assisted reproduction is widely used to manage infertility associated with endometriosis. IVF may enhance the low fecundity associated with advanced endometriosis. Various studies have reported beneficial effects while others have reported poor outcomes. Various factors play confounding role in pregnancy outcomes; factors like size of endometrioma, previous medical treatment, surgical history and type of surgical treatment, time interval between procedure and embryo transfer (ET), and skill of surgeon. The mainstay of treatment for infertility due to endometriosis is IVF. Whether endometriomas need treatment before starting IVF is another topic of debate. When there is reduced response to gonadotropin hyperstimulation, it reflects damage to ovarian reserve and is noted in patients with nonoperated endometrioma. At present, there is deficiency in randomized trials to consider the benefits of surgical treatment with respect to expectant management before IVF-intracytoplasmic sperm injection (ICSI) cycles. Patients with nonoperated unilateral endometrioma undergoing IVF can have a mean reduction of 25% (6–44%) in codominant follicles in the ovaries affected in comparison to the intact ones. Presence of large and multiple cysts in one ovary can further reduce responsiveness to exogenous gonadotropins. Primordial follicles can be seen histologically close to the cyst wall, probably due to the technical difficulties encountered in removing the cyst, in more than 50% of the endometriomas removed.

Pretreatment for 3–6 months with GnRH-a is suggested as it prevents the premature LH surge effect. The outcome of IVF-ET in patient with mild-moderate endometriosis after long protocol with GnRH-a and human menopausal gonadotropin (hMG) stimulation and tubal factor infertility is similar.

Gonadotropin-releasing hormone antagonist could act as a reasonable choice for poor responder patients in IVF cycles as they cause immediate suppression of LH. Prolonged GnRH-a treatment prior to IVF in cases of moderate-severe endometriosis has been associated with increased pregnancy rates (recommendation grade A, evidence e level 1b). A Cochrane review analyzed three randomized controlled trials in women with endometriosis and compared those who received standard protocol versus GnRH agonist for 3–6 month. However, this recommendation is based on only one properly randomized study and called for further research, particularly on the mechanism of action.

Management of severe/deeply infiltrating endometriosis is difficult and IVF with ultra-long or long protocol is mainstay when other treatments have failed. COH for IVF/ICSI is equally effective with both GnRH antagonist and GnRH agonist protocols in terms of implantation and clinical pregnancy rates but COH with GnRH-a may be preferred because of the availability of more metaphase II (MII) oocyte and embryos. There is no evidence of increased cumulative endometriosis recurrence rates after ovarian stimulation for IVF/ICSI in women with endometriosis.

Recommendation: GCPR on Endometriosis—FOGSI

- Controlled ovarian stimulation (COS) using GnRH agonists or antagonists is effective in IVF patients with mild-to-moderate endometriosis and in those with endometrioma who did not undergo surgery [Evidence level A].
- *In vitro* fertilization or ICSI is recommended when tubal function is impaired, advanced age, male infertility [Evidence level GPP].
- *In vitro* fertilization pregnancy rate and ovarian response to stimulation does not change significantly

after surgical management of endometrioma [Evidence level A].

- In women undergoing IVF, stage III and IV is associated with poor implantation and lower clinical pregnancy rate [Evidence level A].
- In women with endometrioma, clinicians may use antibiotic prophylaxis at the time of oocyte retrieval to reduce the risk of ovarian abscess [Evidence level C].
- In severe endometriosis, IVF treatment after surgery does not increase the risk of recurrence [Evidence level B].
- The effectiveness of surgical removal of deeply infiltrating lesions in women undergoing ART with regards to pregnancy outcome is debatable [Evidence level C].

CONCLUSION

In minimal-mild endometriosis, medical treatment of endometriosis does not improve spontaneous pregnancy rates, whereas there is evidence that surgery is beneficial. There is controversial evidence regarding endometrioma removal owing to the potential impact on ovarian reserve.

In moderate-to-severe endometriosis whether surgical excision enhances pregnancy rate or not, RCTs or meta-analyses are needed. IUI is the treatment for minimal-mild endometriosis, doing ovarian stimulation is effective but the role of unstimulated IUI is uncertain.

In vitro fertilization treatment is advised in patient with male factor infertility and tubal factor. Pregnancy rates in tubal infertility are higher than endometriosis disease. Pretreatment for 3–6 months with GnRH agonist should be considered in endometriosis as it increases the rates of clinical pregnancy.

Combined medical, surgical, and ART treatments may benefit women and they should be used judiciously depending on grade and severity of endometriosis.

FUTURE THOUGHTS

Endometriosis treatment is still in developing stage and various improvements in current medication like oral GnRH antagonists and selective estrogen or progesterone receptor modulators need RCT. Especially in light of the fertility issues related to endometriosis, future therapies are being searched for that will manage pain symptoms without suppressing ovulation, or will result in cure rather than just temporary suppression of endometriosis. In this regard, immunomodulators and antiangiogenic agents are of prime interest. Obstacles to this research still involve lack of complete understanding of the pathogenesis and natural history of the disease.

EDITORS' COMMENTS

1. Endometriosis in its various severity is one of the most common and challenging cases faced by any ART clinicians.
2. Both ectopic and eutopic endometria from patients with endometriosis differ from normal endometrium this can be attributed to changes in the immunology cell adhesion molecules, protein production and gene expression, angiogenesis, steroids and cytokine production.
3. Oxidative stress and decrease in number of granulosa cells, increase in apoptosis in "S" phase, and toxic ovarian micro environment due to chocolate cyst/long standings endometriomas make oocyte quality a major cause of concern in ART cycles.
4. Decision to operate or not is a major debate in endometriosis. Evidence-based guidelines have now come up helping ART clinicians.
5. Dienogest, a newer synthetic oral progestin, has strong progestational and moderate antigonadotropic effect and may be used for medical management for mainly symptoms related to endometrioma and chronic pelvic pain.
6. Recent addition of elagolix (oral GnRH antagonist) is the new drug on block for endometriosis; its efficacy is yet to be tested.

SUGGESTED READING

1. Al-Azemi M, Bernal AL, Steele J, et al. Ovarian response to repeated controlled stimulation in in-vitro fertilization cycles in patients with ovarian endometriosis. Hum Reprod. 2000;15:72-5.
2. Alborzi S, Momtahan M, Parsanezhad ME, et al. A prospective, randomized study comparing laparoscopic ovarian cystectomy versus fenestration and coagulation in patients with endometriomas. Fertil Steril. 2004;82(6):1633-7.
3. Alborzi S, Ravanbakhsh R, Parsanezhad E, et al. A comparison of follicular response of ovaries to ovulation induction after laparoscopic ovarian cystectomy or fenestration and coagulation versus normal ovaries in patient with ovarian endometrioma. Fertil Steril. 2007;88:507-9.
4. Bansal K. Manual of Endometriosis. New Delhi: Jaypee Brothers Medical Publishers (P) Ltd; 2013. pp. 1-2.
5. Bansal K. Manual of Endometriosis. New Delhi: Jaypee Brothers Medical Publishers (P) Ltd; 2013. pp. 42-57.
6. Bansal K. Manual of Endometriosis. New Delhi: Jaypee Brothers Medical Publishers (P) Ltd; 2013. pp. 71-72.
7. Bansal K. Manual of Endometriosis. New Delhi: Jaypee Brothers Medical Publishers (P) Ltd; 2013. pp. 96-99.
8. Bansal K. Manual of Endometriosis. New Delhi: Jaypee Brothers Medical Publishers (P) Ltd; 2013. pp. 193-7.

9. Benaglia L, Somigliana E, Vercellini P, et al. The impact of IVF procedures on endometriosis recurrence. Eur J Obstet Gynecol Reprod Biol. 2010;148:49-52.
10. Benaglia L, Somigliana E, Vighi V, et al. Is the dimension of ovarian endometriomas significantly modified by IVF–ICSI cycles? Reprod Biomed Online. 2009;18:401-6.
11. Benschop L, Farquhar C, van der Poel N, et al. Interventions for women with endometrioma prior to assisted reproductive technology. Cochrane Database Syst Rev. 2010.
12. Cullen TS. Adenomyoma uteri diffusum benignum. Johns Hopkins Hosp Bull. 1896;6:133-7.
13. Demirol A, Guven S, Baykal C, et al. Effect of endometrioma cystectomy on IVF outcome: A prospective randomized study. Reprod Biomed Online. 2006;12:639-43.
14. Dlugi AM, Loy RA, Dieterle S, et al. The effect of endometriomas on in vitro fertilization outcome. J In Vitro Fert Embryo Transf. 1989;6:338-41.
15. Dong X, Wang R, Zheng Y, et al. Surgical treatment for endometrioma does not increase clinical pregnancy rate or live birth/ongoing pregnancy rate after fresh IVF/ICSI treatment. Am J Transl Res. 2014;6(2):163-8.
16. Dunselman GA, Vermeulen N, Becker C, et al. ESHRE guideline: Management of women with endometriosis. Hum Reprod. 2014;29(3):400-12.
17. Endometriosis: Diagnosis and Management. Society of Obstetricians and Gynecologists of Canada. JOGC. 2010;32(7):S4.
18. Exacoustos C, Zupi E, Amadio A, et al. Laparoscopic removal of endometriomas: Sonographic evaluation of residual functioning ovarian tissue. Am J Obstet Gynecol. 2004;191:68.
19. Garcia-Velasco JA, Mahutte NG, Corona J, et al. Removal of endometriomas before in vitro fertilization does not improve fertility outcomes: A matched, case-control study. Fertil Steril. 2004;81:1194-7.
20. Geber S, Ferreira DP, Spyer Prates LF, et al. Effects of previous ovarian surgery for endometriosis on the outcome of assisted reproduction treatment. Reprod Biomed Online. 2002;5: 162-6.
21. Gelbaya TA, Gordts S, D'Hooghe TM, et al. Management of endometrioma prior to in vitro fertilization: Compliance with ESHRE guidelines. Reprod Biomed Online. 2010;21(3):325-30.
22. Genbacev OD, Prakobphol A, Foulk RA, et al. Trophoblast L-selectin-mediated adhesion at the maternal fetal interface. Science. 2003;299:405-8.
23. Hachisuga T, Kawarabayashi T. Histopathological analysis of laparoscopically treated ovarian endometriotic cysts with special reference to loss of follicles. Hum Reprod. 2002;17: 432-5.
24. Hart R, Hickey M, Maouris P, et al. Excisional surgery versus ablative surgery for ovarian endometriomata: A Cochrane review. Hum Reprod. 2005;20(11):3000-7.
25. Ho HY, Lee RK, Hwu YM, et al. Poor response of ovaries with endometrioma previously treated with cystectomy to control ovarian hyperstimulation. J Assst Reprod Genet. 2002;19:507-11.
26. Holoch KJ, Lessey BA. Endometriosis and infertility. Clin Obstet Gynecol. 2010;53(2):429-38.
27. Hornstein MD, Yuzpe AA, Burry KA, et al. Prospective randomised double-blind trial of 3 versus 6 months of nafarelin therapy for endometriosis associated pelvic pain. Fertil Steril. 1995;63:955-62.
28. Hughes E, Brown J, Collins JJ, et al. Ovulation suppression for endometriosis. Cochrane Database Syst Rev. 2007;18(3): CD000155.
29. Inkanen H, Kujansuu E. In vitro fertilization in patients with ovarian endometrioma. Acta Obstet Gynecol Scand. 2000;79:119-22.
30. Jacobson TZ, Duffy JM, Barlow D, et al. Laparoscopic surgery for subfertility associated with endometriosis. Cochrane Database Syst Rev. 2010.
31. Kampe D, Sahl AC, Schweppe K-W. Pra- und postoperative Endometriosetherapiemit GnRH-Agonisten in Depotform: drei- versus sechsmonatige Behandlungsdauer. Zentralbl Gynakol. 2003;125:304.
32. Kao LC, Germeyer A, Tulac S, et al. Expression profiling of endometrium from women with endometriosis reveals candidate genes for disease-based implantation failure and infertility. Endocrinology. 2003;144:2870-81.
33. Klinkert ER, Broekmans FJM, Looman CWN, et al. Expected poor responders on the basis of an antral follicle count do not benefit from a higher starting dose of gonadotropins in IVF treatment: A randomized controlled trial. Hum Reprod. 2005;20:611-5.
34. Kriplani A, Devi R. Good Clinical Practice Recommendations on Endometriosis-FOGSI, 2016.
35. Kuivasaari P, Hippeläinen M, Anttila M, et al. Effect of endometriosis on IVF/ICSI outcome: Stage III/IV endometriosis worsens cumulative pregnancy and live-born rates. Hum Reprod. 2005;20(11):3130-5.
36. Lebovic DI, Mueller MD, Taylor RN. Immunobiology of endometriosis. Fertil Steril. 2001;75:1-10.
37. Lessey BA, Castelbaum AJ, Sawin SW, et al. Aberrant integrin expression in the endometrium of women with endometriosis. J Clin Endocrinol Metab. 1994;79:643-9.
38. Marcoux S, Maheux R, Berube S. Laparoscopic surgery in infertile women with minimal or mild endometriosis. Canadian Collaborative Group on Endometriosis. N Engl J Med. 1997;337:217-22.
39. National Collaborating Centre for Women's and Children's Health (UK). Fertility: Assessment and Treatment for People with Fertility Problems. London, UK: RCOG Press; 2004..
40. Nothnicle WB. Novel targets for the treatment of endometriosis. Expert Opin Ther Targets. 2004;8(5);459-71.
41. Opøien HK, Fedorcsak P, Byholm T, et al. Complete surgical removal of minimal and mild endometriosis improves outcome of subsequent IVF/ICSI treatment. Reprod Biomed Online. 2011;23(3):389-95.
42. Pabuccu R, Onalan G, Kaya C. GnRH agonist and antagonist protocols for stage I–II endometriosis and endometrioma in in vitro fertilization/intracytoplasmic sperm injection cycles. Fertil Steril. 2007;88:832-9.
43. Ragni G, Somigliana E, Benedetti F, et al. Damage to ovarian reserve associated with laparoscopic excision of

endometriomas: A quantitative rather than a qualitative injury. Am J Obstet Gynecol. 2005;193:1908.
44. Royal College of Obstetricians and Gynaecologists. The investigation and management of endometriosis (green-top guideline; no. 24). London, England: RCOG; 2006:3.
45. Sampson JA. Peritoneal endometriosis due to the menstrual dissemination of endometrial tissue into the peritoneal cavity. Am J Obstet Gynecol. 1927;14:422-69.
46. Schenken RS, Asch RH, Williams RF, et al. Etiology of infertility in monkeys with endometriosis: Luteinized unruptured follicles, luteal phase defects, pelvic adhesions, and spontaneous abortions. Fertil Steril. 1984;41:122-30.
47. Somigliana E, Infantino M, Benedetti F, et al. The presence of ovarian endometriomas is associated with a reduced responsiveness to gonadotropins. Fertil Steril. 2006;86:192-6.
48. Somigliana E, Ragni G, Benedetti F, et al. Does laparoscopic excision of endometriotic ovarian cysts significantly affect ovarian reserve? Insights from IVF cycles. Hum Reprod. 2003;18:2450-3.
49. Suganuma N, Wakahara Y, Ishida D, et al. Pretreatment for ovarian endometrial cyst before in vitro fertilization. Gynecol Obstet Invest. 2002;54(Suppl 1):36-40.
50. Suginami H, Yano K. An ovum captures inhibitor (OCI) in endometriosis peritoneal fluid: An OCI-related membrane responsible for fimbrial failure of ovum capture. Fertil Steril.1988;50:648-53.
51. The Practice Committee of the American Society for Reproductive Medicine. Endometriosis and infertility. Fertil Steril. 2004;81:1441-6.
52. Tsoumpou I, Kyrgiou, M, Gelbaya TA, et al. The effect of surgical treatment for endometrioma on in vitro fertilization outcomes: A systematic review and meta-analysis. Fertil Steril. 2009;92:75-87.
53. Verma S. Evidence linked treatment for endometriosis-associated infertility. Apollo Med. 2012;9(3):184-92.
54. Von Rokitansky C. Ueber Uterusdrusen-Neubildung in Uterus- und Ovarial-Sarcomen. Ztschr KK Gesellsch der Aerzte zu Wien. 1860;37:577-81.
55. Winkel CA. Evaluation and management of women with endometriosis. Obstet Gynecol. 2003;102:397-408.
56. Yanushpolsky EH, Best CL, Jackson KV, et al. Effect of endometriomas on oocyte quality, embryo quality, and pregnancy rates in in vitro fertilization cycles: A prospective, case-controlled study. J Assist Reprod Genet.1998;15:193-7.
57. Yap C, Furness S, Farquhar C. Pre- and postoperative medical therapy for endometriosis surgery. Cochrane Database Syst Rev. 2004;(3):CD003678.

24

CHAPTER

Recurrent Implantation Failure

Hrishikesh Pai, Unnati Mamtora

INTRODUCTION

Recurrent implantation failure (RIF) is one of the most common and challenging entities encountered by a fertility clinician in his practice. It is often depressing and saddening for both the patients and the clinicians themselves to deal with. It is said to occur after repeated attempts of embryo transfer fail to achieve a desirable pregnancy due to lack of implantation.

The most common cause of recurrent *in vitro* fertilization (IVF) failure is implantation failure. Repeated IVF failure refers to failure to achieve pregnancy after several IVF attempts. Poor response to ovarian stimulation, poor embryo quality, advanced maternal age, and uterine factors are relatively common causes of recurrent IVF failures. Recurrent implantation is a subset/subgroup of RIF. There are no well-set criteria to define implantation failure. Implantation is the attachment of the embryo to the luminal surface of lining of the endometrium of the uterus. It in turn involves various steps like adhesion, invasion, and vascularization. We clearly see and understand that for successful implantation, the embryo, the endometrial lining, and its interplay have a crucial and important role.

There is no definitive consensus on the definition of RIF.

Recurrent implantation failure is defined as the failure of successful implantation after the transfer of four or more good quality embryos in three or more attempts of embryo transfer in a woman aged less than 40 years of age.

Implantation is said to be successful after evidence of gestational sac in uterine cavity on ultrasonography. Implantation failure may be thus of two types, one in which the beta human chorionic gonadotropin (β-hCG) is detected positive, often called as a biochemical pregnancy but no evidence of gestational sac or second one, in which β-hCG is negative.

There are many causes of RIF which include both embryonic and maternal causes:

- *Embryonic causes*:
  - Genetic
  - Poor embryo quality (egg/sperm)
  - Male factor contribution.
- *Maternal causes*:
  - Age
  - Anatomical
    - Congenital anomalies
    - Acquired (septum/polyp/fibroids/adhesions)
  - Endometrial function
  - Thrombophilia and connective tissue disorder
  - Immunological (altered adhesion molecule, Th2/Th1 ratio).

Successful implantation may be hampered if the embryo is disordered. The quality of the embryo, the number of embryos, the stage of the embryo, and the storage protocol used play an important determining factor in achieving a successful pregnancy.

The embryo of a superior quality increases the probability of getting a successful pregnancy. A good quality embryo is defined as the one which has all the cells equal in size, regular margins without fragmentation.

Maternal factors include the anatomical/uterine factor and immunological factor.

Uterine factors may either be due to congenital anomalies in the uterus or due to the acquired factors.

While major of the congenital anomalies are due to fusion defect in the Mullerian ducts, the septate uterus is the most common anatomical factor. The uterine septal abnormalities are associated with reduction in the implantation rates and increased miscarriage rates. Most common reason is due to altered anatomy and the compromised blood flow secondary to the septum. Various studies conducted have shown to have better pregnancy rates and implantation rates with reduced miscarriage rates after corrective surgery of septate uterus.

The *Hoxa 10* and *Hoxa 11* genes are proposed to be regulatory genes in the functional endometrium for implantation. Hoxa genes are said to be regulatory genes in the Mullerian duct development. These are said to be altered in RIF.

In contrast to septate uterus, bicornuate uteri have good pregnancy rates and implantation rates but increased incidences of miscarriage and preterm delivery.

ACQUIRED UTERINE ABNORMALITIES

The acquired uterine pathologies include the endometrial polyps, intrauterine fibroids, and intrauterine adhesions. These pathologies often go unrecognized in 25–50% of the patients.

The submucosal uterine fibroids result in increased contractility, cytokine derangement, decreased blood supply, and chronic inflammation. The submucosal fibroids are associated with decreased pregnancy rates and implantation rates with increased miscarriage rates. (Bernard et al 2000; Farhi et al.,1995; Narayan and Goswamy, 1994; Varasteh et al., 1999).

Intramural Fibroids

Intramural fibroids have a controversial role on the IVF outcome. There is contrasting evidence according to the studies conducted in the past regarding the role of submucosal fibroids and pregnancy rates. Metwally et al. (2011) in his analysis concluded that the evidence available is weak due to the heterogeneity and methodology used in the studies.

Women with intramural fibroids have reduced implantation rates as compared with those without one. Myomectomy did not improve pregnancy rates in a study conducted by Petris et al. (2009).

Endometrial polyps: Endometrial polyps affect implantation rates after embryo transfer too and removal of polyp improves the pregnancy rates in these women.

Intrauterine adhesions may occur secondary to intrauterine infections or prior surgery like an emergency curettage following a missed abortion. Their incidence in women with RIF is approximately 8.5%. Treating the intrauterine adhesions improves the pregnancy rates in these patients.

Hydrosalpinges

Hydrosalpinges affect the implantation rates and have a major role in RIF. Many theories have been proposed to explain their role. Some signify the fluid in the hydrosalpinx has embryo toxic effect, impairs implantation and also might have a flushing effect on the embryo.

Removal of hydrosalpinges restored the levels of leukemia inhibiting factor and integrins. After removal of the hydrosalpinx following salpingectomy, the pregnancy rates and live birth rates improved significantly in a Scandinavian study.

Immunological Factors and Thrombophilic Conditions

There is no proper consensus derived from the presently available evidence in literature. Many studies have been conducted but none of them have been able to guide about the role of the immunological investigations and treatment in RIF.

The role of thrombophilic conditions in relation to RIF still remains to be determined. Thrombophilia has a definitive role in recurrent pregnancy losses and such cases seem to be benefited from the use of heparin and aspirin. However, the studies conducted in relation with RIF give controversial results, whereas others could not confirm it (Hill and Scott., 2000; Hornstein et al., 2000; Kowalik et al., 1997).

Investigations

Blood investigations like ovarian function tests [anti-Müllerian hormone (AMH), antral follicle count (AFC), and basal follicle-stimulating hormone (FSH)] to rule out compromised ovarian function in women with RIF.

Karyotyping: Incidence of couples with abnormal karyotype in RIF is approximately 2.5% which is higher than the general population.

Others include pelvic ultrasonography, hysteroscopy, and combined hysterolaparoscopy.

Management

Management of RIF requires a holistic approach. Couples need to be reviewed by a senior reproductive medicine specialist, a senior embryologist, and a counselor. A total review on all the details about the previous history paper, diagnosis, investigation, and management should be noted and further plan and management should be done accordingly.

Counseling regarding lifestyle modification, cessation of smoking, and alcohol consumption should be taken into consideration.

A total review of the previous ovarian stimulation protocol should be considered. A small group of women having poor response to the stimulation protocol may require increase in dose of gonadotropin. A few poor responder patients and patients above age of 35 years get benefited from adding LH.

Also, ultra-long protocol is beneficial in women with endometriosis and adenomyosis which increases the pregnancy rates in IVF/intracytoplasmic sperm injection (ICSI) cycles.

SPERM DNA FRAGMENTATION

In cases where male factor infertility is the cause of RIF and sperm DNA fragmentation is high, medical treatment may be considered along with addition of oral antioxidants.

Spermatozoa with low levels of DNA damage can be selected. Use of newer laboratory technologies like Annexin-V column, techniques like intracytoplasmic morphologically selected sperm injection (IMSI), use of CLASS technology (confocal light absorption scattering spectroscopy), and use of high magnification ICSI to identify vacuoles on the surface of spermatozoa, will help in getting good quality for sperm fertilization. More randomized controlled trials are required to confirm the above technologies.

The level of the DNA damage is much lower in the spermatozoa in the testicles as compared to the ones in the ejaculated samples and the epididymis

And hence the testicular spermatozoa may be useful over the ejaculated ones in patients of RIF with high DNA fragmentation. But we need more randomized controlled trials for the same.

Embryo quality and the stage at which the embryos are transferred play a crucial role in achieving successful implantation.

Blastocyst transfer improves the results in patients with RIF and this has been supported by many studies including one meta-analysis (Papanikolaou et al. 2008). The synchronicity between the embryo and the endometrium is improved by blastocyst transfer (Blake et al. 2007); and so does the effect of sequential transfer or a double transfer. Various studies have been conducted which state that sequential transfer improves the implantation rates, pregnancy rates, live birth rates, and also causes reduction in the miscarriage rates. It improves the window of implantation and also has the benefits of endometrial scratching effect (D3+D5) transfer.

Assisted Laser Hatching

An intrinsic abnormality in the embryo and the blastocyst is associated with thickening of the zona pellucida. This can be tackled by artificial thinning or breaching of the zona pellucida to improve the implantation rates and pregnancy rates in RIF patients (ASRM, 2008). Though there is no risk of damage to the individual blastomeres and the embryos, there is increased risk of monozygotic twinning.

It is proposed that assisted hatching is useful in poor prognosis patients, in women above the age of 38 years, in poor embryo quality embryos, and multiple failed attempts of previous IVF cycles (ASRM practice guidelines, 2008).

Preimplantation Genetic Diagnosis

There is a lot of controversy regarding the role of preimplantation genetic diagnosis in RIF. Mosaicism detected in a single blastomere cannot be applied to the whole embryo. Hence, we require more randomized controlled trials to recommend the use of preimplantation genetic diagnosis in RIF.

Comparative genomic hybridization and single-nucleotide polymorphism micro arrays provide blastocyst cytogenetic in detailed manner. This helps in selecting normal euploid embryos.

Metabolomics: The metabolomic changes in the culture medium (amino acids, proteins, consumption of oxygen) can be used and measured and thus are useful for embryo selection.

Embryo Transfer

Embryo transfer plays a key role in the successful implantation process. The technique of transfer, the catheter used, the experience of the clinician, and ultrasound-guided procedure play an important role. The details of the previous transfer should be viewed as to understand if any difficulties were encountered during the procedure. Acute anteversion of uterus, acute retroversion of uterus, and cervical stenosis are few reasons for difficult transfer. Adequate partial filling of bladder before the procedure, proper patient position, acutely flexed thighs, and ultrasound-guided procedure are some of the steps that help in improving the ease of the procedure. Ultrasound-guided procedures improve the clinical pregnancy rates and live birth rates (Abou-Setta et al., 2007). A trial embryo transfer or a mock transfer may be done prior to actual transfer day. Aspiration of the cervical mucus is proposed to improve the pregnancy rates; however, studies done by Letterie et al. (2003) contradict this belief.

There is insufficient evidence if bed rest after embryo transfer improves the success rates.

If all the above fail, then transfer into the fallopian tube [zygote intrafallopian transfer (ZIFT)] but many randomized controlled trials conducted failed to demonstrate any evidence that above might improve the implantation rates or not. We need more randomized controlled trails to define the role in RIF.

Pre-ART (assisted reproductive technique) hysteroscopy: Demirol and Gurgan (2004) have established evidence that hysteroscopy improves results in patients with RIF. Corrective surgery may be performed in the same sitting and these patients may be benefitted by doing the same.

Thin Endometrium

Tackling the thin endometrium improves the result in patients with RIF. Many novel techniques like endometrial scratching, instillation of granulocyte colony-stimulating factor (GCSF), and platelet-rich plasma (PRP) may be useful.

The evidence available is too small and we need more randomized controlled trials for the same.

Empirical Therapies

Aspirin

There is good evidence to prove that aspirin should not be used in patients with RIF.

Heparin

Patients who test positive for antiphospholipids, antinuclear or beta glycoprotein I antibodies did not show any improvement in implantation rates and pregnancy rates after giving heparin therapy (Stern et al., 2003).

The therapy is not justified according to the present data availability (ASRM 2008).

GAMETE DONATION AND SURROGACY

If the implantation fails after several attempts and application of the above improvements in the treatment, gamete donation and surrogacy options should be explored. Gamete donation in case of embryo as causative factor and in cases of uterus being at fault surrogacy might come to rescue. When all the above fail, adoption should be discussed and offered as the last resort.

EDITORS' COMMENTS

1. Recurrent implantation failure is one of the most challenging situations for any ART clinician in his clinic practice.
2. Meticulous retrospective analysis of gametes, procedures, QA, and QC in laboratories, etc. could reveal simplest possible solution or lacunas in treatment cycle and is of utmost importance for further management.
3. Numerous treatment options are available for RIF; one can take an approach to trying everything as a cocktail or be evidence-based in treating the patient keeping into consideration the financial, psychological and time constraints.

SUGGESTED READING

1. Abou-Setta AM, Al-Inany HG, Mansour RT, et al. Soft versus firm embryo transfer catheters for assisted reproduction: A systematic review and meta-analysis. Hum Reprod. 2005;20:3114-21.
2. Akrakis E, Pantos K. The outcomes of hysteroscopy in women with implantation failures after in-vitro fertilization: Findings and effect on subsequent pregnancy rates. Curr Opin Obstet Gynecol. 2010;22:339-43.
3. Balasch J, Vidal E, Penarrubia J, et al. Suppression of LH during ovarian stimulation: Analysing threshold values and effects on ovarian response and the outcome of assisted reproduction in down-regulated women stimulated with recombinant FSH. Hum Reprod. 2001;16:1636-43.
4. Bartoov B, Berkovitz A, Eltes F, et al. Pregnancy rates are higher with intracytoplasmic morphologically selected sperm injection than with conventional intracytoplasmic injection. Fertil Steril. 2003;80:1413-9.
5. Bernard G, Darai E, Poncelet C, et al. Fertility after hysteroscopic myomectomy: Effect of intramural myomas associated. Eur J Obstet Gynecol Reprod Biol. 2000;88:85-90.
6. Blake D, Farquhar C, Johnson N, et al. Cleavage stage versus blastocyst stage embryo transfer in assisted conception. Cochrane Database Syst Rev. 2007;CD002118.
7. Bosteels J, Weyers S, Puttemans P, et al. The effectiveness of hysteroscopy in improving pregnancy rates in subfertile women without other gynaecological symptoms: A systematic review. Hum Reprod Update. 2010;16:1-11.
8. Clark DA, Stricker RB. Is intravenous immunoglobulins (IVIG) efficacious in early pregnancy failure? A critical review and meta-analysis for patients who fail in vitro fertilisation and embryo transfer (IVF). J Assist Reprod Genet. 2006;23:113.
9. Coulam C, Kaider B, Kaider AS, et al. Antiphospholipid antibodies associated with implantation failure after IVF/ET. J Assist Reprod Genet. 1997;14:603-60.
10. Daftary GS, Taylor HS. Implantation in the human: The role of HOX genes. Semin Reprod Med. 2000;18:311-20.
11. Das M, Holzer HE. Recurrent implantation failure: Gamete and embryo factors. Fertil Steril. 2012;97:1021-7.
12. Dawood A, Al-Talib A, Tulandi T. Predisposing factors and treatment outcome of different stages of intrauterine adhesions. J Obstet Gynaecol Can. 2010;32:767-70.
13. Demirol A, Gurgan T. Effect of treatment of intrauterine pathologies with office hysteroscopy in patients with recurrent IVF failure. Reprod Biomed Online. 2004;8:590-4.

14. Dirckx K, Cabri P, Merien A, et al. Does low-dose aspirin improve pregnancy rate in IVF/ICSI? A randomized double-blind placebo controlled trial. Hum Reprod. 2009;24:856-60.
15. Fragouli E, Lenzi M, Ross R, et al. Comprehensive molecular cytogenetic analysis of the human blastocyst stage. Hum Reprod. 2008;23(11):2596-608.
16. Gelbaya TA, Kyrgiou M, Li TC, et al. Low-dose aspirin for in vitro fertilization: A systematic review and meta-analysis. Hum Reprod Update. 2007;13:357-64.
17. Glass KB, Green C, Fluker MR, et al. Multicenter randomized controlled trial of cervical irrigation at the time of embryo transfer. Fertil Steril. 2000;73(Suppl 1):S31.
18. Greco E, Iacobelli M, Rienzi L, et al. Reduction of the incidence of sperm DNA fragmentation by oral antioxidant treatment. J Androl. 2005;26:349-53.
19. Greco E, Scarselli F, Iacobelli, M, et al. Efficient treatment of infertility due to sperm DNA damage by ICSI with testicular spermatozoa. Hum Reprod. 2005;20:226-30.
20. Grimbizis GF, Camus M, Tarlatzis BC, et al. Clinical implications of uterine malformations and hysteroscopic treatment results. Hum Reprod Update. 2001;7:161-74.
21. Guerif F, Bidault R, Gasnier O, et al. Efficacy of blastocyst transfer after implantation failure. Reprod Biomed Online. 2004;9:630-6.
22. Hershlag A, Paine T, Cooper GW, et al. Monozygotic twinning associated with mechanical assisted hatching. Fertil Steril. 1999;71:144-6.
23. Hill JA, Scott RT. Immunologic tests and IVF: 'Please, enough already.' Fertil Steril. 2000;74:439-42.
24. Hornstein MD, Davis OK, Massey JB, et al. Antiphospholipid antibodies and in vitro fertilization success: A meta-analysis. Fertil Steril. 2000;73:330-3.
25. Isidori AM, Pozza C, Ganfrilli D, et al. Medical treatment to improve sperm quality. Reprod Biomed Online. 2006;12:704-14.
26. Jakab A, Sakkas D, Delpiano E, et al. Intracytoplasmic sperm injection: A novel selection method for sperm with normal frequency of chromosomal aneuploidies. Fertil Steril. 2005;84:1665-73.
27. Kaider BD, Price DE, Roussev RG, et al. Antiphospholipid antibody prevalence in patients with IVF failure. Am J Reprod Immunol. 1996;35:388-93.
28. Lavergne N, Aristizabal J, Zarka V, et al. Uterine anomalies and in vitro fertilization: What are the results? Eur J Obstet Gynecol Reprod Biol. 1996;68:29-34.
29. Letterie G, Marshall L, Angle M. Intrauterine reflux of media during cervical irrigation at embryo transfer. Fertil Steril. 2003;79:1444-5.
30. Mains L, Van Voorhis BJ. Optimizing the technique of embryo transfer. Fertil Steril. 2010;94:785-90.
31. Marek D, Langley M, Gardner DK, et al. Introduction of blastocyst culture and transfer for all patients in an in vitro fertilization program. Fertil Steril. 1999;72:1035-40.
32. Marrs R, Meldrum D, Muasher S, et al. Randomized trial to compare the effect of recombinant human FSH (follitropin alfa) with or without recombinant human LH in women undergoing assisted reproduction treatment. Reprod Biomed Online. 2004;8:175-82.
33. McNamee P, Huang T, Carwile A, et al. Significant increase in pregnancy rate achieved by vigorous irrigation of endocervical mucus prior to embryo transfer with the Wallace catheter in an IVF-ET program. Fertil Steril. 1997;68(Suppl 1):S208-9.
34. Metwally M, Farquhar CM, Li TC. Is another meta-analysis on the effects of intramural fibroids on reproductive outcomes needed? Reprod Biomed Online. 2011;23:2-14.
35. Papanikolaou EG, Kolibianakis EM, Tournaye H, et al. Live birth rates after transfer of equal number of blastocysts or cleavage-stage embryos in IVF. A systematic review and meta-analysis. Hum Reprod. 2008;23:91-99.
36. Phelps JY, Figueira-Armada L, Levine AS, et al. Exogenous luteinizing hormone (LH) increases estradiol response patterns in poor responders with low serum LH concentrations. J Assist Reprod Genet. 1999;16:363-8.
37. Qublan HS, Eid SS, Ababneh HA, et al. Acquired and inherited thrombophilia: Implication in recurrent IVF and embryo transfer failure. Hum Reprod. 2006;21:2694-8.
38. Raga F, Bauset C, Remohi J, et al. Reproductive impact of congenital Mullerian anomalies. Hum Reprod. 1997;12:2277-81.
39. Richlin SS, Ramachandran S, Shanti A, et al. Glycodelin levels in uterine flushing and in plasma of patients with leiomyomas and polyps: Implications for implantation. Hum Reprod. 2002;17:2742-7.
40. Said TM, Grunewald S, Paasch U, et al. Advantage of combining magnetic cell separation with sperm preparation techniques. Reprod Biomed Online. 2005;10:740-6.
41. Sallam HN, El-Kassar Y, Hany Abdella Rahman A, et al. Glucose consumption and total protein production by preimplantation embryos in women with the polycystic ovary syndrome. Fertil Steril. 2006;86(Suppl 3):S462-3.
42. Schieve LA, Meikle SF, Peterson HB, et al. Does assisted hatching pose a risk for monozygotic twinning in pregnancies conceived through in vitro fertilization? Fertil Steril. 2000;74:288-94.
43. Schoolcraft WR, Fragouli E, Stevens I, et al. Clinical application of comprehensive chromosomal screening at the blastocyst stage. Fertil Steril. 2010;94:1700-6.
44. Sharif K, Afnan M, Lenton W. Mock embryo transfer with a full bladder immediately before the real transfer for in-vitro fertilization treatment: The Birmingham experience of 113 cases. Hum Reprod. 1995;10:1715-8.
45. Shokeir TA, Shalan HM, El-Shafei MM. Significance of endometrial polyps detected hysteroscopically in eumenorrheic infertile women. J Obstet Gynaecol Res. 2004;30:84-9.
46. Souza Setti A, Ferreira RC, Paes de Almeida Ferreira Braga D, et al. Intracytoplasmic sperm injection outcome versus intracytoplasmic morphologically selected sperm injection outcome: A meta-analysis. Reprod Biomed Online. 2010;21:450-5.

47. Spiewankiewicz B, Stelmachow J, Sawicki W, et al. The effectiveness of hysteroscopic polypectomy in cases of female infertility. Clin Exp Obstet Gynecol. 2003;30:23-5.
48. Stern C, Chamley L, Norris H, et al. A randomized, double-blind, placebo-controlled trial of heparin and aspirin for women with in vitro fertilization implantation failure and antiphospholipid or antinuclear antibodies. Fertil Steril. 2003;80:376-83.
49. Strandell A, Lindhard A, Waldenstrom U, et al. Hydrosalpinx and IVF outcome: A prospective, randomized multicentre trial in Scandinavia on salpingectomy prior to IVF. Hum Reprod. 1999;14:2762-9.
50. Suganuma R, Yanagimachi R, Meistrich ML. Decline in fertility of mouse sperm with abnormal chromatin during epididymal passage as revealed by ICSI. Hum Reprod. 2005;20:3101-8.
51. Sunkara SK, Khan KS. Adenomyosis and female fertility: A critical review of the evidence. J Obstet Gynaecol. 2012;32: 113-6.
52. Taylor H. The role of HOX genes in human implantation. Hum Reprod Update. 2000;6:75-79.
53. Tomas C, Tikkinen K, Tuomivaara L, et al. The degree of difficulty of embryo transfer is an independent factor for predicting pregnancy. Hum Reprod. 2002;17:2632-5.
54. Tremellen K, Russell P. Adenomyosis is a potential cause of recurrent implantation failure during IVF treatment. Aust NZ J Obstet Gynaecol. 2011;51:280-3.

25

CHAPTER

Recurrent Pregnancy Loss: What's New

Mala Arora

INTRODUCTION

Recurrent miscarriage (RM) is a profound personal tragedy experienced by couples seeking parenthood and is an equally challenging task for the attending obstetrician. Miscarriage is defined as the spontaneous loss of pregnancy before the fetus reaches viability and therefore, includes all pregnancy losses from the time of conception until 20 weeks of gestation. RM may also be referred as recurrent pregnancy loss (RPL) and recurrent spontaneous miscarriage (RSM).

DEFINITION

Royal College of Obstetricians & Gynecologists (RCOG) (UK) defines RPL as three or more consecutive pregnancy losses at 20 weeks or less or with fetal weight of less than 500 grams. American College of Obstetrics and Gynecologists (ACOG) defined it as two or more spontaneous miscarriages for clinical purposes. American Society of Reproductive Medicine (ASRM) defines RPL as two or more failed clinical pregnancies, which should be documented by either ultrasound or histopathological examination. None of the definitions include biochemical pregnancies, ectopic pregnancies, or pregnancy of uncertain location.

Sporadic miscarriages occur in 25% of pregnancies. A woman may have three sporadic miscarriages during her obstetric career, but if these are interspersed with viable births, they are not classified as RMs.

Primary aborters are women who have no previous pregnancy that progressed to viability and secondary aborters are women who have one or more pregnancies that have proceeded beyond 20 weeks' gestation.

For research purposes, the definition of RM is three or more consecutive losses and RCOG recommends investigations after three consecutive losses. However, ASRM practice guidelines state that, in the clinical scenario, evaluation should be considered following two consecutive miscarriages, especially with advanced maternal age >35 years. In patients that conceive with assisted reproductive technology (ART) procedures, early investigations are warranted. One sporadic miscarriage does not warrant detailed investigations as the chances of a subsequent normal birth are high.

INCIDENCE

Although spontaneous miscarriage occurs in around 15–25% of pregnancies, RMs (as per definition of three or more consecutive pregnancy losses) affect 0.4–1% of couples and as per two consecutive losses affects 5% of couples.

Recurrence Risk

The risk of recurrence is influenced by various factors, which includes maternal age, parental and fetal karyotypes, gestation age of previous loss, and various laboratory parameters (Table 1). The risk of miscarriage is higher (25–57%) in less than 6 weeks gestation and reduces to 2–3% in gestation above 10 weeks. Chromosomal analysis may offer an explanation in only 50% of cases.

ETIOLOGY

The causes of RM are listed in Box 1. The list is exhaustive and investigations are expensive. More than one factor may

TABLE 1 Risk of miscarriage with number of prior miscarriages.

	Number of prior miscarriages	*Percentage risk of recurrence in next pregnancy*
Women with one live born infant	0	12%
	1	24%
	2	26%
	3	32%
	4 or more	40–50%
Women with no live infant	2 or more	40–45%

Source: Arora M, Konje J (Eds). Recurrent Pregnancy Loss. New Delhi: Jaypee Brothers Medical Publishers; 2007.

BOX 1 Causes of recurrent miscarriage.

Lifestyle factors
- Maternal age >35 years
- Maternal obesity BMI >30
- Paternal age

Immunological—autoimmune
- Primary antiphospholipid syndrome
- Secondary antiphospholipid syndrome [Systemic lupus erythematosus (SLE)]
- Autoimmune thyroiditis

Immunological—alloimmune (classified as unexplained)
- Abnormalities of cytokine production—lack of shift of Th1 to Th 2 response
- Lack of alpha V beta 3 integrin
- Increased levels of tumor necrosis factor-alpha (TNF-α) in the endometrium
- Increased uterine natural killer cells
- Lack of endometrial plasticity due to lack of stem cells

Genetic
- Fetal trisomy, polyploidy, monosomy
- Parental balanced translocations, inversions, deletions, duplications
- Skewed inactivation of X chromosome
- Single gene defects, e.g. alpha thalassemia major, Rett syndrome, etc.
- Epigenetic modifications in the embryo

Hormonal
- Polycystic ovarian syndrome
- Luteal phase defects
- Hyperandrogenism
- Hypothyroidism/hyperthyroidism
- Hyperprolactinemia
- Low AMH/poor ovarian reserve
- Adrenal hyperplasia/Addison disease
- Deficiency of Vitamin D
- Uncontrolled diabetes mellitus

Anatomical
- Müllerian abnormalities, septate uterus
- Myomas—submucous, intramural
- Uterine synechiae and polyps
- T-shaped uterus
- Cervical incompetence

Contd...

Contd...

Inherited thrombophilia
- Antithrombin III deficiency
- Deficiency of protein C and protein S
- Activated protein C resistance (APCR)
- Factor V Leiden mutation
- Methyl tetrahydrofolate *(MTHFR)* gene homozygosity
- Prothrombin gene mutation
- Plasminogen activator inhibitor (PAI)
- Hyperhomocysteinemia

Semen factors
- High sperm DNA fragmentation index
- Y chromosomal abnormalities
- Sperm aneuploidies
- Male accessory gland infections (MAGI)

Infections
- Genital tract infections like bacterial vaginosis (BV), early female genital tuberculosis (FGTB), and chlamydia
- Systemic infections like syphilis, Lyme disease, toxoplasmosis, brucellosis
- Male accessory gland infections (MAGI)

Maternal systemic conditions
- Hypertension
- Chronic renal disease
- Chronic pulmonary disease
- Heart disease
- Severe rhesus sensitization

Miscellaneous
- Endocrine disrupters in environment
- Smoking, alcohol, drugs
- Exposure to irradiation
- Exposure to environmental toxins, pesticides, DDT, dry cleaning chemicals
- Exposure to anesthetic gases

Idiopathic

After exclusion of all above factors, a large proportion of miscarriages shows no apparent etiological factor. It is the authors' belief that majority of these miscarried fetuses may have subtle genetic defects like single gene disorders that will be missed on routine karyotyping but will be diagnosed by newer techniques like next generation sequencing (NGS).

(AMH; anti-Müllerian hormone; DDT: dichlorodiphenyltrichloroethane)

operate in successive pregnancies, e.g. early miscarriages due to any cause may be coupled with a late miscarriage due to cervical incompetence. On the other hand, early miscarriages may be coupled with a late fetal demise in patients with either congenital or acquired thrombophilia.

Figure 1 shows percentage-wise distribution of etiology of recurrent miscarriages.

The mechanism of pregnancy loss in various conditions is discussed further in text.

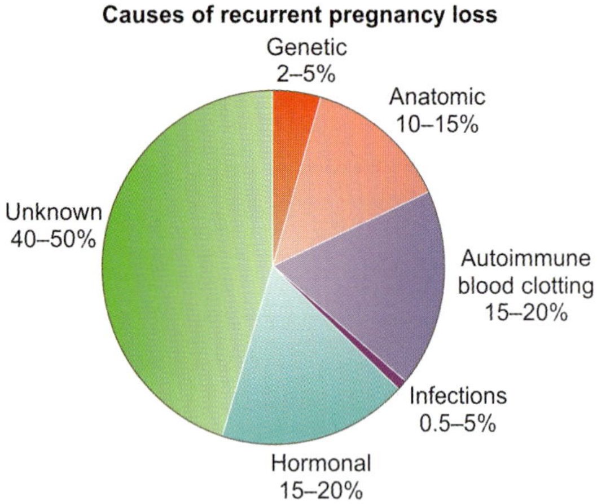

Fig. 1: Percentage-wise distribution of etiology of recurrent miscarriages.

Genetic Causes

Genetic Abnormalities in Karyotypically Normal Parents

Various studies demonstrate that at least 50% of clinically recognized pregnancy loss results from a cytogenetic abnormality, of which 51% show autosomal trisomies, 22% show polyploidy, 19% show monosomy, 4% show translocations, and the rest are unclassified genetic defects. The autosomal trisomies commonly encountered are those of chromosomes 3, 4, 9, 13-16, 19, 21, and 22.

Genetic Abnormalities in Karyotypically Abnormal Parents

Women may have structural chromosomal abnormality in the following forms:

- Deletions and duplications produce large chromosomal defects, which may cause severe phenotypic anomalies, thus individuals with these anomalies rarely reproduce.
- Dicentric and ring chromosomes are mitotically unstable, so the chances of offspring acquiring these anomalies are very small.
- In balanced translocations in men, the reproductive fitness is only slightly diminished. In spite of their good reproductive performance, these individuals show a significant decrease in live births and a significant increase in both fetal death and interval infertility; hence, they will present with RM.
- In unbalanced translocations in men, not only is there productive fitness greatly decreased but the risk of abnormal offspring is also increased.
- In single gene defects, diagnosis can only be made by a detailed family history coupled with fluorescent PCR testing.

Hormonal Disorders

A multitude of endocrinal disorders can cause RM.

Polycystic ovarian syndrome is one of the most common endocrinal abnormalities affecting female reproductive performance. Besides infertility, it presents higher risks of first- and second-trimester miscarriages.

Factors associated with a high miscarriage rate are hyperandrogenism, hyperinsulinemia, and/or ovulatory dysfunction that accompany high levels of luteinizing hormone and low levels of progesterone.

Women with poorly controlled type 1 (insulin-dependent) diabetes mellitus with glycosylated hemoglobin (HbA1C) levels greater than four standard deviations above the mean had a higher pregnancy loss rate. Well-controlled diabetes had pregnancy loss rates similar to those of nondiabetics. Apart from frank diabetes, syndrome X, which comprises impaired glucose tolerance test (GTT), hypertension, hypertriglyceridemia, and a procoagulant state with increased coronary heart disease, could also potentially cause RPL.

Abnormal maternal thyroid functions have been implicated as a cause of RM. However, mild or subclinical thyroid dysfunction is not associated with RM, as it more often leads to infertility, but increased levels of thyroid peroxidase and/or microsomal antibodies have been associated with RM. In autoimmune thyroid disease (AITD), the risk of miscarriage was the same whether the status was hypothyroid or euthyroid, indicating that AITD negatively affects fetal implantation. Hence, all women with positive thyroid antibodies should be treated with a low dose of thyroxine replacement to suppress thyroid autoimmunity and achieve a favorable maternal and perinatal outcome.

Hyperprolactinemia usually causes infertility due to luteolysis; however, in partially treated cases, the picture may change to early pregnancy loss due to corpus luteum deficiency.

Although rare, the patient with an untreated late onset congenital adrenal hyperplasia may have an increased chance of RM owing to hyperandrogenism. On the other hand, incipient Addison disease will also cause RMs; the patient often has low blood pressure and hyperpigmentation.

Poor ovarian reserve, diagnosed by low levels of anti-Müllerian hormone (AMH) and a poor antral follicle count, remains an important factor responsible for RM, owing to increased rate of aneuploidy in oocytes. Women with AMH levels below 1 ng/mL not only experience difficulty in conceiving but also have a higher rate of pregnancy loss due to a higher rate of aneuploidy in the embryo.

Anatomic Abnormalities

Anatomic abnormalities of the uterus and cervix are amenable to surgery. An estimated 15% of couples (one in six) with RM have an anatomic abnormality of the uterus as the primary cause. These abnormalities include the following:

- Defects of Müllerian fusion, which include septate uterus, unicornuate uterus, and bicornuate uterus with unequal uterine horns
- Acquired anatomical defects, such as, submucous or intramural myomas, endometrial polyps, and uterine synechiae
- *Small tubular uterine cavity*: This may be congenital, secondary to diethylstilbestrol exposure in utero or genital tuberculosis.
- Cervical incompetence, which is diagnosed by visualizing the cervix with an empty bladder on transvaginal ultrasound scan and assessing the width at the internal os as well as the cervical length from internal to external os. It may be a congenital weakness or secondary to repeated cervical dilatation. It is also associated with unicornuate or bicornuate uteri.

Although women with primary RMs are more likely to have anatomical abnormalities, recent study indicates that the uterus needs evaluation even in cases of secondary RMs.

Table 2 frequency of various anatomical abnormalities (Jaslow & Kutteh, 2013).

TABLE 2 Frequency of various anatomical abnormalities.

Comparison of uterine anomalies
Primary RM compared with secondary RM

	Primary RM (n = 479)	*Secondary RM (n = 425)*	*p-value*
All uterine anomalies	22.8 (109)	15.8 (67)	0.009
Congenital anomalies	8.8 (42)	4.5 (19)	0.011
Bicornuate uterus	1.0 (5)	0.5 (2)	NS
Didelphic uterus	0.2 (1)	0.2 (1)	NS
Septate uterus	6.3 (30)	3.1 (13)	0.028
T-shaped uterus	0.4 (2)	0.2 (1)	NS
Unicornuate uterus	0.8 (4)	0.5 (2)	NS
Acquired anomalies	14.6 (70)	11.8 (50)	NS
Adhesions	4.0 (19)	4.2 (18)	NS
Fibroid(s)	7.3 (35)	5.4 (23)	NS
Polyp(s)	4.0 (19)	2.4 (10)	NS

Values are % occurrence (n)

(NS: nonsignificant; RM: recurrent miscarriage)

Source: Jaslow CR, Kutteh WH. Effect of prior birth and miscarriage frequency on the prevalence of acquired and congenital uterine anomalies in women with recurrent miscarriages: a cross sectional study. Fertil Steril. 2013;99(7):1916-22.

Immunological Causes

Antiphospholipid antibody syndrome (APS) is the most common immunological cause of RM. Antibodies are directed against negatively charged phospholipids, which are the major constituents of trophoblast. These antibodies can cause placental thrombosis, infarction, impaired trophoblastic function, and abnormal placentation, and thus may lead to pregnancy-induced hypertension, intrauterine growth retardation (IUGR), intrauterine fetal death (IUD), and RM. Pregnancy loss usually occurs in the mid-trimester between 14 weeks and 18 weeks; however, both early first-trimester losses and late third-trimester losses can occur. There is usually an ultrasound confirmation of a viable pregnancy prior to the pregnancy loss in most first-trimester losses.

The diagnosis of APS is made by the presence of one clinical criterion and one laboratory criterion, which must be positive on two occasions 3 months apart.

Clinical criteria include the following:

- One or more unexplained deaths of a morphologically normal fetus of more than 10 weeks' gestation documented by ultrasonography or direct examination.
- One or more preterm births at or before 34 weeks' gestation due to severe pre-eclampsia or placental insufficiency with evidence of IUGR.
- Three or more consecutive miscarriages before 10 weeks' gestation with no maternal hormonal, anatomic abnormalities, normal maternal and paternal chromosomes, and other causes of recurrent losses being ruled out.

Laboratory criteria include detection of any of the following:

- Lupus anticoagulant by dilute Russel viper venom time (DRVVT), activated partial thromboplastin time (APTT), or partial thromboplastin time (PTT)
- Anticardiolipin (ACL) antibodies immunoglobulin G (IgG)/IgM
- Antiphospholipid (aPL) antibodies IgG/IgM
- Anti-beta 2 glycoprotein antibodies.

Autoimmune disorders, such as systemic lupus erythematosus, and systemic sclerosis are associated with RM, and are often classified as secondary antiphospholipid syndrome (or SAPS). The mechanism of loss and the treatment are the same as those for primary APS.

Treatment with steroids is not recommended based on current evidence. A combination of low-dose aspirin, i.e. ≤100 mg and unfractionated/low-molecular-weight heparin currently gives the best pregnancy outcome. Heparin is not only an anticoagulant, but it also has a potent complement inhibitory action which is beneficial in preventing complement-mediated damage in APS syndrome. Aspirin should be started preconceptually and heparin after a positive pregnancy test and continued until the time of delivery. Postpartum thromboprophylaxis is recommended for 2 weeks to prevent deep vein thrombosis.

Thrombophilias

These are rare inherited disorders that predispose an individual to venous and arterial thrombosis. They cause inadequate placental circulation owing to thrombosis in the placental vasculature, and lead to adverse pregnancy outcomes like IUGR, IUD, and placental abruption. They are not commonly associated with recurrent early miscarriages. However, late miscarriages and IUD may be encountered. Congenital thrombophilias include the following:

- *Activated protein C resistance (APCR) due to Factor V Leiden mutation*: A single missense mutation of the Factor V gene can cause 90% cases of APCR and is present in 5% of the UK population.
- *Deficiency of antithrombin III*: This occurs in 32–51% patients with thrombophilia.
- *Deficiency of protein C and protein S*: In patients with thrombophilia, 22–26% have protein C deficiency, while 12–17% have protein S deficiency.
- Prothrombin gene mutation G 20210A leads to elevated levels of prothrombin and is present in 2% of the UK population.
- Homozygosity for the thermolabile mutation of *MTHFR* gene with or without hyperhomocysteinemia.
- Homozygous genotype for plasminogen activator inhibitor (PAI) is also associated with RMs.

Hyperhomocysteinemia

Homocysteine is an amino acid that is synthesized in the body from methionine. Its normal levels are 4–15 μmol/L. High homocysteine levels result from genetic mutations that cause enzyme deficiency or dietary deficiency of vitamin B6, B12, and folic acid that are cofactors essential for the functioning of the enzyme that metabolizes it to cysteine. Homocysteine levels normally decrease during pregnancy, but high levels are associated with placental vascular thrombosis and placental abruption.

Homocysteine levels may be lowered by administration of vitamin B_6, B_{12}, and folic acid. Its association with RMs is not proved but when levels are more than 30 μmol/L, it may cause a thrombogenic state and result in RMs.

The risks of adverse pregnancy outcomes in thrombogenic states are depicted in Table 3.

TABLE 3 Risks of adverse pregnancy outcomes in thrombogenic states.

High risk	*Medium risk*	*Low risk*
Antiphospholipid syndrome	Protein C deficiency	Heterozygosity for Factor V Leiden mutation
	Protein S deficiency	Heterozygosity for *Prothrombin* gene mutation
Antithrombin III deficiency	Homozygosity for Factor V Leiden mutation	Hyperhomocysteinemia 13–30 μmol/L
Hyperhomocysteinemia >30 μmol/L	Homozygosity of *Prothrombin* gene mutation	
	Combined Heterozygosity for Factor V Leiden and *Prothrombin* gene mutation	

Systemic Conditions

Severe maternal illness, such as, essential hypertension, cardiac disease, chronic pulmonary disease, and chronic nephritis, are important causes of RMs. Pregnancy in a rhesus-sensitized woman with a high titer of anti-D antibodies will also result in RPLs.

Systemic infections like syphilis were an important cause of RMs in the past and are re-emerging in the human immunodeficiency virus (HIV) positive population. Currently, Lyme disease and toxoplasmosis can result in repetitive losses. Bacterial infections acquired from dairy products, like brucella abortus, also cause RM.

Genital Infections

Genitourinary tuberculosis is classically associated with infertility, but in its latent form, can also cause recurrent ectopic pregnancy, biochemical pregnancies as well as miscarriages. Bacterial vaginosis and chlamydia trachomatis infections are implicated in RMs, recurrent preterm labor, and preterm premature rupture of membranes.

Miscellaneous Causes

Smoking, alcohol intake, and the use of recreational drugs will cause RM. Other factors include prolonged exposure to irradiation, anesthetic gases, pesticides, and other environmental toxins. Of increasing importance is the presence of endocrine disrupters that are emanated by plastic devices in our environment.

Idiopathic

In 50% of cases, the cause of RMs is not clearly elucidated at present. Implantation is a complex process that involves synchronization of endometrial maturity with fertilization. Successful implantation involves expression of *HOXA10* genes in the endometrium, formation of pinopodes, as well as the presence of anti-inflammatory cytokines such as interleukins 4, 6, and 10, leukemia inhibiting factor (LIF), and transforming growth factor beta (TGF-β). A disturbance in any of the above processes will lead to early pregnancy losses. Absence of the cytokine LIF in the endometrium is associated with RMs in the knockout mouse model but its exact role in humans is yet to be elucidated. Other cytokine abnormalities (such as increased levels of inflammatory cytokines, i.e. TNF-α) in the endometrium are the subject of current research in RMs. Measurement of levels of TNF-α in the peripheral blood, during the luteal phase of the cycle or during early pregnancy, has been recommended by some. These are classically raised in graft rejection and may be marginally raised in fetal rejection. However, the test is not standardized for clinical use during pregnancy yet.

An increased number of natural killer cells (NKCs) in the endometrium will lead to embryolysis. Increased numbers of NKCs result from an abnormal maternal immune response to the foreign antigenic makeup of the embryo and are hence termed alloimmune cause of RPL. Measurement of NKC subsets in peripheral blood has also been recommended by some. However, its correlation to the uterine NKC population is still not established. NKC population in the endometrium can be quantified during the luteal phase of the menstrual cycle with a pipelle biopsy. Immunohistochemistry and/or flow cytometry can be employed to identify the CD 69 positive NK cells. The test has been developed for clinical use but needs to be standardized across laboratories. Immune potentiation may help a small subset of these patients with alloimmune causes or immune rejection of the fetal allograft.

Autoimmunity is also known to affect embryogenesis by altering the endometrial environment. In a recent study, 515 patients with idiopathic RMs and no overt autoimmune disease, and a control group, were screened for autoantibodies. The results were as follows: anti-thyroglobulin antibody was positive in 21.2% in RM group versus 7.8% in the control group. Antimitochondrial antibody was positive in 4.8% in RM group versus 0.5% in control group.

In short, any one antibody was positive in 28.3% in RM group versus 14.5% in the control group. Similarly, another study reported deficiency of IgG subclass in women with RM compared with controls, while yet another study reported micro-RNA mutations diagnosed by PCR amplification in the idiopathic RM group (n = 200) versus fertile controls (n = 300) with an odds ratio of 2.98 and CI of 1.40–2.81 and a p value of 0.0001.

These studies point out that a variety of unrelated pathologies may be responsible for idiopathic RM and investigating this group fully may not be clinically feasible at present but should be possible in the near future.

Hence, RPL may occur due to a variety of causes, some well understood and others less so. Some are treatable, such as immunological, hormonal, anatomical causes as well as thrombophilias. An abnormal cytokine environment may be responsible for some of the hitherto unexplained RMs.

EVALUATION, WORKUP, AND TREATMENT

Ideally, the couple should be seen together at a dedicated RM clinic and given accurate information to facilitate decision making about future pregnancies. Clearly written patient leaflets are recommended to provide information that the couple can take home. Various guidelines have been proposed for the evaluation of RMs by various academic societies. Individualization of management options according to the workup should be done when managing RPL.

History

A careful history should include details of the previous losses (pattern, trimester, and characteristics), preceding infertility and its management, past history suggestive of acute or chronic infections, endocrinological disorders (thyroid dysfunction, hyperprolactinemia, diabetes mellitus, thrombosis), APL, and other autoimmune disorders should be noted. Prior medication history and consumption of recreational drugs, caffeine, alcohol, and cigarette smoking should be noted. Prior gynecological surgery is relevant.

Physical Examination

Obesity, hirsutism, acanthosis, thyroid enlargement, and galactorrhea are obvious indicators of the cause. A pelvic examination should be carried out to exclude infections and to look for possible anatomic abnormalities.

Transvaginal Ultrasound Scan

Uterine evaluation is required in all patients with RMs. This will diagnose Müllerian abnormalities, submucous myomas, adenomyosis, and endometrial hyperplasia. If indicated, further evaluation is performed with the help of transvaginal three-dimensional (3D) and 4D scan which diagnoses all uterine abnormalities comfortably. It is noninvasive and has a high sensitivity and specificity in experienced hands. Sonohysteroscopy is the procedure of scanning after saline infusion of the uterine cavity. This will help diagnose intracavity lesions like polyps and adhesions. Hysterosalpingography involves exposure of the ovaries to radiation but provides a visual record of the uterine cavity and tubal patency. It is valuable in confirming Müllerian anomalies like unicornuate uterus. Hystero/laparoscopy is not only the gold standard for diagnosis but also allows remedial action at the same time like excision of polyp, adhesions, submucous myomas, and uterine septum. Difficult cases may be performed under laparoscopic vision to avoid perforations.

The Algorithm for Workup

Checking for hormonal abnormalities, screening for antiphospholipid syndrome, and evaluation of the uterine cavity is recommended after two consecutive miscarriages. Fetal karyotype evaluation is recommended after the second or third consecutive miscarriage. Products of conception (POC) obtained from early nonviable pregnancies via a dilatation and evacuation may not be suitable for karyotyping but can be analyzed by fluorescence *in situ* hybridization (FISH), which classically analyzes five chromosomes, i.e.13, 18, 21, X, and Y. In RPL cases, extending this to 7 or 8 chromosomes is preferable. Some authors recommend three rounds of FISH to analyze all 24 chromosomes for copy number variation. For subtle genetic defects, next generation sequencing (NGS) or microarray for complete genomic hybridization (CGH) may be indicated. Flowcharts 1 and 2 show the algorithm for genetic workup in RM.

Flowchart 1: Initial evaluation of recurrent miscarriage.

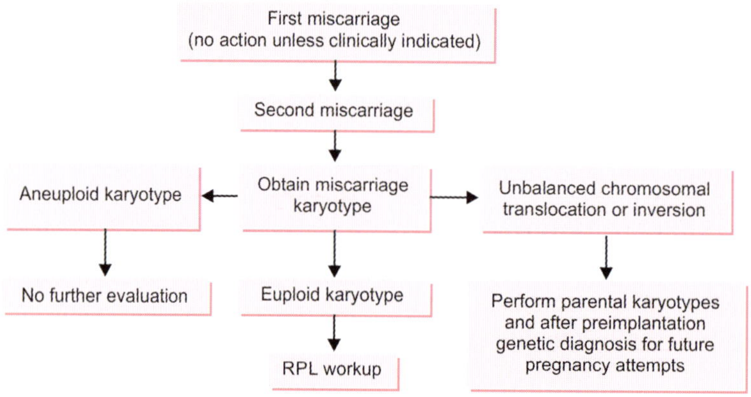

(RPL: recurrent pregnancy loss)

Source: Brezina PR, Ke RW, Kutteh WH. Preimplantation genetic screening: a practical guide. Clin Med Insights Reprod Health. 2013;7:37-42.

Flowchart 2: Full recurrent pregnancy loss (RPL) workup.

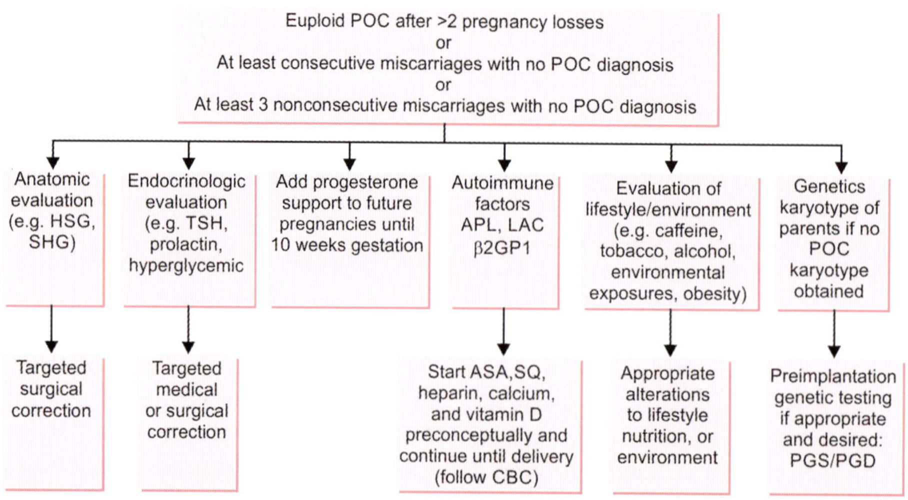

(APL: antiphospholipid; ASA: aspirin; β2GP1: beta-2 glycoprotein 1; CBC: complete blood count; HSG: hysterosalpingogram; LAC: lupus anticoagulant; POC: products of conception; PGD: preimplantation genetics diagnosis; PGS: preimplantation genetic screening; SHG: sonohysterogram; TSH: thyroid-stimulating hormone)

Source: Brezina PR, Ke RW, Kutteh WH. Preimplantation genetic screening: a practical guide. Clin Med Insights Reprod Health. 2013;7:37-42.

For a full workup, all the possible causes have to be looked into.

Treatment

Anatomical Causes

The treatment often involves corrective hysteroscopic surgery. Resection of the septum may be done with the use of cautery or rarely with hysteroscopic scissors. Excision of submucous myoma is performed with the resectoscope. Adhesion bands and polyps are excised with the help of hysteroscopic scissors. Rarely, correction of bicornuate uterus requires a Strassman operation. Repeated implantation in the smaller horn of a bicornuate uterus may require excision of the rudimentary horn by laparoscopy/laparotomy. Disabling implantation in a rudimentary horn by placing an intrauterine contraceptive device (IUCD) in it may also be a viable noninvasive treatment option to prevent miscarriages.

Cervical Insufficiency

Prenatal diagnosis can be done with a hysterosalpingogram. Serial cervical sonographic surveillance should be offered in the pregnant women with history of second-trimester pregnancy loss and a cervical length of less than 25 mm is considered significant. Progesterone therapy (vaginal or parenteral) is recommended and cervical cerclage may be offered if cervical length is less than 1.5 cm. However, there is no conclusive evidence that prophylactic cerclage reduces the risk of pregnancy loss and preterm delivery in women at risk of preterm birth or mid-trimester loss due to infective causes or multiple gestations. Most often cervical dilatation may be the result of a sterile inflammatory response (SIRS) at the decidual membrane interface that causes release of prostaglandins. Cervical incompetence may be prevented by avoiding forceful manual dilatation of the cervix and resorting to medical evacuation rather than surgical. Preterm rupture of membranes is prevented by diagnosing and treating subclinical endocervical infections and bacterial vaginosis. Probiotics may be more effective than antibiotics in many instances as there is an overgrowth of vaginal commensals that do not grow on routine cultures. Progesterone therapy is recommended for short cervical length >1.5 cm, provided the internal os is closed. Progesterone can be administered long term as daily vaginal gel/suppositories or weekly progesterone depot injections.

HORMONAL CAUSES

Luteal Phase Deficiency

There is controversy whether this entity actually exists. Absence of corpus luteum formation at the 6 weeks scan is sometimes documented. Earlier the diagnosis was based on result of a phased endometrial biopsy, however this is not recommended as a diagnostic modality any more. Poor echogenic change in the endometrium, low levels of serum progesterone in the mid-luteal phase (<10 ng/mL), and a short luteal phase is considered diagnostic. A recent Cochrane review evaluating 15 trials concluded that routine administration of progesterone to all women with RPL had considerable benefit. However, recently concluded randomized multicentric PROMISE study concluded that pregnancy outcome was not affected by progesterone administration. However, the progesterone supplementation was started at 6 weeks of pregnancy in the PROMISE trial and not during the luteal phase.

Thyroid Dysfunction

The American Thyroid Association recommends serum thyroid-stimulating hormone (TSH) measurement for targeted screening and includes history of preterm delivery or miscarriage as one of the indication. TSH values >2.5 IU/L are considered abnormal during pregnancy. The Endocrine Society recommends that patients with RPL should be treated to maintain TSH levels between 1.0 mIU/mL and 2.5 mIU/mL in first trimester and up to 3 and 3.3 mIU/mL in second and third trimesters, respectively. For TSH levels between 2.5 mIU and 10 mIU, levothyroxine is recommended in the starting dose of 50 μg/day. The mechanism of pregnancy loss may be autoimmune or epigenetic rather than a hormonal deficiency.

Abnormal Glucose Metabolism

Screening with HbA1c levels is recommended for all women with RMs. This has replaced the oral glucose tolerance test in the first trimester. Weight reduction, diet alteration, and lifestyle modification are first steps in the management. Oral hypoglycemic agents like metformin are safe to prescribe during pregnancy in borderline cases. However, strict glycemic control is required in the first trimester to prevent congenital anomalies and insulin is often required. Patient education and counseling and initiation of self-blood glucose monitoring (SBGM) along with self-injections of insulin improves pregnancy outcome. Maintaining a diary of weekly blood sugar series fasting and postprandial with insulin dosage administered helps the clinician to fine-tune the glycemic control.

Strict glycemic control is desirable prior to pregnancy with HbA1c levels less than 7 in patients with overt diabetes.

Table 4 shows frequency of abnormal tests in RPL.

TABLE 4 Frequency of abnormal tests in recurrent pregnancy loss (RPL).

		Frequency of abnormal tests in 1,020 women with RPL			
Control	*Number of prior losses*	*2 (n= 447)*	*3 (n = 343)*	*≥4 (n = 230)*	*p-value (2, 3, or 4)*
0.4%	Parental genetics	2.8%	5.4%	5.2%	NS
7.5%	Anatomy	18.7%	18.2%	16.7%	NS
0.5%	Lupus anticoagulant	5.0%	2.9%	1.9%	NS
6.7%	Anticardiolipin	15.6%	13.1%	17.1%	NS
3.9%	TSH	8.1%	6.5%	6.2%	NS
6.9%	HbA1c	14.1%	16.3%	17.4%	NS

(HbA1c: glycosylated hemoglobin; NS: nonsignificant; TSH: thyroid-stimulating hormone)

Infections

The role of infection in RPL is unclear. Toxoplasmosis, rubella, cytomegalovirus, herpes, and listeria infections are not implicated in RPL and hence routine TORCH test is not recommended. Most patients with RPL are not benefitted by extensive workup for detecting infective etiology. Bacterial vaginosis is a risk factor for preterm delivery and a strong risk factor for late miscarriages. In symptomatic women, testing and treatment of bacterial vaginosis is indicated by checking the vaginal pH, which will be greater than 6 and looking for clue cells in vaginal secretions. The results of screening and treatment trials in asymptomatic women however are inconsistent.

IVF and Preimplantation Genetic Screening

Most early miscarriages show genetic abnormalities in the implanting embryo. Although this may be a sporadic event in embryogenesis and is not often repeated, patients with advanced maternal age and poor ovarian reserve will benefit by fast tracking to IVF with the possibility of trophectoderm biopsy of the blastocyst which will confirm the genetic makeup of the embryo. Chromosomal analysis may be performed with FISH for five chromosomes (13, 18, 21, X, and Y) CGH for all 23 chromosomes or NGS for quicker results.

In cases where there are no normal embryos formed, the option of donor oocytes or embryos should be explored. In cases of balanced translocations in the parents, substitution with donor gametes may be required, although many cases of spontaneous normal embryogenesis and pregnancy are reported after multiple miscarriages.

UNEXPLAINED RECURRENT MISCARRIAGE

A significant proportion of cases of RM remain unexplained despite detailed workup. Supportive care without pharmacological intervention in a dedicated RPL care offers an excellent prognosis for future pregnancy outcome. These women can be reassured that the prognosis for a successful future pregnancy with supportive care alone is in the region of 75%. The value of psychological support in improving pregnancy outcome cannot be overemphasized.

Immune potentiation may be achieved by the following methods:

- *Lymphocyte immune therapy (LIT)*: This involves injection of husband's/third party leukocytes subcutaneously in the mother. This therapy does not have the approval of United States Food and Drug Administration (US FDA), and its benefits are to date unproven. Besides, it carries the potential hazard of transmitting communicable diseases as well as a small risk of graft versus host reaction. Hence, LIT therapy is currently considered empirical.
- *Correction of low Vitamin D levels*: Vitamin D deficiency is endemic in India. Besides contributing positively to bone health, vitamin D is a potent immune potentiator, hence its deficiency should be corrected in all individuals.
- *Intravenous immunoglobulins (IVIGs)*: They have a role in women with isolated IgG subclass 1-4 deficiency. IgG levels were estimated in 160 patients of RM and 160 controls. In the RM group, 16 patients showed a deficiency of IgG which is when corrected with IgG administration 200 mg/kg/month throughout pregnancy. This resulted in a successful pregnancy outcome in >90% of cases. Use of IVIG in other autoimmune/alloimmune conditions is largely empirical.
- *Intralipids*: It is an extract of soy lecithin that was developed in Sweden for total parenteral nutrition. It demonstrated effective immune modulation in mice and has been used in a small number of humans with recurrent implantation failure and idiopathic RM with

promising results. However, there are no randomized controlled trials as yet to prove its superiority over placebo.

A Cochrane review of immunotherapy for RM by Porter, which was conducted in 2006, and included 28 trials of high quality, that used paternal cell immunization, third party donor leukocytes, trophoblast membrane, and IVIGs, concluded that various forms of immunotherapy did not show significant benefit over placebo. There has been no review on vitamin D and intralipid use.

- *Granulocyte colony stimulating factor (GCSF)*: In a randomized controlled trial, subcutaneous administration of GCSF in a dose of 1 µg/kg body weight/day administered from 6th postovulatory day and repeated every alternate day has shown to improve clinical pregnancy rates in unexplained RMs.
- *TNF-α blockers*: Although the diagnostic test for high TNF-α levels as the cause of miscarriage is not robust, some people have tried using TNF-α blockers with a variable response in patients with RM associated with high TNF-α levels in the peripheral blood. These are expensive molecules with no data on fetal safety as yet and need to be used with extreme caution. However, in patients with rheumatoid arthritis with high TNF-α levels these drugs have been used successfully. Ratio of interferon (IFN) beta to IFN alpha, if high, will predict a poor response to TNF-α inhibitors. These are classified as category B drugs in pregnancy. The molecules that have been used during pregnancy are:
  - Infliximab
  - Etanercept
  - Adalimumab
  - Certolizumab.

However, its use in pregnancy is limited to a few patients suffering from severe inflammatory bowel disease. Certolizumab is used and its use is stopped in the second trimester as it crosses the placenta and will cause IUGR.

In a review of use of anti-TNF-α blockers during pregnancy of rheumatology patients, 58 case reports/case series were analyzed and the review concluded that the use of TNF-α blockers does not increase the rate of congenital malformations nor does it increase the chances of any other adverse pregnancy outcomes.

PROGNOSTIC FACTORS IN EARLY PREGNANCY TRANSVAGINAL SCAN

Abnormalities of the gestational sac between 4 weeks and 6 weeks of pregnancy will be predictive of pregnancy outcome. Some abnormal features that may be encountered are:

- No gestational sac visible with a serum beta hCG level of 1,500 IU/L or more signifies pregnancy of uncertain location.
- No visible yolk sac with a mean sac diameter (MSD) of 8 mm or more signifies a pseudosac which is seen in ectopic pregnancy.
- No visible fetal pole with a MSD of 16 mm or more signifies anembryonic pregnancy.
- Irregular shape of gestational sac is associated with missed miscarriage.
- Thin choriodecidual reaction <3 mm signifies poor implantation.
- Large yolk sac >10 mm or calcification in the yolk sac is associated with fetal demise.
- Sac position too low in the cavity may be seen in scar ectopic/cervical ectopic pregnancy.
- Oligoamniotic sac MSD – CRL ≤5 mm signifies poor trophoblastic invasion.
- Early growth retardation MSD–CRL ≤4 mm.
- Slow increase in sac diameter <0.7 mm/day. Normal increase is 1.2 mm/day
- Absent fetal cardiac activity with a fetus of CRL 6 mm or more.
- Fetal bradycardia of less than 85 beats/min at 6 weeks or more.
- Subchorionic hemorrhage of >40% of the sac volume.

Corrective action can be taken if above abnormalities are diagnosed in early pregnancy. This includes progesterone support and other treatment modalities indicated.

Prognosis

With appropriate medical therapy and continued psychological support, the prognosis for women with RM is good. Lund in his study on 987 women with RPL found that the chances of achieving a live birth within 5 years of initial evaluation were 80% in women less than 30 years of age and around 60–70% for women aged 31–40 years (Fig. 2).

SUMMARY

Majority of miscarriages are sporadic and thought to result from genetic abnormalities of the embryo, which are influenced by maternal age. Dilemmas exist in defining RPL; however, most researchers are of the opinion that for epidemiological purposes it should be defined as three consecutive losses. In the clinical setting though, a thorough physical examination and testing is recommended after two consecutive miscarriages. In almost 50% cases of RPL, the cause remains unexplained and pharmacological intervention is not recommended. Immunotherapy needs

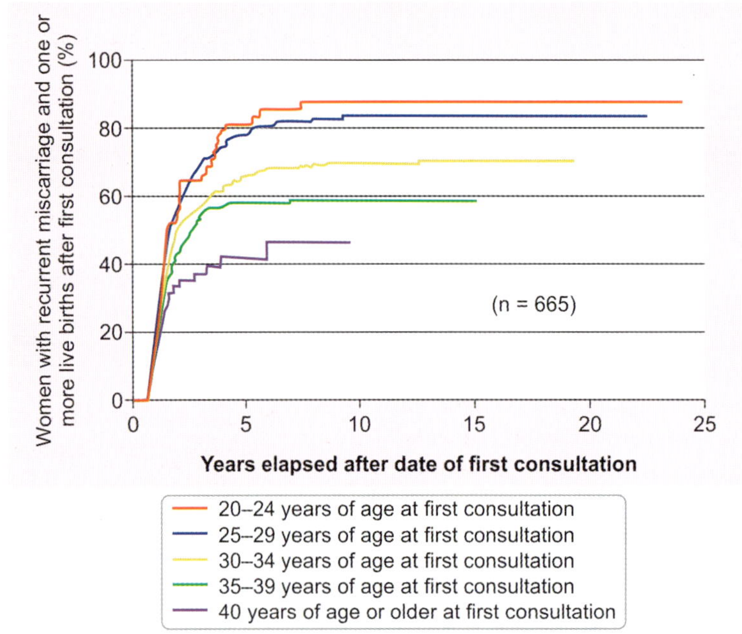

Fig. 2: Prognosis of recurrent pregnancy loss based on maternal age and current diagnostic and treatment strategies.
Source: Lund M, Kamper-Jorgensen MK, Nielsen HS, et al. Prognosis for live birth in women with recurrent miscarriage—what is the best measure of success? Obstet Gynecol. 2012;119:37-43.

to be evaluated by multicentric randomized controlled trials. Tender loving care, reassurance, and stress-relieving therapies like acupressure, acupuncture, yoga, and meditation are supportive therapies that go a long way in reducing stress and should be recommended for all patients with RPL.

EDITORS' COMMENTS

1. Genetic abnormality is an important cause for RPL. Traditional karyotyping of the parents and over and above chromosomal microarray karyotyping is of importance as it enables the detection of losses and/or gains of chromosomal material that are submicroscopic.
2. Immunological factors and immunotherapy has a role in indicated patients. Maternal killer-cell immunoglobulin-like receptor (KIR) and fetal human leukocyte antigen-C (HLA-C) typing in future could open doors to diagnosis in RPL.
3. Basic causes like bacterial vaginosis should not be forgotten.

SUGGESTED READING

1. ACOG (2013). FAQ100. [online] Available from www.acog.org [Last Accessed July, 2019].
2. Arora M (Ed). Hyperhomocysteinemia in Pregnancy. Elsevier ECAB; 2012.
3. Arora M, Konje J (Eds). Recurrent Pregnancy Loss. New Delhi: Jaypee Brothers Medical Publishers; 2007.
4. Arora Mala, Basu HK. Non-surgical management of uterus didelphys. Saudi Med J. 1989;10(1):141-2.
5. Arora S (Ed). A Practical Guide to First trimester of Pregnancy. Valia Ajay Practical Tips for Ultrasound. New Delhi: Jaypee Brothers Medical Publishers; 2014.
6. Bhattacharya S. Recurrent miscarriage: should the definition be revised? In: Arora M (Ed). World Clinics Obstetrics & Gynecology, Volume 1, Number 1. New Delhi: Jaypee Brothers Medical Publishers; 2011.
7. Boui J, Boui A, Lazar P. Retrospective and prospective epidemiological studies of 1500 karyotyped spontaneous human abortions. Teratology. 1975;12(1):11-26.
8. Brezina PR, Ke RW, Kutteh WH. Preimplantation genetic screening: a practical guide. Clin Med Insights Reprod Health. 2013;7:37-42.
9. Bussen S, Steck T. Thyroid antibodies in euthyroid non pregnant women with recurrent spontaneous abortions. Hum Reprod. 1995;10:2938-40.
10. Clark DA. Intralipid as treatment for recurrent unexplained abortion. Am J Reprod Immunol. 2013;32(4):290-3.
11. Coomarasamy A, Williams H, Truchanowicz E, et al. PROMISE trial: A randomized trial of progesterone in women with recurrent miscarriages. N Eng J Med. 2015;373:2141-8.
12. De Groot L, Abalovich M, Alexander EK, et al. Management of thyroid dysfunction during pregnancy and postpartum: An Endocrine society clinical practice guideline. J Clin Endocrinol Metab. 2012;97:2543-65.

13. Dopoulos PG, Templeton AA, Fisk N, et al. The frequency of chromosomal anomalies in human preimplantation embryos after in vitro fertilization. Hum Reprod. 1987;4:91-8.
14. Ernest JM, Marshburn PB, Kutteh WH. Obstetric antiphospholipid antibody syndrome- an update on pathophysiology and management. Semin Reprod Med. 2011;29(6):522-39.
15. Gilnoer D, Soto MF, Bourdoux P, et al. Pregnancy in patients with mild thyroid abnormalities: maternal and neonatal repercussion. J Clin Endocrinol Metab. 1991;73:421-7.
16. Gispert JP, Chaparro M. Safety of anti-TNF agents during pregnancy and breast feeding in women with inflammatory bowel disease. Am J Gastroenterol. 2013;108(9):1426-38.
17. Gomez R. Ultrasonographic examination of uterine cervix is better than cervical digital examination as a predictor of the likelihood of premature delivery in patients with preterm labor and intact membranes. Am J Obstet Gynecol. 1994;171:956-64.
18. Haas DM, Ramsy PS. Progestogen for preventing miscarriage. Cochrane Database Systematic Rev. 2008;(2):CD003511.
19. Harrison P. Blood test predicts TNF inhibitor response in RA patients. Am Coll Rheumatol. 2014.
20. Jacobs PA. Structural rearrangements of chromosomes in men. In: Hook EB, Porter IM (Eds). Population Cytogenetics. New York: Academic Press; 1977. pp. 81-97.
21. Jaslow CR, Kutteh WH. Effect of prior birth and miscarriage frequency on the prevalence of acquired and congenital uterine anomalies in women with recurrent miscarriages: a cross sectional study. Fertil Steril. 2013;99(7):1916-22.
22. Lata K, Dutta P, Sridhar S, et al. Thyroid autoimmunity and obstetric outcomes in women with recurrent miscarriage: a case control study. Endocrine Connect. 2013;2(2):118-24.
23. Lathi RB, Gray Hazard FK, Heerema-McKenney A, et al. First trimester miscarriage evaluation. Semin Reprod Med. 2011;29(6):463-9.
24. Lund M, Jorgensen MK, Nielsen HS, et al. Prognosis for live birth in women with recurrent miscarriage - what is the best measure of success? Obstet Gynecol. 2012;119:37-43.
25. Manfredi G, Aera D, Ligouri R. Overcoming RSM in women suffering from IgG subclass deficiency: high efficacy of low dose IvIg treatment. Eur Ann Allergy Clin Immunol. 2015;4793:91-4.
26. Mumusoglu S, Beksac MS, Ekiz A, et al. Does presence of antibodies without autoimmune disease and hereditary thrombophilia have an effect on RPL? J Matern Fetal Neonatal Med. 2016;29(14):2352-7.
27. Nielson OH, Loftus EV Jr, Jess T. Safety of TNF alpha inhibitors during IBD pregnancy: a systematic review. BMC Med. 2013;11:174.
28. O'Brien J. Cervical causes of preterm labor. World Clin Obstet Gynecol. 2012;2(1).
29. Ota K, Dambaeva S, Han AR, et al. Vit D deficiency may be a risk factor for recurrent pregnancy losses by increasing cellular immunity and autoimmunity. Hum Reprod. 2014; 29(2):208-19.
30. Piercy NC. Thromboembolic disease. Obstetric Medicine, 1st volume. London: Martin Dunitz; 2002. pp. 42-4.
31. Porter TF, La Coursiere Y, Scott JR. Immunotherapy for recurrent miscarriage. Cochrane Database Systematic Rev. 2006;(2):CD000112.
32. Practice Committee of the American Society for Reproductive Medicine. Definitions of infertility and recurrent pregnancy loss. Fertil Steril. 2008;89:1603.
33. Practice Committee of the American Society for Reproductive Medicine. Aging and infertility in women. Fertil Steril. 2006;86(5 Suppl):S248-52.
34. Praveen F, Agrawal S. Recurrent miscarriage and micro RNA among North Indian women. Reprod Sci. 2015;22(4):410-5.
35. Rai RS. Antiphospholipid syndrome and recurrent miscarriages. J Post Grad Med. 2002;48:3-4.
36. Regan L, Owen EJ, Jacobs HS. Hypersecretion of luteinizing hormone, infertility and miscarriage. Lancet. 1990; 336(8724): 1141-4.
37. Robertson L, Wu O, Langhorne P, et al. Thrombophilia in pregnancy: a systematic review. Br J Haematol. 2006;132: 171-96.
38. Royal College of Obstetricians and Gynecologists (2011). The investigation and treatment of couples with recurrent first-trimester and second-trimester miscarriage. Green-top Guideline No. 17. [online] Available from www.rcog.org.uk [Last Accessed July, 2019].
39. Salat-Baroux J. Recurrent spontaneous abortions. Reprod Nutr Dev. 1988;28(6B):1555-68.
40. Scarpellini F, Sbracia M. Use of granulocyte colony stimulating factor for the treatment of unexplained recurrent miscarriage: a randomized controlled trial. Hum Reprod. 2009;24(11): 2703-8.
41. Stirrat GM. Recurrent miscarriage. Lancet. 1990;336(8716): 673-5.
42. Wilcox AJ, Weinberg CR, O'Connor JF, et al. Incidence of early loss of pregnancy. N Engl J Med. 1988;319(4):189-94.
43. Zaveroni I, Bonini L, Fantuzzi M, et al. Hyperinsulinemia, obesity and AQ syndrome X. J Intern Med. 1994;235:51-6.

26

CHAPTER

Fertility Preservation: Newer Concepts

Nalini Mahajan

INTRODUCTION

Reproductive compromise may occur as a result of treatment with gonadotoxic drugs, radiotherapy (RT), immunological disease, or genetic conditions, and also in women, due to advancing age. Progress in assisted reproductive technology (ART) has brought hope to these young men and women by making it possible to preserve their gametes, for use at a later date. Fertility preservation (FP) has become a "quality-of-life" issue and the "standard of care" for cancer survivors and noncancer patients at risk of decreased fertility.

Cancer survivorship is steadily increasing due to early detection and improved multimodality treatments, leading to a growing need for FP. European and US data suggest that long-term survival in children and adolescents diagnosed with cancer is around 80% (Hudson, 2010). A recent study estimated that 1 in 530 young adults between the ages of 20 years and 39 years is a childhood cancer survivor (Ward et al., 2014). Even in the developing countries like India, cancer survivorship is increasing despite poor resources [Indian Cancer Registry (ICR)]. FP is also being adopted increasingly for patients on cytotoxic drugs for nonmalignant disorders and genetic issues leading to reduced fertility. The one area where gamete preservation has seen a dramatic increase is in "social freezing", i.e. FP in women wanting to delay childbearing for social reasons.

This chapter will touch upon the basic aspects of FP and the promising techniques, which may well become the future of FP.

EFFECT OF CHEMOTHERAPY AND RADIOTHERAPY ON GONADS

Cytotoxic chemotherapy (CT) causes cell death or prevents cell growth generally through inhibitory microtubule functions, protein functions, or DNA synthesis. Unfortunately, this action is not limited to cancer cells alone and can be quite disastrous to the metabolically active gonadal cells. Cytotoxic agents produce DNA abnormalities and oxidative damage in the somatic as well as germ cells leading to apoptosis.

Females

Effect of Chemotherapy

Ovarian effects: There is a reduction in ovarian reserve because of apoptosis of the growing follicles and fibrosis of stromal blood vessels. Furthermore, resting follicles are activated and undergo subsequent apoptosis, leading to a "burn-out" effect (Meirow, 2001; Anderson RA, 2006). The degree of ovarian damage is related to the dose and type of chemotherapeutic agent used, age of the patient, and the baseline ovarian reserve. Gonadotoxicity is greatest with alkylating agents such as cyclophosphamide (Cy) (Zavos et al., 2016; Meirow et al., 1999) which is responsible for the highest age-adjusted odds ratio of ovarian failure, followed by other drug families (Meirow et al., 2010). The prepubertal ovary has a larger primordial pool and is therefore less susceptible to CT agents while a poorer ovarian reserve in older women increases their risk of premature ovarian failure (POF) (Meirow et al., 2009). *The clinical manifestations range from complete amenorrhea to premature menopause and varying degree of infertility.*

Effect on oocytes: Most cytotoxic drugs are mutagenic and teratogenic to oocytes exposed during maturation (Di Giacomo, 2005). In humans, the oocyte maturation phase lasts approximately 6 months (Meirow, 2005). It is therefore recommended that conception should be delayed for 6 months after completing gonadotoxic treatments. FP techniques are best carried out prior to CT; however, if a delay is unavoidable then a wait of 6 months after treatment is mandatory. FP should not be performed between treatment cycles (Chung, 2013). A precise safety interval between CT and oocyte collection is yet to be established.

Effect of Radiotherapy

Unlike CT, effects of RT are seen on both the ovary and the uterus.

Ovary and oocytes: A median lethal dose (LD50) of <2 Gray (Gy) damages the oocyte. Age of the patient and dose of ovarian exposure determines the damage. The fertility window is determined by the size of the ovarian primordial follicle pool and radiation dose received at the time of treatment. Following total body irradiation (TBI) of 10–15.75 Gy, 90% of patients have been reported to have ovarian failure. With total abdominal irradiation of 20–30 Gy during childhood, 97% of women develop ovarian failure (Wallace et al., 2005).

Uterine effect: Uterine growth starts at puberty and is completed almost 7 years after menarche, i.e. around the age of 20 years (Holm et al., 1995). An increase in uterine blood flow is also seen during puberty (Laursen EM et al., 1996). Radiation exposure causes fibrosis, reduces vascularity, and decreases endometrial sensitivity to hormonal stimulation. These effects are responsible for infertility and adverse reproductive events like increase in miscarriages and premature labor. Direct radiation causes endometrial atrophy and lowers the uterine volume. The threshold dosage for causing significant uterine damage is as follows: in adults 12 Gy (TBI) and in childhood >25 Gy. Dose above this causes an irreversible damage to uterus (Larsen et al., 2004).

Males

Effect of Chemotherapy and Radiotherapy

Testis is highly susceptible to the effects of CT and RT throughout life. The prepubertal testis is especially vulnerable as there is a constant regeneration of early germ cells, somatic cells, and maturation of Leydig cells (Jahnukainen et al., 2011).

Low-dose chemotherapy and radiotherapy: Deplete the developing spermatogonia in the adult and pubertal testes. Clinical effects range from *temporary oligospermia to azoospermia*.

High doses of chemotherapy and radiotherapy: These may lead to apoptosis of spermatogonial stem cells (SSCs) and thereby causing complete depletion of SSC pool and seminiferous tubules leading to *Sertoli cells only (SCO) syndrome* (de Rooij et al., 2002), *permanent azoospermia, and sterility*.

Majority of males undergo a normal puberty and most produce normal adult levels of testosterone (Jahnukainen et al., 2011, Heikens et al.,1996).

Drug, dose, and duration of exposure: The extent of damage is related to the type of drug, dose, and duration of CT and RT. Alkylating agents are the most damaging and multiple doses appear to cause more harm. For Cy, the threshold dose for infertility is between 7.5 g/m^2 and 9 g/m^2 (Ridola et al., 2009; Meistrich et al., 1992). A dose of 19–20 g/m^2 of Cy may lead to permanent sterility. Scattered RT doses of 0.1 Gy may lead to temporary cessation of spermatogenesis. A dose of 2–3 Gy can cause long-term azoospermia and doses higher than 6 Gy can deplete the SSC pool resulting in permanent infertility (Rowley et al., 1774; Centola et al., 1994). Fractionated RT appears to increase germ cell toxicity by activating reserve cells (Ash P, 1980). A fractionated total dose of 1.2 Gy is found to be a threshold dose after which permanent testicular damage is possible. Higher doses are required to cause Leydig cells damage.

FERTILITY PROTECTION AND PRESERVATION

Fertility Protection Females

The added stress and strain of FP procedures could be well avoided if drugs were available to protect the gonads against the ill effect of CT. Though there is ongoing research to develop such agents, the only drug available for clinical use so far is the long-acting gonadotropic-releasing hormone agonist (GnRHa). Ovarian protection is thought to be conferred by creating a:

- Hypogonadotropic state similar to that seen in the prepubertal ovary
- Reduced ovarian blood flow due to hypoestrogenic status
- Direct effect on ovary (GnRH receptors are found in ovary)
- Upregulation of antiapoptotic molecules such as sphingosine-1-phosphate (S1P) in the ovary
- Prevention of gonadotoxicity on oogonial stem cells (Ataya et al., 1995; Roness et al., 2014; Blumenfeld, 2016).

The drug is given at least a week prior to CT to reduce damage caused by follicular activation due to its "flare effect", and it should be continued till 2 weeks after completion of therapy. Use of GnRH analog decreases the rate of premature menopause in breast cancer (BC) patients, though its effect on fertility protection is controversial) (Blumenfeld et al., 2015; Lambertini et al., 2015; Munhoz et al., 2016). This protective effect is yet not proven for patients with ovarian cancer and lymphoma (Del Mastro et al., 2014; Demeestere et al., 2016).

Recommendations on Use of GnRHa

The 2nd International Consensus Guidelines for Breast Cancer in Young Women (BCY2) support the use of GnRHa in all premenopausal BC patients who have to undergo CT and are interested in ovarian function and/or FP irrespective of the hormone receptor (HR) status of their disease. American Society of Clinical Oncology (ASCO) guidelines 2013 state that there is insufficient evidence to recommend use.

Fertility Protection Males

Gonadotropin-releasing hormone analog co-administration during CT to conserve fertility has not been found to be useful in men (Shetty and Meistrich, 2005).

FERTILITY PRESERVATION TECHNIQUES (FLOWCHARTS 1 AND 2)

Fertility preservation techniques in females (Flowchart 2):
- Embryo cryopreservation
- Oocyte cryopreservation
- Ovarian tissue cryopreservation (OTC)
- *In vitro* maturation (IVM).

Embryo and Oocyte Cryopreservation

Embryo cryopreservation by vitrification is a time-tested technique; however, it requires involvement of the husband or partner. The need for reproductive autonomy has increased the use of oocyte vitrification for FP. Both procedures require ovarian stimulation (OS) from day 2 of the menstrual cycle (MC) and oocyte retrieval; therefore, a period of approximately 12–14 days is required before CT. The preferred protocol is the antagonist protocol with a GnRH-a trigger for oocyte maturation, as it is shorter and decreases the risk of ovarian hyperstimulation syndrome (OHSS). To avoid delay in CT, a random start protocol has been introduced where OS is started at any time of the MC without compromising the outcome (Cakmak et al., 2013). Literature suggests that age is the only factor that contributes to a decrease in the number of oocytes

Flowchart 1: Fertility preservation in males.

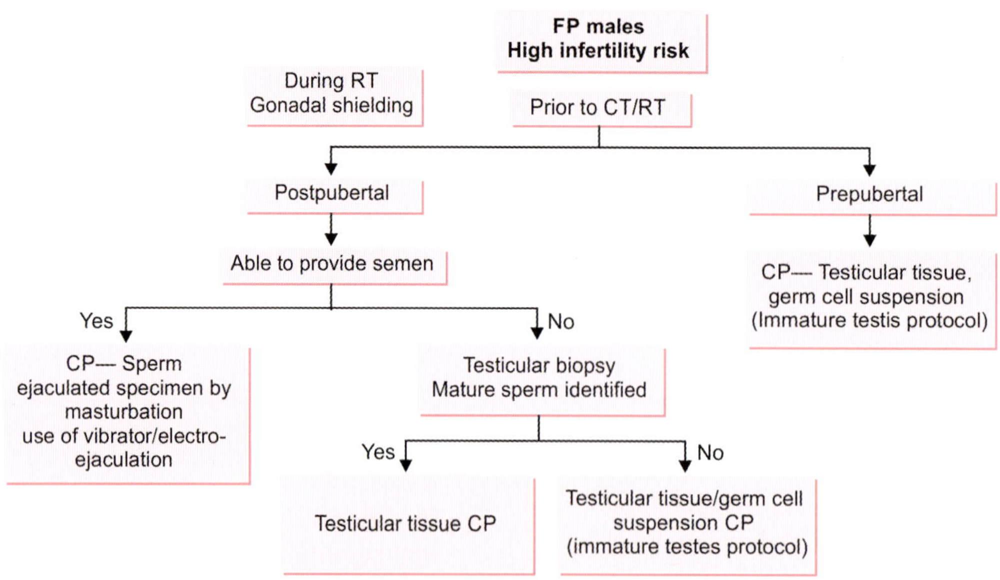

(FP: fertility preservation; CT: chemotherapy; CP: cryopreservation; RT: radiotherapy)

Flowchart 2: Fertility preservation techniques in females.

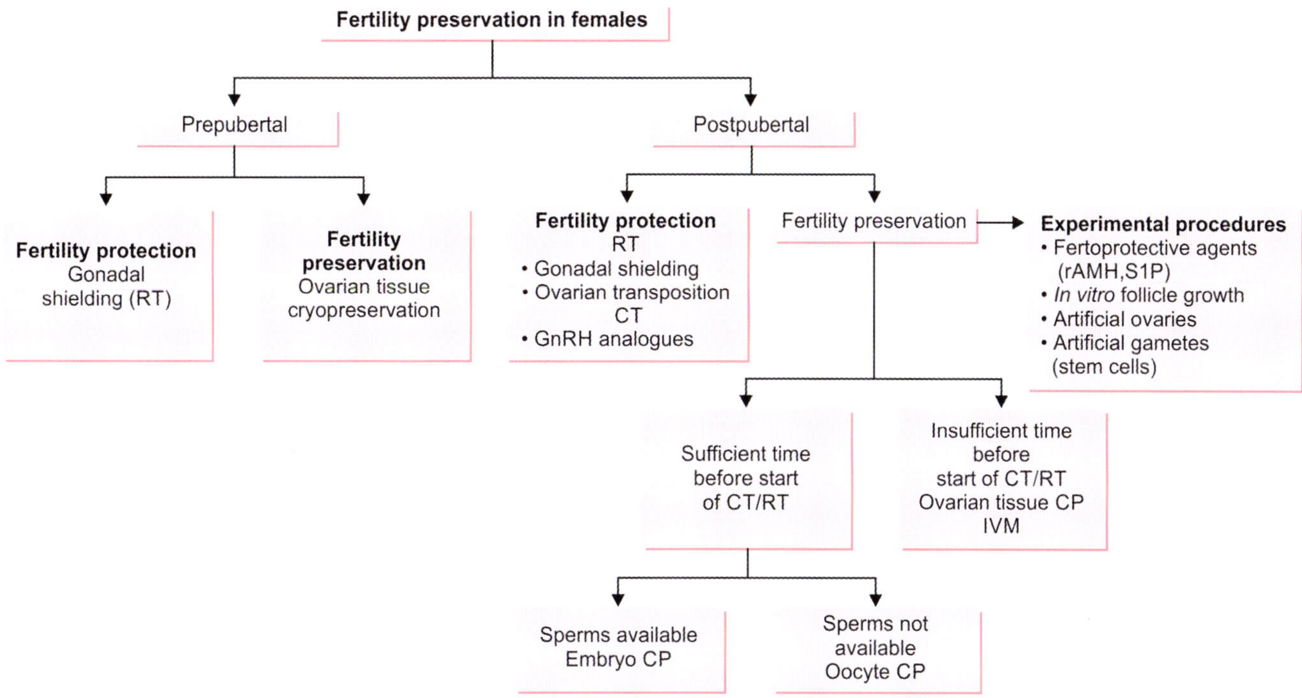

(S1P: sphingosine-1-phosphate; IVM: *in vitro* maturation; CT: chemotherapy; RT: radiotherapy; CP: cryopreservation)

recovered in oncological patients, though there are concerns about a pre-existing reduced ovarian reserve in patients with BRCA mutations and lymphoma (Oktay et al., 2010; Lawrenz B et al., 2012).

Supraphysiological estradiol (E2) levels achieved during OS have raised concerns in hormone-sensitive cancers. This has been addressed effectively by the addition of letrozole, an aromatase inhibitor, along with gonadotropins during OS. It is given from the start of OS in a dose of 2.5–5 mg daily and continued till after oocyte retrieval, until the E2 levels normalize. Use of letrozole does not appear to affect the oocyte number or fertilization rate (Oktay et al., 2015). Tamoxifen, a selective estrogen receptor modulator (SERM), has also been used during OS in hormone-sensitive BC patients. Tamoxifen is routinely used to improve survival rates in HR positive BC (Meirow et al., 2014).

ART Results Using Cryopreserved Gametes

Live birth rates similar to nononcological patients have been reported using cryopreserved embryos (Dolmans et al., 2015; Oktay et al., 2015). Successful oocyte freezing requires a skilled embryologist as human oocytes are highly prone to ice crystal formation and damage by cryoprotectants. Using vitrified thawed oocytes, an overall survival rate of 85.2% (95% CI 83.2–87.2) was reported by Cobo et al., 2015. The author also estimated an oocyte-to-baby rate of 6.5%; the probability increases progressively with a plateau being reached at 25 years.

In Vitro Maturation

Immature oocytes are retrieved from unstimulated ovaries and are matured in the laboratory for 30 hours, before fertilization. This procedure has not witnessed universal success as *in vitro* oocyte maturation is technically challenging. Improved culture techniques have led to better pregnancy rates (PRs) in appropriately selected patients (Grynberg et al., 2013). PRs/embryo transfer varies from 0% to 36% and spontaneous abortion rate between 17% and 63% (Holte et al., 2007). Studies assessing the health risks of children conceived after IVM have also been reassuring. The advantage of IVM is that it can be performed when delay in CT is not possible; additionally, no gonadotropin stimulation is required and therefore can be used in estrogen-sensitive tumors.

Cryopreservation of Ovarian Tissue

Cryopreservation of ovarian tissue (OTC) involves removal of ovarian cortical tissue rich in primordial follicles and cryopreservation by slow freezing or vitrification (a more recent technique) after tissue preparation. Collection of ovarian tissue and retransplantation can both be performed laparoscopically. Reimplantation of tissue is preferentially in the pelvic cavity (orthotopic); however, heterotopic transplantation can be carried out if required. Reports of pregnancies achieved after ovarian tissue transplantation are increasing and a live birth rate of 23% has been reported (Van der Ven, 2016). One of the major advantages of the procedure is that it can be done in patients requiring urgent CT, OS is not required, gonadal function is preserved, and a subsequent spontaneous conception is possible. Success of transplantation depends on the patients' age, baseline ovarian reserve, and expertize of the surgeon and cryobiologist performing the procedure. Ovarian function generally resumes between 60 days and 240 days post-transplant and lasts for up to 7 years (Kim SS, 2012). It is the only technique available for preserving fertility in prepubertal girls.

One of the major concerns with ovarian tissue transplantation is the risk of tumor reseeding. Based on the available data, the risk for different malignancies was estimated as follows: high risk—leukemia, moderate risk—gastrointestinal cancers, and low risk—BC, sarcomas of the bone and connective tissue, gynecological cancers, and Hodgkin's and non-Hodgkin's lymphoma (Rosendahl et al., 2013).

Whole Ovary Preservation

An entire ovary with its vascular pedicle can be preserved, though it is technically challenging requiring a vascular anastomosis at transplantation (Donnez et al., 2005).

Criteria for Ovarian Tissue Banking

International Society for Fertility Preservation (Kim et al., 2012) and Edinburgh criteria laid down the following criteria for ovarian tissue banking:

- *Age*: Under 37 years (may be individualized based on the status of ovarian reserve)
- *Ovarian function*: Premenopausal by follicle-stimulating hormone (FSH), antral follicle count (AFC), or anti-Müllerian hormone (AMH)
- *Communication with oncologists*: Cancer treatment plan, prognosis
- *When embryo freezing or oocyte freezing is not indicated*: Delaying cancer treatment is not acceptable, hormonal stimulation is not permitted, ART is not allowed
- Prepubertal girls who do not have any other options
- High risk for POF (when significant loss of ovarian follicles is anticipated with cancer therapy)
- Informed consent from adult patients
- Informed consent from parents/guardians as well as informed assent from minors, if the patient is less than 18 years
- Physically and mentally healthy enough for surgery
- Desires to have a child in the future (preferably before the age 50)
- Should understand experimental nature and potential risks of cancer cell transmission.

Edinburgh selection criteria for ovarian cortex cryopreservation:

- Age <35 years
- A realistic chance of surviving for more than 5 years
- More than 50% risk of developing POF after treatment
- No previous CT or RT if aged >15 years at diagnosis but mild gonadotoxic CT acceptable if age <15 years
- Informed consent
- Negative human immunodeficiency virus (HIV), hepatitis B, and syphilis serology
- Not pregnant and no existing children.

FUTURE DIRECTIONS

Technologies in the field of reproductive and regenerative medicine are evolving at an incredibly fast pace. Many experimental therapies have evolved for follicular growth and generation of gametes from stem cells (Table 1). At this point, they remain experimental and should only be carried out in the context of a research trial.

Females

New Fertoprotective Agents

Drugs with antiapoptotic properties and those that prevent follicular activation are being researched. Agents like imatinib, S1P, granulocyte colony-stimulating factor, tamoxifen, and thyroid hormone T3 are antiapoptotic and have been shown to reduce follicle loss in animals (Kim et al., 2016). One of the major concerns is that they may counteract or reduce the apoptotic effect of CT on cancer cells. Other agents that show promise are AS101, an immune modulator that acts on the PI3K/PTEN/AKT follicle activation pathway, and the AMH. AMH is produced by granulosa cells of small-growing follicles and is a negative regulator of follicle activation. AMH knock-out mice demonstrated accelerated primordial follicle recruitment and growth, resulting in exhaustion of the ovarian follicle pool (Durlinger et al., 1999). Replacement of negative regulator, AMH, at the time of Cy treatment prevents CT-induced follicle activation and loss of the ovarian reserve. AMH acts independently of the PI3K pathway. One advantage of AMH over other agents is that it is as an endogenous hormone and activity is limited

TABLE 1 Non-oncological conditions requiring fertility preservation.

Autoimmune causes	• Systemic lupus erythematosus • Rheumatoid arthritis • Inflammatory bowel disease • Behçet's disease • Pemphigus vulgaris • Glomerulonephritis (steroid resistant) • Eosinophilic granulomatosis
Hematopoietic stem cell transplantation	• Sickle cell anemia • Thalassemia major • Aplastic anemia
Medical conditions causing premature ovarian insufficiency (POI)	• Mosaic Turner syndrome • Fragile X mental retardation 1 • Endometriosis • Benign ovarian tumors • Ovarian oophoritis • Galactosemia • Beta-thalassemia
Male genetic disorders	• Klinefelter syndrome
Testicular damage	
Gender reassignment procedures	
Severe body trauma requiring surgical intervention	

Source: Martinez F; International Society for Fertility Preservation–ESHRE–ASRM Expert Working Group. Update on fertility preservation from the Barcelona International Society for Fertility Preservation-ESHRE-ASRM 2015 expert meeting: indications, results and future perspectives. Fertil Steril. 2017;108(3):407-15.e11.

to the ovary so the possibility of side effects is reduced (Roness, et al., 2016). Clinical applicability of these agents will depend on their ability to prevent follicular loss without interfering with cancer treatment.

Ovarian Activation

Immature primordial follicle activation has been achieved by interrupting the Hippo signaling pathway and treating ovarian tissue with AKT3 activators before transplantation. Hippo signaling pathway is interrupted mechanically by cutting the ovarian tissue into small fragments (Hsueh et al., 2015). This leads to an increase in downstream CCN growth factors and BIRC apoptosis inhibitors, which promote follicular growth. Incubation of ovarian cortical tissue with phosphatase and tensin homolog (PTEN) inhibitors and phosphatidylinositol-3-kinase (PI3K) stimulators activates dormant primordial follicles by increasing oocyte AKT activity to promote nuclear exclusion of FOXO3, thus preventing its suppression of primordial follicle growth (Kawamura et al., 2013). Live births have been reported in patient with premature ovarian insufficiency (POI) using a combination of these techniques (Kawamura et al., 2013; Suzuki et al., 2015). This technique could also prove useful in prepubertal girls.

In Vitro Follicular Growth

In vitro culture and growth of immature follicles to achieve complete maturation is challenging in humans, though successful animal experiments have been conducted (Telfer and Zelinski, 2013). One of the greatest advantages of this procedure would be to avoid or minimize the risk of reseeding cancer cells since ovarian follicles are surrounded by a basal membrane, excluding them from the stromal environment, capillaries, and nerves (Luyckx et al., 2013). Three-dimensional (3D) culture methods using alginate gel mimic the in vivo environment and have met with greater success. They preserve cell-cell interaction which is critical for oocyte growth and maturation (McLaughlin and Telfer, 2010; Skory et al., 2015). Xiao et al. (2015) have reported development of mature MII oocytes in humans; however, it remains to be seen if such oocytes are competent to produce healthy offspring. There are also concerns about establishment and maintenance of genomic imprinting in human oocytes grown *in vitro*.

Artificial Ovaries

Grafting of preantral follicles enzymatically isolated from frozen-thawed ovarian tissue and embedded in a 3D matrix along with other ovarian cells is referred to as an "artificial ovary" (Luyckx et al., 2013). This allows follicles to develop in a micro-environment akin to the ovarian environment (Kim et al., 2016). Ovarian stromal cells secrete numerous factors that regulate primordial-to-primary follicle transition and are recruited by growing follicles to differentiate into steroid-secreting theca cells required for follicle development and ovulation (Knight and Glister, 2006; Magoffin et al., 2005). Endothelial cells have also been added for proper vascularization of the artificial ovary (Dath et al., 2011). Ovarian cells (stromal and endothelial) can be isolated from a fresh ovarian biopsy (cortex and/or medulla) once the patient is disease-free. These cells isolated from fresh ovarian tissue can be combined with follicles obtained from cryopreserved cortex and would not require malignant cell purging (Soares et al., 2015). When transplanted, they can restore endocrine function in addition to fertility (Kim et al., 2016).

Males

Surveys performed in cancer survivors have shown that though 80% of cancer survivors consider parenthood, only 10% of them are comfortable with use of donor sperm or choose adoption (Wyns et al., 2015). For most couples, a genetic link with their child holds immense importance.

Cryopreservation of Immature Testicular Tissue and Germ Cell Suspension

Fertility preservation in prepubertal males poses a problem because their seminiferous tubules contain only SSCs, which are the diploid precursors of spermatozoa. Cryobanking of ITT or germ cell suspension can be offered to these patients. A controlled slow freezing procedure using dimethyl sulfoxide as the main cryoprotectant is used for cryopreservation of small ITT fragments (2–4 mm^3). Tissue is taken from one testis only with sampling limited to less than 5% of the testicular volume (Wyns et al., 2015; Picton et al., 2015). The integrity of the SSC niche that regulates stem cell self-renewal and differentiation is found to be well preserved (Wyns et al., 2008; Ogawa et al., 2005). To obtain mature gametes, the tissue needs to be transplanted back into the testis or IVM can be carried out. Autotransplantation carries the risk of reseeding malignant cells and requires careful screening. SSCs (whole testicular biopsy or isolated SSCs) are cultured in 3D systems that resemble the in vivo situation (Picton et al., 2015). However, the fertilizing ability of in vitro-cultured sperm is yet to be established.

Artificial Gametes from Stem Cells

Pluripotent stem cells (PSCs), including induced pluripotent stem cells (iPSCs), have the capacity to differentiate into all three germ layers and have been used as a cell source in regenerative medicine. As an alternative to gamete donation, embryonic stem cells or iPSC have been used to produce gametes (Vassena et al., 2015).

Spermatozoa

Zhou et al. (2016) have reported live birth after generation of mouse spermatid-like cells. Correct epigenetic reprogramming is essential for the development of functional gametes in general. It would seem that normal methylation patterns of imprinted genes are obtained when gametogenesis is resumed in in vivo conditions (Hayashi et al., 2011; Nakaki et al., 2013) giving rise to healthy offspring. Ramathal et al. (2014) transplanted human iPSC from azoospermic and normospermic males into the testis of sterile mouse and demonstrated signs of early spermatogenesis. Hayashi et al. (2011) were successful in producing healthy mouse offspring after transplanting in vitro produced primordial germ cell (PGC) cells. These experiments underpin the importance of the testicular niche in normal spermatogenesis. Despite intensive research and successful reports by some scientists, this technology is still not validated for clinical application.

Oocytes

Research on oocyte production has yet not met with success. Lacham-Kaplan et al. (2006) demonstrated that mouse embryonic stem cells (mESCs) are able to form follicle-like structures with oocyte-like cells, but they were not able to progress into meiosis. Using the mouse model, Hayashi et al. (2011) used PGCs obtained from female epiblast stem cells (EpiLCs) to derive immature oocytes. These were subsequently matured and fertilized in vitro leading to the birth of healthy and fertile offspring in foster mothers. The second-generation PGCs unfortunately were not completely normal, producing fragile and misshapen oocytes, sometimes lacking supporting granulosa cells. Fertilization of these artificial oocytes leads to formation of abnormal pronucleus and lower implantation rates.

SUMMARY

The Expert Working Group—European Society for Human Reproduction and Embryology-American Society for Reproductive Medicine (ESHRE-ASRM) 2015 expert meeting (Martinez et al., 2017) made the following recommendations:

- Several oncological and nononcological diseases may affect current or future fertility, either due to the disease itself or to gonadotoxic treatment, and need an adequate FP approach. These patients should be counseled regarding potential fertility loss and should be referred to fertility specialists to discuss options for FP and current results.
- Women wishing to postpone maternity and transgender individuals before starting hormone therapy or undergoing surgery to remove/alter their reproductive organs should also be counseled accordingly.
- Embryo and oocyte cryopreservation are first-line FP methods in postpubertal women. Metaphase II oocyte cryopreservation (vitrification) is the preferred option.
- Cumulative evidence for restoration of ovarian function and spontaneous pregnancies after ART following orthotopic transplantation of cryopreserved ovarian tissue supports its future consideration as an open clinical application.

- Semen cryopreservation is the only established FP technique in men.
- Testicular tissue cryopreservation should be recommended in prepubertal boys even though fertility restoration strategies by autotransplantation of cryopreserved testicular tissue have not yet been tested for safe clinical use in humans.
- The establishment of international registries on the short- and long-term outcomes of FP techniques is strongly recommended.

CONCLUSION

Fertility preservation has become the standard of care for patients at risk of losing their reproductive potential due to cancer treatment, immunological disease, or genetic make-up. Offering FP counseling is mandatory, though many oncologists are still reluctant to refer patients to the reproductive specialists. For postpubertal women, oocyte and embryo freezing is available and is an established technique. It needs to be performed before CT and requires a time period of 2 weeks. In women where there is an urgency to start CT and in prepubertal girls, ovarian tissue freezing may be offered. OTC requires laparoscopy both for removal and transplantation of tissue; however, it does offer the possibility of spontaneous conception subsequently and restoration of endocrine secretion. As more and more births are being reported, it has lost the experimental tag in some countries. However, it is important to screen the tissue before transplantation to avoid reseeding of malignant cells. In males, semen cryopreservation is the gold standard. In case it is not possible to collect an ejaculated semen sample, testicular tissue is frozen. For the prepubertal male, freezing of ITT and germ cell suspension can be offered but currently regeneration of mature sperm is in the experimental stage. In the future, IVM of gametes may be possible in humans using 3D reconstruction of ovary/testis. Stem cell therapies are not clinically validated at present and should not be used outside research protocols to maintain safety. A lot of work is going on to develop safe fertoprotective drugs which can be given concomitantly with CT, thus eliminating the need for preservation of gametes in oncofertility.

EDITORS' COMMENTS

1. Fertility preservation is very important yet underutilized branch of ART, due to its lack of awareness and integration required from members of different Medical Societies.
2. It is sometimes a very valuable option to have future children from one's own gametes is timely advised.
3. Various societies across the world have been formed which are working in this subject such as the Oncofertility Consortium, International Society of Fertility Preservation (ISFP), Fertility Preservation Society of India, etc.
4. Oocyte banking, OTCP, and testicular tissue cryopreservation are now the most common forms of techniques.
5. Ovarian tissue cryopreservation is a modern procedure for fertility preservation, requiring surgeries and meticulous tissue preparation and long-term storage.
6. Also, in young prepubertal women with cancer, induction of puberty post-treatment with cryopreserved ovarian tissue is an option.
7. Testicular tissue cryopreservation should be recommended in prepubertal groups but the functional restoration of cryopreserved samples is a challenging task.

SUGGESTED READING

1. Anckaert E, De Rycke M, Smitz J. Culture of oocytes and risk of imprinting defects. Hum Reprod Update. 2013;19:52-66.
2. Anderson RA, Themmen AP, Al-Qahtani A, et al. The effects of chemotherapy and long-term gonadotrophin suppression on the ovarian reserve in premenopausal women with breast cancer. Hum Reprod 2006;21:2583-92.
3. Ash P. The influence of radiation on fertility in man. The British Journal of Radiology. 1980;53:271-8.
4. Ataya K, Rao LV, Lawrence E, et al. Luteinizing hormone-releasing hormone agonist inhibits cyclophosphamide-induced ovarian follicular depletion in rhesus monkeys. Biol Reprod. 1995;52(2):365-72.
5. Blumenfeld Z, Evron A. Endocrine prevention of chemotherapy-induced ovarian failure.Curr Opin Obstet Gynecol. 2016;28(4):223-9.
6. Blumenfeld Z, Zur H, Dann EJ. Gonadotropin-releasing hormone agonist cotreatment during chemotherapy may increase pregnancy rate in survivors. Oncologist. 2015;20(11):1283-9.
7. Cakmak H, Katz A, Cedars MI, et al. Effective method for emergency fertility preservation: random-start controlled ovarian stimulation. Fertil Steril. 2013;100(6):1673-80.
8. Centola GM, Keller JW, Henzler M, et al. Effect of low-dose testicular irradiation on sperm count and fertility in patients with testicular seminoma. Journal of Andrology. 1994;15:608-13.
9. Chung K, Donnez J, Ginsburg E, et al. Emergency IVF versus ovarian tissue cryopreservation: decision making in fertility preservation for female cancer patients. Fertil Steril. 2013;99:1534-42.

10. Cobo A et al. Six years' experience in ovum donation using vitrified oocytes: report of cumulative outcomes, impact of storage time, and development of a predictive model for oocyte survival rate. Fertil Steril. 2015;104(6):1426-34.
11. Dath C, Dethy A, Van Langendonckt A, et al. Endothelial cells are essential for ovarian stromal tissue restructuring after xenotransplantation of isolated ovarian stromal cells. Hum Reprod. 2011;26:1431-39.
12. De Rooij DG, van de Kant HJ, Dol R, et al. Long-term effects of irradiation before adulthood on reproductive function in the male rhesus monkey. Bio Reprod. 2002;66(2):486-94.
13. Del Mastro L, Ceppi M, Poggio F, et al. Gonadotropin- releasing hormone analogues for the prevention of chemotherapy-induced premature ovarian failure in cancer women: systematic review and meta-analysis of randomized trials. Cancer Treat Rev. 2014;40:675-83.
14. Demeestere I, Brice P, Peccatori FA, et al. No evidence for the benefit of gonadotropin-releasing hormone agonist in preserving ovarian function and fertility in lymphoma survivors treated with chemotherapy: final long-term report of a prospective randomized trial. J Clin Oncol. 2016; 34(22):2568-74.
15. Di Giacomo M, Barchi M, Baudat F, et al. Distinct DNA-damage-dependent and -independent responses drive the loss of oocytes in recombinant defective mouse mutants. Proc Natl Acad Sci USA. 2005;102:737-42.
16. Dolmans MM, Hollanders de Ouderaen S, Demylle D, Pirard C. Utilization rates and results of long-term embryo cryopreservation before gonadotoxic treatment. J Assist Reprod Genet. 2015;32(8):1233-7.
17. Donnez J, Dolmans MM, Martinez-Madrid B, et al. The role of cryopreservation for women prior to treatment of malignancy. Curr Opin Obstet Gynecol 2005;17:333-8.
18. Durlinger AL, Kramer P, Karels B, et al. Control of primordial follicle recruitment by anti-Mullerian hormone in the mouse ovary. Endocrinology. 1999;140:5789-96.
19. Grynberg M, El Hachem H, de Bantel A, et al. In vitro maturation of oocytes: uncommon indications. Fertil Steril. 2013;99(5):1182-8.
20. Hayashi K, Ohta H, Kurimoto K, et al. Reconstitution of the mouse germ cell specification pathway in culture by pluripotent stem cells. Cell. 2011;146:519-32.
21. Heikens J, Behrendt H, Adriaanse R, et al. Irreversible gonadal damage in male survivors of pediatric Hodgkin's disease. Cancer. 1996;78:2020-24.
22. Holm K, Laursen EM, Brocks V, et al. Pubertal maturation of the internal genitalia: an ultrasound evaluation of 166 healthy girls. Ultrasound in Obstetrics & Gynecology. 1995;6(3): 175-81.
23. Holte TO, Norderhaug IN. In vitro maturation of oocytes within assisted reproduction. Oslo, Norway: Knowledge Centre for the Health Services at The Norwegian Institute of Public Health (NIPH); 2007[Internet].
24. Hsueh AJ, Kawamura K, Cheng Y, Fauser BC. Intraovarian control of early folliculogenesis. Endocr Rev. 2015;36:1-24.
25. Hudson MM. Reproductive outcomes for survivors of childhood cancer. Obstet Gynecol 2010;116:1171-83.
26. Indian Cancer Registry. Consolidated Report of the PBCRs: 2001-2004. Available from: www.icmr.nic.in/ncrp/cancer_reg.htm.
27. Jahnukainen K, Ehmcke J, Hou M, et al. Testicular function and fertility preservation in male cancer patients. Best Pract Res Clin Endocrinol Metab. 2011;25(2):287-302.
28. Kawamura K, Cheng Y, Suzuki N, et al. Hippo signaling disruption and Akt stimulation of ovarian follicles for infertility treatment. Proc Natl Acad Sci USA. 2013;110(43):17474-9.
29. Kim SS, Donnez J, Barri P, et al. Recommendations for fertility preservation in patients with lymphoma, leukemia, and breast cancer. J Assist Reprod Genet. 2012;29(6):465-8.
30. Kim SS. Assessment of long term endocrine function after ovarian transplantation of frozen-thawed human ovarian tissue to the heterotopic site: 10 year longitudinal follow-up study. J Assist Reprod Genet. 2012;29:489-93.
31. Kim SY, Kim SK, Lee JR, Woodruff TK. Toward precision medicine for preserving fertility in cancer patients: existing and emerging fertility preservation options for women. J Gynecol Onco. 2016;27(2):e22.
32. Knight PG, Glister C. TGF-beta superfamily members and ovarian follicle development. Reproduction. 2006;132: 191-206.
33. Lacham-Kaplan O, Chy H, Trounson A. Testicular cell conditioned medium supports differentiation of embryonic stem cells into ovarian structures containing oocytes. Stem Cells. 2006;24:266-73.
34. Lambertini M, Ceppi M, Poggio F, et al. Ovarian suppression using luteinizing hormone-releasing hormone agonists during chemotherapy to preserve ovarian function and fertility of breast cancer patients: a meta-analysis of randomized studies. Ann Oncol. 2015;26(12):2408-19.
35. Larsen EC, Schmiegelow K, Rechnitzer C, et al. Radiotherapy at a young age reduces uterine volume of childhood cancer survivors. Acta Obstetricia et Gynecologica Scandinavica. 2004;83(1):96-102
36. Laursen EM, Holm K, Brocks V, et al. Doppler assessment of flow velocity in the uterine artery during pubertal maturation. Ultrasound in Obstetrics and Gynecology. 1996;8(5):341-45.
37. Lawrenz B, Fehm T, von Wolff M, et al. Centers of Ferti-PROTEKT Network. Reduced pretreatment ovarian reserve in premenopausal female patients with Hodgkin lymphoma or non-Hodgkin-lymphoma—evaluation by using antimüllerian hormone and retrieved oocytes. Fertil Steril. 2012;98(1):141-4.
38. Loren AW, Mangu PB, Beck LN, et al. American Society of Clinical Oncology. Fertility preservation for patients with cancer: American Society of Clinical Oncology clinical practice guideline update. J Clin Oncol. 2013;31(19):2500-10.
39. Luyckx V, Dolmans MM, Vanacker J, et al. First step in developing a 3D biodegradable fibrin scaffold for an artificial ovary. J Ovarian Res. 2013;25;6(1):83.
40. Magoffin DA. Ovarian theca cell. Int J Biochem Cell Biol. 2005;37:1344-9.

41. Martinez F; International Society for Fertility Preservation–ESHRE–ASRM Expert Working Group. Update on fertility preservation from the Barcelona International Society for Fertility Preservation-ESHRE-ASRM 2015 expert meeting: indications, results and future perspectives. Fertil Steril. 2017;108(3):407-15.e11.
42. Masciangelo R, Bosisio C, Donnez J, et al. Safety of ovarian tissue transplantation in patients with borderline ovarian tumors. Hum Reprod. 2018;33(2):212-9.
43. McLaughlin M, Telfer EE. Oocyte development in bovine primordial follicles is promoted by activin and FSH within a two-step serum-free culture system. Reproduction. 2010; 139:971-8.
44. Meirow D, Biederman H, Anderson RA, et al. Toxicity of chemo- therapy and radiation on female reproduction. Clin Obstet Gynecol 2010;53:727-39.
45. Meirow D, Lewis H, Nugent D, et al. Subclinical depletion of primordial follicular reserve in mice treated with cyclophosphamide: clinical importance and proposed accurate investigative tool. Hum Reprod. 1999;14(7):1903-7.
46. Meirow D, Nugent D. The effects of radiotherapy and chemotherapy on female reproduction. Hum Reprod Update 2001;7:535-43.
47. Meirow D, Raanani H, Maman E, et al. Tamoxifen co-administration during controlled ovarian hyperstimulation for in vitro fertilization in breast cancer patients increases the safety of fertility-preservation treatment strategies. Fertil Steril. 2014;102(2):488-95.e3.
48. Meirow D, Schiff E. Appraisal of chemotherapy effects on reproductive outcome according to animal studies and clinical data. J Natl Cancer Inst Monogr. 2005;(34):21-5.
49. Meirow D, Wallace WH. Preservation of fertility in patients with cancer. N Engl J Med. 2009;360:2682-3.
50. Meistrich ML, Wilson G, Brown BW, et al. Impact of cyclophosphamide on long-term reduction in sperm count in men treated with combination chemotherapy for Ewing and soft tissue sarcomas. Cancer. 1992;70:2703-12.
51. Munhoz RR, Pereira AA, Sasse AD, et al. Gonadotropin-releasing hormone agonists for ovarian function preservation in premenopausal women undergoing chemotherapy for early-stage breast cancer: a systematic review and meta-analysis. JAMA Oncol. 2016;2(1):65-73.
52. Nakaki F, Hayashi K, Ohta H, et al. Induction of mouse germ-cell fate by transcription factors in vitro. Nature. 2013;501: 222-26.
53. Nayernia K, Nolte J, Michelmann HW, et al. In vitro-differentiated embryonic stem cells give rise to male gametes that can generate offspring mice. Dev Cell. 2006;11(1):125-32.
54. Ogawa T, Ohmura M, Ohbo K. The niche for spermatogonial stem cells in the mammalian testis. Int. J. Hematol. 2005;82: 381-88.
55. Oktay K, Kim JY, Barad D, et al. Association of BRCA1 mutations with occult primary ovarian insufficiency: a possible explanation for the link between infertility and breast/ovarian cancer risks. J Clin Oncol. 2010;28(2):240-4.
56. Oktay K, Turan V, Bedoschi G, et al. Fertility preservation success subsequent to concurrent aromatase inhibitor treatment and ovarian stimulation in women with breast cancer. J Clin Oncol. 2015;33(22):2424-9.
57. Paluch-Shimon S, Pagani O, Partridge AH, et al. Second international consensus guidelines for breast cancer in young women (BCY2). Breast. 2016;26:87-99.
58. Picton HM, Wyns C, Anderson RA, et al. ESHRE task force on fertility preservation in severe diseases. A European perspective on testicular tissue cryopreservation for fertility preservation in prepubertal and adolescent boys. Hum Reprod. 2015;30(11):2463-75.
59. Ramathal C, Durruthy-Durruthy J, Sukhwani M, et al. Fate of iPSCs derived from azoospermic and fertile men following xenotransplantation to murine seminiferous tubules. Cell Rep. 2014;7:1284-97.
60. Ridola V, Fawaz O, Aubier F, et al. Testicular function of survivors of childhood cancer: a comparative study between ifosfamide- and cyclophosphamide-based regimens. European Journal of Cancer. 2009;45:814-8.
61. Roness H, Kalich-Philosoph L, Meirow D. Prevention of chemotherapy-induced ovarian damage: possible roles for hormonal and non-hormonal attenuating agents. Hum Reprod Update. 2014;20:759-74.
62. Roness H, Kashi, O, Meirow D. Prevention of chemotherapy-induced ovarian damage. Fertil Steril. 2016;105: 20-9.
63. Rosendahl M, Greve T, Andersen CY. The safety of transplanting cryopreserved ovarian tissue in cancer patients: a review of the literature. J Assist Reprod Genet. 2013;30(1):11-24.
64. Rowley MJ, Leach DR, Warner GA, et al. Effect of graded doses of ionizing radiation on the human testis. Radiation Research. 1974;59:665-78.
65. Shetty G, Meistrich ML. Hormonal approaches to preservation and restoration of male fertility after cancer treatment. J Natl Cancer Inst Monogr. 2005;34:36-9.
66. Sklar C. Reproductive physiology and treatment-related loss of sex hormone production. Med Pediatr Oncol. 1999;33:2-8.
67. Skory RM, Xu Y, Shea LD, Woodruff TK. Engineering the ovarian cycle using in vitro follicle culture. Hum Reprod 2015;30:1386-95.
68. Soares M, Sahrari K, Chiti MC, et al. The best source of isolated stromal cells for the artificial ovary: medulla or cortex, cryopreserved or fresh? Hum Reprod. 2015;30(7):1589-98.
69. Suzuki N, Yoshioka N, Takae S, et al. Successful fertility preservation following ovarian tissue vitrification in patients with primary ovarian insufficiency. Hum Reprod. 2015;30(3):608-15.
70. Telfer EE, Zelinski MB. Ovarian follicle culture: advances and challenges for human and nonhuman primates. Fertil Steril. 2013;99:1523-33.
71. Van der Ven H, Liebenthron J, Beckmann M, et al. FertiPROTEKT network. Ninety-five orthotopic transplantations in 74 women of ovarian tissue after cytotoxic treatment

in a fertility preservation network: tissue activity, pregnancy and delivery rates. Hum Reprod. 2016;31(9):2031-41.

72. Vassena R, Eguizabal C, Heindryckx B. Stem cells in reproductive medicine: ready for the patient? Hum Reprod. 2015;30:2014-21.
73. Wallace WH, Thomson AB, Saran F, et al. Predicting age of ovarian failure after radiation to a field that includes the ovaries. Int J Radiat Oncol Biol Phys. 2005;62:738-44.
74. Wallace WHB, Smith AG, Kelsey TW, et al. Fertility preservation for girls and young women with cancer: a population-based validation of criteria for ovarian tissue cryopreservation. Lancet Oncol 2014;15:1129-36.
75. Ward E, DeSantis C, Robbins A, et al. Childhood and adolescent cancer statistics, 2014. CA Cancer J Clin 2014; 64:83-103.
76. Wyns C, Collienne C, Shenfield F, et al. Fertility preservation in the male pediatric population: Factors influencing the decision of parents and children. Hum Reprod. 2015;30:2022-30.
77. Wyns C, Van Langendonckt A, Wese FX, et al. Long-term spermatogonial survival in cryopreserved and xenografted immature human testicular tissue. Hum Reprod. 2008;23: 2402-14.
78. Xiao S, Zhang J, Romero MM, et al. In vitro follicle growth supports human oocyte meiotic maturation. Sci Rep. 2015;5:17323.
79. Zavos A, Valachis A. Risk of chemotherapy-induced amenorrhea in patients with breast cancer: a systematic review and meta-analysis. Acta Oncol 2016;55:664-70.
80. Zhou Q, Wang M, Yuan Y, et al. Complete meiosis from embryonic stem cell-derived germ cells in vitro. Cell Stem Cell. 2016;18:330-40.

27

CHAPTER

Third-party Reproduction

Molina Patel, Nayana H Patel

INTRODUCTION

Third-party reproduction, also referred to as donor-assisted reproduction, is defined as an alternative human reproduction technique in which DNA or pregnancy is provided by a third party, that is, a person other than the prospective parents, who will raise the resulting baby.

The American Society for Reproductive Medicine (ASRM) defines it as follows:

Arrangements in which intended parents collaborate with gamete donors and/or gestational carriers (GCs) are referred to as "third-party reproduction".

There are four different types of third-party reproduction arrangements, which at the same time allow combinations between them:

1. Egg donation
2. Sperm donation
3. Embryo donation/adoption
4. Surrogacy.

EGG DONATION

Egg donation has revolutionized fertility for many women whose egg reserve has diminished in both quality and quantity. The acceptance of either of the gametes, from another individual for procreation is understandably a difficult decision for any couple. The first pregnancy resulting from egg donation was reported in 1984 by Trounson and colleagues. Since then, with the advent of advanced *in vitro* fertilization (IVF) options, egg donation has helped many women struggling with infertility to conceive.

Indications of Donor Oocyte

Egg donation is often used for women whose ovaries have either been surgically removed or are functioning poorly. The various indications are listed in Table 1.

Counseling of Donors and Recipients

All patients and their partners require a detailed explanation of the procedures involved in egg donation and counseling on the moral, ethical, and legal implications.

TABLE 1 Indications of egg donation.

Ovarian dysfunction	*Normal ovarian function*
• *Premenopausal*: – Poor ovarian responders – Diminished ovarian reserve – Premature ovarian failure (includes genetic, autoimmune, iatrogenic causes, surgical oophorectomy, etc.) – Previous ART failure – Unexplained • *Postmenopausal* – Oncology related chemoradiotherapy – Genetic – Unexplained	• Genetic transmittable disorder – Autosomal/sex chromosomal related • Recurrent pregnancy loss – With/without recurrent aneuploidy • Same sex couples • Research • Inaccessible ovaries • Older women with reduced ovarian reserve/diminished oocyte quality • Female survivors of cancer in childhood and adolescence treated with bone marrow transplant including total body irradiation (TBI), X-ray therapy, or chemotherapy • Ovarian resistance syndrome

(ART: assisted reproductive technology)

- Implications counseling
- Support counseling
- Therapeutic counseling.

Who are Egg Donors?

There are several ways of obtaining donor eggs which are as follows:

Anonymous Donors

Anonymous donors include women who are not known to the recipient(s). Donors may be found through egg donation programs or through agencies.

Known (Directed Donors)

Directed donors include women who are known to the recipient(s). The donor is generally a close relative or friend. In some instances, recipients advertise directly for donors in newspapers or on the internet. In these circumstances, the recipient(s) and the donor are known to each other in a limited way, and meet without an intermediary program or agency. Recipients should be cautious if recruiting donors directly without having an intermediary program or agency screen donors or without seeking legal counsel.

In Vitro Fertilization Programs

Women undergoing IVF may agree to donate their excess eggs to infertile patients. Using spare oocytes has its advantages like:

- Donor does not have to suffer additional risk.
- Egg sharing reduces the cost of treatment.

However, the disadvantages are as follows:

- Donation of oocytes from an infertile woman has lesser success rates.
- When the best oocytes are used for the donor, the outcome for the subsequent recipient may be suboptimum.

Given the paucity of donors, alternative sources of donor oocytes using emerging technologies need to be explored like:

- *In vitro* maturation of eggs
- Oocyte vitrification and cryopreservation
- Egg banks
- Use of preimplantation genetic screening (PGS)
- Ovarian rejuvenation techniques using bone marrow concentrates/stem cells
- Optimizing treatment of male infertility to counter-balance the egg subfertility.

Selection and Screening of Oocyte Donors According to the Indian Council of Medical Research

- Donors should be healthy, well screened, and in the age-group of 21–35 years.
- Relevant information regarding the donor, such as, age, height, weight, blood group, educational qualifications, profession, and color of the skin and the eyes must be recorded.
- Detailed history should be taken to rule out hereditary disease and to exclude individuals who might be at high risk for human immunodeficiency virus (HIV), sexually transmitted infections, or other infections that might be transmissible via gamete donation.
- Basic investigations should include endocrine profile [follicle-stimulating hormone (FSH), luteinizing hormone (LH), estradiol levels, serum thyroid-stimulating hormone (serum TSH), prolactin, and serum progesterone], blood profile, screening for sexually transmitted diseases [like HIV, hepatitis B/C, hepatitis C virus (HCV), syphilis, gonorrhea, chlamydia], detailed pelvic ultrasound examination, genetic karyotyping, and hemoglobin electrophoresis to rule out conditions such as thalassemia.
- Psychological evaluation and counseling for the oocyte donor and her partner. In circumstances involving known donors, this counseling should be offered to the donor and her partner, as well as the recipient and her partner.
- The donor must be informed that the offspring will not know her identity.
- A written and informed consent should be taken according to ICMR guidelines.
- It is advisable that a single person donates not more than six times with a gap of 3 months between subsequent egg retrievals.
- Additional testing can be performed based on the ethnicity of the donors.

Evaluation of Recipient(s)

- Evaluation of the recipient(s) is similar to that of couples undergoing routine IVF.
- They must be counseled and explained in detail of the procedure and its legal, moral, and ethical implications.
- The physician should obtain a comprehensive medical history from the recipient and her partner (if there is one).
- In addition, the assessment of the female partner will include a comprehensive gynecologic history and complete physical examination. She should have an

assessment of ovarian reserve (when appropriate), blood type and Rh, and rubella and cytomegalovirus (CMV) testing.
- Evaluation of her uterine cavity with a hysterosalpingogram (HSG), sonohysterogram (SHG), or hysteroscopy.
- If the female recipient is over the age of 45 years, a more thorough evaluation with assessment of cardiac function, risk for pregnancy-related hypertension, and gestational diabetes should be considered.
- A consultation with a high-risk obstetrical specialist is recommended to discuss the impact of advanced maternal age on pregnancy, as well as any medical conditions that may affect a pregnancy.
- The assessment of the male partner (if there is one) should include a semen analysis, blood type and Rh factor, and genetic-carrier screening as indicated. All intended recipients (female and male) should be screened for syphilis, hepatitis B and C, and HIV-1/2.

Selection and Screening of Egg Recipient (Table 2)

- Hormonal profile
- Hepatitis B surface antigen (HbsAg), HIV, blood group and Rh factor (BGRh), Pap smear
- Transvaginal sonography (TVS)—to see for pelvic pathology and assess mock cycle
- Hysterosalpingogram/hysteroscopy
- Medical conditions—heart disease, hypertension, diabetes mellitus (DM)
- Counseling
- Male partner assessment.

Evaluation of the Partner of the Oocyte Recipient

- Semen analysis for male partners
- Blood type and Rh factor
- Serologic test for syphilis
- Hepatitis B surface antigen
- Hepatitis B core antibody [immunoglobulin G (IgG) and IgM]
- Hepatitis C antibody and NAT
- HIV-1 (AB and NAT), HIV-2 AB testing
- Appropriate genetic screening and testing based on history counseling.

Cycle Management

There are two ways of preparing the donor using this technique:

1. GnRH agonist protocol
2. GnRH antagonist protocol

TABLE 2 Selection and screening of egg recipient.

Test/consultation	*When needed*
Hysterosalpingogram, saline hysterosonography, or hysteroscopy	Within 2 years
Pap smear	Within 1 year
Mammogram	Within 5 years if recipient is between ages 35 and 40, within 2 year if she is 51 years or older
Fasting glucose level	Within 3 years if anyone in recipient's immediate family or two or more people among her relatives have diabetes, if she is obese, or if she has had diabetes while pregnant
Test/consultation	When needed
Electrocardiogram	Within the year if recipient is aged 40 years or more
Total cholesterol level	Within the year if a parent or sibling of the recipient has/had a total >240 mg/dL, if members of her family developed premature (<55 years) cardiovascular disease, if she has diabetes, or if she smokes
Test/consultation	When needed
Preconceptual counseling	If recipient is aged 35 years or more, with an obstetrician, to review risks of pregnancy
General medical screening	If recipient is aged 45 years or more, or gets short of breath, has a heart murmur, or has an abnormal electrocardiogram, a high total cholesterol, or blood in her stools
Psychological counseling	Recommended for all

GnRH Agonist Protocol

Preparation of the donor: The donor is treated with a period of long downregulation with the gonadotropin-releasing hormone (GnRH) analog, leuprolide or buserelin, for up to 2 weeks, after which the serum levels of estradiol, LH, and progesterone are measured. A baseline pelvic scan is conducted and then follicular stimulation can begin with recombinant FSH/human menopausal gonadotropin (hMG), etc. (150 IU or 225 IU daily, depending on various clinical parameters and hormone profile).

Monitoring of the follicles is done using TVS and blood hormone profile and dose adjustments are made accordingly. When we can see at least three follicles of 17 mm with normally rising estradiol levels, a suitable trigger like human chorionic gonadotropin (hCG) 10,000 IU is given 34–36 hours before the intended time of oocyte retrieval.

Note: The aim being optimal stimulation with prevention of the ovarian hyperstimulation syndrome (OHSS), tailored

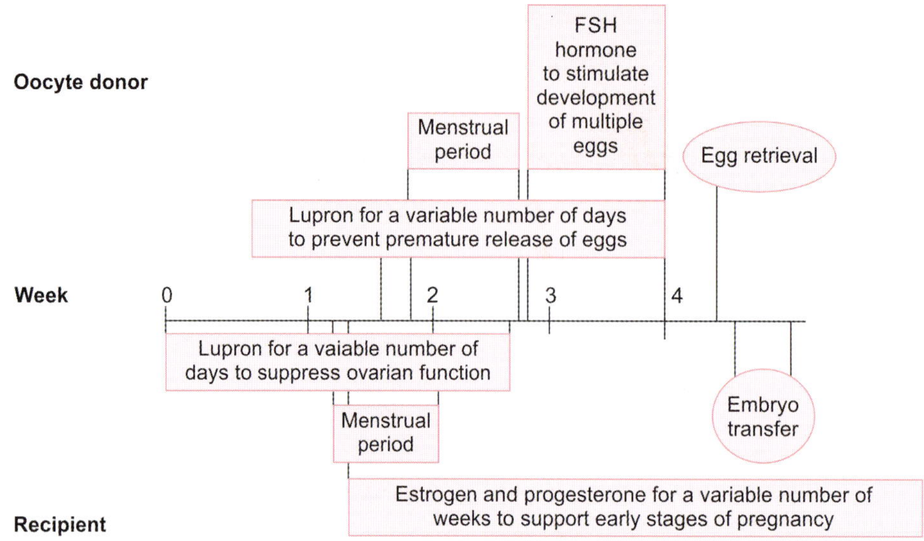

Fig. 1: Agonist protocol.
(FSH: follicle-stimulating hormone)

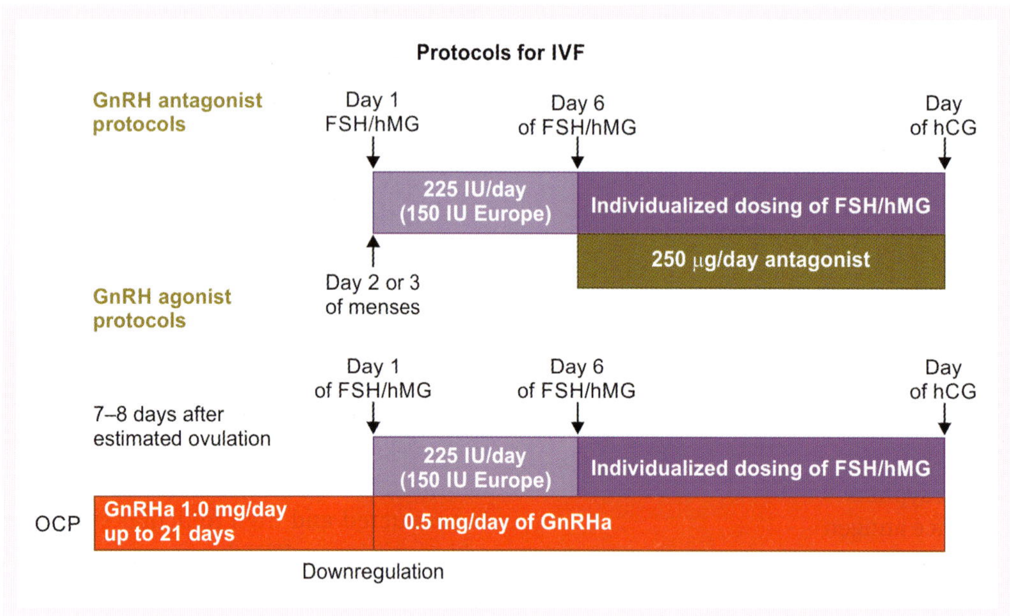

Fig. 2: Antagonist protocol.
(FSH: follicle-stimulating hormone; GnRHa: gonadotropin-releasing hormone agonist; hCG: human chorionic gonadotropin; hMG: human menopausal gonadotropin; IVF: *in vitro* fertilization)

protocols for every individual donor should be the norm. In donors at risk of OHSS, the use of the antagonist protocol, and with replacement of the hCG trigger with recombinant LH or GnRH agonists (only in an antagonist protocol cycle) helps in prevention of OHSS (Figs. 1 and 2).

GnRH Antagonist Protocol

After evaluating the baseline levels of S estradiol, LH and progesterone, and conducting a pelvic scan, follicular stimulation can begin depending on various clinical

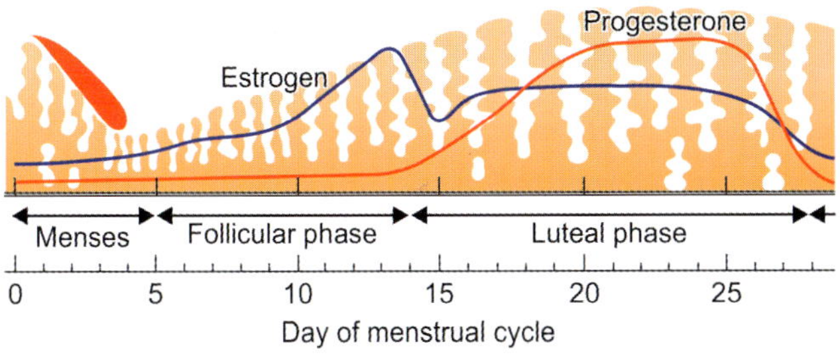

Fig. 3: Hormone profile of endometrium in the preparation of the recipient for embryo transfer.

Flowchart 1: Preparation of the recipient for embryo transfer.

Endometrial preparation (fresh/frozen cycle)

- Nonfunctional ovaries
- *Functional ovaries*
  - Natural cycles
  - Modified natural cycles
  - HRT with/without downregulation
  - CC/letrozole prepared endometrium

(CC: clomiphene citrate; HRT: hormone replacement therapy)

parameters. The GnRH antagonist is added as per two protocols

1. *Fixed protocol*: GnRH antagonist is added on the Day 6 of stimulation irrespective of size of the follicles.
2. *Flexible protocol*: GnRH antagonist is added when the follicles reach a size of 12–14 mm.

Advantages of using GnRH antagonist protocol:

- Decreases the duration of ovarian stimulation days
- Reduces the incidence of OHSS.

Key points to remember while stimulating a donor:

- Preferably antagonist cycle
- Ovarian hyperstimulation syndrome prevention
- Optimal oocyte number around 10–15 (minimum 7)
- Safety and wellbeing of donor
- Complication free stimulation and oocyte retrieval procedure.

Preparation of the Recipient for Embryo Transfer (Fig. 3 and Flowchart 1)

- Endometrial preparation is the most optimal step in third-party cycles.
- Endometrial preparation of the recipient is modeled on the natural menstrual cycle.
- The higher success rate of donor cycle is attributed highly to the endometrial preparation techniques and trying to optimize window of implantation (WOI).
- The implantation window is defined as that period when the uterus is receptive for implantation of the free-lying blastocyst.
- This period of receptivity is short and results from the programmed sequence of the action of estrogen and progesterone on the endometrium.
- In cycles where endogenous hormonal activity is suppressed or absent, the optimal time for embryo transfer (ET) lies between luteal Days +3 to +5, where luteal Day +1 is the first day of exogenous progesterone treatment.
- In the human, blastocyst apposition begins about LH Day +6 and is complete by LH +10).

Aim is to get recipient's menstruation 2 days (1–2 days) before the donor or simultaneously for synchronization.

- Synchronize the donor and recipient cycle by GnRH agonist or progesterone.
- When both donor and recipient are downregulated, recipient starts estrogen and donor starts ovarian stimulation 2–3 days later.

Women with Nonfunctioning Ovaries

- *Hormone replacement therapy—estradiol valerate*:
  - 6–8 mg daily, fixed or variable dose regimen
  - Starting 2–3 days before stimulation of the donor
  - Transdermal estrogen 0.2–0.4 mg
  - Ideally, 12–14 days of estrogen.
- *Progesterone replacement*:
  - Injectable 100 mg daily
  - Vaginal pessaries 200 mg three times a day
  - Starting on the day of OPU or when the endometrium ≥8 mm
  - Transfer according to the embryo staging.

Women with Functioning Ovaries

- Natural cycle
- Hormone replacement therapy (HRT) cycle
- Semi-HRT cycle
- Gonadotropin-releasing hormone agonist (GnRHa) + HRT cycle
- Clomiphene citrate/aromatase inhibitors.

Natural cycle:

- No HRT supplementation to be given
- To decide follow-up based on cycle length
- ET to be evaluated along with follicular growth strictly from Day 8 to Day 10 of cycle

- Ovulation cannot be missed (LH kit can be used in midcycle or daily ultrasound).

Transfer is planned on LH surge + 7 days or Ovulation +5 days.

Modified natural cycle: No HRT treatment is given. To decide the follow-up based on cycle length:
- Endometrium and follicular growth meticulously evaluated
- With ET ≥8 mm and follicle ≥18 mm, hCG trigger (5,000 IU/10,000 IU) is given
- Ovulation is checked
- Transfer is planned hCG + Day 7.

Clomiphene citrate/letrozole induced endometrium: Oral ovulogens are sometimes used to stimulate development of follicle which would cause natural development of endometrium. hCG can be given at follicle ≥18 mm and adequate ET can be planned accordingly.

Endometrial Receptivity

Endometrial receptivity is the window of time when the uterine environment is conductive to embryo acceptance and subsequent implantation.

Endometrial receptivity can be assessed by:
- Transvaginal USG
- Color Doppler
- Recently using three-dimensional (3D)/4D USG
- Hormonal evaluation
- Endometrial thickness (>7 to <14 mm)
- Endometrial pattern (triple-line pattern)
- Endometrial and subendometrial blood flow (within zone 3)
- Uterine artery resistance index/pulsatility index (RI/PI).

Complications with Oocyte Donation

Complications associated with oocyte donation are given in Table 3.

Pregnancy Rates with Egg Donation Program

Pregnancy rates in oocyte donation program are better when compared to use of own oocytes. Reasons for higher success rates may be due to:
- No risk of hyperestrogenism
- Controlled ovarian hyperstimulation (COH) results in abnormal endometrial development
- High level of estrogen seen in COH may cause premature luteolysis
- Pituitary downregulation with GnRHa is detrimental to luteal phase
- Ovarian aspiration disrupts granulosa cells
- Better control of window receptivity.

TABLE 3 Complications of oocyte donors.

	Short-term	*Long-term*	*Fertility-related*
Donor	*Recipient*		
OHSS	*Medical complications in pregnancy*:	Oncologic—breast/uterine/ovarian	Future sub/infertility
Ovarian torsion	Miscarriage	Psychological effect on offspring	Premature menopause
Pain	Aneuploidy		
Anesthesia related	Multiple pregnancies		
Bleeding	Premature births		
Infection	Placental pathology		
	Hypertensive disorders		

(OHSS: ovarian hyperstimulation syndrome)

EMBRYO DONATION

- It is defined as the giving—generally without compensation—of embryos remaining after one couple's IVF to either another person or couple for implantation or to research.
- Where it is given for the purpose of implantation, the donation is followed by the placement of those embryos into the recipient woman's uterus to facilitate pregnancy and childbirth in the recipient.
- This is a relatively simple, safe, and cost-effective procedure compared to oocyte donation or IVF.
- The selection, screening, and counseling of embryo donors and recipients is essentially the same as oocyte and sperm donors. Embryo donation can be a controversial process from both an ethical and a legal standpoint. Of paramount importance is that informed consent and counseling be provided to both the donors of the embryos and the recipient(s).

Indications for Embryo Donation Program

- Menopausal and perimenopausal women with subfertile partner
- Recurrent IVF failures
- Carriers of genetic or chromosomal abnormalities like germ cell disease, etc.
- Financial constraints
- Untreatable infertility in one/both partners.

Pregnancy following embryo donation depends on the quality of the embryos that were frozen, the age of the woman who provided the eggs, and the number of embryos transferred.

SPERM DONATION

The use of donor sperm has been practiced for over a century, although the first published reports of such were in 1945. Since the late 1980s, with the emergence of HIV, donor insemination (DI) has been performed only with frozen and quarantined sperm to allow for time to test the donors. Food and Drug Administration (FDA) and ASRM guidelines recommend that sperm be quarantined for at least 6 months before being used.

Contrary to what happens in the case of women, sperm quality and quantity do not change over the years so dramatically. Thus, delayed fatherhood is not a major reason when it comes to diagnosing male infertility.

Nevertheless, today's lifestyle habits do contribute greatly to the production of poor-quality sperm. Damaged sperm parameters, i.e. sperm motility, sperm count, and/or sperm morphology are the main causes behind the most common causes of male infertility.

Indications for Donor Sperm

Donor sperm can be used in the following:

- Genetic diseases or anomalies
- Obstructive and nonobstructive azoospermia, which may be congenital or acquired
- Severe azoospermia [congenital absence of the vas deferens (CBAVD) or vasectomy]
- Severe oligozoospermia
- Ejaculatory dysfunction
- Medical and/or surgical procedures (cancer treatments, vasectomy)
- Absence of a male partner (single women/lesbian couples)
  - Donor insemination may be used if the female is Rh-sensitized and the male partner is Rh-positive.
  - Donor insemination often is used in the treatment for a single woman who desires a pregnancy but who lacks a male partner.

Selection of Sperm Donors

- The main qualities to seek in selecting a donor for therapeutic donor insemination (TDI) are an assurance of good health status and the absence of known genetic abnormalities.
- The assisted reproductive technology (ART) banks shall obtain semen from males between 21 and 45 years of age, both inclusive, and cannot donate semen more than 25 times (ART Bill, 2015).
- In the event that the man intending to act as sperm donor is married, the consent of his spouse shall be required before he may act as sperm donor (ART Bill, 2015).
- He should be screened for psychological evaluation and all diseases transmitted via semen as well as for genetically transmitted diseases.

SURROGACY

This marvel of reproductive technique dates back to ancient times. Surrogacy, also known as surrogate motherhood, is a fertility treatment in which a woman other than the intended mother carries the pregnancy to term and delivers the baby for the intended parents. This technique is the one involving a greater degree of complexity from the ethical, psychological, moral, and technical points of view.

There exist two types of surrogacy:

1. *Partial, straight, or traditional surrogacy*: The surrogate contributes the eggs, and therefore is the genetic mother of the resulting child. It is done via intrauterine insemination (IUI), using the sperm of the intended father or from a donor.
   The ICMR does not allow traditional surrogacy in India.
2. *Full, host, or gestational surrogacy*: The surrogate, in this case named GC, just carries the pregnancy and therefore she is not the biological mother of the child. The eggs are contributed by the intended mother or an egg donor.
   The gestational surrogate has no genetic link to the fetus she is carrying. Despite the requirement for IVF to create embryos, the utilization of a gestational surrogate, legally, is a lower risk procedure and is the more common approach conducted in most countries. If implantation happens, then by contract agreement, the surrogate woman carries the pregnancy till term in a normal course of events.

Gestational surrogacy can be of two types:

1. *Commercial surrogacy arrangement*: This is when the surrogate is paid and compensated for her services, over and above her medical expenses.
2. *Altruistic surrogacy arrangement*: This is when the surrogate is given no financial gain for carrying a child. Only realistic out of pocket expenses are covered by the intended parents.

Current Status of Surrogacy in India

- On August 24, the Union cabinet approved the Surrogacy (Regulation) Bill, 2016.

- The bill proposes a ban on commercial surrogacy.
- Restricting "ethical" and "altruistic surrogacy" to legally-wedded infertile Indian couples, who have been married for at least 5 years.

The 228th report of the Law Commission had recommended prohibiting commercial surrogacy and allowing ethical altruistic surrogacy by enacting a suitable legislation. So, the "Surrogacy (Regulation) Bill, 2016" was introduced in the Lok Sabha on 21 November in 2016 and was referred to the Parliamentary Standing Committee on Health and Family Welfare in January 2017. The Cabinet, on March 22, 2018, gave its approval for moving official amendments in a bill which aims at banning commercial surrogacy, allowing altruistic surrogacy to needy infertile couples and its effective regulation in the country.

Indications of Surrogacy

These are shown in Table 4.

Steps in Surrogacy

Proper patient selection:

- Source of surrogate (ART bank)
- Proper selection and screening of the surrogate
- Intensive counseling—the key factor
- Proper controlled ovarian stimulation and IVF technique
- Preparing the surrogate
- Synchronizing the cycles of the surrogate and the genetic mother
- Window period for embryo transfer
- Taking care of the legalities and financial contracts
- Transparency of the whole arrangement.

Screening of the Surrogate

According to ICMR:

- The surrogate should be in the age group of 21–35 years.
- Tested for blood group, HIV, HBsAg, HCV, and Venereal Disease Research Laboratory (VDRL).
- A thorough medical history and extensive medical testing and physical examination.
- A complete personal and sexual history to exclude individuals who might be at high risk for sexually transmitted infections.
- Psychological evaluation and counseling by a qualified professional is recommended for the surrogacy and her partner, and immediate family.
- The surrogate should be well informed about the procedure and the possible complications.
- The surrogate should be free from any medical conditions, hereditary disorders, hemoglobinopathies, infectious diseases, and personal addictions like smoking or alcohol consumption.

TABLE 4 Indications of surrogacy.

Patients with uterus	*Patients without a uterus*
Repeated miscarriages/pregnancy loss	Mullerian agenesis (e.g. MRKH syndrome)
Repeated IVF failures—nonreceptive uterus	Hysterectomized (for gynecological indications like large fibroids, cancers, etc.)
Women with medical conditions, in which pregnancy is contraindicated (e.g. chronic kidney disease, Eisenmenger syndrome, etc.)	Hysterectomized for obstetric purposes (for PPH, uterine rupture)

(MRKH: Mayer-Rokitansky-Küster-Hauser; PPH: postpartum hemorrhage)

Counseling

The role of counseling is of utmost importance in surrogacy arrangement. This is to prepare all parties contemplating in this last resort treatment regarding the psychological, social, legal, and emotional aspects. Counseling ensures that they be confident and comfortable with their various decisions, and have trust in each other.

Couples should also be informed realistically about the failures of the treatment. Legal considerations and financial obligations are to be discussed carefully. An attorney knowledgeable in reproductive law may also be consulted, whenever the need arises.

Counseling for the couple:

- The medical and psychological risks of surrogacy
- Potential psychological risk to the child
- The chances of having a multiple pregnancy
- The possibility that the host may wish to retain the child after birth
- The importance of obtaining legal advice.

Screening for the Surrogate

- A physical examination and pap smear
- Infective disease testing
- Hysteroscopy
- A mock cycle
- Psychological testing and evaluation.

Counseling for the Surrogate

- The full implications of undergoing treatment by IVF surrogacy
- The possibility of multiple pregnancy

- The possibility of her family and friends being against her having treatment
- The medical risks associated with pregnancy and delivery
- The implications of guilt on both sides if the host should spontaneously abort a pregnancy
- The possible effect on her own children for acting as a surrogate
- The possibility that the host may face a sense of bereavement when she gives the baby to the commissioning couple.

ICMR CODE OF PRACTICE, AND ETHICAL CONSIDERATIONS IN GESTATIONAL SURROGACY (SALIENT POINTS)

- A child born through surrogacy must be adopted by the genetic (biological) parents, unless they can establish by genetic (DNA) fingerprinting that the child is theirs.
- Advertisements regarding surrogacy should not be made by the ART clinic. The responsibility of finding a surrogate mother, through advertisement or otherwise, should rest with the couple, or a registered agency.
- Legal papers regarding the contract agreement should be made by a lawyer, and as per the rules of the court.
- Payments to surrogate mothers should cover all genuine expenses associated with the pregnancy. Documentary evidence of the financial arrangement for surrogacy must be available. The ART center should not be involved in this monetary aspect.
- A relative, a known person, as well as a person unknown to the couple may act as a surrogate mother for the couple. In the case of a relative acting as a surrogate, the relative should belong to the same generation as the woman desiring the surrogate. The consent of the surrogate's spouse is essential in all cases.
- A surrogate mother should not be over 45 years of age.
- No woman may act as a surrogate more than thrice in her lifetime.
- Sex selection at any stage after fertilization, or abortion of the fetus of any particular sex should not be permitted, except to avoid the risk of transmission of a genetic abnormality assessed through genetic testing of biological parents or through preimplantation genetic diagnosis (PGD).
- A surrogate mother carrying a child biologically unrelated to her must register as a patient in her own name. The birth certificate shall be in the name of the genetic parents.
- The surrogate mother must relinquish in writing all parental rights concerning the offspring and vice versa.

REPRODUCTIVE TOURISM

Regulations governing oocyte/sperm donation and surrogacy greatly vary from country to country. As a result, there exists a huge disparity in not only the spectrum of services, but the cost at which they are available to the infertile couple.

Due to these differences, we have witnessed the birth of fertility tourism, also known as reproductive tourism. This concept is defined as the process of traveling abroad to undergo a fertility treatment.

Singles and couples who opt for this option are usually forced to do so because of the restrictions they find in their own country, or because the process or part of it does not accommodate their needs.

DISCLOSURE TO CHILDREN

There exist many opinions regarding this issue, but the truth is that it depends on each family. Nonetheless, the ASRM considers that disclosure might be beneficial for the child for various reasons, including:

- Knowing your biological origins reinforces your autonomy.
- Understanding your identity improves your decision-making skills.
- Parents are able to build a relationship with the child based on openness and honesty.
- Knowing your genetic heritage allows you to deal more accurately with severe health problems.
- It helps protect the child against later inadvertent consanguinity.

On the other hand, those who are against disclosure argue that it would subject the child to a psychological turmoil, thereby affecting his long-term capacity of developing social skills. Nevertheless, researchers have found a greater interaction and skills between child and mothers who opted for third-party reproduction than naturally conceived. More studies in this respect are needed to draw conclusive evidence.

CONCLUSION

Third-party reproduction provides many couples an opportunity to make their dream of having a child a reality. The comprehensive nature of the screening and counseling for all parties is designed to meet the needs of all involved. As third-party reproduction continues to be widely used, care must be taken to adhere to and broaden our understanding of the ethical, moral, legal, and psychological aspects of practicing third-party reproduction.

EDITORS' COMMENTS

1. In any form of third party reproduction, counseling and documentation (in terms of proper informed consent form) play an immensely vital role.
2. The comprehensive nature of screening for all parties should be designed to meet the needs of all involved.
3. Using a gestational carrier is both emotionally and medically a complex process that requires careful evaluations by medical and legal professionals to ensure that the entire procedure is satisfactory and smooth for the intended parents as well as the carrier.
4. Protocols and laws of different countries relating to third-party reproduction are different and that should be strictly taken into account.

SUGGESTED READING

1. American Society for Reproductive Medicine. Guidelines for oocyte donation. Fertil Steril. 2002;77:S6-S8.
2. Deonandan R, Green S, van Bienum A. Ethical concerns for maternal surrogacy and reproductive tourism. J Med Ethics. 2012;38:742-5.
3. ESHRE task force on Ethics and the Law. Gamete and embryo donation. Hum Reprod. 2002;17:1407-8.
4. Practice Committee of the American Society for Reproductive Medicine and the Practice Committee for the Society of Assisted Reproductive Technology. Recommendations for gamete and embryo donation: a committee opinion. Fertil Steril. 2013;99:47-52.

28

CHAPTER

Laparoscopic-assisted Uterus Retrieval from Live Organ Donors for Uterine Transplant: The Next Step in Infertility and a Giant Leap in Surgery

Shailesh Puntambekar, Sambit Nanda

INTRODUCTION

By the time the article is published the first live baby from the first laparoscopic-assisted uterine transplant was delivered on 18th October 2018 indicating the ultimate success of the surgical procedure. However this article only deals with the surgical aspects and principles and thought process and protocol behind the uterine transplant and not with the antenatal period which followed later. The details of the antenatal and postnatal period is discussed in another article under the heading of high-risk obstetric care of uterine transplant pregnant women and not in this article which focuses on minimally invasive gynecology.

The year 2017 was signalized by a remarkable achievement in the field of "Minimally Invasive Gynecology", the unraveling of the mysterious and puzzling phenomenon of uterine transplant, which doubtless any practicing laparoscopic surgeon will ever forget. Advances in the field of infertility have evolved with a steady time and pace answering most challenges faced in clinical practice. However even after systematically addressing various factors of infertility and its challenges, the treatment of absolute uterine factor infertility (AUFI) has remained an enigma. The worldwide incidence of AUFI has been estimated to be predominant in 1 in 500 infertile women. The incidence in India can be higher considering the prevalence of genital tuberculosis and cervical malignancy in fertile age groups.

The successful live birth from human uterine transplant first occurred in 2014 which opened newer modalities of management of AUFI apart from the conventional surrogacy and adoption. Pregnancy remains the distinctive and singular objective of uterine transplant thus making the analogy that the uterus can be removed once desired parity has been achieved to prevent long-term adverse effects of immunosuppression. Minimally invasive techniques have been applied to various vital organ transplants, i.e. kidney and liver with successful outcomes. The first laparoscopic-assisted uterine transplant was conducted in May 2017 in Galaxy Care Hospital, Pune, India which has added another feather to the cap of laparoscopy. A team of doctors from China performed the world's first robotic-assisted uterine transplant surgery emphasizing on the benefits of minimally invasive methods of procurement of the uterus.

FORMULATION OF TEAM AND PATIENTS

The uterine transplant team at Galaxy Care Hospital was a crew of 12 members comprising of a laparoscopic surgeon, gynecologists, vascular surgeon, transplant surgeon, assisted reproductive technology specialist, a high risk obstetrician, a neonatologist, anesthesiologists, intensivists, a psychiatrist, a transplant counselor and a transplant coordinator. Screening and selection of candidates with infertility was done by strict adherence to the Montreal criteria guidelines. In order to reduce risks/complications and improve or maximize the outcome these candidates were further screened and reduced to two candidates with AUFI being selected for surgery (Table 1). The first AUFI candidate being an MRKH syndrome patient with nonfunctioning rudimentary uterine buds while the second candidate was a case secondary infertility with Grade 4 Asherman's syndrome. The individual candidates' kin (mother) would be the donor for the transplant surgery.

TABLE 1 Patients summary.

	Donor and Recipient history			
	Donor 1	*Donor 2*	*Recipient 1*	*Recipient 2*
Age, Year	5	2	21	26
Parity	4, all vaginal births	3, all vaginal births	–	Primipara with neonatal death, 2 missed abortions
Years married	–	–	3	8
Menstrual function	Normally menstruating	Normally menstruating	–	Amenorrhea for 2 years
Body mass index, kg/m^2	21.5	21	19.5	20
Blood group	O positive	B positive	B positive	AB positive
Pathology	–	–	Mayer-Rokitansky-Küster-Hauser syndrome, no associated renal abnormalities	Asherman's syndrome, grade IV
History	Not significant	Not significant		Disseminated intravascular coagulation and postpartum hemorrhage in first pregnancy; 2 dilatation and curettage, uterine perforation on check curettage, laparotomy done for the same
HLA crossmatch	–	–	4/6	3/6

PRESURGICAL PROCEDURES

On selection of the candidates for the transplant surgery, various presurgical procedures had to be undertaken as the part of the plan. The transplanted uterus may or may not behave in an identical physiological manner as a normal uterus. Interactions with immunosuppressive medications may hinder the action of fertility enhancing drugs which may be needed once transplant has been successful. However to circumvent this obstacle, prior to surgery *in vitro* fertilization (IVF) procedures were done to both candidates to extract secondary oocytes and create embryos for embryo transfer postsurgery. IVF for these candidates would help achieving higher chances of successful pregnancies as seen even in normal uteruses. *In vitro* fertilization for recipients was done 4 weeks before the uterine transplant surgery according to the recommendations of the transplant committee (Box 1).

Oocyte retrieval was done using the antagonist protocol followed by IVF which yielded four embryos from the first recipient (candidate) and eight embryos from the second recipient (candidate). All embryos were frozen till they reached day 3 of life. The recovery of the ovaries was noted on USG after 2 weeks.

BOX 1 Patient workup.

Preoperative investigations for donors and recipients

- *Complete blood count*: Hemoglobin, polymorphonuclear leukocytes, total white blood cell count, platelets
- Blood group
- HLA crossmatch
- Karyotyping
- *Kidney function*: Creatinine, blood urea nitrogen
- *Liver function*: SGPT, SGOT, alkaline phosphatase, bilirubin, total proteins, albumin
- *Electrolytes*: T3, T4, thyroid-stimulating hormone
- Thyroid profile
- *Blood sugar*: Fasting and postprandial, HbA1C
- Lipid profile
- Homocysteine
- HIV/HBsAg/hepatitis C virus
- Epstein-Barr virus
- Toxoplasma
- Rubella
- Syphilis
- Herpes
- Cardiolipin antibodies
- TPO antibodies
- Protein C and S
- Urine routine
- Vaginal swab for culture
- Pap smear
- Electrocardiography
- *Imaging studies*: Ultrasound pelvis, color Doppler, magnetic resonance imaging of the pelvis, chest X-ray, 2D-ECHO, carotid Doppler

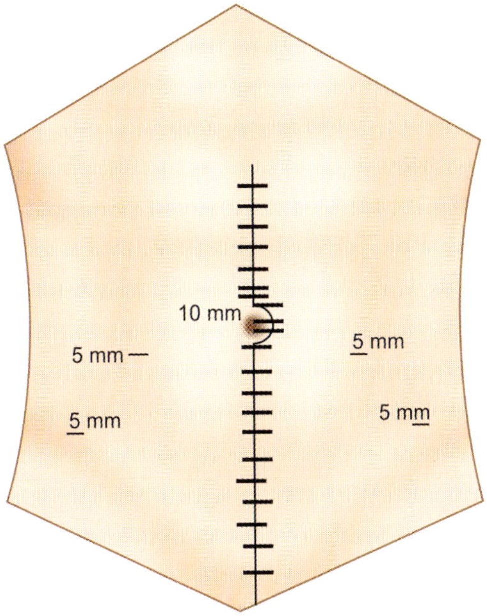

Fig. 1: *Port positions and incisions*: This image shows the port positions during the laparoscopy-assisted dissection of the donor uterus. The Midline incision was taken later during the retrieval of the donor uterus to proceed for bench surgery. The same port positions and incision has been replicated the recipient as well. The port position for the laparoscopic preparation of uterine bed (Neovagina) for the donor uterus and the midline incision for the anastomosis of vessels.

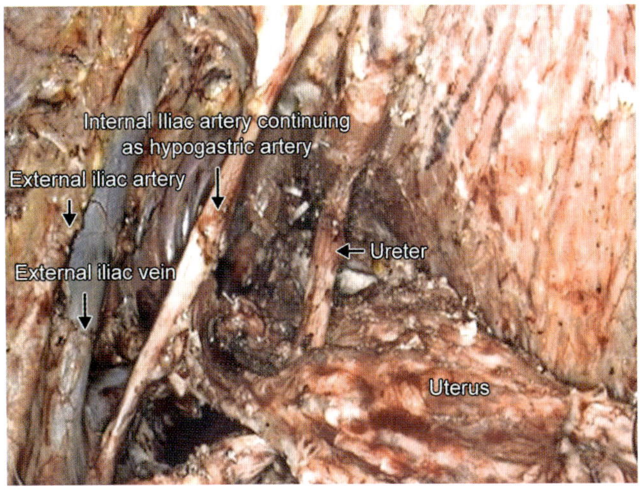

Fig. 2: *Vessels and structures during dissection*: This image displays the degree of dissection done on the donor uterus prior to retrieval. The external as well as the internal iliac arteries have been completely denuded. The internal iliac artery can be seen giving of the uterine artery branch and continuing further as the obliterated hypogastric artery. The ureter can be seen clearly under the uterine artery. The uterine even can be seen under the ureter and running parallel to the uterine artery.

Uterine Transplant Surgery

The uterine transplant surgery was orchestrated by the donor and the recipient surgery being conducted simultaneously in separate operating rooms. Both recipients were provided with intravenous antibiotic and antifungal coverage. Plasmapheresis and antithymocyte globulin (2.5 mg/kg) was given 12 hours prior to surgery to prevent any foreseeable immunologically mediated reactions posttransplant.

Donor Surgery

The patient position and the port placement were done in a standardized manner. The patient as placed in modified lithotomy position under general anesthesia. Pneumoperitoneum was created with a Verres needle through the palmer's point. Ports placement was as shown in Figure 1.

The surgery begins with the left infundibulopelvic ligament skeletonized up to the pelvic brim. The ovarian artery and vein were dissected up to their entry into infundibulopelvic ligament. This is followed by retroperitoneal dissection. The left pararectal and paravesical spaces dissected up to levator ani muscle. The pouch of Douglas was dissected. The rectovaginal space was dissected up to levator ani muscle. The key step in this surgery is ureteric dissection.

The left ureter was completely lateralized and separated from all surrounding structures. Thus, completely denuding the ureter in the pelvis. The ureter was separated from the level of uterine artery crossing-over up to its insertion into bladder. This is followed by skeletonization of the anterior branch of the internal iliac artery and the uterine artery. This dissection is followed up to the obliterated hypogastric artery. Arborization of both the uterine artery and the vein is seen around the ureter. These minor vessels were carefully ligated or clipped and separated. Internal iliac artery distal to origin of uterine artery was ligated. The lateral branches were ligated and clipped. This is followed by sequential clipping and separation of venous structures around the uterus. The internal iliac vein was dissected from the origin to the insertion of uterine veins followed by the lateral ilioinguinal and obturator vein followed by the vaginal veins and pudendal veins. The entire vein distal to the insertion of uterine vein was ligated. A good pedicle length of uterine vein is thus obtained. External iliac artery and vein were skeletonization followed by ilio-obturator lymphadenectomy was done for better visualization of internal iliac vessels. Mirroring of steps repeated on right side (Fig. 2).

A uterosacral cuff is created and dissected by resecting the uterosacrals approximately 2–2.5 cm away from the attachment to uterus to facilitate their plication to the uterosacral of recipients. Rectovaginal space dissection is done to separate the rectum completely from the entire posterior vaginal wall. Thus the supports to the uterus have been released from its attachment to the pelvic wall, and a colpotomy has to be done before clamping the vessels which increases the chance of hemorrhage as the vascular supply is intact. In the process of controlling hemorrhage there is a chance of damage to rectum during posterior colpotomy. However, no complication or morbidity was seen in the patients postoperatively due to rectal dissection. Levator ani with covering endopelvic fascia was visualized on both sides of the rectum. The Mackenrodt's/cardinal ligament was not dissected because the vessels travel through this ligament. Anterior colpotomy was done by separating the vagina anteriorly from posterior surface of bladder to get approximately 1.5 cm of vagina and posteriorly from rectum. The entire uterus was suspended on the bilateral infundibulopelvic ligament with ovarian vessels and bilateral parametrium consisting of uterine arteriovenous complex.

At this stage, the uterus is ready to be retrieved from the donor. The retrieval is facilitated by steady sequential clamping of the vascular structures and swift retrieval and deliver to the transplant surgeons waiting to check organ and its vascularity at bench surgery. Vascular clamps were applied bilaterally on internal iliac artery, uterine vein and ovarian artery and vein only after performing a 7 cm abdominal incision, thus keeping warm ischemia time less than 5 minutes. Bilateral oophorectomy was performed for both donors. Retrieval of the uterus was done through abdominal incision to prevent infection or trauma to the harvested vessels that could happen if removal by vaginal route. Prior to clamping of uterine artery and internal iliac artery, 5,000 µg unfractionated heparin intramuscular (IM) was given uterine veins were clamped at the point of entry into internal iliac vein. The uterus retrieved from donor with vascular supply and transported on a tray of ice slush for bench surgery and handed over to vascular and transplant surgeons. The vaginal vault sutured with Vicryl (polyglactin 910) 2-0 with continuous interlocking sutures. Bilateral DJ stenting done under cystoscopic guidance because of devascularization of ureters. The abdomen closed in layers with a drain kept *in situ*. Intraoperative blood loss in both donor patients was 100 mL which is added advantage of minimal invasive surgery. Dissection of donor has been completed.

Bench Surgery

The main aim of this surgery is to check the vascular integrity of the uterus at a microscopic level. The transplant surgeon with the help of operating loupes magnification and operation theater lights would examine the artery and vein and flush custodial solution through the artery and look for the outflow through the vein to denote intact vascularity without any thrombosed vessels inside the uterus. Secondly, it is of paramount importance to rule out and close all leaks from both the artery and vein so as to prevent bleeding during reanastomosis (Table 2). Bleeding during reanastomosis becomes a crisis where blood tends to flood the operative field and any amount of cauterization to achieve hemostasis would be at the cost of hampering the blood supply to the donor uterus. Thus the structural integrity is checked at the bench surgery.

The harvested uterus is received on a sterile trolley in tray full of ice slush to maintain a hypothermic environment while the bench surgery is being commenced in a separate operation room. Bilaterally internal iliac and ovarian vessels were identified, dissected, skeletonized, terminal openings prepared kept ready for anastomosis. Nearly 1,000 mL custodial solution was infused through bilateral uterine and ovarian pedicles. In first case ovarian pedicles had significantly small bilateral ovarian veins and in second case pedicles had only veins and right ovarian artery which was in confluence of 4–5 small pedicles.

Throughout the procedure the uterus was kept surrounded by custodial solution and ice slush and custodial solution was infused through the organ until returning fluid clear of blood. After checking and ruling out all anastomotic leaks the bench surgery is completed and the harvested uterus is now shifted to the recipient operating theater.

TABLE 2 Bench surgery details.

Bench surgery		*Findings at the end of bench surgery*				
		B/L uterine artery with anterior division of internal iliac artery (cm)	*B/L uterine vein (cm)*	*B/L ovarian artery (cm)*	*B/L ovarian vein (cm)*	*Bench surgery time (min)*
Recipient 1	Pedicle length	8.5	9	11	11	45
Recipient 2	Pedicle length	9	10	4	11	34

(B/L: bilateral)

Recipient Surgery

Simultaneously the recipient surgery was started prior to retrieval of the uterus. By the time the uterus is retrieved, the bed for the transplanted uterus has been created laparoscopically and ready to open the abdomen to facilitate transplant and restore the vascularity as soon as possible. The vascular dissection should not be initiated till the recipient bed has been made ready in the separate operating room in a fine-tuned synchronized and coordinated manner. Standard laparoscopic port placement as mentioned above was done under epidural and general anesthesia.

Recipient 1: The retroperitoneal dissection is done by an incision over the peritoneum is starting from the sacral promontory towards the common iliac vessels, along the external iliac vessels till the peritoneum covering the round ligament. An anterior peritoneal incision was taken over the uterovesical fold and coronally over the band connecting two buds. The retroperitoneum was accessed and external iliac vessels were exposed and fibrofatty tissues cleared for anastomosis. The right ureter exposed along its entire pelvic length from pelvic brim to the right ureteric tunnel. Similar steps repeated on left side.

An impression of the neovagina is made over the pelvic peritoneum by inserting a probe vaginally. A transverse incision was made over the vaginal protrusion. Bladder and rectum dissected and pushed off the vaginal impression. An adequate margin for potential vaginal suturing was created by carefully pushing off the bladder and the rectum. The incision was opened and extended transversely after identifying and protecting the ureter on either side. The ventral band was incised and surrounding tissue was dissected up to bladder in front and rectum behind. Stay suture was taken over the round ligament and vagina. A prolene suspension stitch was taken over anterior longitudinal ligament over sacral promontory for uterosacral anchorage. Once the bed was made and cleared, abdomen opened in layers with a vertical midline incision. The bench prepared uterus was transported to the recipient's operating room on an ice slush tray on sterile trolley. The donor uterus was put in the pelvic cavity with normal anatomic orientation; bilateral uterine and ovarian vessels were oriented for anastomosis. Bilateral internal iliac and ovarian vessels were anastomosed to the external iliac vessel using a 7-0 prolene suture in a continuous fashion under operating loupes.

Intravenous methylprednisolone 500 mg was given just before uterine reperfusion. Once vascular anastomosis was complete and functional vaginal sutures were tied to the donor vaginal reciprocal sites. An anchoring prolene stitch was taken from the uterosacral ligaments of donor to the promontory. Round ligaments were tied to their respective counterparts. All anastomosis sites were checked for potency and flow of blood across anastomosis. All were working satisfactorily with balanced flow. Bleeding from the sutured vaginal margins was tackled by taking hemostatic sutures. Blood loss was approximately 1 L, which was due to the revascularization of transplanted uterus. The patient was transfused intraoperatively with 4 pints of blood (Fig. 3).

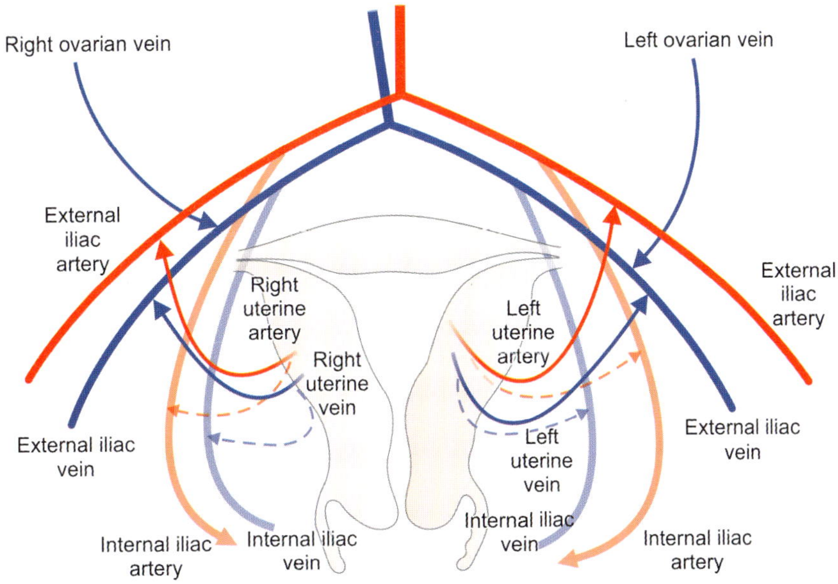

Fig. 3: *Re-anastomosis of vessels*: This is a schematic diagram of the re-anastomosis of the vessels as planned for this uterine transplant. The uterine artery dissected at the origin is anastomosed to the external iliac artery. While the uterine vein dissect is anastomosed to the external iliac vein.

Recipient 2: A 5 mm Visiport was inserted through the Palmer's point. The remaining port positions were as mentioned above. Total laparoscopic hysterectomy was performed with routine steps except for the following modifications. The round ligaments were tied close to the uterus and kept long. Ovarian pedicles were tied, developed and taken cephalad. They were anchored to the peritoneum in lateral gutters above the pelvic brim on both sides. Uterosacral ligaments were cut close to the uterus to maintain adequate length for joining the transplanted uterus. Fallopian tubes on both sides were excised. Stay sutures were placed on the uterosacral and Mackenrodt's ligaments. Ureters were dissected and lateralized to keep them out of anastomotic area. The vascular bed was prepared for anastomosis and abdomen opened with vertical midline incision. The rest of the procedure of uterine anastomosis were similar to that described above.

The possible reason for blood loss from the sutured vaginal margin in the recipient was discussed after the first case. We concluded that the small veins in cervicovesical fascia were responsible for the bleed from sutured vaginal margins after the revascularization of the uterus. To prevent this, we sutured the cervicovesical fascia and Denonvilliers' fascia to the donor vaginal edges with 4-0 Vicryl continuous sutures before vessel clamping, which cause these veins to retract into the fascia. An anchoring cervical prolene stitch was performed from the uterosacral ligament of the donor to the promontory. Round ligaments were tied to their retrospective counterparts. All anastomosis sites were checked for potency and flow of blood. Balanced perfusion was noted in the uterus with no leak at any anastomotic site. The intraoperative blood loss was 300 mL and the patient did not require any intraoperative blood transfusion. Thus the uterine transplant surgery was completed.

POSTOPERATIVE PROCEDURES

Both donors and recipients were transferred to isolation intensive care unit (ICU) for better monitoring and later shifted to a ward. The recipients were kept for 1 week while the donors were shifted after 24 hours. Barrier nursing was provided and aseptic precautions were taken. Antithrombotic prophylaxis was given to the donors for 48 hours while the recipient received it for a longer duration owing to their exposure to immunosuppressive medication.

Donors

The postoperative course of the donors remained uneventful without any additional care provided as compared to routine hysterectomy. The donors were shifted out of the ICU after 24 hours. Urinary catheters removed on postoperative day 3. Their hospital stay was uneventful discharged after 1 week. Double J stents were removed after 6 weeks. Bilateral oophorectomy was done for both donors to prevent postoperative avascular necrosis *in situ* after ovarian vessel dissection and harvest. The donors were started on hormone replacement therapy by our endocrinologist.

Recipients

Tacrolimus was the primary or the cornerstone immunosuppression started orally postoperatively as soon as bowel peristalsis was regained. Prednisolone 20 mg/day, mycophenolate mofetil 720 mg twice a day, and valganciclovir were also added as an adjunct as well as to prevent any opportunistic infections. Serial monitoring of tacrolimus levels along with other vital parameters were done every day until discharge.

Visual inspection of cervix and the vaginal suture on postoperative Day 3 demonstrated a healthy and pink cervix. Hysteroscopy-guided cervical biopsy (vaginoscopy without distension media) was taken on postoperative day 4 and sent for histopathology and immunohistochemistry examination. Office hysteroscopy was done using a 1.9-mm, 30°, and forward oblique Bettocchi hysteroscope. No local or regional anesthesia was used. No distension media was used. No signs of rejection were seen in either recipient. Surveillance with hysteroscopy-guided cervical biopsies was taken on days 7, 14, and 21.

For the first recipient, patient with Mayer-Rokitansky-Küster-Hauser syndrome, the hysteroscopic cervical biopsy done on postoperative day 7 showed slough on the cervix, and the histopathology showed increased leukocytosis. She was given a stepped-up dose of steroids and higher antibiotics. A repeat hysteroscopic cervical biopsy showed reversal of phenomenon, a healthy cervix and no signs of rejection on histopathology. The dose of the steroids was tapered accordingly. Ultrasound scans and color Doppler for uterine artery flow were done every day for a week. Subsequently, the scans were done on alternate days until discharge. All scans showed a good flow in both uterine arteries. After a steady serum tacrolimus levels, with no clinical signs or symptoms of rejection, subsequent cervical biopsies suggestive of healthy cervix and uneventful postoperative period for more than 72 hours, the recipients were discharged after 1 month stay in the hospital. Follow-up was maintained every 3 weeks after discharge. The follow-ups included inspection of the cervix, hysteroscopy-guided cervical biopsy, measuring of tacrolimus levels, and color Doppler for uterine artery flow (Fig. 4).

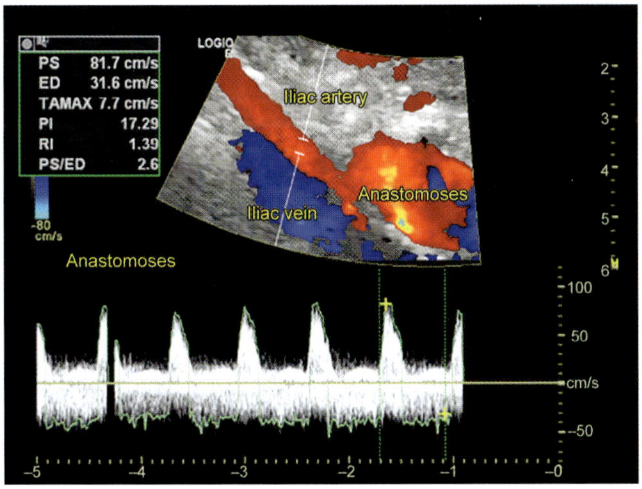

Fig. 4: Doppler image of iliac vessels and anastomoses.

Both recipients remained healthy even after discharge without medical supervision. There were no signs of rejection or any kind of complications in the recipients. The first recipient attained her menarche after 34 days with scanty flow that lasted for 3 days. The second recipient had her first menstruation after 48 days in similar manner. She had her second menses after an interval of 30 days that lasted for 4 days with average flow (3–4 pads per day). Both patients have attained their sixth menstrual cycle after operation at the time of writing this report. Office hysteroscopy with normal saline solution as the distention medium was done for both the recipients as a method of assessment of graft rejection after 3 months post-transplant. In the first recipient minimal slough was seen on the endometrium, which was removed by hysteroscopy-guided endometrial and cervical biopsies were also taken. The histopathology showed mild signs of rejection in the form of increased leukocytosis. Antibiotics coverage and increased doses of steroid cover was given. A repeat hysteroscopy after 10 days showed a healthy endometrium and no signs of rejection on histopathology. Intraopterative and postoperative parameters are summarized in Table 3.

DISCUSSION

Organ procurement remains the cornerstone of any transplant surgery. The entire surgery narrows down to how delicately and easily with minimal handling can the organ be retrieved. Hence, the surgical procedure to the living donor has to be safe, the least disruptive to minimize surgical risks and morbidity, and at the same time allow for minimal tissue handling, proving better quality of the harvested organ. This has given way to the introduction of minimal invasive techniques for organ procurement. Laparoscopic kidney and liver live donor retrieval for transplant have been established and become standardized worldwide. Decreased morbidity associated with laparoscopic procurement of these vital organs has even led to an increase in live organ donation. To our knowledge this is the first ever report of laparoscopic-assisted uterus retrieval for uterus transplant. Laparoscopic retrieval offers all the benefits of minimal invasive surgery. It shortens the operative time, thereby minimizing surgery related complications. Our retrieval time for the donor surgeries was significantly less than the previously reported time (Table 3). Uterus retrieval is more complex compared to other vital organ retrieval and need surgeons with superior surgical skills and a high level of preparation. The dissection of uterine and ovarian vessels to adequate lengths is essential so as to anastomose without tension to the external iliac vessels. This is achievable only if a minimum length of 8 cm needed. Compared with the renal vessels the caliber of uterine vessels is 7 mm and those of ovarian vessels are of <5 mm. Thus, to achieve length as well as larger diameter the internal iliac artery and veins have to be dissected and removed from the origin at the bifurcation. Thus, surgeons with higher dexterity are warranted. We dissected the entire length of anterior division of the internal iliac artery and vein from the bifurcation downward. All the branches and tributaries distal to the origin of the uterine artery and insertion of the uterine vein were clipped and ligated laparoscopically. Three-dimensional endoscopy system was used for enhanced and excellent visualization and minimal handling of vessels and good magnification especially helpful during the vascular dissection phase of the entire uterus retrieval. All the small branches were dissected and coagulated using the Harmonic Ace scalpel (Johnson and Johnson). The bench surgery time (cold ischemia) for first patient was 45 minutes and for the second patient 34 minutes.

Laparoscopic kidney retrieval from live donors has been proven to be feasible and less morbid. This has encouraged live donation rates. Similarly, we anticipate a rising trends in live donation of organs once the procedure becomes standardized. Laparoscopic retrieval for uterus transplant offers all the benefits of minimally invasive surgery. Our case being the index case worldwide needs larger series studies to compare it with open surgery like every other surgery has to undergo a comparison when the minimally invasive leap is taken. This however may not be feasible to carry out in our institution, because this is a complex surgery and will require more cases to prove that laparoscopy decreases morbidity in comparison with laparotomy. A magnified

TABLE 3 Operative summary.

	Intraoperative and postoperative summary														
	Intraoperative						*Postoperative*								
	Operative time (hr)	*Bench time (cold ischemia) (min)*	*First warm ischemia (min)*	*Second warm ischemia (min)*	*Blood loss (mL)*	*Blood transfusion*	*Isolation ICU stay (days)*	*Per oral feeds*	*Ward stay (days)*	*Tacrolimus levels*	*Cervical biopsy*	*Postdischarge cervical biopsy*	*Blood reports*	*Uterine artery Doppler*	*Menstruation attained*
Donor 1	4	45	>5		~100	–	1	Second day	7	–	–		Everyday third day	–	–
Recipient 1	4		–	30	1000	4 pints	7	Second day	14	Every third day	Postoperative days 4, 7, 14, 21	3 weekly	Everyday	Everyday day for 1 week Alternate day until discharge On every follow-up	After 34 days
Donor 2	4	34	>5		~100	–	1	Second day	7	–	–		Everyday third day		–
Recipient 2	4		–	30	300	–	7	Second day	14	Every third day	Postoperative days 4, 7, 14, 21	3 weekly	Everyday	Everyday for 1 week Alternate day until discharge On every follow-up	After 48 days

visualization of the vessels, a better dissection, a shorter operative time (4 hours compared with 14 hours in the Swedish cases) and early bowel recovery are some of the benefits offered. The retrieval incision was performed last to avoid packing of bowels. Even in general surgery many procedures like radical nephrectomy and low anterior resection and Whipple's procedure are laparoscopy assisted and never fully laparoscopic. We feared that vaginal retrieval would lead to infection of the vessels, especially fungal.

Our vast experience of laparoscopic radical hysterectomy has helped us understand pelvic anatomy better and enabled better dissection for vessel harvest. This has also been instrumental in helping us standardize our procedure, the Pune technique, which has led to good reproducibility of the procedure and better outcomes. Similarly, standardization of the technique of laparoscopic retrieval of donor uterus will give it the potential of reproducibility and widespread acceptance. It will also help the progression of uterus transplant from a novel procedure to a mainstream treatment offered to patients with AUFI. From the experience of previously reported human uterus transplants the main cause of failure has been attributed to thromboembolism. The surgical technique of vessel retrieval is directly related to the risk of thromboembolism. Our belief is that, organ and vessel handling during harvesting can lead to microcirculatory disturbances after reperfusion, leading to thromboembolism. Laparoscopy helps to minimize vessel handling, thereby decreasing intimal damage and thus can prevent thromboembolism. Venous drainage is another aspect related to uterine thromboembolism. During our preparation period in trial cases of uterus harvesting from donor (during bench surgery) we used methylene blue mapping of the ovarian vessels. Dye pushed form one ovarian vessel was seen to circulate and drain into the contralateral ovarian vessel. Thus, in addition to the uterine venous anastomosis, the anastomosis of the ovarian vein will help to decrease uterine congestion and improve the venous drainage. The main challenge of venous anastomosis is the small caliber of vessels. A good vascular surgeon with experience in coronary bypass can easily overcome this difficulty, as was seen in our cases. In our first case, the recipient had bleeding from the sutured vaginal edges after the reperfusion of the uterus. In our second patient, we sutured the recipient's cervicovesical fascia and Denonvilliers' fascia to the donor's vagina, which prevented bleeding from the vaginal anastomosis site. This we believe is the most important step. Most of the literature also raises concern over the elasticity and the pliability of the anastomosed vessels during pregnancy. The space required for the uterus to expand in pregnancy is less. Taking the ovarian anastomosis higher provides adequate space for the uterus to expand cranially, minimizing any strain to the vascular anastomosis. We did a hysteroscopy for both recipients as a method of surveillance for graft rejection.

Routine cervical biopsy requires traction on the anterior lip of cervix with a Vulsellum, which could disrupt our suture line on the transplanted uterus. Thus we used hysteroscopic guidance to cause under vision and minimally handling of the transplanted uterus. With office hysteroscopy all possible angles and sides of the cervix can be visualized and biopsy taken under direct vision distention medium was used in view of aseptic precautions to prevent retrograde transmission of vaginal flora into the uterus. We did not encounter any cervical stenosis. We believe that office hysteroscopy along with cervical biopsy gives better chances of finding the earliest sign of graft rejection and is a far superior method for surveillance of graft rejection. Although invasive, no complication was noted that could be attributed to hysteroscopy. Anatomical variability of the internal iliac veins makes the dissection of the internal iliac vein more extensive and thus the procedure morbid. In the future, if the surgery can duplicated/reproducible with only uterine arteries and ovarian veins, it will eliminate the need for the extensive dissection of the internal iliac veins, thus making this procedure safe. We believe that only the utero-ovarian vessels are enough for good vascularization of the entire uterus.

In conclusion, minimally invasive techniques for uterus retrieval are the future of uterus transplant. With many teams taking up uterine transplant trials, in the near future uterus transplant may become a mainstay procedure offered to women with AUFI. Live birth rather than successful surgery will be the real proof needed to show that minimally invasive surgical techniques can be successful for uterine transplant.

The first successful live birth of the uterine transplant baby was done on 18th October 2018 at Galaxy Care laparoscopy Hospital Pune. And the rest is history.

EDITORS' COMMENTS

1. In spite of selected successful cases around the world uterine transplant has gained good popularity in ART.
2. Continued advances in transplantation techniques, improved methods for immunosuppression, and advances in IVF technology can put an end to absolute uterine factor infertility (AUFI).
3. A multidisciplinary team comprising of gynecologists, ART clinicians, vascular surgeons, immunologists, etc.

with profound knowledge of surgical guidelines and postoperative anticipated complications, and advanced operative setup are needed for this major surgical procedure.

4. After the first ambitious case of uterine transplant by the author in 2018, the bar of expectations has been truly raised. The first resultant live birth after uterine transplant will create a new ray of hope for couples with AUFI.
5. Religious acceptance, medicolegal framework, post of safety, and cost of procedure are few concerns that might come in the way of making this option for wider masses of patients.

SUGGESTED READING

1. Brännström M, Bokström H, Dahm-Kähler P. One uterus bridging three generations: first live birth after mother-to-daughter uterus transplantation. Fertil Steril. 2016;106:261-6.
2. Brännström M, Johannesson L, Bokström H, et al. Livebirth after uterus transplantation. Lancet. 2015;385:607-16.
3. Brännström M. Uterus transplantation and beyond. J Mater Sci Mater Med. 2017;28:70.
4. Brosens I, Ghaem-Maghami S, Pijnenborg R. Uterus transplantation in the human: a complex surgical, medical and ethical challenge. Hum Reprod. 2013;28:292-3.
5. Cauchy F, Schwarz L, Scatton O, et al. Laparoscopic liver resection for living donation: where do we stand? World J Gastroenterol. 2014;20:15590-8.
6. Erman Akar M, Ozkan O, Aydinuraz B, et al. Clinical pregnancy after uterus transplantation. Fertil Steril. 2013;100:1358-63.
7. Fageeh W, Raffa H, Jabbad H, et al. Transplantation of the human uterus. Int J Gynaecol Obstet. 2002;76:245-51.
8. Grace GA, Devaleenal DB, Natrajan M. Genital tuberculosis in females. Indian J Med Res. 2017;145:425-36.
9. Johannesson L, Järvholm S. Uterus transplantation: current progress and future prospects. Int J Womens Health. 2016; 8:43-51.
10. Jones BP, Saso S, Yazbek J, et al. Uterine transplantation: past, present and future. BJOG. 2016;123:1434-8.
11. Lefkowitz A, Edwards M, Balayla J. Ethical considerations in the era of the uterine transplant: an update of the Montreal Criteria for the Ethical Feasibility of Uterine Transplantation. Fertil Steril. 2013;100:924-6.
12. Milliez J. Uterine transplantation FIGO Committee for the Ethical Aspects of Human Reproduction and Women's Health. Int J Gynaecol Obstet. 2009;106:270.
13. Ozkan O, Akar ME, Ozkan O, et al. Preliminary results of the first human uterus transplantation from a multiorgan donor. Fertil Steril. 2013;99:470-6.
14. Puntambekar S, Telang M, Kulkarni P, et al. Laparoscopic-Assisted Uterus Retrieval From Live Organ Donors for Uterine Transplant: Our Experience of Two Patients. J Minim Invasive Gynecol. 2018;25:622-31.
15. Puntambekar SP, Palep RJ, Puntambekar SS, et al. Laparoscopic total radical hysterectomy by the Pune technique: our experience of 248 cases. J Minim Invasive Gynecol. 2007;14:682-9.
16. Rampersad C, Patel P, Koulack J, et al. Back-to-back comparison of mini-open vs. laparoscopic technique for living kidney donation. Can Urol Assoc J. 2016;10:253-7.
17. Ratner LE, Ciseck LJ, Moore RG, et al. Laparoscopic live donor nephrectomy. Transplantation. 1995;60:1047-109.
18. Sreedevi A, Javed R, Dinesh A. Epidemiology of cervical cancer with special focus on India. Int J Womens Health. 2015;7:405-14.
19. Testa G, Koon EC, Johannesson L, et al. Living donor uterus transplantation: a single center's observations and lessons learned from early setbacks to technical success. Am J Transplant. 2017;17:2901-10.
20. Wei L, Xue T, Tao KS, et al. Modified human uterus transplantation using ovarian veins for venous drainage: the first report of surgically successful robotic-assisted uterus procurement and follow-up for 12 months. Fertil Steril. 2017;108:346-56.

29

CHAPTER

Regenerative Medicine in Infertility

Nayana H Patel, Molina Patel

INTRODUCTION

Regenerative medicine is considered a novel frontier of medical research as it holds the promise of engineering damaged tissues and organs by stimulating the body's own repair mechanisms to functionally heal previously irreparable tissues or organs. The term "regenerative medicine" in generally applied to the multidisciplinary approach to disease management, encompassing tissue and organ culture, bioengineering, and the use of natural and engineered tissues to repair or regenerate human tissues or to enhance function of existing tissues or organs. The term "regenerative medicine" was first used in 1992 by Leland Kaiser, who in an article on hospital administration stated that, "A new branch of medicine will develop that attempts to change the course of chronic disease and in many instances will regenerate tired and failing organ systems".

When nearly 72.4 million people or one in six couples experience fertility problems due to one or multiple reasons, some of which are still incurable even after advancements in assisted reproduction treatment, regenerative medicine is considered to be as new dawn for treatment of male and female infertility.

Over the past two decades, scientists have advanced the field of reproductive tissue engineering to restore normal sexual function and preserve fertility in both female and male patients. Stem cells and platelet-rich plasma (PRP) are being widely used as a tool of regeneration for improving human health by restoring the function of cells and tissues that are damaged due to degeneration and/or injury and treating patients with severe reproductive system disorders, such as congenital abnormalities, cancer, trauma, infection, inflammation, and iatrogenic injuries.

Results of many studies indicate that stem cells and PRP have potential to restore fertility by effective treatment of ovarian rejuvenation, increasing endometrial thickness, improving development of embryo *in vitro*, helping in implantation of embryo in patient with recurrent implantation failure (RIF), increasing the motility of sperm, reversing the damage to the testis, etc. and has potential to generate functional gametes. The goal of stem cell therapies is to promote cell replacement in organs that are damaged beyond their ability to self-repair.

PLATELET-RICH PLASMA

Platelet-rich plasma therapy has accumulated considerable attention over the last two decades, mainly due to its potential ability in regenerative medicine, including oral and maxillofacial surgery, and sports and veterinary medicine. Platelets as main components of the PRP, contain more than 1,100 different proteins, with numerous post-translational modifications, resulting in over 1,500 protein-based bioactive factors. These factors include immune system messengers, growth factors, enzymes and their inhibitors, and other factors which can participate in tissue repair and wound healing (Figs. 1 and 2).

Platelet-rich plasma has a greater concentration of growth factors than whole blood. PRP contains vascular endothelial growth factor (VEGF), transforming growth factor (TGF), platelet-derived growth factor (PDGF), and epidermal growth factor (EGF). These factors aid in migration, attachment, proliferation, and differentiation of cells and promote accumulation of extracellular matrix (Table 1). Recently, PRP has been applied in various clinical scenarios, such as orthopedics, ophthalmology, and wound

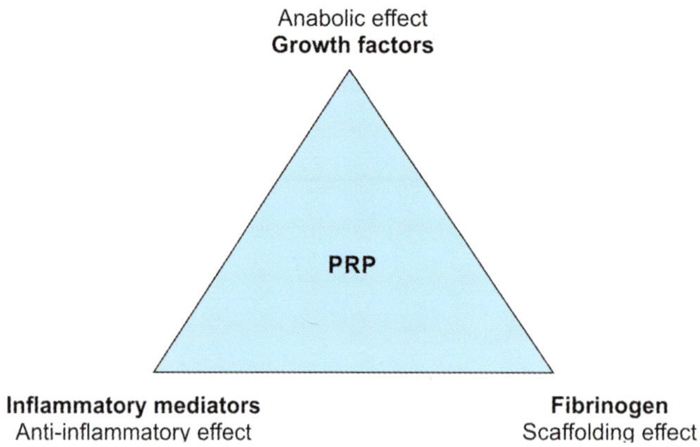

Fig. 1: Constitution of platelet-rich plasma (PRP).

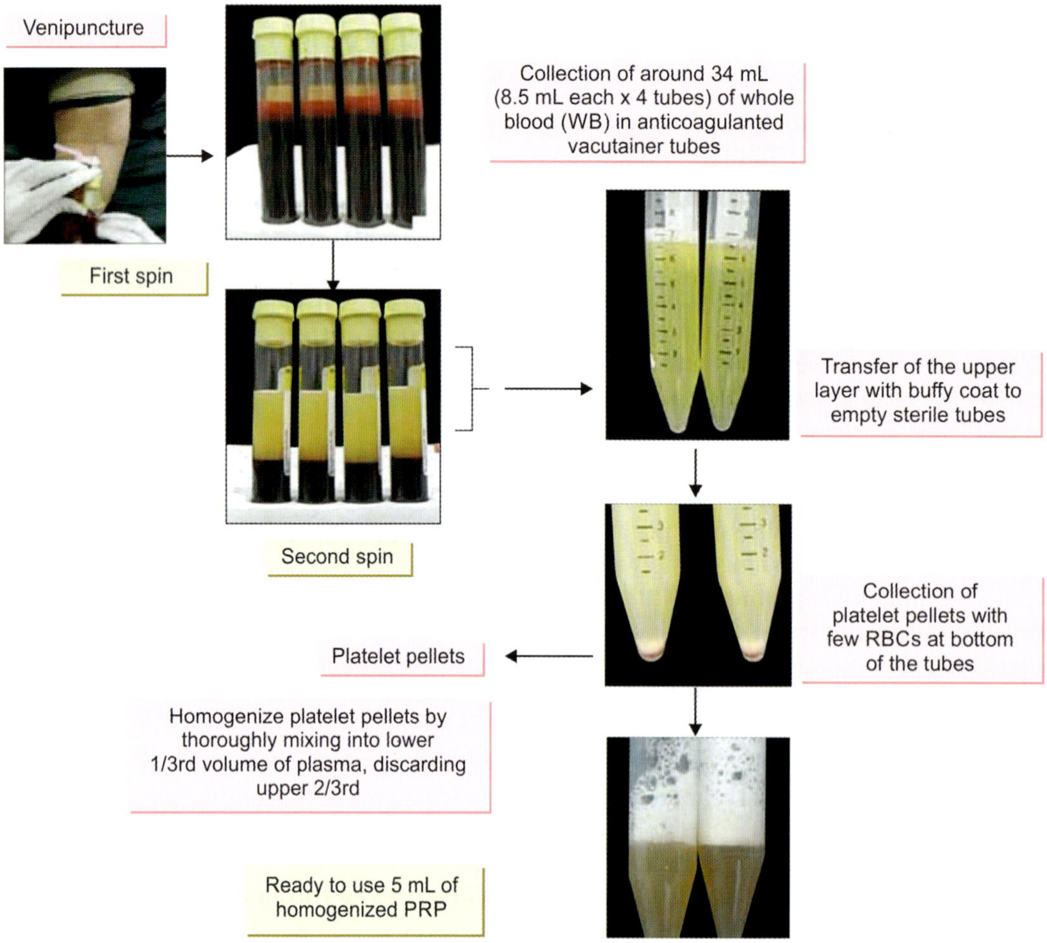

Fig. 2: Platelet-rich plasma (PRP) preparation.
(RBC: red blood cell)

TABLE 1 Growth factors in platelet rich plasma and their biological functions.

Name	*Abbreviation*	*Function*
Platelet-derived growth factor	PDGF	Enhances collagen synthesis, proliferation of bone cells, fibroblast chemotaxis and proliferative activity, macrophage activation
Transforming growth factor β	TGF-β	Enhances synthesis of type 1 collagen, promotes angiogenesis, stimulates chemotaxis of immune cells, inhibits osteoclast formation and bone resorption
Vascular endothelial growth factor	VEGF	Stimulates angiogenesis, migration and mitosis of endothelial cells, increases permeability of the vessels, stimulates chemotaxis of macrophages and neutrophils
Epidermal growth factor	EGF	Stimulates cellular proliferation, differentiation of epithelial cells, promotes cytokine secretion by mesenchymal and epithelial cells
Insulin-like growth factor	IGF	Promotes cell growth, differentiation, recruitment in bone, blood vessel, skin and other tissues, stimulates collagen synthesis together with PDGF
Fibroblast growth factor	FGF	Promotes proliferation of mesenchymal cells, chondrocytes and osteoblasts, stimulates the growth and differentiation of chondrocytes and osteoblasts

healing to improve the tissue regeneration. Also, usefulness of PRP in treatment of infertility is being accessed.

STEM CELLS

In recent years, stem cell research has emerged as an important area of biomedical science. It has potential applications in varied areas of biomedicine including developmental biology, disease modeling, tissue engineering, drug development, and toxicity testing. Stem cells are undifferentiated cells that are present in the embryonic, fetal, and adult stages of life and give rise to differentiated cells that are building blocks of tissue and organs. In the postnatal and adult stages of life, tissue-specific stem cells are found in differentiated organs and are instrumental in repair following injury to the organ. Due to their unlimited source and high differentiation potential, stem cells are considered as potentially new therapeutic agents for the treatment of infertility.

The major characteristics of stem cells are:

- Self-renewal (the ability to extensively proliferate)
- Clonality (usually arising from a single cell)
- Potency (the ability to differentiate into different cell types).

Totipotent or Omnipotent Cells

Cells which can differentiate into cells of any lineage including extraembryonic tissue are termed as totipotent cells such as zygote.

Pluripotent Stem Cells

Cells which are able to differentiate into any cell type but not into embryonic tissue.

Flowchart 1: Classification of stem cells.

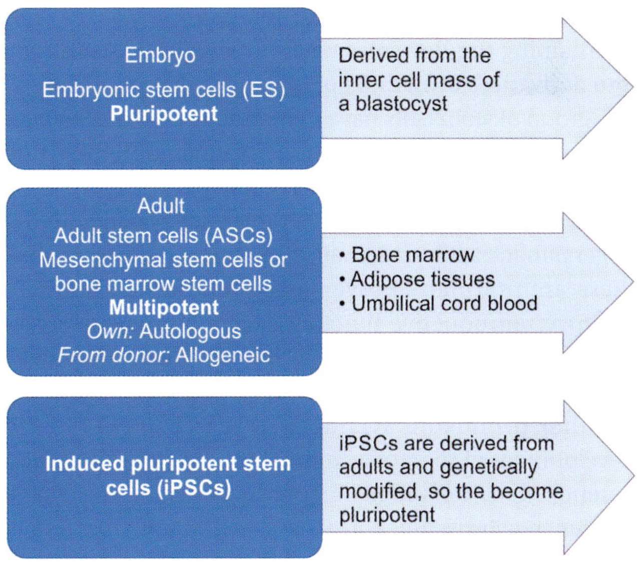

They can differentiate into cells that arise from the three germ layers—ectoderm, endoderm, and mesoderm—from which all tissues and organs develop.

Commonly, stem cells are derived from two main sources:

- Early embryos [embryonic stem cells (ESCs)]
- Adult tissue (adult stem cells) (Flowchart 1).

Embryonic stem cells are pluripotent stem cells derived from the inner cell mass of the blastocyst which are donated by couples who have completed their families via assisted reproduction. They are pluripotent and have potential to form derivatives of all three embryonic germ layers. Use of these cells has lots of ethical issues and many countries prohibit the use of healthy blastocysts for research purpose. The other sources of ESC are single blastomere biopsy (SBB), isolation of cells from poor quality embryos which are not considered for transfer, or embryos which found genetically aberrant by preimplantation genetic screening (PGS).

Mesenchymal stem cells (MSCs) are most common adult, multipotent stem cells. They can be derived from bone marrow, adipose tissue, Wharton jelly, umbilical cord blood, and peripheral blood. MSCs are characterized by specific surface cell markers.

Induced pluripotent stem cells (iPSCs) are adult somatic cells that have been genetically reprogrammed to an ESC-like state by being forced to express genes and factors important for maintaining the defining properties of ESCs. iPSCs share similar characteristics with ESCs: exhibiting morphology of ESCs, expressing ESCs markers, having normal karyotype, expressing telomerase activity, and maintaining the developmental potential to differentiate into derivatives of all three primary germ layers. Although this group of stem cells have tremendous potential to cure many disorders, their application in humans is limited due to technical and ethical reasons (Table 2).

To date, stem cell-based therapies are available to the larger public mostly in domain of clinical trials. Specifically, there are not many proven stem cell-based means to improve reproductive function except autologous adult bone marrow-derived CD113+ hematopoetic stem cells which are granted "Orphan Drug Designation" (ODD). Another promising avenue of research includes the development of therapies from adult stem cells of limited potency in the treatment of reproductive tract alterations, such as erectile dysfunction or damaged endometrial lining.

With development in the field of regenerative medicine for treatment of infertility, future of patient-specific stem cell therapies, sperm sorting, egg selection, and even organ repair and replacement with bioengineered tissues is no longer only in the realm of science fiction.

General Strategies for Stem Cell Replacement

There are at least three different therapeutic concepts for cell replacement that can be envisaged. One therapeutic approach involves direct administration of stem cells. The cells may be administered directly into the damaged organ, where they can differentiate into the desired cell type. On the other hand, stem cells may be injected systemically since they have the capacity to home in on damaged tissues by following gradients of cytokines and chemokines released by the diseased organ. Moreover, a second approach involves transplantation of differentiated cells derived from stem cells. For example, pancreatic islet cells can be generated from stem cells before transplantation into diabetic patients, and cardiomyocytes can be generated to treat ischemic heart disease. Lastly, a third approach involves stimulation of endogenous stem cells to facilitate repair. This goal might be accomplished by administration of appropriate growth factors and drugs that amplify the number of endogenous stem/progenitor cells and/or direct them to differentiate into the desired cell types. Therapeutic stimulation of precursor cells is already a clinical reality in the hematopoietic system, where factors such as erythropoietin, granulocyte colony-stimulating factor (GCSF), and granulocyte-macrophage colony-stimulating factor are used to increase production of specific blood elements. In addition to these strategies for cell replacement, a number of other approaches could involve stem cells for *ex vivo* or *in situ* generation of tissues, a process termed

TABLE 2 Potential advantages and disadvantages of stem cells in regenerative medicine.

Stem cells	*Advantages*	*Disadvantages*
ESCs	Pluripotent; high telomerase activity	Ethical concerns; malignant potential; difficult to control; may require many steps to differentiate into desired cell type; immune rejection
MSCs	No ethical or moral concerns; low malignant potential; avoiding allogeneic immune rejection	Limited flexibility; multipotent; difficulty to be maintained in cell culture for long periods
Stem cell from extraembryonic tissues	No ethical or moral concerns; reducing risk of tumorigenicity	Limited flexibility; multipotent
iPSCs	No ethical or moral concerns; patient-specific cells	Use of viral vectors to introduce genes; malignant potential
Spermatogonial stem cells	No ethical or moral concerns	Relatively small numbers in testis; difficulty to be maintained in cultures; immune rejection

(ESCs: embryonic stem cells; iPSCs: induced pluripotent stem cells; MSCs: mesenchymal stem cells)

tissue engineering. Stem cells are also excellent candidates as vehicles for cellular gene therapy. Finally, transplanted stem cells may exert paracrine effects on damaged tissues without the differentiation and replacement of lost cells.

Strategies for Transplantation of Stem Cells

- Undifferentiated or partially differentiated stem cells may be injected directly into the target organ or intravenously.
- Stem cells may be differentiated *ex vivo* before injection into the target organ.
- Growth factors or other drugs may be injected to stimulate endogenous stem cell populations.

Stem cell transplantation is not a new concept but rather is already a part of established medical practice. Hematopoeitic stem cells (HSCs) are responsible for the long-term repopulation of all blood elements in recipients of bone marrow transplants, and hematopoietic stem cell transplantation is the gold standard against which other stem cell transplantation therapies will be measured. Transplantation of differentiated cells is also a clinical reality and donated organs and tissues are often used to replace damaged tissues. However, the need for transplantable tissues and organs far outweighs the available supply and organ transplantation has limited potential for some tissues, such as the brain. Stem cells offer the possibility of a renewable source of replacement cells for virtually all organs (Fig. 3).

APPLICATION OF REGENERATIVE MEDICINE IN INFERTILITY (TABLE 3)

Regenerative Medicine for Female Infertility

Female infertility is complex area and many conditions alone or in combination can deteriorate state of female fertility starting from absence of uterus, primitive quality of oocytes, thin endometrium, exhausted/compromised ovaries due to age, and other factors or disorders contribute to infertility directly or indirectly. Among these, effectiveness of regenerative medicine has been evaluated for many conditions.

A pioneering work by White et al. has identified a rare population of mitotically active germ cells in human ovaries that can be purified and cultured *in vitro* to form spontaneous oocytes.

Augment

The treatment developed by Massachusetts-based Ovascience, Augment aims to revitalize old and poor quality eggs by giving them a power boost. An egg's energy comes from mitochondria, tiny "battery packs" that weaken by age (Fig. 4).

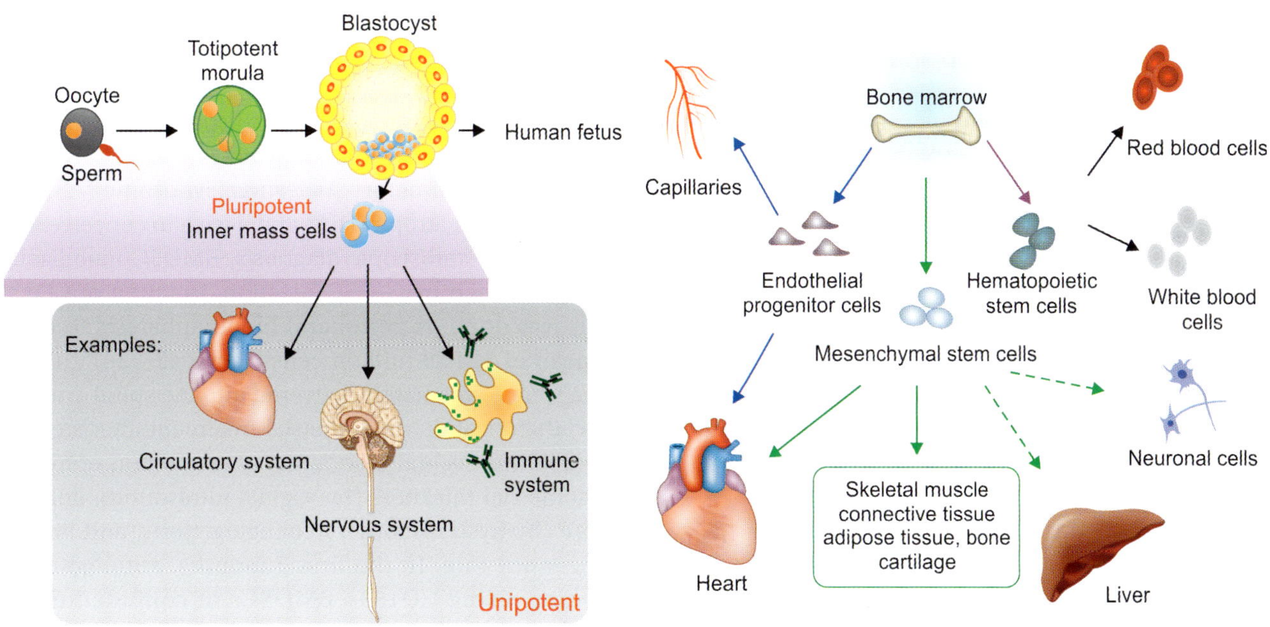

Fig. 3: Schematic representation of the loss of potency as development and cell differentiation occurs.
Source: Adapted from Vassena R, Eguizabal C, Heindryckx B, et al. Stem cells in reproductive medicine: Ready for the patient? Hum Reprod. 2015;30(9):2014-202.

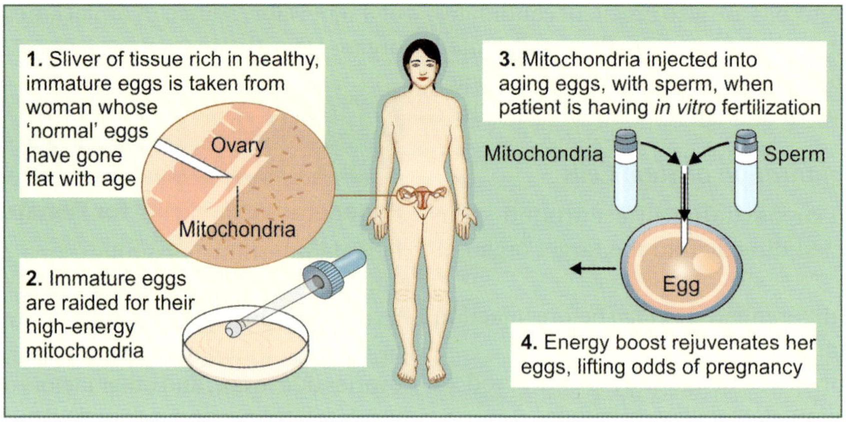

Fig. 4: How fertility is given a boost?

TABLE 3 Application of regenerative medicine in male and female infertility.

Egg	*Sperm*
Oocyte derived germ cells	Improvement in semen quality
Augment	Restore functions in testis
Ovarian rejuvenation and reversal of menopause	Erectile dysfunction in diabetes mellitus
Endometrium regeneration	
Endometrial thickness	
Growth of embryo and implantation of embryo	

Many women in their 40s who turn to donor eggs would be able to use their own instead. Younger patients could also benefit, with early research suggesting the technique could boost the odds of pregnancy fivefold.

The technique is already under trial in Turkey, Dubai, and Canada, where the world's first Augment baby was born in summer 2015.

Ovarian Rejuvenation and Reversal of Menopause

Sfakianoudis's team has found that PRP seems to rejuvenate older ovaries, and presented some of their results at the European Society of Human Reproduction and Embryology (ESHRE) annual meeting in Helsinki, Finland.

- The team was able to collect oocytes and fertilize them from a woman whose menopause had established 5 years ago, at age of 40. For the treatment, they injected PRP into ovaries of the patient and 6 months after, she experienced her first period since menopause. Thus, PRP is found to be effective in reversal of menopause and initiation of folliculogenesis.
- Two live births have been reported after stem cell ovarian autologous transplantation of mobilized-bone marrow-derived stem cells (BMDSCs) in poor responder women in trial (registration number: NCT02240342) done by Herraiz et al., (2016) and presented at ESHRE, 2016.
- Clinical trial, The ROSE (Rejuvenation of Premature Ovarian Failure with Stem Cells, Registration No: NCT02696889), is planned to evaluate the efficiency of BMDSC therapy on ovarian function recovery in patients with idiopathic and other types of premature ovarian failure (POF).

Endometrium Regeneration

Study by Santamaria et al. (2016) suggests that CD133+ BMDSC autologous cell therapy may be useful in treating patients with refractory Asherman syndrome (AS) and/or endometrial atrophy (EA) and a wish to conceive. After the initial hysteroscopic diagnosis, BMDSC mobilization was performed by G-CSF injection, isolation of CD133+ cells was done by peripheral blood apheresis to obtain a mean of 124.39 million cells (range 42–236), the cells then were immediately delivered into the spiral arterioles by catheterization. Endometrial treatment after stem cell therapy was evaluated in terms of restoration of menses, endometrial thickness (by vaginal ultrasound), adhesion score (by hysteroscopy), neoangiogenesis, and ongoing pregnancy rate. In the first 3 months, autologous cell therapy, using CD133+ BMDSCs in conjunction with hormonal replacement therapy, increased the volume and duration of menses as well as the thickness and angiogenesis processes of the endometrium while decreasing intrauterine adhesion scores.

Endometrial Thickness

Adequate endometrial thickness is a crucial factor for implantation and pregnancy. Thin endometrium could be the reason for cancellation of embryo transfer *in vitro* fertilization (IVF) cycle. Several methods have been defined for endometrial preparation but there is not any conclusive method yet. Intrauterine infusion of G-CSF has been studied in recent time but inconsistent results have been reported. Autologous PRP promotes endometrial growth and improves pregnancy outcome during IVF. Intrauterine infusion of PRP found to improve the endometrial thickness in women with thin endometrium. In study by Chang et al. (2015), increase in endometrial thickness after infusion of PRP was found in all the five patients, which suggested that intrauterine infusion of PRP represents innovative approach for the thin endometrium with poor response to conventional therapy. In another study by Zadehmodarres et al. (2017), total 10 patients with history of FET cancellation due to thin endometrium were recruited. With the indication of inadequate endometrium growth, all the participants needed PRP in the treatment cycle. After 48 hours of first PRP treatment, increased endometrial thickness was noted and this reached to more than 7 mm after the second PRP in all patients. Embryo transfer was then carried out for all of them. Five patients were pregnant and in four of them the pregnancy progressed normally.

Growth of Embryo

In study by Consiglio et al. (2015), culture of embryo in medium supplemented with platelet concentrate (PC) improved the growth and quality of developed embryos in bovine model. The *in vitro* results from the study showed that 5% of PC and 5% of fetal calf serum (FCS) increased the rate of blastocysts compared with the control containing 10% FCS only (43.04% vs 35.00%, respectively). The immune-histochemical study exposed more proliferating nuclei in the treated uterine horn compared to the control one. After intrauterine insemination in red blood cells (RBCs) (repeat breeder cow), the percentage of pregnant cows in the control group was 33.33% compared to 70% of the treated animals. However, such study in human model shall be proposed to check the effectiveness of such culture methods.

Implantation of Embryo

Nazari et al. (2016) had studied 20 women with a history of RIF who were candidates for frozen-thawed embryo transfer. Intrauterine infusion of 0.5 mL of PRP that contained platelet four to five times more than peripheral blood sample was performed 48 hours before blastocyst transfer. 18 participants were pregnant with one early miscarriage and one molar pregnancy. Sixteen clinical pregnancies were recorded and their pregnancies are ongoing. According to this study, PRP was found effective in improvement of pregnancy outcome in RIF patients.

Regenerative Medicine for Male Infertility

Effectiveness of regenerative medicine has been evaluated to treat many conditions that lead to male infertility among which many showed prominent results.

Improvement of Semen Quality

In trial NCT02708537, researchers at the IVI Bilbao and BTI Vitoria clinics in Spain are testing the effect of PRP rich in growth factors on quality of sperm by adding it into a sample of semen. Positive result of this study will be immensely useful in improvement of quality of sperm.

Restore Functions of Testes

Study by McLean (2008) states that successful transplantation and donor-derived spermatogenesis in recipient animals can lead to the restoration of fertility in infertile male mice. In combination with spermatogonial stem cell culture, transplantation technique can also be used for the purpose of generating transgenic animals through the male germline. In study by Valeriy et al. (2014), infusion of PRP found to induce morphofunctional mice testes following doxorubomycine hydrochloride exposure.

Erectile Dysfunction in Diabetes Mellitus

Bahk et al. found that human umbilical cord blood stem cell therapy has positive effects on erectile dysfunction in diabetes mellitus. Seven type 2 diabetic patients with complaint of erection failure for at least 6 months despite using medication and who were currently awaiting penile prostheses, had participated in the study. Except for impotence and diabetes mellitus, all other laboratory results were normal. A total of 1.5 × 107 human umbilical cord blood stem cells were infused into the corpus cavernosum. No immunosuppressive measures were taken in any of the patients. The mean age was found to be 69.5 years (range 57–87 years). Morning erections were regained in three subjects within 1 month, and for all except one by the 3rd month, and maintained for more than 6 months. Stem cells and unknown humoral factors of human umbilical cord blood stem cells mediate mechanisms that contribute to these positive effects.

FUTURE PROSPECTS OF REGENERATIVE MEDICINE

Stem Cell-derived Oocytes

Though stem cell-based tactics for ovarian regeneration and oocyte production have been proposed as upcoming clinical therapies for treating infertility in women, there has been a dilemma regarding the presence of ovarian stem cells in adult mammalian ovaries. Research studies in past claimed identification of functional oogonial stem cells in the postnatal ovary of several different species including humans. Now, there is progressively increasing experimental evidence on their existence. The work by Hayashi et al. (2012) showed that mouse stem cells could be differentiated in an *in-vitro/in-vivo* system into oocyte-like cells that are capable of being fertilized by spermatozoa and generating normal progeny. Usefulness of such experiment for human stem cells remains to be seen. However, this advancement is a crucial step forward in generating functional *de novo* oocytes from human iPSCs obtained from female patients rendered sterile by medical interventions, POF, or exposure to toxicants.

Stem Cells for Male Gametes

Hubner et al. (2003) first reported the successful derivation of gametes from mouse ESCs *in vitro*. Afterward, different studies with mouse ESCs have shown the ability to make functional spermatozoa capable of giving rise to live offspring after use of intracytoplasmic injection. Differentiation of male germ cells from human ESC has also been demonstrated. Similarly, studies with human ESCs have revealed the ability to differentiate *in vitro* into advanced spermatogenic stages, including round spermatids which are not capable of fertilizing oocytes in high-order mammals.

Study by Tamadon et al. (2015) found that transplanted bone marrow mesenchymal stem cells (BM-MSCs) could successfully induce spermatogenesis in seminiferous tubules of hamster with azoospermia. Therefore, BM-MSCs can be an attractive candidate in cell transplantation of azoospermia. Hermann et al. (2012) found that spermatogonial stem cell transplantation into rhesus testes regenerates spermatogenesis and produces functional sperm. Drusenheimer and co-workers, showed that human BM-MSCs (hBM-MSCs) could transdifferentiate into putative male germ cells that could sustain sperm production.

Japanese group at Kyoto University, were working for differentiation of ESC from mouse, and to form functional spermatogonial cells in vitro and in vivo having capacity to fertilize mouse oocyte.

ISSUES RELATED TO USE OF STEM CELLS

Use of stem cells in regenerative medicine holds promise for improving human health by restoring the function of cells and tissues that are damaged due to degeneration and/or injury. Like all other medical innovations, basic and translational research in the field not only requires a sound scientific rationale, but also needs to take into consideration ethical, legal, and social norms. Apart from challenges of selecting the appropriate stem cells for a particular condition, there are important concerns related to the use of embryos for creating human embryonic stem cell (hESC) lines as these may lead to commoditization of human cells and tissues. Further, there are challenges related to gene editing/modification, human germ-line engineering, and reproductive cloning. Besides, the robust technologies are being developed for deriving pluripotent stem cells from a variety of sources which may be easily accessible for clinical applications, often without rationale. The potential danger of tumorigenicity of stem cells, considering their capacity for unlimited proliferation, possible risk of contamination and genomic changes arising due to *in vitro* manipulations, and limitations related to immunological tissue incompatibility between individuals are all areas of serious concern. All of these pose an inherent risk of exploitation of individuals particularly those belonging to the underprivileged groups. Hence, the guidance for stem cell research, development, and its possible application in the frame of clinical trial is felt essential.

CURRENT STATUS OF STEM CELLS IN INDIA

- For treating patient with stem cells in India, guidelines are given by National Guideline for Stem Cells Research Indian Council of Medical Research and Department of Biotechnology, 2017.
- Therapeutic use of stem cells other than proven indications shall be treated as investigational and conducted only in the form of a clinical trial after obtaining necessary regulatory approvals from Drug Controller General of India (DCGI), Institutional Committee for Stem Cell Research (IC-SCR), and National Apex Committee (NAC).
- Procurement of biological material as a source of stem cells is subject to approval by IC-SCR and Institutional Ethics Committee (IEC).
- Prior to procurement of biological material for isolation of stem cells, it is mandatory to obtain audio-visual

informed consent from the voluntary donor as per the Central Drugs Standard Control Organisation (CDSCO) guidelines dated January 9th, 2014 (Schedule Y).

CONCLUSION

Research in regenerative medicine including stem cells is a growing field which currently holds great promise despite the numerous technical, procedural, and regulatory challenges. Though some stem cell based therapies are showing positive signs in the limited number of patients receiving treatment, such applications are still far from routine and the regulatory landscape. Unfortunately, there is a flourishing industry offering unproven and often unsafe stem cell-based "therapies", also affecting the field of reproductive medicine, often leaving both the physician and the patients unsure about their options. To achieve the long-term goal of routine clinical application of regenerative medicine in ART will require close collaboration between academia, clinicians, regulators, tissue engineers, and industries. Government authorities shall encourage such research, though under control of regulations for the safety and wellbeing of the participants involved, to expand the horizon of regimens for incurable conditions.

Regardless of the source of the stem cells used in regenerative strategies, a number of generic problems must be overcome for the development of successful clinical applications. Methods must be devised to reliably generate large numbers of specific cell types, to minimize the risk of tumor formation or proliferation of inappropriate cell types, to ensure the viability and function of the engrafted cells, to overcome immune rejection when autografts are not used, and to facilitate revascularization of regenerated tissue. Each organ system also will pose tissue-specific problems for stem cell therapies.

KEY NOTES

- Regenerative medicine definitely holds bright future in the field of medicine and infertility as it is the most advanced form of treatment for male and female infertility. The potential clinical applications of putative ovarian-derived stem cells are apparent. The development of techniques will allow prolongation of the window of fertility for women to meet the needs of future populations and their delay in childbearing.
- The protocols for isolation and culture of germline stem cells (GSCs) must be optimized further. In meantime, production of germ cells from ESCs or iPSCs is another possible alternative for treatment of infertility.
- The ethical and logistical need to keep up with technology should be accelerating as the science progresses.
- Clinicians need to be ready to answer their patients' questions and also participate in the ongoing discussions of ethics, patient needs, and acceptable use that will inevitably follow these technological advancements. More clinical trials with use of regenerative medicine should be encouraged as it seems to have potential to be future regimen for many infertility-related problems.

CLINICAL STUDIES AT AKANKSHA HOSPITAL AND RESEARCH INSTITUTE

- *Ovarian Rejuvenation Data*: 45 cases
- *Effects of PRP on implantation and pregnancy in patients undergoing IVF*: A pilot study, wherein the study population was 100 [Study: 50 and Control (without PRP): 50].

The final results showed impressive results—the clinical pregnancy rates were higher with 35.7% in the study group and 23.7% in control group (without PRP).

- *Testicular rejuvenation at Akanksha Hospital and Research Institute*: 5 cases
- *Bone marrow-derived aspiration of internal artery stem cells for thin endometrium*: 3 cases

EDITORS' COMMENTS

1. Regenerative medicine definitely holds bright future in the field of medicine and infertility as it is the most advanced form of treatment for male and female infertility. The potential clinical applications of putative ovarian-derived stem cells are apparent. The development of techniques will allow prolongation of the window of fertility for women to meet the needs of future populations and their delay in childbearing.
2. The protocols for isolation and culture of GSCs must be optimized further. In meantime, production of germ cells from ESCs or iPSCs is another possible alternative for treatment of infertility.
3. The ethical and logistical need to keep up with technology should be as accelerating as the science progresses.

Conflict of interest: None.

SUGGESTED READING

1. Bahk JY, Jung JH, Han H, et al. Treatment of diabetic impotence with umbilical cord blood stem cell intracavernosal transplant: preliminary report of 7 cases. Exp Clin transplant. 2010;8(2):150-60.

2. Boswell SG, Cole BJ, Sundman EA, et al. Platelet-rich plasma: a milieu of bioactive factors. Arthroscopy. 2012;28(3):429-39.
3. Chang Y, Li J, Chen Y, et al. Autologous platelet-rich plasma promotes endometrial growth and improves pregnancy outcome during in vitro fertilization. Int J Clin Exp Med. 2015;8(1):1286-90.
4. Hayashi K, Ogushi S, Kurimoto K, et al. Offspring from oocytes derived from in vitro primordial germ cell-like cells in mice. Science. 2012;338(6109):971-5.
5. Hermann BP, Sukhwani M, Winkler F, et al. Spermatogonial stem cell transplantation into rhesus testes regenerates spermatogenesis producing functional sperm. Cell Stem Cell. 2012;11(5):715-26.
6. Herraiz S, Buigues A, Díaz-García C, et al. Fertility rescue and ovarian follicle growth promotion by bone marrow stem cell infusion. Fertil Steril. 2018;109(5):908-18.
7. Hubner K, Fuhrmann G, Christenson LK, et al. Derivation of oocytes from mouse embryonic stem cells. Science. 2003;300(5623):1251-6.
8. Kessler JA. Applications of stem cell biology in clinical medicine. Harrison's Principles of Internal Medicine, 19th edition. New York: McGraw-Hill Education; 2014.
9. Lange-Consiglio A, Cazzaniga N, Garlappi R, et al. Platelet concentrate in bovine reproduction: effects on in vitro embryo production and after intrauterine administration in repeat breeder cows. Reprod Biol Endocrinol. 2015;13:65.
10. Macrae F. Turbocharged IVF that'll help older women conceive: Cells taken from other parts of the ovary will boost poor quality eggs leading to greater chance of pregnancy. Daily Mail. January 25th, 2016.
11. McLean DJ. Spermatogonial stem cell transplantation, testicular function, and restoration of male fertility in mice. In: Hou SX, Singh SR (Eds). Germline Stem Cells. Totowa, NJ: Humana Press; 2008. pp. 149-62.
12. Mouhayar Y, Sharara FI. Modern management of thin lining. Middle East Fertil Soc J. 2017;22(1):1-12.
13. Nayernia K, Nolte J, Michelmann HW, et al. In vitro-differentiated embryonic stem cells give rise to male gametes that can generate offspring mice. Develop Cell. 2006;11(1):125-32.
14. Nazari L, Salehpour S, Hoseini S, et al. Effects of autologous platelet-rich plasma on implantation and pregnancy in repeated implantation failure: A pilot study. Int J Reprod Biomed. 2016;14(10):625-8.
15. Reed-Maldonado AB, Lue TF. The current status of stem-cell therapy in erectile dysfunction: A review. World J Men's Health. 2016;34(3):155-64.
16. Santamaria X, Cabanillas S, Cervello I, et al. Autologous cell therapy with CD133+ bone marrow-derived stem cells for refractory Asherman's syndrome and endometrial atrophy: a pilot cohort study. Hum Reprod. 2016;31(5):1087-96.
17. Tamadon A, Mehrabani D, Rahmanifar F, et al. Induction of spermatogenesis by bone marrow-derived mesenchymal stem cells in busulfan-induced azoospermia in hamster. Int J Stem Cells. 2015;8(2):134-45.
18. Valeriya Z, Kuleshova O, Kholodkova O. Platelet-rich plasma induces morphofunctional restoration of mice testes following doxorubomycine hydrochloride exposure. J Exp Clin Med. 2014;31(3):183-7.
19. Vassena R, Eguizabal C, Heindryckx B, et al. Stem cells in reproductive medicine: Ready for the patient? Hum Reprod. 2015;30(9):2014-21.
20. White YA, Woods DC, Takai Y, et al. Oocyte formation by mitotically active germ cells purified from ovaries of reproductive-age women. Nature Med. 2012;18(3):413-21.
21. Zhao XY, Li W, Lv Z, et al. Viable fertile mice generated from fully pluripotent iPS cells derived from adult somatic cells. Stem Cell Rev. 2010;6(3):390-7.

30

CHAPTER

Quality Control in Embryology Laboratory

Priya Kannan

INTRODUCTION

Assisted reproductive technology, when introduced about 40 years ago, was considered an experimental procedure. From then to now, it has evolved into an established therapeutic management for the treatment of infertility. This can be largely attributed to the vast improvements in the culture systems, introduction of newer techniques that are better and safer, and of course the ongoing research into better understanding of the factors that influence pregnancy, which in turn translates into routine clinical applications.

Another important aspect that has majorly contributed to the improvements and stability of the results in fertility programs are attention to details in the embryology laboratory, stringent quality control programs, introduction of regulatory requirements, and setting of professional standards for embryology professionals.

IMPORTANCE OF QUALITY MANAGEMENT

Quality control is the basic level of quality management, concerned with controlling the quality of a product by identifying problems or defects, and involves processes such as inspecting, testing, checking, and others. Another important aspect of quality management is quality assurance which is a proactive process and is preventive in nature and aims at preventing nonconformities from occurring. It recognizes flaws in the processes. It is based on the realization that quality can be improved and organization management is at the core of quality assurance. The ambit of quality management has expanded to quality improvement. Hence, the present day quality management system (QMS) takes into consideration all aspects of the system.

Although the implementation of QMS involves finances and manpower and could be a burden to the management, it immensely helps a successful in vitro fertilization (IVF) program. Quality management prevents uncontrolled deviation in the processes and thus ensuring consistency of results. Essential elements of quality management are standard operating protocols, communication, training, risk management, and validation.

QUALITY MANAGEMENT IN IVF LABORATORY

To improve results in an IVF program, it is most imperative to implement quality management in the IVF laboratory, which is the heart of any IVF program. IVF is governed by biology of the oocyte and the sperm. Hence, the function of the IVF laboratory is to provide optimal environment (culture system) for the gametes and embryos and also to protect them from external adverse factors. It is extremely important to understand that stress on the gametes and embryos as a result of suboptimal culture conditions can alter gene expression and introduce epigenetic changes that can have adverse effects from birth weight to behavioral changes.

Hence, it is important to understand the biology and then breakdown the processes, establish controls, identify key performance indicators (KPI), and monitor the process. For an IVF laboratory, this involves:

- Designing of IVF laboratory

- Maintenance of culture systems
- Proper handling of gametes and embryos.

The IVF laboratory process was eloquently distributed into three areas by Dr Mortimer (Table 1).

It is important to monitor each process and equipment using indicators and compare them to the set benchmarks.

QUALITY CONTROL OF CULTURE SYSTEMS

Culture system is the most important part of the IVF laboratory, the quality of which is directly proportional to the reproductive outcomes from any IVF laboratory. Three very important physiochemical parameters to maintain in the culture system are temperature, pH, and osmolality. These determine the quality of the culture system.

Temperature

Human meiotic spindle is sensitive to alterations in temperature and there is alteration of the spindle in cooler temperatures with limited recovery after rewarming. Situations where changes in temperature can occur are during follicular aspiration, manipulations of gamete and embryo, and during embryo transfer. Hence, maintenance of temperature at 37°C during in vitro manipulation is important for normal fertilization and optimal embryo development. Ideally, apart from measuring the external temperatures in the heated stages, incubators, etc. temperature in the culture dish should be measured.

pH

The pH varied from one commercial culture to another, ranging between 7.2 and 7.4. The pH of the media is maintained by bicarbonate buffer and regulated by the CO_2 dissolved in the culture medium, which is in turn dependent on the partial pressure of CO_2 in the incubator air (Henderson-Hasselbalch equation). It is recommended to check the pH of each new batch of culture media after equilibration.

Osmolality

The osmolality of the commercially available culture media ranges from 255 mOsm/kg to 298 mOsm/kg. With the developments in methods of culture such as single step media, where there is extended culture without media change, monitoring of osmolality has come into focus. However, this is yet to be implemented in routine practice.

To measure outcomes, we need series of benchmarks or indicators that would measure a specific step or process or an element. Performance indicators (PIs) are objective

TABLE 1 Three areas of in vitro fertilization laboratory process.

Process	*Control*	*Factors*	*Requirements*
Inputs	Gametes	COI	Nuclear maturation
		OPU	Suction pressure, temperature
		Sperm collection and processing	Temperature, prevention of iatrogenic damage, senescence
	Contact materials	OPU needles	Bore, nontoxicity
		Semen collection jars	Sterility, nontoxicity
		Plastics—tubes and dishes	Sterility, nontoxicity
		Culture media	Formulations, sterility, endotoxins
Realization	Laboratory environment	Air quality	Particulates and microbes
	Culture system	Light	VOCs
		Incubators	Spectral sensitivity
			Temperature
			pCO_2, pO_2
			Humidity
			VOCs
			Calibration
			Malfunction
	Laboratory process	Methodology	Selection, SOPs
		Personnel	Training, skill, competence
		Insemination	Washed sperm concentration
		Handling and assessment conditions	Temperature, medium, pH, osmolarity
Outputs		Zygotes, embryos, blastocysts	Developmental competence

(COI: controlled ovarian induction; OPU: ovum pick-up; SOP: standard operating procedure; VOC: volatile organic compound)

measures for evaluating critical healthcare domains (patient safety, effectiveness, equity, patient-centeredness, timeliness, and efficiency). KPIs are essential for assessment of the following:

- Establishing minimum standards for proficiency
- Monitoring ongoing performance within a QMS
- Introduction of new technique or process
- External quality assurance
- Benchmarking and quality improvement.

Key performance indicators are robust, reliable, and incorporated into the routine work flow. In general, the results of a series of KPIs will provide an adequate overview of the most important steps in the IVF laboratory process. It is suggested that each laboratory must develop their own KPIs.

The following are the KPIs in an IVF laboratory as suggested by the Vienna consensus of 2017. The discussions identified three different types of indicators: Reference indicators (RIs), PIs, and KPIs.

1. Reference indicators were related to the oocytes coming into the laboratory, and so were proxy indicators of the response to ovarian stimulation (Table 2).
2. Performance indicators were those for which data should be documented and stored, even if they are not routinely reported in a control chart (Table 3).
3. Key performance indicators were those related to the "core business" of the ART laboratory (Table 4).

TABLE 2 Reference indicators for identifying performance of the ART laboratory.

Reference indicator	*Calculation*	*Benchmark value*
Proportion of oocytes recovered (stimulated cycles)	No. of oocytes retrieved × 100/No. of follicles on day of trigger	80–95% of follicles measured
Proportion of MII oocytes at ICSI	No. of MII oocytes at ICSI × 100/No. of COC retrieved	75–90%

(ART: assisted reproductive technology; COC: cumulus-oocyte complex; ICSI: intracytoplasmic sperm injection; MII: metaphase II)

KEY PERFORMANCE INDICATORS FOR ASSISTED REPRODUCTIVE TECHNOLOGY PROGRAM

The results of any program must be subgrouped based on the female partners' age. More subgroups can be made based on other variables such as third party reproduction, procedures, etc. For each group, the following should be calculated:

- Biochemical pregnancy rate [>100 IU of serum beta human chorionic gonadotropin (hCG), 14 days post-embryo transfer]
- Clinical pregnancy rate (gestational sac on ultrasound)
- Ongoing pregnancy rate (presence of fetal heart pulsation on ultrasound by 7 weeks)
- Implantation rate (number of gestational sacs at 7 weeks ultrasound per embryos transferred, in percentage)
- Early pregnancy loss rate (proportion of positive serum beta hCG that fail to show gestational sac on ultrasound)
- Multiple pregnancy rate (number of pregnancies with more than one gestational sac on 7 weeks ultrasound).

QUALITY CONTROL OF IVF LABORATORY ENVIRONMENT

Air quality of the IVF laboratory has been proven to be an important factor determining the success of an ART program starting from the landmark publication of Cohen and his colleagues in 1997. Many studies have since been published on the effect of air quality on IVF laboratory outcome. Hence, the emphasis is on clean room designs for

TABLE 3 Performance indicators for the ART laboratory.

Performance indicator	*Calculation*	*Competency value*	*Benchmark value*
Sperm motility postpreparation (for IVF and IUI)	Progressively motile sperm × 100/All sperm counted	90%	≥95%
IVF polyspermy rate	No. of fertilized oocytes with >2 PN × 100/No. of COC inseminated	<6%	
1PN rate (IVF)	No. of 1 PN oocytes × 100/No. of COC inseminated	<5%	
1PN rate (ICSI)	No. of 1 PN oocytes × 100/No. of MII oocytes injected	<3%	
Good blastocyst development rate	No. of good quality blastocysts on Day 5 × 100/No. of 2 PN/2 PB oocytes on Day 1	≥30%	≥40%

(ART: assisted reproductive technology; COC: cumulus-oocyte complexes; ICSI: intracytoplasmic sperm injection; IVF: *in vitro* fertilization; IUI: intrauterine insemination; PB: polar body; PN: pronucleus)

TABLE 4 KPIs for the ART laboratory.

Key performance indicator (KPI)	*Calculation*	*Competency value*	*Benchmark value*
ICSI damage rate	No. of damaged or degenerated × 100/All oocytes injected	≤10%	≤5%
ICSI normal fertilization rate	No. of oocytes with 2PN and 2PB × 100/No. of MII oocytes injected	≥65%	≥80%
IVF normal fertilization rate	No. of oocytes with 2PN and 2PB × 100/No. of COC inseminated	≥60%	≥75%
Failed fertilization rate (IVF) cycles	No. of cycles with no evidence of fertilization × 100/No. of stimulated IVF	<5%	
Cleavage rate	No. of cleaved embryos on day 2 × 100/No. of 2PN/2PB oocytes on Day 1	≥95%	≥99%
Day 2 embryo development rate	No. of 4-cell embryos on day 2 × 100/No. of normally fertilized oocytes*	≥50%	≥80%
Day 3 embryo development rate	No. of 8-cell embryos on day 3 × 100/No. of normally fertilized oocytes	≥45%	≥70%
Blastocyst development rate	No. of blastocysts day 5 × 100/No. of normally fertilized oocytes	≥40%	≥60%
Successful biopsy rate	No. of biopsies with DNA detected × 100/No. of biopsies performed	≥90%	≥95%
Blastocyst cryosurvival rate	No. of blastocysts appearing intact × 100/No. of blastocysts warmed	≥90%	≥99%
Implantation rate (cleavage stage)†	No. of sacs seen on ultrasound × 100/No. of embryos transferred	≥25%	≥35%
Implantation rate (blastocyst stage)†	No. of sacs seen on ultrasound‡ × 100/No. of blastocysts transferred	≥35%	≥60%

*Defined as oocytes with 2PN and 2PB on Day 1.

†Based on total number of embryos transferred to all patients in the reference group, not just to those for whom an implantation occurred.

‡Definition reached after discussion, as some felt that number of fetal heart beat detected/number of embryos transferred was a more meaningful indicator.

(ICSI: intracytoplasmic sperm injection; MII: metaphase II; PB: polar body; PN: pronucleus)

an IVF laboratory. The parameters that need to be controlled are (1) volatile organic compounds (VOCs), (2) airborne microbes, and (3) airborne chemically active substances.

Air quality regulations may differ from one country to another. It can vary from ISO (International Standards Organization) 7 to 8 or EU GMP (European Good manufacturing practice) D to C. Monitoring of air quality needs to be done both in rest and in activity.

The Cairo consensus on the IVF laboratory environment and air quality has recommended the following:

- ISO Class 7/GMP Grade B "in operation"/Grade C "at rest"
- Air changes per hour (ACH) of 10–15/hours, including three fresh air changes per hour, which can be obtained by installing high efficiency particulate air (HEPA) filters or mobile filtration units
- *Particulates*: Less than 352,000 particles larger than 0.5–10 μm/m^3 (equivalent to <10,000 such particles per cubic foot)
- *Microorganisms*: Less than 10 cfu/m^3 and less than 2 spores/m^3 at rest
- *Volatile organic compounds*: Total VOCs less than 500 μg/m^3 (~ 400–800 ppb total VOC, depending on molecular species); less than 5 μg/m^3 aldehydes.
- *Overpressure*: Ideal target is +38 to +50 Pa in the IVF laboratory (recommended minimum +30 Pa).
- *Temperature*: Maintained within the range of 20–24°C
- *Humidity*: Room relative humidity should be between 40% and 45%.

Daily measurement of VOC, temperature, relative humidity in the IVF lab is recommended. There should be regular preventive maintenance of the air purification systems, such as filter replacement, maintenance of records of the filter change date, and the batch numbers.

QUALITY CONTROL OF EQUIPMENT

Assessment of equipment performance and malfunction are important components of quality control of laboratory equipment. All the equipment in the IVF laboratory needs to be checked, serviced, and calibrated at regular intervals. Equipment drift is a definitive entity and hence calibration of IVF laboratory equipment with independent sensors needs to be done. It is also imperative to make sure that the independent sensors have been calibrated. Real time monitoring (RTM) of equipment has been in vogue in recent years, through modern web-based systems with the present availability of inexpensive wireless technology, internet, and smart phones. It is presently possible to connect equipment independent sensors for temperature, gas levels, VOCs, and liquid nitrogen (LN2) levels. This can warn the concerned person about a crisis in the laboratory, such as unexpected failure of equipment or malfunctioning, thus providing greater stability and reliability. A major advantage of the RTM is the remote accessibility.

An important aspect of quality control is daily monitoring of equipment and assessing its performance.

Equipment performance

Every equipment has a definitive set of parameter to be checked on a daily basis such as the following:

- *Laminar air flow (LAF)*: Temperature of the working surfaces, air quality
- *Incubator*: Measurement of gases, temperature, pH, humidity
- *Test tube warmer*: Temperature
- *Storage dewar*: LN_2 levels.

Individual equipment should have a separate sheet which needs to be filled every month for analysis.

Sample record of daily maintenance sheet for LAF:
LAF—(Number)

Date	Time	Technique	Temperature		Adjustments	Sign
			Inbuilt	External		
			Range			

Sample record of daily maintenance sheet for incubator:
Incubator—(Number)

Date	Time	Technique	Temperature		CO_2		Adjustments	Sign
			Inbuilt	External	Inbuilt	External		
			Range		Range			

More information such as O_2, pH can be added as and when required.

Sample record of daily maintenance sheet for incubator:
Dewar—(Number)

Date	Technique	LN_2 level	Refilling
		Range	

General laboratory maintenance:

Date	Technique	Lab temp	Lab humidity	VOC	Adjustments	Sign

Witnessing

Witnessing is another important aspect in preventing mishaps in the IVF lab. This can be done using human double witnessing or by using automated witnessing systems. Although human double witnessing systems are more commonly seen presently, it does have its share of flaws which is overcome by the automated systems. To have these as part of routine quality control might be the way in future.

QUALITY CONTROL IVF LABORATORY PERSONNEL

As in any field of medicine, appropriate number of professions with technical proficiency directly influences the outcome. Each country has its own set of regulations to qualify to be trained as clinical embryologist. However, the number of embryologists seems to be similar in various guidelines. It has been recommended that there should be one full time embryologist per 120–150 stimulation cycles per year.

CONCLUSION

It is the desire of all personnel involved in ART for a healthy singleton pregnancy for the patient and everyone strives for the same. At the same time, quality is the standard which in turn translates to safety for the patient. Hence, QMSs are a must in present day ART.

EDITORS' COMMENTS

Fertility centers can benefit greatly by implementing quality control as per quality management system (QMS) standards, regardless of their size and whether they are public or private. This is achieved by routinely measuring how well the output of their processes complies with a set of pre-defined requirements, and how quality policies are implemented, and quality objectives achieved. In other words, the abovementioned elements form the pillars of the QMS.

A QMS makes clear how tasks are supposed to be done because all documents, procedures and the workflow, as well as roles and responsibilities, are clearly defined. Quality management also addresses internal needs, such as the efficient use of resources (materials, human, technology and information), which is directly related to profitability. Such systems also guarantee the involvement of all staff in the process. As a result, improved communication and motivation to excel as a team is ensured. Importantly, a QMS provides tools to monitor what to do, leading inevitably to the continuous improvement of the service as a whole. It then encourages changes, adjustments, and improvements based on facts and not on assumptions, since all data is formally recorded and analyzed. High-quality Fertility Centers should also incorporate robust metrics concerning various dimensions of care, including effectiveness, safety, patient-centeredness, efficiency, timeliness and equity; therefore, they should not rely on a single parameter such as pregnancy rates as a measure of success.

Our clinic has implemented QMS as per the ISO 9001 standards over 10 years ago, and our results have been reassuring in achieving the goals discussed above. We have contributed articles and books[1-3] on the matter concerned and thus invite readers to get further insights on the matter concerned after reading the well-written chapter on QC in embryology laboratory presented here.

REFERENCES

1. Bento FB, Esteves SC, Agarwal A (Eds). Quality management in ART Clinics: A Practical guide. New York: Springer US; 2013. p. 246.
2. Bento FC, Esteves SC. Establishing a quality management system in a fertility center: experience with ISO 9001. MedicalExpress. 2016;3(3):M160302. [online]. Available from http://dx.doi.org/10.5935/Medical Express.2016.03.02. [Last accessed July, 2019].
3. Fischer R, Nakano FY, Roque M, et al. A quality management approach to controlled ovarian stimulation in assisted reproductive technology: the "Fischer protocol". Panminerva Med. 2019;61(1):11-23.

SUGGESTED READING

1. Ecker DJ, Stein P, Xu Z, et al. Long term effects of culture of pre implantation mouse embryos on behaviour. Proc Nat Acad Sci USA. 2004;101:1595-600.
2. ESHRE Guideline Group on good practice in IVF labs, De los Santos MJ, Apter S, et al. Revised guidelines for good practice in IVF laboratories. Hum Reprod. 2016;31(4):685-6.
3. Esteves S, Bento F. Summary evidence for the effect of laboratory air quality on pregnancy outcome in in vitro fertilization. In: Esteves SC, Varghese AC, Worrilow KC (Eds). Clean Room Technology in ART Clinics: A Practical Guide. Boca Raton: Taylor and Francis Group; 2016. pp. 345-52.
4. Kleijkers SH, Mantikou E, Slappendel E, et al. Influence of embryo culture medium (G5 and HTF) on pregnancy and perinatal outcome after IVF: a multicenter RCT. Hum Reprod. 2016;31(10):2219-30.
5. Kohn LT, Corrigan JM, Donaldson MS. To Err is Human: Building a Safer Health System. Washington DC: National Academies Press; 2000.
6. Mortimer D, Cohen J, Mortimer S, et al. Cairo consensus on the IVF laboratory environment and air quality: report of an expert meeting. RBM Online. 2018;36(6):658-74.
7. Mortimer D, Martimer S. Quality control and quality assurance in the IVF laboratory. In: Gardner D, Simon C (Eds). Handbook of In Vitro Fertilisation, 4th edition. Boco Raton: CRC Press; 2018. pp. 291-302.
8. Pickering Sj, Braude PR, Johnson MH, et al. Transient cooling to room temperature can cause irreversible disruption of the meiotic spindle in human oocyte. Fert Steril. 1990;54:102-8.
9. Salinas M, Lopez-Garrigos M, Gutierrez M, et al. Achieving continuous improvement in laboratory organization through performance measurements: a seven-year experience. Clin Chem Lab Med. 2010;48:57-61.
10. Swain JE, Pool TB. Culture media in IVF: Decisions for the laboratory. In: Zsolt PN, Alex CV, Ashok A (Eds). Practical Manual of In vitro Fertilisation: Advanced Methods and Novel Devices. New York: Springer; 2012.
11. The Vienna consensus: report of an expert meeting on the development of art laboratory performance indicators. ESHRE Special Interest Group of Embryology Alpha Scientists in Reproductive Medicine. Human Reprod Online. 2017;2:35.
12. Wang WH, Meng L, Hackett RJ, et al. Limited recovery of meiotic spindle in living human oocytes after cooling-rewarming observed using polarized light microscopy. Human Reprod. 2001;16:2374-8.

31

CHAPTER

Newer Media in Embryology Laboratory

Pankaj Talwar, Pooja Awasthi

INTRODUCTION

The advances in the world of assisted reproduction have been rapid and impressive and the future holds even more. Culture media play a major role in this success. The number of children conceived by assisted reproduction technologies (ART) has reached 5 million as calculated by the International Committee for Monitoring Assisted Reproduction Technologies (ICMART) and presented in European Society of Human Reproduction and Embryology (ESHRE) (Adamson et al., 2012). The great improvement in embryo culture conditions and *in vitro* fertilization (IVF) culture media has been an important part of this success. The IVF and culture of human egg were proposed by Rock and Menkin (1944).

Ludwig and Ringer developed the first tissue culture media nearly 150 years ago, by using simple salt solutions, which was initially based on the chemical properties of blood serum. During the 1970s, the emergence of second generation media came into the existence, aiming to mimic the natural reproductive environment or the back to nature principle.

Culture media are an essential part of a culture system that aims to minimize stress and mimic the natural reproductive condition to gametes and embryos. Culture media provide a balance of ions, energy substrates, and nutrients, safeguarding (securing) the best possible clinical outcomes. Culture media for embryo development must meet the metabolic needs of preimplantation embryos and its composition should be based on the specific developmental stage of the embryo.

THE COMPOSITION OF EMBRYO CULTURE MEDIA

The constituents of culture media play crucial role during embryonic development and are listed below.

Salts

The main components of embryo culture media are salts, which dissociates in aqueous solutions into their inorganic ions. Inorganic ions serve a very large variety of functions in cell and are vital for a vast number of cell physiological processes.

- In establishing the characteristic intracellular environment, (in which K^+ concentrations are higher while Na^+ and Cl^- concentrations are kept low mediated by the ubiquitous Na^+, K^+-ATPase).
- In the maintenance of cell membrane potential.
- Serves as the energy source for the transportation of metabolites and amino acids and others that perform homeostatic functions such as intracellular pH (pHi) regulations.

Osmolality is an estimation of the osmolar concentration of plasma and is proportional to the number of particles per kilogram of solvent; it is expressed as mosmol/kg. The osmolarity of the culture medium must be in the range of 275–290 mosmol/kg.

pH and Buffers

pH is a measure of the acidity or basicness of a substrate. Most culture media utilize a bicarbonate/CO_2 buffer system to keep pH in the range of 7.2–7.4. In the human oocyte/embryo, glycolysis protein conformation, and a number of other critical metabolic and transport processes are regulated by pHi. Regulating pHi is therefore crucial, especially in the early embryo. Extracellular pH (pHe) of the culture medium is generally higher than pHi, but critical factor in establishing pHi.

The ability to regulate pHi varies with cell stage. Morula and blastocyst stage embryos appear to have more rigorous control over their pHi, possibly due to formation of tight-junctions between cells, while denuded mature oocytes lack robust pHi regulatory capacity. The ability to regulate pHi, normally supplied via surrounding cumulus cells. pHi controls several intracellular processes that can impact embryo as well as resulting fetal development.

For procedures performed in room atmosphere, like gamete collection, intracytoplasmic sperm injection (ICSI), cryopreservation, and embryo transfer, many laboratories choose to utilize handling media with reduced bicarbonate levels and inclusion of another pH buffer to maintain the pH outside the incubator. Common buffers are HEPES and MOPS.

HEPES [4-(2-hydroxyethyl)-1-piperazineethanesulfonic acid] is a zwitterion organic chemical buffering agent. HEPES can be utilized as a free acid, or may be conjugated to various salts. HEPES provides no nutritional benefit to the dividing cells. It is added to the media exclusively for extra buffering capacity when the IVF cell culture requires prolonged periods of manipulation outside of a CO_2 incubator.

HEPES is having following characteristics:

- pKa values between 6.0 and 8.0
- High solubility
- Membrane impermeability
- Limited effect on biochemical reactions.

MOPS [3-(N-morpholino)propanesulfonic acid] is a buffer which is a structural analog to MES. Its chemical structure contains a morpholine ring. With a pKa of 7.15 at 20°C, it is very useful for buffering of IVF biologic systems where stable pH is required for a longer period.

Carbohydrates

Culture media that support the development of zygotes up to 8-cells contain pyruvate and lactate. Some commercial media are glucose free, while others add a very low concentration of glucose to supply the needs of the sperm during conventional insemination.

Amino Acids

Supplement of the culture medium with amino acids is necessary for embryo development. Media that support the development of zygotes up to 8-cells are supplemented with nonessential amino acids (NEAAs): Proline, serine, alanine, asparagine, aspartate, glycine, and glutamate. Media that support the development of 8-cell embryos up to the blastocyst stage are supplemented with essential amino acids (EAAs): Cysteine, histidine, isoleucine, leucine, lysine, methionine, valine, argentine, glutamine, phenylalanine, threonine, and tryptophan.

L-glutamine provides nitrogen for NAD, NADPH, and nucleotides and serves as a secondary energy source for metabolism. Taurine acts as an antioxidant, eliminating the extreme effects of cell metabolism.

Antibiotics

Antibiotics are used to minimize the risks of microbial growth. The most commonly used antibiotic is Penicillin. The antibacterial effect of penicillin is attributed to its ability to inhibit the synthesis of peptidoglycan, unique glycoproteins of the bacterial cell wall. Streptomycin and gentamycin, which exert their antibacterial effect by inhibiting bacterial protein synthesis. Regular use of antibiotics for cell culture is not recommended.

Chelators

Chelators are frequently used to control or suppress reactive oxygen species (ROS) levels as embryos develop. However, there is no consensus regarding doses, time of exposure, and proper combinations of antioxidants and chelators in embryo culture.

Ethylenediaminetetraacetic acid (EDTA) is used as a chelator in medium that supports the embryo from the zygote stage to 8-cells and prevents abnormal glycolysis. EDTA probably acts in several ways, including:

- Chelation of heavy metal divalent cations that may be present as trace contaminants in media components and plastic culture ware.
- Impede the enzyme 3-phosphoglycerate kinase, thus reducing glycolytic activity in an early embryo.
- Increased glycolysis in an early embryo seems to be associated with deprived development.

Phenol Red

Large number of the commercially available culture media includes phenol red as a pH indicator, which allows constant monitoring of pH. Phenol red is bright red at pH of 7.4, the optimum pH value for cell culture during the cell growth. It changes color as pH is changed due to the metabolites released by the cells or media contamination.

At low pH levels, phenol red turns the medium yellow, while at higher pH levels it turns the medium purple.

Vitamins

Vitamins are essential for growth and proliferation of cells. Vitamins cannot be synthesized in sufficient quantities by cells and are therefore important supplements required in tissue culture. Media are also enriched with different vitamins making them suitable for a particular cell line.

Macromolecules

Albumin is the most abundant and commonly used protein source for in vitro culture systems of human embryo. In vivo, it serves as a source of the free amino acids and fixed nitrogen to support preimplantation of embryo. It can be extracted from the patient's own serum and commercially available as pooled human serum.

The recombinant form of albumin is a recently developed macromolecule that has been shown to be very effective in mammalian embryo culture. It has several advantages, including batch-to-batch consistency and biological stability; it is free from viral and prion contaminants; and has lower endotoxin levels.

Glycosaminoglycans (GAGs) such as hyaluronan (HA, hyaluronic acid) are found in abundance in the female reproductive tract of several species, including humans and have a role in fertilization, adhesion, and proliferation of several cell types.

Growth Factors

Numerous growth factors are present in the in vivo environment of human embryos. Although very less concentrations are required, but they have a profound effect on tissue growth and differentiation through attachment to factor specific receptors on cell surface. Tables 1 and 2 summarize the expression of growth factors.

ADVANCES IN THE MEDIA

In recent years there has been change in the way media are formulated and several media have been designed to support development up to blastocyst stage such as DM1/2/3, G1/G2 media, potassium simplex optimization medium (KSOM), and Quinn's Advantage. Until recently, embryologists used to prepare their own culture media in house.

In 1984–1985, special media were developed for human IVF. Menezo and his colleagues published a paper, in 1984, describing a new concept in human embryo culture. They suggested adding serum albumin as a source for amino acids. The serum protein ensures that oocytes and embryos do not adhere to the glass surface of the pipette used to manipulate them.

In 1985 Quinn et al. published in the journal Fertility and Sterility a formula entitled human tubal fluid (HTF), which mimics the in vivo environment to which the embryo is exposed. The formulation of HTF was based on the known chemical composition of the fluids in human fallopian tubes as known at that time. This medium is based on a simple balanced salt solution without amino acids; however, the concentration of potassium was adjusted to that measured in the human female reproductive tract. This medium was found to be better compared with earlier media developed. In last decade, there has been major shift away from in house media preparation to commercially produced media manufacturing procedure with strict regulatory and quality control. Currently there are essentially two types of media that are widely used for clinical IVF: sequential culture systems and monoculture systems.

ADVANCES IN OILS

Oil is a term that specifies that the substance is a nonpolar and viscous liquid. Oil creates a barrier between the embryo culture media and air to stop evaporation. This protects gametes and embryos from pH fluctuations, temperature variations, and change in osmolality during ART procedures.

To ensure that it meets high standards of purity, cool chain should be maintained during the transportation. The first step involves the formation of peroxide. Peroxides are very reactive and can do a lot of damage to any cells that they come in contact with. Refined mineral oils or liquid paraffin consists exclusively of saturated hydrocarbons, which improves chemical stability and prevents oxidation of the oils.

Hydrotreating is a process, in which hydrogen, heat, and pressure convert and remove aromatics and unsaturated bonds (sulfur) from the mineral oil. One should check if the fallowing tests were performed on culture oil before using the same.

- Special handling and packaging
- Biocompatibility testing
- Testing for the presence of volatile organic compounds (VOCs) in mineral oil
- Peroxide value determination
- Peroxide toxicity testing.

Mineral oils can absorb VOCs from ambient air during manufacturing, transportation, and storage (when exposed to heat and light) and these VOCs can negatively affect the health of the embryo, therefore utmost handling should be taken. It is also important to minimize the head space of container to prevent oil from oxidation. The rate of oxidation correlates the amount of oxygen that the oil absorbs.

TABLE 1 Expression of growth factors within the reproductive tract in relation to the menstrual cycle.

Oviduct	LIF	Peak from late follicular to mid-luteal phase
	GM-CSF	Peak in late follicular through mid-luteal phase
	HB-EGF	Peak from late follicular to mid-luteal phase
	LIF	Throughout the cycle
	TGF-0	Peak from late follicular to mid-luteal phase
	VEGF	Peak during preovulatory period
Follicular fluid	FGF and fibronectin	Throughout the menstrual cycle
	Insulin-like growth factor-1	
	Insulin-like growth factor-2	
	M-CSF	
Cumulus/granulosa cells	Activin A (stimulated by hCG)	Immature follicles and subsequent to ovulation stimulated by hCG
	FGF	
	Fibronectin primarily in the corona cells	
	Insulin-like growth factor-1	
	Insulin-like growth factor-2 (stimulated by hCG)	
	Inhibin (He et al., stimulated by hCG)	
	LIF	
	M-CSF	
	TGF-0	
	VEGF	
Corpus luteum	Inhibin (stimulated by hCG)	
	VEGF (stimulated by hCG)	
Endometrium	LIF by the luminal epithelial cells	Peak in the luteal phase
	Activin A, by the epithelial cells	Throughout the menstrual cycle
	Colony stimulating factor	Higher in luteal phase
	EGF	Throughout the menstrual cycle except during early follicular phase
	Fibronectin	Throughout the menstrual cycle
	Granulocyte-macrophage colony stimulating factor-8 primarily by the luminal and glandular epithelial cells	Peak in mild-luteal phase
	Heparin-binding epidermal growth factor by the apical surface of the luminal epithelium	Peak just before implantation
	Insulin-like growth factor-1 primarily in the luminal and glandular epithelium	Peak from late follicular to mild-luteal phase
	Insulin-like growth factor-2	During the luteal phase primarily
	Inhibin	Primarily during luteal phase
	PDGF	
	VEGF on the apical surface of the epithelium	

(EGF: epithelial growth factor; FGF: fibroblast growth factor; GM-CSF: granulocyte-macrophage-colony stimulating factor; HB-EGF: heparin-binding epidermal growth factor; hCG: human chorionic gonadotropin; LIF: leukemia inhibitory factor; M-CSF: macrophage colony-stimulating factor; PDGF: platelet-derived growth factor; TGF: transforming growth factor; VEGF: vascular endothelial growth factor)

Volatile organic compounds adversely impact preimplantation embryo development. These volatiles include ketones, toluene, chloroform, isopropanol, and xylene.

Biocompatibility testing for genotoxicity and cytotoxicity should be performed in accordance with ISO 10993, "Biological Evaluation of Medical Devices".

The polycarbon lipid tail of mineral oil contains more unsaturated bonds than the more saturated paraffin oil. This makes mineral oil more unstable and prone to attack by free oxygen radicals and photo-oxidation than paraffin oil.

The paraffin oil is prewashed with human serum albumin (HSA)-containing medium and has very low

TABLE 2 Expression of growth factors by oocyte and the embryo.

Factor	*Oocyte*	*Stage*	*Stage*	*Blastocyst*	*Comments*
TGF-0		+	+	+	
CSF1		+	+		
EGF	I	+	+		
GM-CSF		+	+	+	
HB-EGF	+	+	+	+	
Insulin-like growth factor-1	+	+	+	+	
Insulin-like growth factor-2	+	+	+	+	
LIF	+	+	+	+	
PAF		+	+	+	
PDGF		+	+	+	
Activin A	+	+	+	+	Increased with endometrial cell coculture

(CSF: colony-stimulating factor; EGF: epithelial growth factor; GM-CSF: granulocyte-macrophage-colony stimulating factor; HB-EGF: heparin-binding epidermal growth factor; LIF: leukemia inhibitory factor; PAF: platelet-activating factor; PDGF: platelet-derived growth factor; TGF: transforming growth factor)

endotoxin and peroxide levels and gives better outcomes in ART procedures. Peroxide concentrations have a negative influence on embryos if it is just above 0.02 mEq/kg. A peroxide value specification of ≤ 0.01 mEq/kg has been implemented as a lot-release limit for Cook culture oil while Vitromed culture oil has peroxide value < 0.1 mEq/kg.

TYPE OF EMBRYO CULTURE MEDIA AND CELL CULTURE

The nutritional requirements of the embryo keep changing during development. Several authors have found that the required energy substrates, amino acids, and proteins concentrations differed according to the embryo stage. On the basis of these results, it was established that between *Days 1 and 3 (cleavage stage)*, the quantity of glucose should be reduced or removed if there are no amino acids or EDTA in the medium, in order to avoid the adverse effects of glucose. Lactate, pyruvate, NEAAs, and taurine should be included, but no EAAs at this point. A protein source such as albumin should also be added.

From *Day 3 to Day 5 (blastocyst stage)*, the concentration of glucose and 20 amino acids should be increased. Pyruvate concentration in particular is lower and protein requirements maintained. Change of media at Day 3 is appropriate, since the embryo undergoes a series of changes at this time, such as compaction and activation of the embryonic genome.

As a consequence, sequential media were developed. By contrast, the single-step media is based on letting the developing embryos choose the nutrients as per its requirement. This way it is possible to minimize the stress caused by different culture environments.

Sequential Media

The sequential media were developed to provide the dynamics of embryos nutrition and to mirror the environment of the female reproductive tract. The embryos are exposed to a gradient of nutrients as it passes along the fallopian tube in to the uterus. Sequential media systems are designed initially to provide optimal support for the development of the cleavage stage embryos. The culture media are subsequently changed to allow for optimal conditions for the extended culture to the blastocysts stage. These media systems are formulated to address the changing requirement of the developing embryos, thereby reducing the cellular stress and limiting the need for the embryo to undergo adaptation to grow to the blastocyst stage. Cleaving embryos use pyruvate and lactate as energy sources and NEAAs for protein metabolism. For the 8-cell stage onwards the major energy source is glucose and EAAs are required for protein metabolism (Table 3).

Single Step Media

Single medium formulation is used to support zygote development till the blastocyst stage. Monoculture is based on the principle of allowing the embryo to choose what it wants during preimplantation development. A monoculture system provides continuous support to the

TABLE 3 Commercially available sequential human embryo IVF culture media from different companies.

Culture Media/ Companies	*VITROLIFE (Sweden)*	*COOK Medical (USA)*	*ORIGIO EmbryoGen, BlastGen (Denmark)*	*ORIGIO Sequential (Denmark)*	*SAGE-Quinn's Advantage (Denmark)*	*IRVINE Scientific (France)*
Sperm preparation	Sperm RINSE, G-IVF PLUS	Sydney IVF sperm preparation media	Sperm preparation media origio	Origio sperm preparation medium	Quinn's sperm washing media	Sperm preparation medium Modified sperm washing media
Rinsing/ flushing media	G-RINSE G-MOPS	Cook Sydney Gamete Buffer	Flushing	Flushing	Quinn's advantage medium with HEPES	Modified HTF media with gentamicin HTF media Multipurpose handling medium (MHM)
Cleavage stage media (D2)	G-IVF PLUS	Cook Sydney fertilization	Origio sequential fertilization if ICSI is done shift oocytes to embryoGen	Origio sequential fertilization	Quinn's advantage fertilization medium	Continuous single culture medium-complete (CSCM-C)
Cleavage stage media (D2)	G-1 PLUS	Cook Sydney cleavage	EmbryoGen	Origio sequential cleavage	Quinn's advantage cleavage medium	Complete early cleavage medium (SSS)
Blastocyst stage media (D5)	G-2 PLUS	Cook Sydney Blastocyst	BlastGen	Origio sequential blastocyst	Quinn's advantage blastocyst	Complete multiBlast medium (SSS)
Embryo transfer	G1/G2 PLUS Embryo Glue	Cook Sydney cleavage blastocyst	Blastgen embryoGen	Origio sequential cleavage/blastocyst	Quinn's advantage cleavage/blastocyst	Complete early cleavage medium (SSS) Complete MultiBlast Medium (SSS)

(HTF: human tubal fluid; IVF: *in vitro* fertilization)

embryo throughout extended culture; hence there is no need to refresh the medium.

Single step media like Irvine's continuous single culture medium-complete (CSCM)-C have optimized energy substrates like D-glucose and L-lactate supporting uninterrupted continuous culture. These are designed to reduce ammonium buildup through the use of a stable glutamine source. In addition, they have high Mg^{2+} to Ca^{2+} ratio to limit detrimental stress-induced calcium influx into the embryo. Use of bioactive L-lactate helps in better control of pHi. The medium can also be used for embryo transfer.

In this series Irvine introduces a newer updated version of CSCM-C, that is CSCM-next generation media (CSCM-NX) which contains lower concentration of lactate as compare to CSCM-C. Lactate dehydrogenase (LDH) converts the glucose present in the culture medium to pyruvate and then into lactate, with the concomitant production of NAD^+ from NADH. This reaction is reversible and operates close to equilibrium. Embryos naturally produce two molecules of lactate from one molecule of glucose metabolism, with the increased consumption of glucose, concentration of lactate increases in the culture medium, resulting in a negative impact on embryo metabolism due to reduced pyruvate conversion by LDH and oxidation.

In a 110-patient prospective split-case trial, CSCM-NX had improved blastocyst rates when compared to CSCM. With the lower lactate concentration, CSCM-NX improves blastocyst formation by 18% when compared to continuous single culture (Table 4).

FUTURE OF EMBRYO CULTURE SYSTEM

Embryo Coculture

Embryo coculturing involves growing embryos in a culture medium on top of a layer of granulosa or endometrial cells. This underlying layer of cells provides the embryos with nutritional products while removing toxic substances from the medium, thereby promoting the development of higher quality embryos.

The uterus lining or the walls of the ovarian follicles and the fallopian tube are the most common sources for the "helper" cells used in embryo coculturing. The initial studies of embryo culture took place in animals. Cole and

TABLE 4 Single step embryo culture media for IVF/ICSI.

Culture Media/ Companies/OEM	*Vitrolife*	*Sage/origio*	*Irvine scientific*	*Global*	*Vitromed*
Sperm preparation	Sperm RINSE G-IVF	Sperm preparation media origio	Sperm washing media	GLOBAL W/HEPES	Sperm wash
Oocyte retrieval	G MOPS	Quinn's Advantage medium with HEPES flushing media	Modified htf media with gentamicin HTF media Multipurpose handling medium (MHM)	GLOBAL W/HEPES	HEPES plus
Fertilization media	Insemination to be done in G-IVF PLUS if ICSI is done shift injected oocytes in G-TL directly	Insemination to be done in origo fertilization media. If ICSI is done shift injected oocytes in SAGE 1-step	Continuous single culture medium complete (CSCM-C): this medium is optimized to be used in an uninterrupted culture system without disc change or medium renewal	GLOBAL fertilization, if ICSI is done shift injected oocytes to GLOBAL total	ONESTEP
Cleavage stage media (D2)	G-TL	SAGE 1- step allows uninterrupted culture following IVF or ICSI insemination through to the blastocyst stage, and is ideal for use with time lapse technology	CSCM-C	GLOBAL total	ONESTEP
Blastocyst stage media (D5)	G-TL	SAGE 1-step	CSCM-C	GLOBAL total	ONESTEP
Embryo transfer	G-TL	SAGE 1-step	CSCM-C ↓ CSCM-NX	GLOBAL total	ONESTEP

(HTF: human tubal fluid; ICSI: intracytoplasmic sperm injection; IVF: *in vitro* fertilization)

Paul, in 1965, reported improved rates of blastulation of mouse embryos culture on a HeLa cell lines.

Embryo coculturing should be recommended to only selected patients, who (1) have had unsuccessful IVF cycles in the past and (2) were unable to achieve successful pregnancy through IVF because of the poor embryo quality.

Despite the use of cell type, a coculture system needs three pivotal constituents: (1) embryo, (2) somatic cells, and (3) culture medium. Chosen somatic cells must assist embryonic development and must be reconcilable with the human embryo.

Epithelial cells seem to be most accepted however, debate for the best type of epithelial cell is still going on.

Nowadays, autologous endometrial coculture (AECC) systems have substituted the use of nonhuman or homologous cell types due to their benefit over other cells and availability.

In vivo, these cells are involved in peri-implantation embryonic development. Coculture impact embryo development through number of mechanisms. These incorporate the release of embryo trophic factors as well as the detoxification of the culture medium (by removal of free radicals, heavy metal cations, or metabolic inhibitors). In the coculture system, embryonic feeder cells provide various cytokines and growth factors that will allow the embryo to pass the critical stage of maternal-to-zygotic transition (MZT) permitting for complete development. These factors must be active during the first 3 days of culture to enhance the metabolic activity of the embryo, subsequently increasing its probability to develop and implant.

Paria and Dey reported paracrine/autocrine relationship between transforming growth factor-1 (TGF-1). These secreted factors have been shown to efficiently coordinate with the quality of embryo development, and successive pregnancy outcomes. The detrimental constituents of

TABLE 5 Enhancement of growth by different cells added in coculture.

Cell type	*Enhancement of growth*
Autologous cumulus cell coculture	Increased cell numbers, reduced fragmentation, and increased blastocyst formation
Human oviduct cells	Increased fertilization rates, cell numbers, and implantation rates
Autologous endometrial cells	Reduce fragmentation
Fetal bovine uterine fibroblasts	Reduced embryo fragmentation, increased cell-to-cell adherence, blastomere expansion, zona thickness variation, and improved hatching and increased ongoing pregnancy rates
Buffalo rat liver cells	Increased pregnancy and implantation
Vero (African green monkey kidney) cells	Improved embryo quality, increased cleavage rates, blastocyst formation, and pregnancy rates
Ovarian cancer cell coculture	Increased blastocyst formation

media (hypoxanthine and oxygen metabolites) hamper the embryo development.

Several studies reported the cross-talk between the developing embryo and the maternal endometrium, this activate certain paracrine factors that enhance the possibility of implantation. De los Santos in 1996, documented that a coculture system with human endometrial epithelial cells leads to increased secretion of embryonic paracrine markers and better uterine receptivity by upregulating certain key adhesion molecules. In 2001, Spandorfer et al. reported the presence of leukemia inhibitory factors (LIF) in coculture media and indicated a positive correlation between LIF levels and embryo development and clinical pregnancy rates.

Meta-analysis by Kattal et al. shows a remarkable benefit to coculture with refinements in implantation rate, blastomere number, and in clinical and ongoing pregnancy rates. For now, coculture is an effective method in the arsenal of ART for selected patients (Table 5).

Microfluidics (Fluid Dynamic Embryo Culture Systems)

The complex environment of oviduct's lumen provides a turbulent progressive movement for the oocyte and early embryo. The environment of the tubal/uterine fluid, the chemical composition, and their interaction create a unique environment able to support the development of embryo and modulate gene expression.

The transport initiates due to the flux created by cilia and peristaltic movements by the contraction of smooth muscles and hence this combined action over tubal crypts generates a turbulent flow towards the uterine horn. This flushes out the pathogens and nonmotile sperm, this initiates homogenization of tubal secretion and facilitation of gamete interaction. The range of velocity of tubal flow and frequency is calculated to range from 6.5 μm/sec to 29 μm/sec and 5 Hz to 20 Hz, respectively.

Dynamic fluid devices are not yet available for mass scale use in clinical embryology laboratories. Indeed, such devices for embryo culture have been constructed and they are under evaluation in Institutional Review Board (IRB). Fluid dynamic devices appear to enhance embryo development and they may be innovative resources for clinical and experimental embryology laboratories.

Media in traditional embryo culture are usually held in plastic culture dishes covered with oil to avoid evaporation. This dynamic culture strategy uses the same plate system, but varies from traditional static culture in that, while in the incubator, rotation, or tilting of the platform in which culture dishes are kept creates fluidic movement. This alters the environment in which the embryos cultured.

Platform movement to generate dynamic fluid in human embryo culture was examined recently by Matsuura et al. Reported methods to generate fluid dynamics can be divided into three categories.

1. Platform/dish movements
2. Wave fluid movement
3. Designed fluid dynamics.

CONCLUSION

The evolution of culture media experienced many folds with the significant development in ART. From simple salt solutions with glucose and egg yolk, to very complex solutions, closer to in vivo reproductive fluids.

Continuous changing nutritional requirements of the developing embryo, at every stage, originate the need to develop the sequential media. However, back to nature philosophy advocated the need of single step media.

Both approaches have its pros and cons and it is yet not clear which media offers best "in vitro" outcomes.

Clinical experiences and increased awareness of the safety and regulation exponential increased the quality of IVF media. Defined recombinant and nonprotein supplements are becoming more viable for gamete and embryo manipulation procedures. Dynamic systems are a new field of research, which may potentially help in understanding the physiological requirements of the embryo. Research is being conducted worldwide aiming to optimize the culture conditions to increase the IVF success rates. Microfluidics and dynamic culture systems aim to replenish the media and may move toward an automated and precise IVF "lab-on-a-chip".

EDITORS' COMMENTS

1. Media for embryo culture play a very important role for clinics take home baby rate.
2. Due to less exposure and time laps imaging system, single culture media are proved to be beneficial for embryo growth.
3. Coculture with cumulus cells is also feasible and easy technique which mimics natural environment with good results.

SUGGESTED READING

1. Adamson GD, Zegers-Hochschild F, Ishihara O, et al. ICMART world report: preliminary 2008 data. Hum Reprod. 2012;27(Suppl 2):ii38-ii39.
2. Alegretti JR, Rocha AM, Barros BC, et al. Microfluidic dynamic embryo culture increases the production of top quality human embryos through reduction in embryo fragmentation. Fertil Steril. 2011;96:S58-S59.
3. Arici A, Engin O, Attar E, Olive D. Modulation of leukemia inhibitory factor gene expression and protein biosynthesis in human endometrium. J Clin Endocrinol Metab.1995;80(6):1908-15.
4. Barmat LI, Worrilow KC, Paynton BV. Growth factor expression by human oviduct and buffalo rat liver co-culture cells. Fertil Steril. 1997;67(4):775-9.
5. Beebe D, Wheeler M, Zeringue H, et al. Microfluidic technology for assisted reproduction. Theriogenology. 2002;57(1):125-35.
6. Ben-Chetrit A, Jurisicova A, Casper RF. Co-culture with ovarian cancer cells enhances human blastocyst formation in vitro. Fertil Steril.1996;65(3):664-6.
7. Biggers JD. Thoughts on embryo culture conditions. Reprod Biomed Online. 2000;4 Suppl 1:30-8.
8. Boehm K, Daimon M, Gorodeski I, et al. Expression of the insulin-like and platelet derived growth factor genes in human uterine tissues. Mol Reprod Dev. 1990;27:93-101.
9. Cabrera LM, Bormann CL, Shah CT, et al. Dynamic micro funnel culture enhances mouse embryo development and pregnancy rates. Hum Reprod. 2010;25(3):613-22.
10. Chia CM, Winston RM, Handyside AH. EGF, TGF-alpha and EGFR expression in human preimplantation embryos. Development. 1995;121:299-307.
11. Chobotova K, Spyropoulou I, Carver J, et al. Heparin-binding epidermal growth factor and its receptor ErbB4 mediate implantation of the human blastocyst. Mech Dev. 2002;119(2):137-44.
12. Cohen J, Gilligan A, Esposito W, et al. Ambient air and its potential effects on conception in vitro. Hum Reprod. 1997;12(8):1742-9.
13. Cole R, Paul J. Properties of cultured preimplantation mouse and rabbit and cell strains developed from them. In: Colak D, Wolstenholme GEW (Eds). Preimplantation Stages of Pregnancy. Boston: Little, Brown; 1965. pp. 82-155.
14. Cross JC, Werb Z, Fisher SJ. Implantation and the placenta: key pieces of the development puzzle. Science. 1994;266(5190):1508-18.
15. Cullinan EB, Abbondanzo SJ, Anderson PS. et al. Leukemia inhibitory factor (LIF) and LIF receptor expression in human endometrium suggests a potential autocrine/paracrine function in regulating embryo implantation. Proc Natl Acad Sci USA. 1996;93(7):3115-20.
16. De los Santos MJ, Mercader A, Francés A, et al. Role of endometrial factors in regulating secretion of components of the immune-reactive human embryonic interleukin-1 system during embryonic development. Biol Reprod. 1996;54(3): 563-74.
17. Desai N, Goldfarb J. Growth factor/cytokine secretion by permanent human endometrial cell line with embryotrophic properties. J Assist Reprod Genet. 1996;1(3):546-50.
18. Di Blasio AM, Vigano P, Cremonesi L, et al. Expression of the genes encoding basic fibroblast growth factor and its receptor in human granulosa cells. Mol Cell Endocrinol. 1993;96:R7-R11.
19. Dornte RW. Oxidation of white oils. Indust Eng Chem. 1936;28(1):26-30.
20. Edwards LJ, Williams DA, Gardner DK. Intracellular pH of the mouse preimplantation mouse embryo: effect of extracellular pH and weak acids. Mol Reprod Dev. 1998;50(4):434-42.
21. Elpiniki C, Joyce C. Harper IVF culture media: past, present and future. Human Reproduction Update. 2015;21(1):39-55.
22. Familiari G, Verlengia C, Nottola SA. Heterogeneous distribution of fibronectin, tenascin-C, and laminin immune reactive material in the cumulus-coronal cells surrounding mature human oocytes from IVF-Et protocols—evidence that they are composed of different sub populations: an immunohistochemical assay using scanning confocal laser and fluorescence microscopy. Mol Reprod Dev. 1996;43(3):392-402.
23. Felice P, Pasquale F, Stefano L, et al. Expression and secretion of inhibin and activin in normal and neoplastic uterine tissues. High levels of serum activin A in women with endometrial and cervical carcinoma. J Clin Endocrinol Metab. 1998;83(4):1194-200.
24. Fitzharris G, Siyanov V, Baltz J M. Granulosa cells regulate oocyte intracellular pH against acidosis in preantral follicles by multiple mechanisms. Development. 2007;134(23): 4283-95.
25. Fitzharris G, Baltz J M. Granulosa cells regulate intracellular pH of murine growing oocyte via gap junctions: development of independent homeostasis during oocyte growth. Development. 2006;133(4):591-9.
26. Freeman MR, Whitworth CM, Hill GA. Granulosa cell co-culture enhances human embryo development and

pregnancy rate following in-vitro fertilization. Hum Reprod. 1995;10(2):408-14.

27. Fukui Y, McGowan IT, James RW, et al. Factors affecting the in vitro development to blastocysts of bovine oocytes matured and fertilized in vitro. J Reprod Fertil. 1991;92(1):125-31.
28. Gardner DK. Changes in requirements and utilization of nutrients during mammalian preimplantation embryo development and their significance in embryo culture. Theriogenology. 1998;49(1):83-102.
29. Giudice LC, Lamson G, Rosenfeld RG, et al. Insulin-like growth factor II (IGF-II) and IGF binding proteins in human endometrium. Ann NY Acad Sci. 1991;626:295-307.
30. Giudice LC, Dsupin BA, Jin IH, et al. Differential expression of messenger ribonucleic acids encoding insulin-like growth factors and their receptors in human uterine endometrium and decidua. J Clin Endocrinol Metab. 1993;76(5):1115-22.
31. Gordon JD, Mesiano S, Zaloudek CJ, Jaffe RB. Vascular endothelial growth factor localization in human ovary and fallopian tubes: possible role in reproductive function and ovarian cyst formation. Clin Endocrinol Metab.1996;81:353-9.
32. He Z, Liu H, Mele C, et al. Expression of inhibin/activin subunits and their receptors and binding proteins in human preimplantation embryos. J Assist Reprod Genet. 1999;16: 73-80.
33. Hediger MA, Romero MF, Peng JB, et al. The ABCs of solute carriers: physiological, pathological and therapeutic implications of human membrane transport proteins: introduction. Pflugers Arch. 2004;447(5):465-8
34. Hickman DL, Beebe DJ, Rodriguez-Zas SL, Wheeler MB. Comparison of static and dynamic medium environment for culturing of pre-implantation mouse embryos. Com Med. 2002:52(2):122-6.
35. Hippelein M. Background concentrations of individual and total volatile organic compounds in residential indoor air of Schleswig-Holstein, Germany. J Environ Monit. 2004;6(9):745-52.
36. Hodgson AT, Levin H. Volatile organic compounds in indoor air: a review of concentrations measured in North America since 1990. Berkeley, CA; Lawrence Berkeley National Laboratory; 2003.
37. Hornung D, Lebovic DI, Shifren JL, et al. Vectorial secretion of vascular endothelial growth factor by polarized human endometrial epithelial cells. Fertil Steril. 1998;69(5):909-15.
38. Hu Y, Maxson W, Hoffman D, et al. Co-culture with assisted hatching of human embryos using Buffalo rat liver cells. Hum Reprod. 1998;13(1):165-8.
39. Isachenko E, Maettner R ,Isachenko V, et al. Mechanical agitation during the in vitro culture of human pre-implantation embryos drastically increases the pregnancy rate. Clin Lab. 2010;56:569-76.
40. Isachenko V, Maettner R et al. In vitro culture of human embryos with mechanical micro vibration increases implantation rate. Reprod Biomed Online. 2011;22(6):536-44.
41. Jiang Q, Chen S, Xing F. Expression of epidermal growth factor receptor in human preimplantation embryos. Zhonghua Fu Chan Ke Za Zhi. 2000;35(8):468-9.
42. Kamat BR, Brown LF, Manseau EJ, et al. Expression of vascular permeability factor/vascular endothelial growth factor by human granulosa and theca lute in cells. Role in corpus luteum development. Am J Pathol. 1995;146(1):157-65.
43. Kaplan JH. Biochemistry of Na, K-ATPase. Annu Rev Biochem. 2002;71:511-35
44. Kattal N, Cohen J, Barmat LI. Role of coculture in human in vitro fertilization: a meta-analysis. Fertil Steril. 2008;90(4):1069-76.
45. Kauma SW, Aukerman SL, Eierman D, et al. Colony-stimulating factor-1 and C-FMS expression in human endometrial tissues and placenta during the menstrual cycle and early pregnancy. J Clin Endocrinol Metab. 1991;73: 746-51.
46. Keltz MD, Attar E, Buradagunta S, et al. Modulation of leukemia inhibitory factor gene expression and protein biosynthesis in the human fallopian tube. Am J Obstet Gynecol. 1996;175:1611-9.
47. Kervancioglu ME, Saridogan E, Atasü T, et al. Human fallopian tube epithelial cell co-culture increases fertilization rate in male factor infertility but not in tubal or unexplained fertility. Hum Reprod. 1997;12(6):1253-8.
48. Khoudja RY, Xu Y, Li T, et al. Better IVF outcomes following improvements in laboratory air quality. J Assist Reprod Genet. 2013;30(1):69-76.
49. Kurachi H, Morishige K, Imai T, et al. Expression of epidermal growth factor and transforming growth factor-alpha in fallopian tube epithelium and their role in embryogenesis. Horm Res. 1994;41(1):48-54.
50. Lam PM, Briton-Jones C, Cheung CK, et al. Vascular endothelial growth factor in the human oviduct: localization and regulation of messenger RNA expression in vivo. Biol Reprod. 2003;68(5):1870-6.
51. Lane M, Gardner DK. Ammonium induces aberrant blastocyst differentiation, metabolism, pH regulation, gene expression and subsequently alters fetal development in the mouse. Biol Reprod. 2003;69(4):1109-17.
52. Leach R, Khalifa R, Ramirez N, et al. Multiple roles for heparin-binding epidermal growth factor-like growth factor are suggested by its cell-specific expression during the human endometrial cycle and early placentation. J Clin Endocrinol Metab. 1999;84:3355-63.
53. Leese HJ. Human embryo culture: back to nature. J Assist Reprod Genet. 1998;15(8):466-8.
54. Lighten A, Hardy K, Winston R, et al. Expression of m-RNA for the insulin-like growth factors and their receptors in human preimplantation embryos. Mol Reprod Dev. 1997;47:134-9.
55. Liu Y, Shao M, Fu L, et al. Source profiles of volatile organic compounds (VOCs) measured in China: part I. Atmos Environ. 2008;42(25):6247-60.
56. Loutradis D, John D, Kiessling AA. Hypoxanthine causes a 2-cell block in random-bred mouse embryos. Biol Reprod. 1987;37(2):311-6.
57. Magli M, Gianaroli L, Ferraretti AP, et al. Human embryo coculture: results of a randomized study. Int J Fertil Menopausal Stud. 1995;40:254-9.
58. Mansour R, Aboulghar M, Serour G, et al. Co-culture of human pronucleate oocyte with their cumulus cells. Hum Reprod. 1994;9:1727-9.
59. Massachusetts General Hospital. Normal reference laboratory values. N Engl J Med. 1980;302:37-48.
60. Matsuura K, Hayashi N, Kuroda Y, et al. Improved development of mouse and human embryos using a tilting embryo culture system. Reprod Biomed Online. 2010;20(3):358-64.

61. Menezo Y, Servy E, Veiga A, et al. embryo culture methods and protocols. Methods in molecular biology (Internet). New York: Humana Press; 1980. pp. 231-47.
62. Menezo Y, Elder K. The enhancers of oocyte competence. In: Tosti E, Boni R (Eds). Oocyte Maturation and Fertilization: A Long History for a Short Event. Sharjah: Bentham Science Publishers Ltd; 2011. pp. 64-70.
63. Menezo Y, Testart J, Perrone D. Serum is not necessary in human in vitro fertilization, early embryo culture, and transfer. Fertil Steril. 1984;42(5):750-5.
64. Morbeck DE, Krisher RL, Herrick JR, et al. Composition of commercial media used for human embryo culture. Fertile Sterile. 2014;102:759-66.
65. Morbeck DE, Leonard PH. Culture systems: mineral oil overlay. In: Smith GD, Swain JE, Pool TB (Eds). Embryo Culture: Methods and Protocols. Totowa, NJ; Humana Press; 2012. pp. 325-31.
66. Morishige K, Kurachi H, Amemiya K, et al. Menstrual stage-specific expression of epidermal growth factor and transforming growth factor-alpha in human oviduct epithelium and their role in early embryogenesis. Endocrinology. 1993;133:199-207.
67. Muttukrishna S, Groome N, Ledger W. Gonadotropic control of secretion of dimeric inhibin and activin A by human granulosa-luteal cells in vitro. J Assist Reprod Genet. 1997;14:566-74.
68. Neulen J, Raczek S, Pogorzelski M, et al. Secretion of vascular endothelial growth factor/vascular permeability factor from human luteinized granulose cells is human chorionic gonadotrophin dependent. Mol Hum Reprod. 1998;4(3): 203-6.
69. Neulen J, Yan Z, Raczek S, et al. Human chorionic gonadotropin-dependent expression of vascular endothelial growth factor/vascular permeability factor in human granulosa cell: importance in ovarian hyperstimulation syndrome. J Clin Endocrinol Metab. 1995;80:1967-71.
70. Nieto F, Watkins WB, Lopata A, et al. The effects of co-culture with analogous cryopreserved endometrial cells on human in vitro fertilization and early embryo morphology: a randomized study. J Assist Reprod Genet. 1996;13(5):386-9.
71. Osterlund G, Wramsby H, Pousette A. Temporal expression of platelet-derived growth factor (PGDF)-A and its receptor in human preimplantation embryos. Mol Hum Reprod. 1996;2(7):507-12.
72. Otsuki J, Nagai Y, Chiba K. Damage of embryo development caused by peroxidized mineral oil and its association with albumin in culture. Fertil Steril. 2009;91(5):1745-9.
73. Otsuki J, Nagai Y, Chiba K. Peroxidation of mineral oil used in droplet culture is detrimental to fertilization and embryo development. Fertil Steril. 2007;88(3):741-3.
74. Paltieli Y, Wechselbaum A, Hoffman N, et al. Laser scattering instrument for real time in vivo measurement of ciliary activity in human fallopian tubes. Hum Reprod. 1995;10(7):1638-41.
75. Pampfer s, Arceci RJ, Pollard JW. Role of colony stimulating factor-1 (CSF-1) and other lymphohematopoietic growth factor in pre-implantation development. Bioessays. 1991; 13(10):535-40.
76. Paria BC, Dey SK. Preimplantation embryo development in vitro: cooperative interactions among embryos and role of growth factors. Proc Natl Acad Sci USA. 1990;87(12):4756-60.
77. Pfeifer TL ,Chegini N. Immunohistochemical localization of insulin-like growth factor (IGF-I), IGF-I receptor, and IGF binding proteins 1-4 in human fallopian tube at various reproductive. Biol Reprod. 1994;50:281-9.
78. Phillips KP, Leveille MC, Claman P, Baltz JM. Intracellular pH regulation in human preimplantation embryos. Hum Reprod. 2000;15(4):896-904.
79. Poddar TK, Sirkar KK. Henry's law constant for selected volatile organic compounds in high boiling oils. J Chem Eng Data. 1996;41(6):1329-32.
80. Pool TB. An update on embryo culture for human assisted reproductive technology: media, performance, and safety. Semin Reprod Med. 2005;23(4):309-18.
81. Prince RJ. Base oils from petroleum. In: Mortier RM, Fox MF, Orszulik ST (Eds). Chemistry and Technology of Lubricants. 3rd edition. New York, NY; Springer Dordrecht Heidelberg; 2010. pp. 3-33.
82. Puglia U, Motta PM. A new morpho-functional classification of the fallopian tube based on its three-dimensional myoarchitecture. Histopathol. 2001;16(1):227-37.
83. Quinn P, Kerin JF, Warnes GM. Improved pregnancy rate in human in vitro fertilization with the use of a medium based on the composition of human tubal fluid. Fertil Steril. 1985;44(4):493-8.
84. Quinn P, Margalit R. Beneficial effects of co-culture with cumulus cells on blastocyst formation in a prospective trial with supernumerary human embryos. J Assist Reprod Genet. 1996;13:9-14.
85. Quinn P. Culture systems: sequential. Methods Mol Biol. 2012;912:211-30.
86. Ramasharma K, Li C. Human pituitary and placental hormones control human insulin like growth factor II secretion in human granulosa cells. Proc Natl Acad Sci USA. 1987;84(9):2643-7.
87. Ringer S. Concerning the influence exerted by each of the constituents of the food on the contraction of ventricles. J Physiol Lond. 1982;3:380-93.
88. Rock J, Menkin MF. In vitro fertilization and cleavage of human ovarian eggs. Science. 1944;10:105-7.
89. Roudebush W, Purnell E, Stoddart N, Fleming S. Embryonic platelet-activating factor, temporal expression of the ligand and receptor. J Assist Reprod Genet. 2002;19:72-8.
90. Salmassi A, Zhang Z, Schmutzler AG, et al. Expression of mRNA and protein of macrophage colony-stimulating factor and its receptor in human follicular luteinized granulosa cells. Fertil Steril. 2005;83:419-25.
91. Sato A, Bo M, Otani T, Mochizuki M. Expression of epidermal growth factor-alpha and epidermal growth factor receptor messenger RNA in human endometrium and endometrial carcinoma. Nippon Sanka Fujinka Gakkai Zasshi. 1995;47: 473-78.
92. Schillaci R, Ciriminna R, Cefalu E, et al. Vero cell effect on in-vitro human blastocyst development: preliminary results. Hum Reprod. 1994;9:1131-5.

93. Simon C, Gimeno MJ, Mercader A, et al. Embryonic regulation of integrins beta 3, alpha 4, and alpha 1 in human endometrial epithelial cells in vitro. J Clin Endocrinol Metal. 1997;82(8):2607-16.
94. Sjoblom C, Wikland M, Robertson S. Granulocyte-macrophage colony-stimulating factor (GM-CSF) acts independently of the beta common subunit of the GM-CSF receptor to prevent inner cell mass apoptosis in human embryos. Biol Reprod. 2002;67:1817-23.
95. Smotrich DB, Stillman RJ, Widra EA, et al. Immunocytochemical localization of growth factors and their receptors in human pre-embryos and fallopian tubes. Hum Reprod. 1996;11: 184-90.
96. Spandorfer SD, Navarro J, Levy D, et al. Autologous endometrial co-culture in patients with in vitro fertilization (IVF) failure: correlations of outcome with leukemia inhibiting factor (LIF) production. Am J Reprod Immunol. 2001;46(6):375-80.
97. Stavreus-Evers A, Aghajanova L, Brismar H, et al. Co-existence of heparin binding epidermal growth factor like growth factor and pinopodes in human endometrium at the time of implantation. Mol Hum Reprod. 2002;8(8):765-76.
98. Sugino N, Kashida S, Karube-Harada A, et al. Expression of vascular endothelial growth factor (VEGF) and its receptors in human endometrium throughout the menstrual cycle and in early pregnancy. Reproduction. 2002;123:379-87.
99. Sugino N, Kashida S, Takiguchi S, et al. Expression of vascular endothelial growth factor and its receptors in the human corpus luteum during the menstrual cycle and in early pregnancy. J Clin Endocrinol Metab. 2000;85:3919-24.
100. Swain JE, Lai D, Takayama S, et al .Thinking big by thinking small: application of microfluidic technology to improve ART. Lab Chip. 2013;13(7):1213-24.
101. Swain JE. Optimizing the culture environment in the IVF laboratory: impact of pH and buffer capacity on gamete and embryo quality. Reprod Biomed Online. 2010;18(6):799-810.
102. Tang XM, Rossi MJ, Masterson BJ, Chegini N. Insulin-like growth factor I (IGF-I), IGF-I receptors and IGF binding proteins 1-4 in human uterine tissue, tissue localization and IGF-I action in endometrial stromal and myometrial smooth muscle cells in vitro. Biol Reprod. 1994;50(5):1113-25.
103. Tazuke SI, Giudice LC. Growth factors and cytokines in endometrium, embryonic development, and maternal: embryonic interactions. Semin Reprod Endocrinol. 1996; 14(3):231-45.
104. Torry DS, Holt VJ, Keenan JA, et al. Vascular endothelial growth factor expression in cycling human endometrium. Fertil Steril. 1996;66(1):72-80.
105. Tsai H, Chang C, Hsieh Y, Lo H. Leukemia inhibitory factor expression in different endometrial locations between fertile and infertile women throughout different menstrual phases. J Assist Reprod Genet. 2000;17:415-8.
106. Turner K, Lenton EA. The influence of Vero cell culture on human embryo development and chorionic gonadotropin production in vitro. Hum Reprod. 1996;11:1966-74.
107. Vajta G, Rienzi L, Cobo A, et al. Embryo culture: can we perform better than nature? Reprod Biomed Online. 2010;20(4):453-69.
108. van Ejik MJ, Mandelbaum J, Salat-Baroux J, et al. Expression of leukaemia inhibitory factor receptor subunits LIFR beta and gp130 in human oocytes and preimplantation embryos. Mol Hum Reprod. 1996;2(5):355-60.
109. Wanggeen K, Lalitkumar P, Hambiliki F, et al. Leukaemia inhibitory factor receptor and gp130 in the human fallopian tube and endometrium before and after mifepristone treatment and in the human preimplantation embryo. Mol Hum Reprod. 2007;13(6):391-7.
110. Watson R, Anthony F, Pickett M, et al. Reverse transcription with nested polymerase chain reaction shows expression of basic fibroblast growth factor transcripts in human granulosa and cumulus cells from in vitro fertilisation patients. Biochem Biophys Res Commun. 1992;187(3):1227-31.
111. White E, Popoff T, Ni T. Low lactate culture medium improves the development of human preimplantation embryos in vitro. ESHRE; 2017.
112. Wiemer K, Cohen J, Wiker SR, et al. Co-culture of human zygote on fetal bovine uterine fibroblast: embryonic morphology and implantation. Fertil Steril. 1989;52:503-8.
113. Yao T, Asayama Y. Human preimplantation embryo culture media: past, present, and future. J Mamm. Ova Res. 2016; 33(1):17-34.
114. Yeung WS, Lau EY, Chan ST, et al. Co-culture with homologous oviduct cells improved the implantation of human embryos—a prospective randomized control trial. J Assist Reprod Genet. 1996;13(10):762-7.
115. Yoo H, Barlow D, Mardon H. Temporal and spatial regulation of expression of heparin binding epidermal growth factor like growth factor in the human endometrium, a possible role in blastocyst implantation. Dev Genet. 1997;21:102-8.
116. Zander-Fox DL, Mitchell M, Thompson JG, et al. Alterations in mouse embryo intracellular pH by DMO during culture impair implantation and fetal growth. Reprod Biomed Online. 2010;21(2):219-29.
117. Zhang L, Scott PA, Turley H, et al. Validation of anti-vascular endothelial growth factor (anti VEGF) antibodies for immunohistochemical localization of VEGF in tissue sections: expression of VEGF in the human endometrium. J Pathol. 1998;185(4):402-8.
118. Zhao y, Chegini N. The expression of granulocyte macrophage colony stimulating factor (GM-CSF) and receptors in human endometrium. Am J Reprod Immonol. 1999;42:303-11.
119. Zolti M, Ben-Rafael Z, Meirom R, et al. Cytokine involvement in oocytes and early embryos. Fertil steril. 1991;56(2): 265-72.

32

CHAPTER

Oocyte Quality and Markers

Vijay Mangoli

INTRODUCTION

Like woman...like oocyte!

An oocyte is a mysterious, unsolved entity. This largest single cell of the body possesses tremendous ability of creation of life. It acquires this ability in a stepwise manner during oogenesis which begins as primary oocytes before birth of the girl in the fetal ovary where it undergoes deoxyribonucleic acid (DNA) synthesis and enters meiosis I. The maturity continues as secondary oocytes after onset of puberty. After various stages of prophase I, its growth arrests at dictyotene stage characterized by a nucleus called germinal vesicle. Its maturity process still continues until just before ovulation when an ovum with haploid number of chromosomes having 1N chromatids is released.

Though theoretically this ovum is ready to get fertilized by male gamete—the sperm, there are many factors responsible for a successful fertilization. As fate of an oocyte is ultimately to grow into a fully functional organism, it must prepare itself to regulate numerous cellular and developmental processes. Fertilization is one of the initial events of embryogenesis. Further viable embryonic growth depends upon collective ability of cytoplasm—comprising of various organelles embedded in the cytosol.

In procedures like *in vitro* fertilization (IVF), where ovaries are stimulated aiming to obtain 10–15 oocytes, all of them may not have potential to form a viable embryo.

Here we should not forget contribution of male gamete in embryogenesis which plays an equal and significant role. As it is beyond scope of this chapter, this aspect is discussed in section.

Though growth potential of the retrieved oocytes cannot be accurately predicted, there are certain morphological criteria and other markers which may help us in assessing overall oocyte quality that correlates with fertilization and embryonic growth. Oocyte quality can be assessed by morphology, by analyzing composition of follicular fluid, by means of proteomics—measuring metabolites excreted into the medium during culture and by studying genetic constitution of polar bodies.

Even after 4 decades of successful application of human IVF, morphological evaluation remains single most routinely used method for oocyte assessment—mainly because it is noninvasive, rapid, can be performed as part of routine handling, and has acceptable predictive value.

In IVF, quality of oocytes largely depends upon response of the patient to the stimulation protocol in that particular cycle. Grossly, these responses can be categorized as:

- Good response throughout the cycle
- Initial good response that becomes poor towards the mid-cycle
- Initial poor response that turns out to be better towards mid-cycle, and
- Poor response throughout the cycle.

From first group, one can expect majority of mature, metaphase II (MII) oocytes. Second and third group may produce mixed crop of mature, immature, and atretic oocytes. Fourth group results in more atretic oocytes and many times these cycles may have to be cancelled due to poor response.

TABLE 1 Morphological assessment of oocyte maturity.

Maturity parameter	*Mature*	*Intermediate*	*Immature*	*post mature*	*Atretic*
Cumulus	Fully expanded, even distribution Embedded in mucoid matrix	Slightly expanded, even distribution	Compact, uneven distribution	Scanty	Clumpy/absent
Corona	Radiating, sunburst	Radiating, staggered	Compact, tightly adhered	Uneven, clumpy	Scanty/absent
Ooplasm	Shiny, clear, round even with 1st polar body	Even, slightly dark, without polar body extruded	Dark, uneven, less PV space, with GV	Large PV, with vacuoles	Uneven, dark. Maybe at any stage of maturity
Granulosa cells	Abundant, loose aggregation, regular cytoplasm	Few, compact	Clumped	Scanty clumped, with dark cytoplasm	Dark, clumped/crushed pieces

(GV: germinal vesicle; PV: perivitelline)

MORPHOLOGICAL ASSESSMENT

When preovulatory oocytes are retrieved through ovum pickup procedure, they display various aspects of maturation, integrity, and viability. Their morphological evaluation can be performed at two stages: (1) cellular assessment under stereomicroscope and (2) cytoplasmic and nuclear assessment using inverted microscope.

At present, rapid visual assessment remains the only practical method for maturity evaluation as there is no reliable and quick biochemical testing available to do so. Oocytes are graded by assessing cumulus, corona, granulose cells, and ooplasm. Table 1 illustrates the correlation between these parameters and maturity status.

When conventional IVF is selected as a mode of insemination, the oocytes are exceptionally stripped of cellular matrix layers—cumulus and corona. This is mainly because sufficient numbers of sperms are available to digest these layers and attain more or less "natural" fertilization. In this situation, oocyte maturity which is an indicative of its quality is assessed based on certain cellular parameters. Such evaluation is done using a stereomicroscope with high resolution optics and good depth of field that allows initial screening at different focal planes. This is the simplest method to assess overall quality of the oocytes primarily to decide preincubation time prior to insemination. Also it requires relatively less time to evaluate. However, cellular assessment has its limitations. This evaluation is based only on the investments around the oocyte and may or may not correlate with nuclear maturity. This demands the need of nuclear evaluation. It is bit difficult and tricky to do nuclear evaluation with outer investments intact around the eggs. Some groups do it by placing oocytes in a flat bottom petri dish with little medium in it that spreads the cumulus-corona (CC) complex. Though it allows us to get structural details like polar body (PB) and ooplasm quality to some extent, the oocytes may get osmotic and pH shock if the observation time is prolonged.

For intracytoplasmic sperm injection (ICSI) as mode of insemination, oocytes are denuded for facilitation of nuclear assessment to confirm MII status and also to perform procedure efficiently without blocking injecting needle with cumulus/corona cells. When denuded, they display certain cytoplasmic characteristics typical of their maturity status.

An oocyte can be mature, intermediate, immature, postmature, or atretic.

Mature Oocyte

A mature oocyte is the one that has acquired cellular and genetic capability to get fertilized by a sperm. Under stereomicroscope, a typical mature oocyte display well spreaded cumulus showing a sunburst appearance and a loose coronal layer attached to the zona pellucida (ZP). Occasionally it is possible to visualize presence of first PB. With good quality sperms, such oocytes generally get fertilized resulting in transferrable embryos. At denuded stage, the cytoplasm appears even, shiny, clear, with minimum perivitelline space (PVS), oolemma almost touching inner membrane of ZP, showing a clear, round or slightly oval first PB, and overall optimum diameter ranging from 120 μm to 150 μm (Figs. 1A and B).

Intermediate Oocyte

These oocytes are neither fully mature nor completely immature. They have completed their cytoplasmic maturation, but slightly lagging behind in nuclear maturity. It is a stage postgerminal vesicle breakdown, before first PB is extruded. Such oocytes display less expansion of cumulus

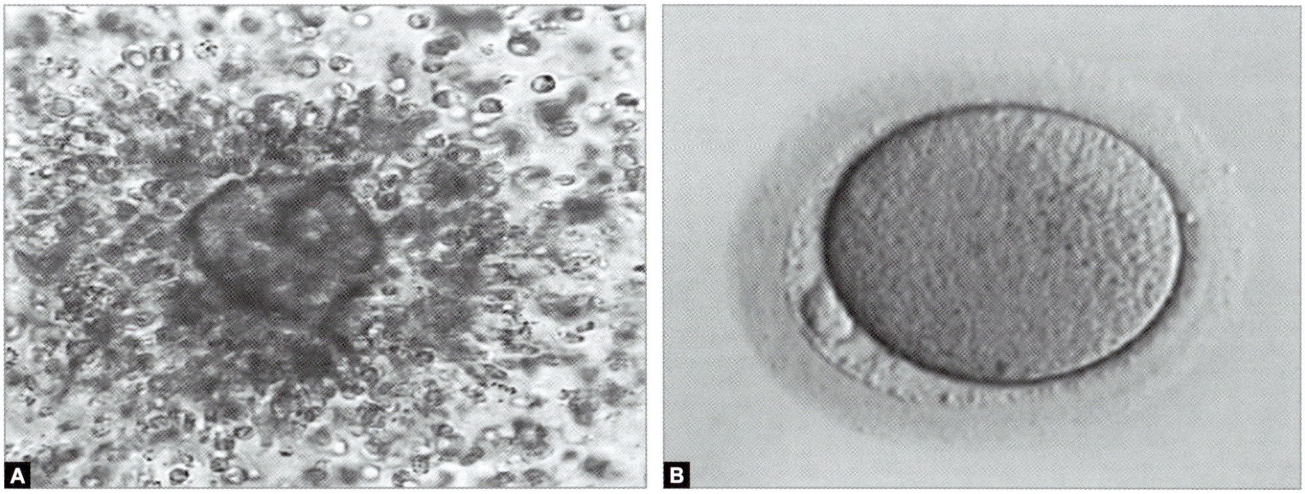

Figs. 1A and B: (A) Mature oocyte, cellular; (B) Mature oocyte, nuclear.

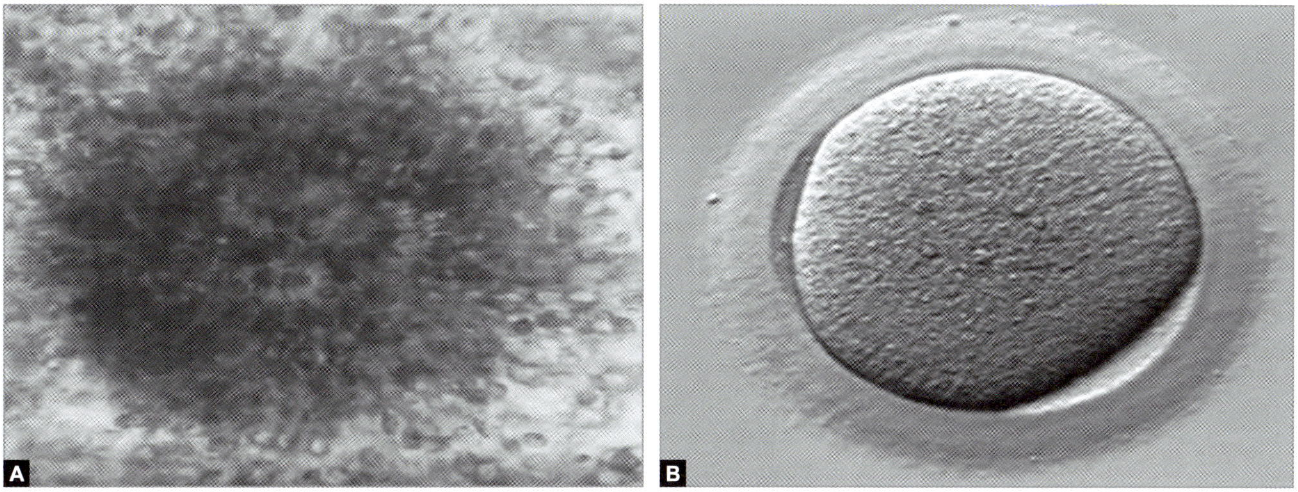

Figs. 2A and B: (A) Intermediate oocyte, cellular; (B) Intermediate oocyte, nuclear.

though evenly distributed. Corona is radiating but staggered with few, compact granulosa cells around. At denuded stage, they display even, with slightly dark ooplasm, without PB extruded. These oocytes usually complete their maturation in 2–6 hours after retrieval and do get fertilized normally (Figs. 2A and B).

Immature Oocyte

These are the oocytes with incomplete cytoplasmic and nuclear maturity. They display compact, unevenly distributed cumulus with tightly adhered corona. Ooplasm is dark, uneven with very thin PVS. Follicular fluid has clumpy granulosa cells. Denuded, they display dark, uneven ooplasm with less PVS with a prominent germinal vesicle. They are not ready for fertilization and may or may not complete their maturation in vitro for further 24 hours. Even if they acquire maturity status of MII and are inseminated next day, they are more likely to result in abnormal fertilization with polyploidy and hampered embryonic growth (Figs. 3A and B).

Postmature

Few oocytes begin their maturity process much earlier in the follicle and by the time they are retrieved, they surpass the

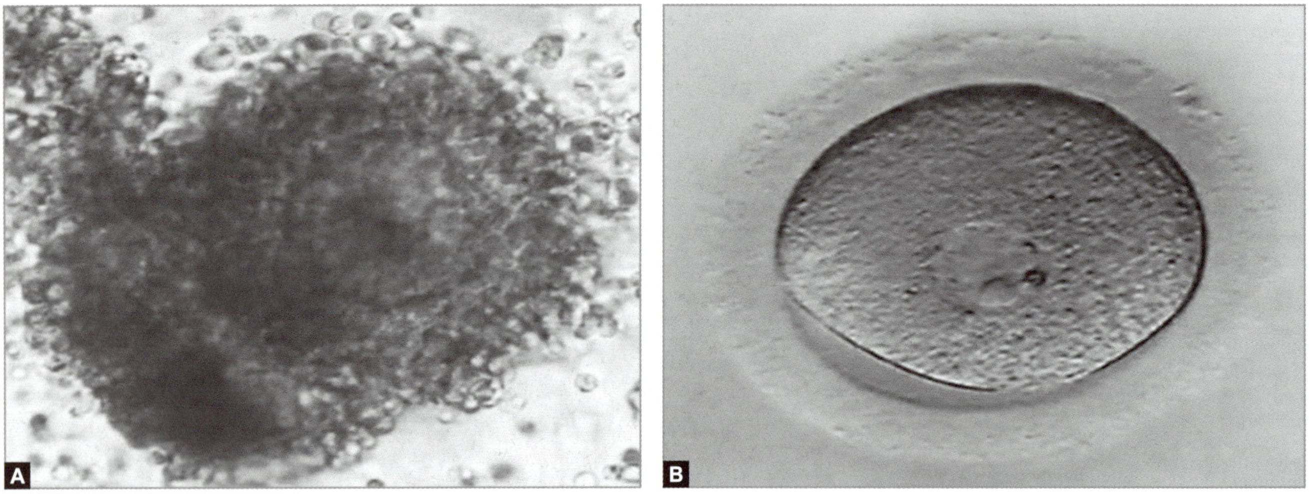

Figs. 3A and B: (A) Immature oocyte, cellular; (B) Immature oocyte, nuclear.

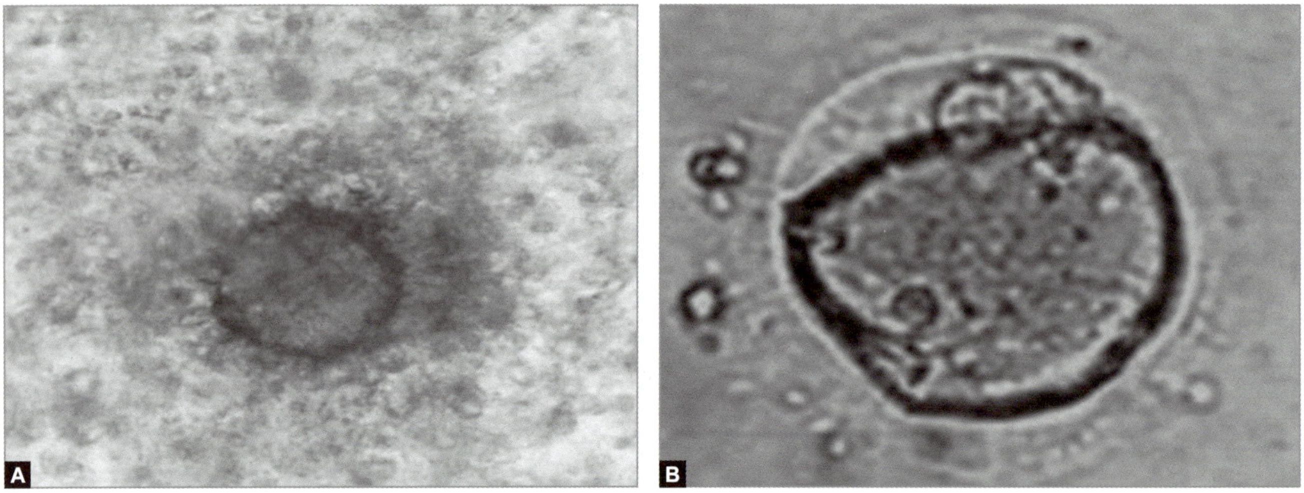

Figs. 4A and B: (A) Postmature oocyte, cellular; (B) Postmature oocyte, nuclear.

optimum timeframe to get fertilized. These oocytes display very scanty or even absent CC complex. They have uneven ooplasm with fragmented PB (Figs. 4A and B).

Atretic

These are the oocytes where maturity process is arrested during oogenesis. This arrest can be at any stage and the exact cause is not known. Generally they display uneven, patchy distribution of cumulus and corona layers. Their cytoplasm may show any of the maturity status from germinal vesicle to fragmented PB (Figs. 5A and B).

During microscopic observation, apart from regular components i.e. zona, oolemma, ooplasm, and PB, oocytes reveal certain features which may or may not contribute to fertilization. For example, slight zona thickness variation or mild ooplasm granularity may be insignificant for fertilization outcome.

However, there are certain abnormalities which adversely affect fertilization. These abnormalities can be categorized in three groups:

1. Intracytoplasmic
2. Extracytoplasmic, and
3. Morphologic.

Intracytoplasmic Abnormalities

This includes presence of:

- Vacuoles
- Smooth endoplasmic reticulum (sER)
- Refractile bodies
- Dark, granular texture of the ooplasm.

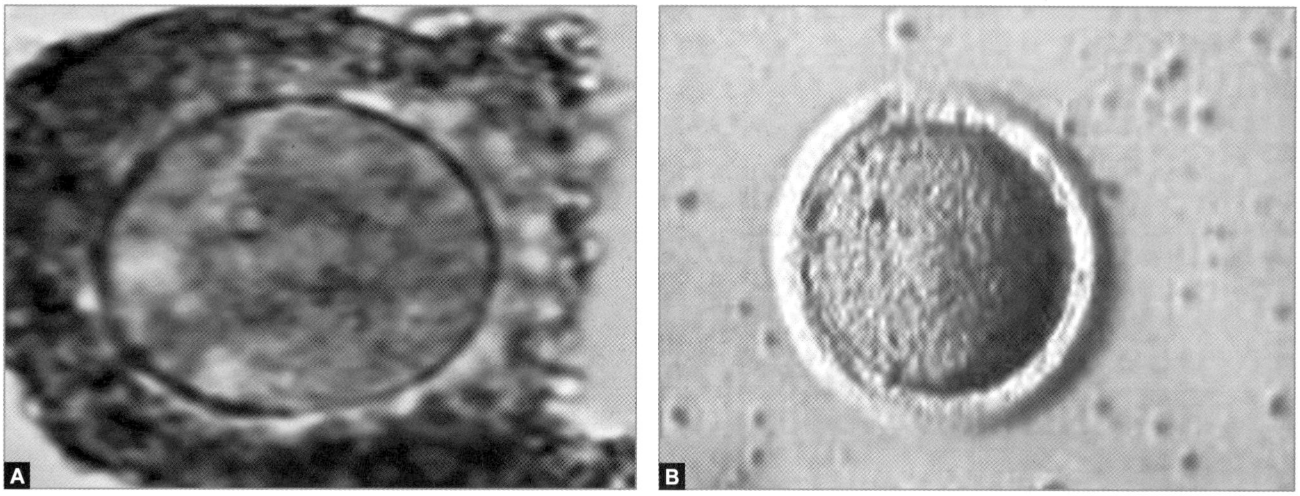

Figs. 5A and B: (A) Atretic oocyte, cellular; (B) Atretic oocyte, nuclear.

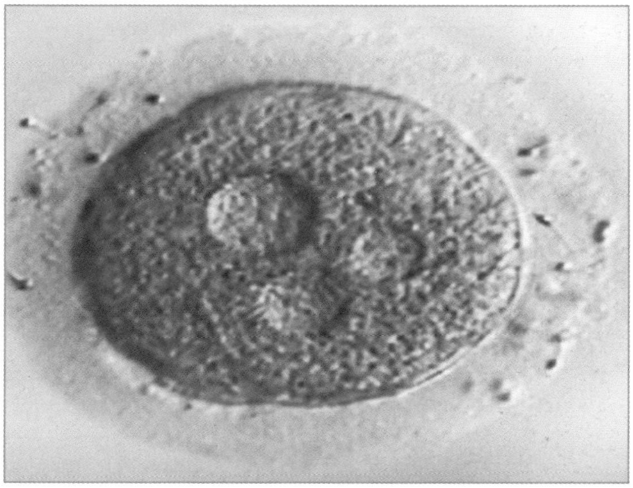

Fig. 6: Oocyte with vacuoles.

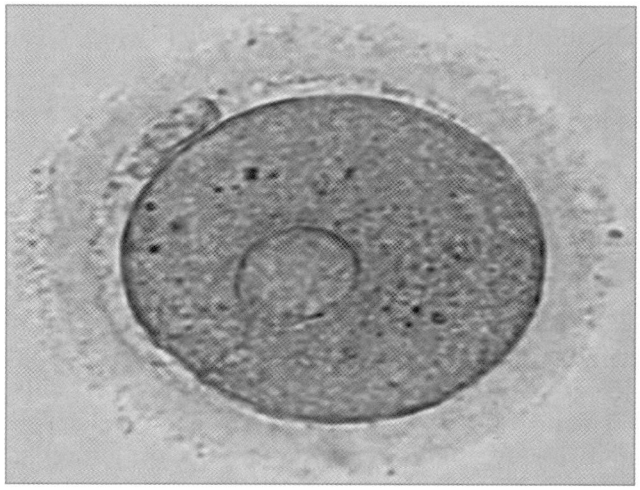

Fig. 7: Oocyte with smooth endoplasmic reticulum.

Vacuoles are membrane bound fluid filled inclusions that may arise spontaneously during oocyte maturation, induced during ICSI procedure or at the time of cell division. 1-2 vacuoles of < 4 μm in diameter may not have significant impact on fertilization; however, larger vacuoles of >14 μm have negative effect on fertilization and subsequent blastocyst formation rates (Fig. 6).

Aggregation of sER is observed only in MII oocytes and has an incidence of 2%. In cycles with affected oocytes the frequency can be as high as 25%. Formation of these structures might correlate with high estradiol levels. During ICSI procedure, if sER aggregation is not disturbed fertilization rate remains unaffected. However, sER aggregation is associated with an impaired blastocyst formation (18%), a lower pregnancy outcome, obstetric problems, and a lower birth weight (Fig. 7).

Refractile body—lipofuscin/refractile inclusions consist of a mixture of lipids and dense granular materials. They can be found in different stages of oocyte maturity. Large lipofuscin inclusions, above 5 μm, are associated with significantly reduced fertilization and unfavorable blastocyst development. Presence of refractile bodies is the single largest cause responsible for failed fertilization in a mature oocyte (Fig. 8).

Central granularity is a morphological feature of the oocyte that is recognized as a large, dark, and spongy granular area in the cytoplasm. This anomaly represents a poor cytoplasmic maturity and is seen in 35% of the oocytes. Granularity has no effect on fertilization rate and embryo development or quality, but it is correlated with an impaired ongoing pregnancy rate of only 13%. Preimplantation genetic diagnosis showed an aneuploidy rate of 52% in

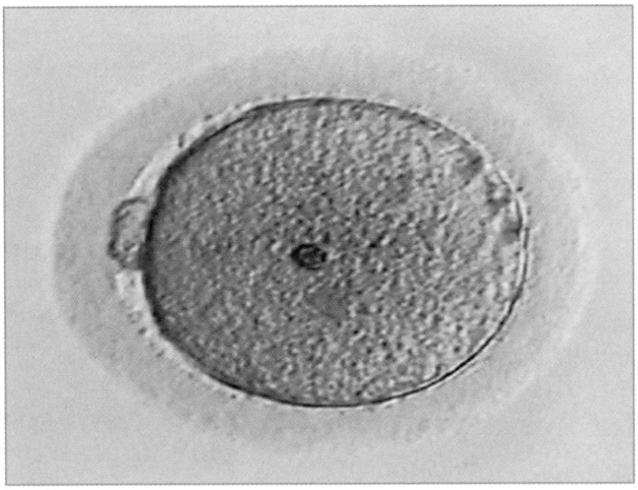

Fig. 8: Oocyte with refractile body.

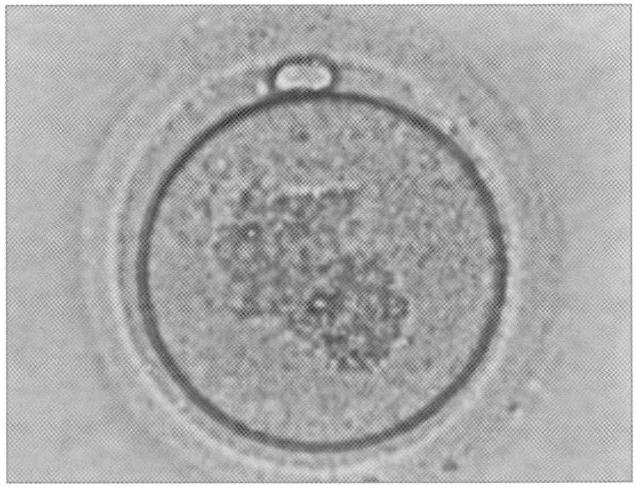

Fig. 9: Oocyte with central granular ooplasm.

blastomeres originating from these oocytes which might explain the high abortion rate (Fig. 9).

Extracellular Abnormalities

Metaphase II oocytes with extracytoplasmic abnormalities:

- Thick, dark, uneven, and irregular ZP
- Large, fragmented, and multiple PB
- Perivitelline debris and wide PVS.

Zona pellucida: Human ZP is the extracellular spherical shell with remarkably uniform thickness of average 15 µm that surrounds the oocyte. It is a protective outer membrane with permeable to enzymes, immunoglobulins, and viruses along with solutions with low molecular weight molecules like Dimethyl sulfoxide (DMSO) and alcohols. ZP dysmorphology has an incidence of 2–5% of all oocytes. Thick zona may hinder fertilization in natural conception or in conventional IVF due to nonbinding of sperm. Thick zona may also adversely affect implantation due to hatching failure thus preventing communication between embryo and uterine lining. Sometimes altered zona structure may lose its ability to prevent polyspermy resulting in polyploidy. Generally, minor variations do not seem to affect fertilization capacity of the oocyte (Fig. 10).

Polar body: Assessment of first PB for size, shape, and extent of fragmentation may be used to determine postovulatory age of the oocyte. As compared to intact PB, fragmented PB is reported to be associated with lower fertilization, blastulation, implantation, and take home baby rates.

However, because the first PB has a very short lifetime, its morphology changes after a few hours of in vitro culture. Therefore, PB morphology assessment may not serve as a reliable marker of oocyte quality and developmental competence (Figs. 11A and B).

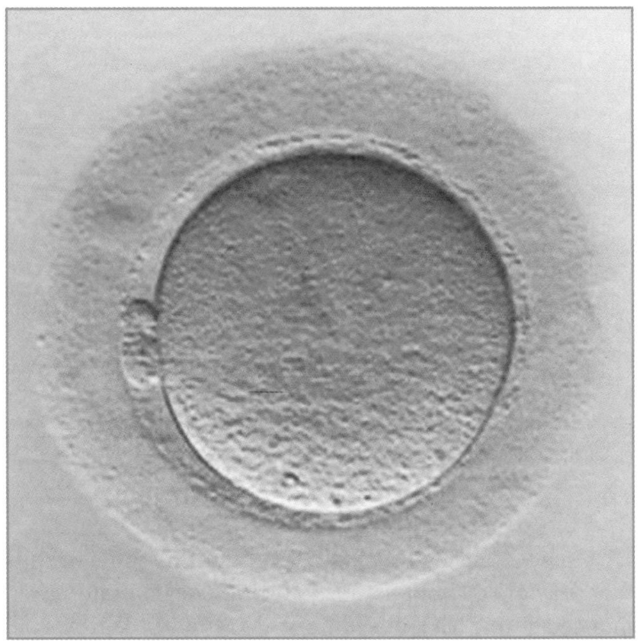

Fig. 10: Metaphase II (MII) oocyte with thick zona.

Perivitelline space: PV abnormalities are among most significant dysmorphisms of oocyte. Large PVS is reported to be associated with aging of oocytes thus resulting in increased aneuploidies. Granular PV is indicative of altered cortical granule reaction capacity and results in polyploidy, oocyte degeneration, and lower fertilization rates (Fig. 12).

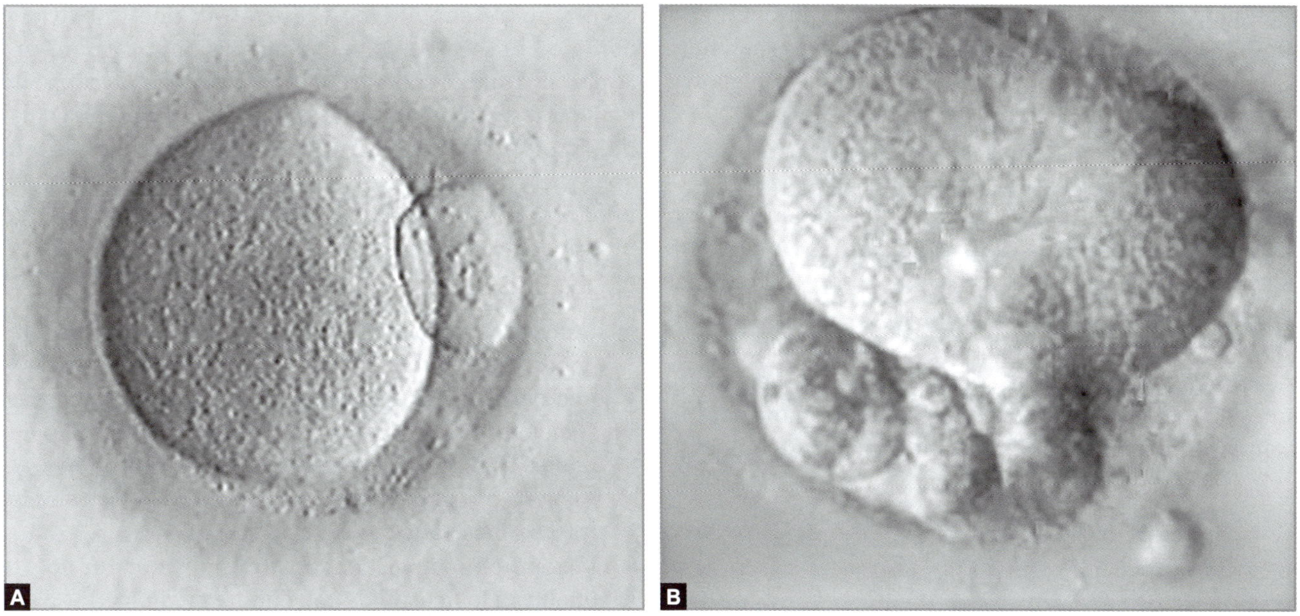

Figs. 11A and B: (A) Oocyte with enlarged polar body; (B) Fragmented polar body.

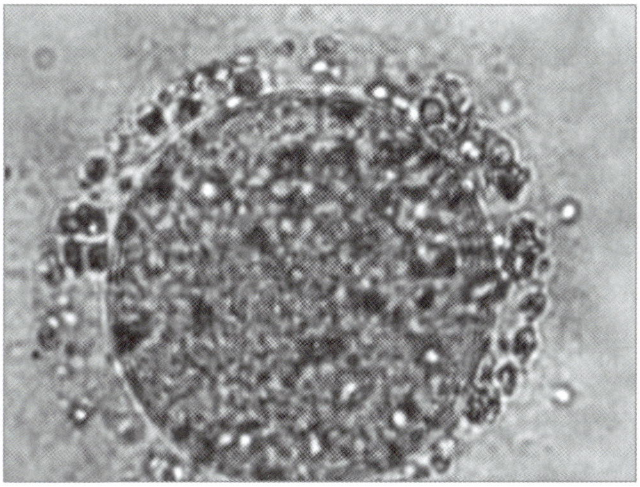

Fig. 12: Perivitelline debris.

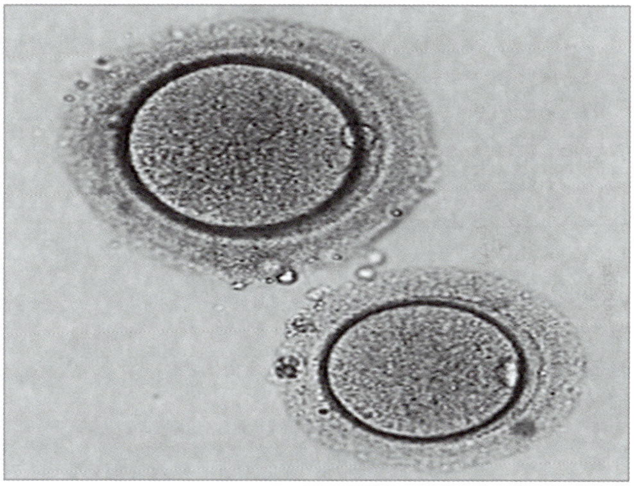

Fig. 13: Normal and giant oocyte.

OOCYTES WITH ABNORMAL SIZE AND SHAPE

This includes:

- Giant oocyte
- Oval shape
- Crescent/abnormal shaped cytoplasm.

Giant Oocyte

Denuded human oocyte has an average diameter of 120 µm. A small proportion (about 0.3%) of the retrieved oocytes have 25–35% larger diameter of up to 200 µms and are called as giant oocytes. Most unfertilized giant oocytes are diploid in nature. Hence, after a sperm nucleus is injected, this extra set of chromosomes results in three pronuclei—a phenomena known as digynic triploidy. This abnormality can be traced only at fertilization check as all further embryonic growth is as normal as that of two pronuclei zygotes. Because they are chromosomally abnormal, such giant oocytes—though reach to grade I blastocyst stage—should not be transferred to avoid fetal complications and miscarriage (Fig. 13).

Oval/Elongated Oocyte

Occasionally elongated or oval shaped oocytes are observed after ovum pickup (OPU). These oocytes most probably result due to altered pressure or squeezing of oocytes in the aspirating needle. They undergo normal fertilization and subsequent cleavage and have same implantation potential as that of spherical oocytes, unless excessive negative pressure tear off the ZP along with cumulus (Fig. 14).

Crescent/Abnormal-shaped Ooplasm

Fertilization potential of such oocytes depends upon extent of abnormality. Mild variation has no adverse effect however, if > 50% of the ooplasm shows abnormal pattern like shrinkage, it adversely affects fertilization and subsequent embryonic growth (Figs. 15A and B).

As mentioned earlier, morphological assessment many times do not represent true growth potential of an oocyte. Cellular and molecular aspects may determine oocyte quality more convincingly. However, due to extreme complex process involved, these evaluations are not applied in routine course. But they form an interesting and popular research topic. At present, cellular and molecular predictors of oocyte quality are intensively studied as they are believed to be more precise and objective indicators of oocyte competence and embryo quality compared to morphological parameters.

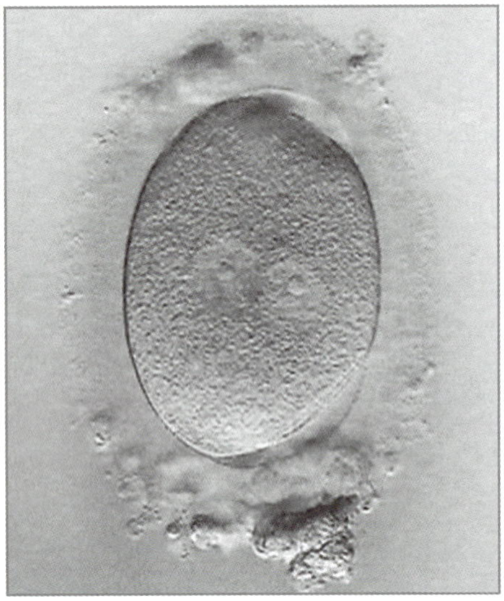

Fig. 14: Elongated oocyte displaying two germinal vesicles.

Subjects that are examined with great interest include:

- Comprehensive analysis of gene expression profiles of oocytes and their associated cumulus cells by using microarray technology
- Genetic constitution and cytogenetic analysis of polar bodies using comparative genomic hybridization
- Analysis of excreted proteins using mass spectrometry (proteomics), and
- Metabolomic investigations for indicators of oocyte quality in follicle fluids and culture medium.

More specific investigations include the mitochondrial status and glucose-6-phosphate dehydrogenase activity in oocytes, apoptosis of follicular cells and levels of the transforming growth factor-β superfamily in follicular fluid. Because most of these tests can be carried out noninvasively, these new approaches are expected to be ideal methods for identifying oocytes destined to produce chromosomally normal and viable embryos with high likelihood for live birth, thus improving the overall efficiency of the IVF process. However, all these investigations are costly, thus are not applicable to all the IVF couples.

As the oocytes are aspirated prior to their spontaneous ovulation, it is a good practice to incubate them for a couple of hours prior to insemination. Trounson et al. have

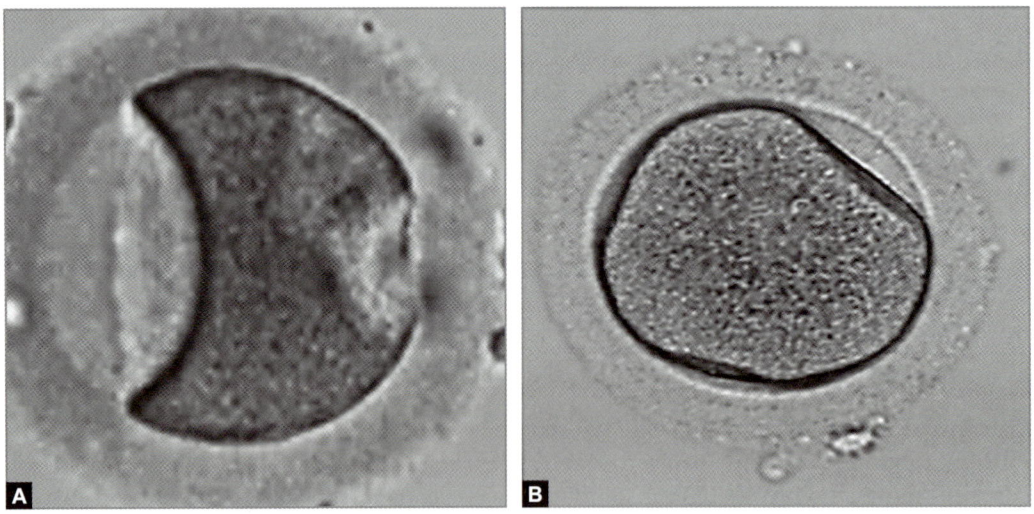

Figs. 15A and B: (A) Crescent ooplasm; (B) Uneven ooplasm.

reported the benefit of delayed insemination on fertilization rates. During early years of IVF, Laufer et al. reported that only 38% oocytes possess first PB immediately after OPU, as compared to 68% after 8 hours of incubation. Another reason for allowing preincubation time is to effectively activate cortical granule reaction that prevents polyspermy. Of course the situation may be different today due to advanced stimulation monitoring and timing of human chorionic gonadotropin (hCG). However, immature oocytes protruding first PB in vitro after 24 hours of incubation have less growth and implantation potential than preovulatory, MII oocytes matured in vivo. Such oocytes, though get fertilized, have decreased potential to withstand freezing-thawing procedure and show higher incidence of polyspermy.

CELLULAR PARAMETERS AND OOCYTE MATURITY

Maturity evaluation based on cellular parameters may be error prone even if all of them are evaluated simultaneously. Particularly, granulosa cells are of little significance when more than one oocyte is aspirated at a time that pools granulose cells from different follicles. Still, a quick observation of this female gamete and the type of cells obtained along with follicular fluid certainly help us in determining extent of their healthiness.

Viability of the oocyte can be assessed at "membrane level" while performing ICSI. Oolemma structure having elasticity confirms quick and auto sealing ability of the egg. An interesting study by Vijay Mangoli et al. illustrates this correlation prominently.

Proteomics may play a crucial role in identifying putative oocyte quality markers from the oocyte proteome and secretome to predict their fertilization, cleavage, and chromosomal competency. High-quality proteins showed abundance of Kelch-like ECH-associated protein 1 (an adaptor for ubiquitin-ligase CUL3), nuclear export factor CRM1, and ataxia-telangiectasia mutated protein kinase. Dystrophin (DMD) was more abundant in low-quality oocytes.

Various components of follicular fluid are suggested as biochemical predictors of oocyte quality. Carpintero NL reported positive correlation high progesterone was correlated with normal fertilization and high estradiol levels were found to be associated with better cleavage pattern as well as pregnancy outcome.

The research is on to develop quick and more precise methods of deciding oocyte maturity by evaluating excreted metabolites from investments around the oocyte and correlating these values with total units of follicle-stimulating hormone (FSH) required by the patient in that cycle. Till then, cellular observations remains the single quickest practical way of oocyte maturity assessment.

EDITORS' COMMENTS

1. Importance of oocyte grading is a proven concept in assisted reproductive technology (ART) treatment, good quality of oocyte gives good fertilization and embryo development.
2. Oocyte morphology markers should be considered as one of the main parameters in ART settings.
3. Also, more data regarding different abnormality of oocyte and its genetic impact on embryo cultured from it is required and all the future research is nowadays created towards oocyte markers.
4. Oocyte quality is also one of the important markers in quality assurance (QA) and quality control (QC) of any ART clinic.

SUGGESTED READING

1. Braga DP, Setti AS, Figueira Rita de, et al. Influence of oocyte dysmorphisms on blastocyst formation and quality. Fertil Steril. 2013;100(3):748-54.
2. Carpintero NL, Suárez OA, Mangas CC, et al. Follicular steroid hormones as markers of oocyte quality and oocyte development potential. J Hum Reprod Sci. 2014;7(3):187-93.
3. De Sutter P, Dozortsev D, Qian C, et al. Oocyte morphology does not correlate with fertilization rate and embryo quality after intracytoplasmic sperm injection. Hum Reprod. 1996;11:595-7.
4. Ebner T, Balaban B, Moser M, et al. Automatic user-independent zona pellucida imaging at the oocyte stage allows for the prediction of preimplantation development. Fertil Steril. 2010;94(3):913-20.
5. Ebner T, Moser M, Sommergruber M, et al. First polar body morphology and blastocyst formation rate in ICSI patients. Hum Reprod. 2002;17:2415-8.
6. Ebner T, Moser M, Sommergruber M, et al. Occurrence and developmental consequences of vacuoles throughout preimplantation development. Fertil Steril. 2005;83:1635-40.
7. El Shafie M, Sousa M, Windt ML, et al. An Atlas of the Ultrastructure of Human Oocytes: A Guide for Assisted Reproduction. New York: Parthenon Publishing Group; 2000.
8. Kahraman S, Yakin K, Donmez E, et al. Relationship between granular cytoplasm of oocytes and pregnancy outcome following intracytoplasmic sperm injection. Hum Reprod. 2000;15:2390-3.
9. Laufer N, Tarlatzis BC, Naftolin F. In vitro fertilization: state of ART. Semin Reprod Endocrinol. 1984;2:197.
10. Mangoli V, Mangoli R. Gamete and embryo assessment in IVF. In: Desai S, Parihar M, Allahabadia G (Eds). Update on Infertility. New Delhi: B I Publications Pvt Ltd; 2004. pp. 1249.

11. Mangoli V, Mangoli R. Morphological assessment of oocyte and embryo. In: Rao KA (Ed). Principles and Practice of Assisted Reproductive Technology. New Delhi: Jaypee Brothers Medical Publishers (P) Ltd; 2014. pp. 992-1002.
12. Mangoli V, Mangoli R. Oocyte grading, handling, maturity evaluation. In: Trivedi P (Ed). Heart & Soul of ART. New Delhi; Jaypee Brothers Medical Publishers (P) Ltd; 2004.
13. Otsuki J, Nagai Y, Chiba K. Lipofuscin bodies in human oocytes as an indicator of oocyte quality. J Assist Reprod Genet. 2007;24:263-70.
14. Otsuki J, Okada A, Morimoto K, et al. The relationship between pregnancy outcome and smooth endoplasmic reticulum clusters in MII human oocytes. Hum Reprod. 2004;19:1591-7.
15. Powell MD, Manandhar G, Spate L, et al. Discovery of putative oocyte quality markers by comparative ExacTag proteomics. Proteomics Clin Appl. 2010;4(3):337-51.
16. Revelli A, Delle Piane L, Casano S, et al. Follicular fluid content and oocyte quality: from single biochemical markers to metabolomics. Reprod Biol Endocrinol. 2009;7:40.
17. Trounson AO, Mohr LR, Wood C, et al. Effect of delayed insemination on in vitro fertilization culture, and transfer of human embryos. J Reprod Fertil. 1982;64:285-94.
18. Verlinsky Y, Lerner S, Illkevitch N, et al. Is there any predictive value of first polar body morphology for embryo genotype or developmental potential? Reprod Biomed Online. 2003;7: 336-41.

33

CHAPTER

Influence of Controlled Ovarian Stimulation on Oocyte Quality

Matheus Roque

INTRODUCTION

Infertility is defined as a couple's failure to conceive after 12 months of regular and unprotected sexual intercourse, and it affects approximately 15% of couples in reproductive age (ASRM, 2012). Assisted reproductive technology, such as in vitro fertilization (IVF) and intracytoplasmic sperm injection (ICSI) is, nowadays, one of the most used treatments for the condition. It has been estimated that, in developing countries, ART accounts for 1–3% of annual births (Santos et al., 2010). One essential step in an ART treatment cycle is the COS, which includes the use of exogenous gonadotropins, aiming at the development and maturation of multiple follicles and oocytes, enabling the selection of one or more embryos to be transferred, while surplus embryos can be cryopreserved, which will lead to an increase in cumulative live-birth rates (LBRs) as it can allow for multiple embryo transfers (Siristatidis et al., 2013; Humaidan et al., 2016; Alviggi et al., 2016). The ideal COS should allow clinicians to obtain an adequate number of good-quality eggs while simultaneously minimizing the adverse drug reactions and cycle cancellations that result from a high or poor response (Loutradis et al., 2012).

Recently, several concerns about the possible deleterious effects of ovarian stimulation on oocyte and embryo quality, endometrial receptivity, and perinatal outcomes have been raised (Santos, 2010). Baart et al. (2007) demonstrated that embryos formed in stimulated cycles have higher rates of aneuploidy when compared to embryos of unstimulated cycles. Besides, data from large registries have shown that rates of live births increase progressively as the number of eggs aspirated in an IVF cycle increases. However, this improvement reaches a plateau around 10–15 aspirated eggs. Conversely, from a certain amount of eggs, this rate goes down, and this decrease could be related to a reduction in oocyte/embryonic quality due to excessive ovarian stimulation. Moreover, as much higher is the ovarian response to ovarian stimulation, the higher the risk of the development of the ovarian hyperstimulation syndrome (OHSS) (Sunkara et al., 2011). With this data, a group of experts went on to advocate that the best for the patients would be to perform a mild ovarian stimulation, where satisfactory clinical results and a decrease in the risks of OHSS development would be obtained, thus increasing the safety of treatments (Nargund and Frydman, 2007; Verberg et al., 2009). However, all these data correlating the number of eggs aspirated to the clinical results of the IVF treatments are considering a fresh embryo transfer. Thus, we cannot determine if the worsening of the results would be related to an effect of the ovarian stimulus over the oocyte/embryo quality or the endometrium.

In this way, it is of fundamental importance that we adequately evaluate the possible deleterious effects of the COS during an IVF cycle. To establish the best protocol of treatment to be implemented to assisted reproduction patients, we need to determine if the possible deleterious effect of COS is over the embryo, endometrium, on both, or if COS does not present any of their harmful effects. Moreover, we need to take into account all the advances that have occurred in the last years regarding the techniques of embryonic and oocyte cryopreservation.

The primary goal of this chapter is to make a critical evaluation of the evidence correlating the effect of ovarian stimulation on oocyte quality, embryonic, and on the results of assisted reproduction treatments, trying to find a balance between efficacy and safety of COS.

DOES OVARIAN STIMULATION EXERT AN EFFECT ON OOCYTE/EMBRYO QUALITY?

The use of gonadotropins during ovarian stimulation leads to the development of several follicles in one IVF cycle. However, part of these follicles that develop during an ovarian stimulation were follicles that naturally evolved into atresia (Pellicer et al., 1988). Thus, we could hypothesize that multifolicular development may be associated with lower oocyte quality and less embryonic development, and this concern has long existed (Testart et al., 1986, Pellicer et al., 1989). Pellicer et al. (1989) evaluated three groups of patients considering the number of retrieved oocytes. The evaluation of oocyte quality was performed indirectly through the complex cumulus-oocyte appearance, fertilization rates, morphological quality, and embryo implantation rate. It was observed that fertilization rates were higher in the two groups with a lower number of aspirated eggs (between 1–5 and 6–10) than the group with the highest number (≥11), and conversely, the rate of implantation was lower in the group with the highest number of aspirated eggs. The total doses of gonadotropins used to achieve an optimal response were lower in patients with a better ovarian response. Thus, it is suggested that the effects on fertilization and embryo quality would not be directly related to excessive ovarian stimulation, but probably to the ovarian response presented by the patient (Pellicer et al., 1989). However, these results referring to implantation rates were obtained in cycles with fresh embryo transfer, where the supra-physiologic hormonal levels observed during the COS may affect the endometrial receptivity and could impair the clinical outcomes (Ubaldi et al., 1997; Kolibianakis et al., 2002; Horcajadas et al., 2005; Labarta et al., 2011).

Studies have also evaluated the correlation between the ovarian stimulation regimen and the rates of embryo aneuploidy and suggested that the ovarian stimulation performed during an IVF treatment would affect the proportion of euploidy embryos (Munné et al., 1997; Katz-Jaffe et al., 2005). Moreover, it has been suggested that superovulation may induce genomic imprinting disorders (Sato et al., 2007). Baart et al. (2007) randomly assigned patients to undergo a mild stimulation in a gonadotropin-releasing hormone (GnRH) antagonist protocol or a conventional high-dose gonadotropin in a GnRH agonist protocol. In the long agonist protocol, the patient was stimulated with fixed 225 IU per day of recombinant follicle-stimulating hormone (rFSH); in the mild antagonist approach, the patients were stimulated with fixed 150 IU of rFSH per day. The group that performed a mild stimulation presented lower aneuploidy rate. However, fewer oocytes and embryos were obtained in the mild approach group. In this way, the average number of chromosomally normal embryos were the same when comparing both groups. The authors suggested that the differences in the aneuploidy rates among the groups could be related to the effect of ovarian stimulation on mitotic segregation errors, leading to an increase in these errors with increasing dose of gonadotropins (Baart et al., 2007).

Thus, as high chromosomal abnormalities have been found in human embryos derived from IVF treatments, it is also essential to evaluate the prevalence of aneuploidy in embryos, resulting from unstimulated cycle IVF treatment. Verpoest et al. (2008) assessed the incidence of numerical chromosomal abnormalities, using preimplantation genetic testing for aneuploidy (PGT-A) with fluorescence in situ hybridization (FISH) technology for chromosomes X, Y, 13, 16, 18, 21, and 22 in thirty women with a mean age of 31.4 years that underwent ICSI treatment in an unstimulated cycle (natural cycle). They found in these young reproductive age patients an aneuploidy rate of 36.4% (Verpoest et al., 2008). Labarta et al. (2012) compared these chromosomal abnormalities in oocyte donors with a mean age of 25.4 years submitted to an unstimulated cycle and the next stimulated cycle using the same sperm donor sample for both cycles, to exclude the interindividual variability in the aneuploidy rates. They performed unstimulated cycle in 185 patients and were able to do PGT-A in 51 of them, and found a 35.3% aneuploidy rate. They compared these rates in a stimulated cycle from 46 of the donors that performed the previous treatment. The mean total dose of gonadotropin used during the stimulated cycle was 2,230 IU, the mean serum estradiol levels on the trigger day were 2,707 pg/mL, and the mean number of retrieved oocytes was 17.8. The aneuploidy rate during these stimulated cycles was 40.6%. When comparing to natural cycle, there was no significant difference between the rates, with risk difference of 5.8 (95% confidence interval (CI) = –20.6; 9.0) and a relative risk of 1.17 (95% CI = 0.77; 1.77; $p = 0.45$) concluding that the ovarian stimulation does not significantly increase the embryo aneuploidy rates when comparing with an unstimulated cycle during an IVF treatment (Labarta et al., 2012).

Interestingly, in a retrospective cohort study evaluating 1,122 IVF cycles, Sekhon et al. (2017) performed trophectoderm biopsy and polymerase chain reaction (PCR) and correlated the aneuploidy rates with the total dose of gonadotropin used during COS. There was no significant association between cumulative gonadotropin dose and odds of aneuploidy [adjusted odds ratio (OR) = 1.049;

$p = 0.232$] in patients with normal ovarian response to stimulation. However, in patients requiring prolonged COS (over 12 days of stimulation), there were elevated odds of aneuploidy with increasing cumulative gonadotropin dose (adjusted OR = 1.20; $p < 0.0001$). These findings raise the hypothesis that the correlation between ovarian stimulation and embryo aneuploidy is not directly related to the intensity of the ovarian stimulus or total dose of gonadotropins used during the stimulus. It may be related to the pattern of ovarian response and the profile of each patient. Thus, the concept of ovarian sensitivity index (OSI) has emerged that performs the combination of gonadotropin dose and ovarian response to the treatment. In theory, the OSI may address the ovary condition, and as much more oocytes can be retrieved with less dose of gonadotropin, the better the patient's outcomes (Huber et al., 2013). Recently, Labarta et al. (2017) accessed whether a higher ovarian response to the same starting dose of gonadotropin during ovarian stimulation may generate more euploid embryos. Moreover, they also addressed whether the higher consumption of gonadotropin per egg obtained in an IVF treatment is associated with a fewer number of euploid embryos. The authors evaluated the cycles of oocyte donors with starting doses of gonadotropin of 150 IU or 75 IU. They found that the aneuploidy rate did not increase with ovarian response or total gonadotropin consumption. Furthermore, the number of euploid embryos available for transfer increases as the number of retrieved oocytes increases (Labarta et al., 2017). However, these data from Labarta et al. (2017) study was based on PGT-A performed by FISH analysis. Recently, it was published in a retrospective study performing PGT-A in more than 4,000 Day 5 and Day 6 blastocyst using single-nucleotide polymorphism (SNP) technology. The objective of this was to evaluate if there was a correlation between the total dose of gonadotropin consumption during an IVF cycle and aneuploidy rates. They found that an independent factor related to the aneuploidy rate was the female age. Considering patients within the same age group, there was no statistical difference in aneuploidy rates regardless of the total dose of gonadotropin consumption during COS (Barash et al., 2017).

There are some interesting data from studies in polycystic ovary syndrome (PCOS) patients that correlate with this concept of the ovarian pattern being responsible for oocyte alteration and not the COS per se. Wood et al. (2007) compared normal ovulatory women to PCOS women to examine whether the alterations in follicle growth and the intrafollicular environment affect gene expression and also the oocyte development in PCOS patients. They performed COS with GnRH analog and rFSH in normal ovulatory and PCOS patients and observed differences in the gene expression profiles when comparing these two groups of patients. They observed that although the oocytes from normal ovulatory and PCOS women are morphologically identical and of high quality, they exhibit different gene expression profiles. They identified 15 genes involved in the meiotic/mitotic cell cycle pathway that in PCOS patients exhibited altered mRNA abundance. These differentially expressed genes are involved in spindle dynamics, homologous recombination/chromosome alignment, cell-cycle checkpoint, and centrosome function (Wood et al., 2007).

Taking all these data into account, it seems that even if we consider that increasing gonadotropin dosage and/or the cohort of retrieved oocytes may increase the embryo aneuploidy, the more significant number of euploid embryos obtained in these situations may compensate for the possible increase in aneuploidy (Orvieto et al., 2017). Thus, it is of fundamental importance to evaluate the effect of the number of retrieved oocytes in IVF outcomes to assess if or not performing a conventional ovarian stimulation instead of using low doses of gonadotropin to optimize the number of retrieval oocytes during one IVF cycle may benefit the patients.

DOES THE NUMBER OF RETRIEVED OOCYTES AFFECT THE IVF OUTCOMES?

With the advent of protocols with GnRH antagonists, the implementation of gentle procedures to ovarian stimulation was possible (Fauser and Devroey et al., 2005).

In the last decade, the discussion and use of the mild approach for ovarian stimulation have become increasingly popular, claiming to reduce the potentially adverse effects of multifollicular ovarian stimulation over IVF effectiveness and safety (risk of OHSS), improving the embryo's quality, and also, the implantation potential (Orvieto et al., 2017). Some previous studies claimed that high-dosage gonadotropins could affect the clinical pregnancy rates (Wennerholm et al., 1997; Källén et al., 2005).

It has been a matter of debate what the ideal number of oocytes to be retrieved to optimize the IVF outcomes would be. Aiming to evaluate the association between egg number and live birth during IVF treatment and trying to identify the ideal number of oocytes to be retrieved after one COS for cycle optimizations, Sunkara et al. (2011) evaluated the data from IVF cycles performed in the United Kingdom (UK) from 1991 to 2008. After evaluating more than 400,000 IVF cycles, they found a relationship between the number of retrieved oocytes and the LBR, independently, on patients' ages, suggesting that the number of oocytes to be retrieved to maximize live birth is around 15. Over this number, there is a plateau in LBR, and after a higher number of oocytes, the LBR decreased (Sunkara et al., 2011). However, these data are based on fresh embryo transfer cycles.

When evaluating fresh transfer cycle, the ovarian stimulation may affect the clinical outcomes. However, the decrease in implantation and LBRs during a fresh cycle, such as those presented by Sunkara et al. (2011) are not related to the effects of COS over the embryo but over the endometrium. Since the late 1990s, some studies associate supraphysiologic hormone levels during COS with endometrial histologic advancement and diminished implantation. One study from 1999 compared endometrial biopsy in women undergoing stimulation for IVF to normal ovulatory women with proven fertility and showed a premature expression of the expected histologic pattern, estrogen receptors, and pinopodes (Develioglu et al., 1999). Subsequent studies continued to show receptivity impairment in stimulated cycles due to histologic advancement, glandular-stromal dyssynchrony, genomic dysregulation, an increased frequency of endometrial waves, and more (Shapiro et al., 2016; Lawrenz et al., 2017; Ruiz-Alonso et al., 2013; Zhu et al., 2012). Studies performing a histological evaluation of the endometrium and endometrial dating found that when the endometrial advancement is more than 3 days, no pregnancies are achieved in a fresh cycle (Ubaldi et al., 1997; Kolibianakis et al., 2002). The techniques to evaluate the endometrial receptivity have evolved and nowadays it is possible to perform the analysis of endometrial gene expression profile. It has been suggested that when comparing stimulated to a natural cycle, there are over 200 genes related to implantation that present different expression, suggesting that ovarian stimulation affects the endometrial receptivity (Horcajadas et al., 2005). Moreover, cycles with supraphysiologic levels of P4 (>1.5 ng/mL) on the trigger day present around 140 genes related to implantation that are up- or downregulated when comparing to patients with lower P4 levels (Labarta et al., 2011). However, these results, in general, were observed in patients presenting a hyper response (Horcajadas et al., 2005; Labarta et al., 2011) or supraphysiologic hormonal levels (Ubaldi et al., 1997; Kolibianakis et al., 2002; Labarta et al., 2011) during OS.

Thus, if the COS may exert a detrimental effect over the endometrium, we need to find an alternative to avoid these possible deleterious effects. Although fresh embryo transfer is the norm in IVF treatments, the results of cycles with frozen embryos have been improving progressively over the last years. Historically, as the first IVF baby was born 40 years ago, embryos were freshly transferred to the uterus, after 2–5 days in culture (Gerris et al., 2003). The first live birth after frozen-thawed embryo transfer (FET) resulted from slow-freeze (1984), followed by vitrification later (1990). Data from the Centers for Disease Control and Prevention (CDC) from 1997 to 2011 show that LBRs from FET cycles have increased over the past 14 years for women of all ages. Relative increases in the LBRs of around 86% can be observed from 1997 to 2011 for women under the age of 35 years (Wong et al., 2014). With the improvements in COS and culture conditions, more good transferable embryos are obtained, allowing the surplus embryos to be cryopreserved and potentially increasing the cumulative outcomes per COS (Wong et al., 2014). Thus, after these historical marks, the development of cryopreservation has led to an improvement in efficacy, with cumulative LBRs close to 70% over a 5-year period (Pinborg et al., 2009; Wong et al., 2014). The possibility of freezing the surplus embryos during an IVF cycle or even the cryopreservation of all the embryos for a deferred embryo transfer makes us consider another critical outcome in assisted reproduction treatments, known as cumulative rates per stimulated cycle. The cumulative outcomes are probably the best way to evaluate the efficacy of any specific strategy during an IVF treatment (Maheshwari et al., 2015).

In contrast, from what was done by Sunkara et al. (2016), Ji et al. (2013) evaluated 2,455 women undergoing IVF and correlated the number of retrieved oocytes and euploidy rates. They found that although the risks increased with more than 15 oocytes retrieved in a fresh cycle, there are no differences in clinical outcomes when evaluating the cumulative LBR. With a greater number of retrieved oocytes, the higher the cumulative outcomes are (Ji et al., 2013). These are the same findings from Drakopoulos et al., 2017. This result is also the same as Drakopoulos et al. (2016), concluding that the cumulative LBR significantly increases the chance of being successful. They found no effect of COS over the embryo quality, which can be seen when evaluating the cumulative LBRs. Recently, it has been proposed the concept of one-and-done approach, where the COS is focusing on the retrieval of the maximal number of oocytes that could better help the couples in reaching their goal. With all the improvements in cryopreservation that have occurred in the last years, one COS with a high number of retrieved oocytes would be an optimal way to program an IVF treatment (Vaughan et al., 2017).

CONCLUSION

The gonadotropin dose or the ovarian stimulation intensity alone during COS is not responsible for the decrease in oocyte quality and clinical outcomes. However, the patient's profile and ovary pattern may be responsible for the poorer outcomes during an IVF treatment. Thus, when evaluating the cumulative outcomes per oocyte retrieval, it would be more beneficial to the patient to obtain a higher number of oocytes than focusing on limiting the number of retrieved oocytes. Thus, when evaluating IVF patients that will be submitted to a COS, we should focus on performing the best ovarian stimulation to achieve the highest chance of a live birth per ovarian stimulation.

KEYNOTE

One essential step in an assisted reproductive technology (ART) treatment cycle is the controlled ovarian stimulation (COS). Recently, several concerns about the possible deleterious effects of ovarian stimulation on oocyte and embryo quality, endometrial receptivity, and perinatal outcomes have been raised. To establish the best protocol of treatment to be implemented to assisted reproduction patients, we need to determine if the possible deleterious effect of COS is over the embryo, endometrium, on both, or if COS does not present any of their harmful effects.

KEY POINTS

- During an IVF treatment and COS, the oocyte quality and competence are related to the patient's profile and ovary pattern and not to the intensity of ovarian stimulation or the total dose of gonadotropin used.
- Instead of considering the total dose of gonadotropin used during COS and trying to correlate to the outcomes, it is more useful to consider the total dose of gonadotropin per oocyte retrieved.
- The most important predictive factor related to embryo aneuploidy is the woman's age.
- Mild approaches for ovarian stimulation focusing on obtaining a lower number of oocytes:
  - Improved use of retrieved oocytes
  - Lower absolute number of euploid embryos
  - Lower cumulative outcomes per oocyte retrieval.
- Conventional approaches for ovarian stimulation focusing on obtaining the highest number:
  - Higher absolute number of euploid embryos
  - Higher cumulative outcomes per oocyte retrieval.

EDITORS' COMMENTS

In this well-written and comprehensive chapter, Dr Roque demystify the association between oocyte quality and intensity of ovarian stimulation. Dr Roque's observations are consistent with our recently published data showing that female age is the most relevant factor consistently affecting the likelihood of oocyte and embryo euploidy.[1,2] The older the patient the lower the probability of the resulting blastocyst be euploid. Thus a possible way to increase the chances of having at least one euploid embryo for transfer in a given patient, in particular those of advanced age, would be by increasing the oocyte number by adequate dosing and gonadotropin regimen. In our 2018 study, the decrease in the probability of blastocyst euploidy followed an age-dependent binomial distribution, progressing with every year of female age, from 1.2% to 24.5% in 28–44-year-old women ($p < 0.0001$) (Esteves et al., 2018). The minimum number of blastocysts needed to obtain at least one euploid blastocyst for transfer was computed for different probabilities and female ages. At the age of 28 years, a total of three blastocysts is required to obtain at least one euploid blastocyst with 90% probability, whereas it is 4, 5, 6, 9, 16, and 29 for ages 35, 37, 39, 41, 43, and 45, respectively. Furthermore, in our 2019 study, we developed a predictive model to estimate the minimum number of metaphase II oocytes needed to achieve at least one euploid blastocyst for transfer in a given infertile couple undergoing IVF/ICSI. The model uses female age and type of sperm used for IVF/ICSI as the primary predictors of blastocyst euploidy (Esteves et al., 2019).

SC Esteves, Campinas, Brazil

REFERENCES

1. Esteves SC, Carvalho JF, Martinhago CD, et al. Estimation of age-dependent decrease in blastocyst euploidy by next generation sequencing: development of a novel prediction model. Panminerva Med. 2018;61(1):3-10.
2. Esteves SC, Carvalho JF, Bento FC, Santos J. A Novel Predictive Model to Estimate the Number of Mature Oocytes Required for Obtaining at Least One Euploid Blastocyst for Transfer in Couples Undergoing in vitro Fertilization/Intracytoplasmic Sperm Injection: The ART Calculator. Front Endocrinol (Lausanne). 2019;10:99.

SUGGESTED READING

1. Baart EB, Martini E, Eijkemans MJ, et al. Milder ovarian stimulation for in-vitro fertilization reduces aneuploidy in the human preimplantation embryo: a randomized controlled trial. Hum Reprod. 2007;22:980-8.
2. Barash OO, Hinckley MD, Rosenbluth EM, et al. High gonadotropin dosage does not affect euploidy and pregnancy rates in IVF PGS cycles with single embryo transfer. Hum Reprod. 2017;32:2209-17.
3. Develioglu OH, Hsiu JG, Nikas G, et al. Endometrial estrogen and progesterone receptor and pinopode expression in stimulated cycles of oocyte donors. Fertil Steril. 1999;71:1040-7.

4. Drakopoulos P, Blockeel C, Stoop D, et al. Conventional ovarian stimulation and single embryo transfer for IVF/ICSI. How many oocytes do we need to maximize cumulative live birth rates after utilization of all fresh and frozen embryo? Hum Reprod. 2016;31:370-6.
5. Fauser BC, Devroey P. Why is the clinical acceptance of gonadotrophin-releasing hormone antagonist cotreatment during ovarian hyperstimulation for in vitro fertilization so slow? Fertil Steril. 2005;83:1607-11.
6. Gerris J, De Neubourg D, De Dutter P, et al. Cryopreservation as a tool to reduce multiple birth. Reprod Biomed Online. 2003;7:286-94.
7. Horcajadas JA, Riesewijk A, Polman J, et al. Effect of controlled ovarian hyperstimulation in IVF on endometrial gene expression profiles. Mol Hum Reprod. 2005;11:195-205.
8. Huber M, Hadziosmanovic N, Berglund L, et al. Using the ovarian sensitivity index to define poor, normal, and high response after controlled ovarian hyperstimulation in the long gonadotropin-releasing hormone-agonist protocol: suggestions for a new principle to solve an old problem. Fertil Steril. 2013;100:1270-6.
9. Ji J, Liu Y, Tong XH, et al. The optimum number of oocyte in IVF treatment: an analysis of 2,455 cycles in Chine. Hum Reprod. 2013;28:2728-34.
10. Källén B, Finnström O, Nygren KG, et al. In vitro fertilization (IVF) in Sweden: risk for congenital malformations after different IVF methods. Birth Defects Res A Clin Mol Teratol. 2005;73:162-9.
11. Katz-Jaffe MG, Trounson AO, Cram DS. Chromosome 21 mosaic human preimplantation embryos predominantly arise from diploid conceptions. Fertil Steril. 2005;84:634-43.
12. Kolibianakis E, Bourgain C, Albano C, et al. Effect of ovarian stimulation with recombinant follicle-stimulating hormone, gonadotropin releasing hormone antagonists, and human chorionic gonadotropin on endometrial maturation on the day of oocyte pick-up. Fertil Steril. 2002;78:1025-9.
13. Labarta E, Martinez-Conejero JA, Alamá P, et al. Endometrial receptivity is affected in women with high circulating progesterone levels at the end of the follicular phase: a functional genomics analysis. Hum Reprod. 2011;26:1813-25.
14. Labarta E, Bosch E, Alamá P, et al. Moderate ovarian stimulation does not increase the incidence of human embryo chromosomal abnormalities in in vitro fertilization cycles. J Clin Endocrinol Metab. 2012;97:E1987-94.
15. Labarta E, Bosch E, Mercader A, et al. A higher ovarian response after stimulation for IVF is related to a higher number of euploid embryos. BioMed Res Int. 2017;2017:5637923.
16. Lawrenz B, Fatemi HM. Effect of progesterone elevation in follicular phase of IVF-cycles on the endometrial receptivity. Reprod Biomed Online. 2017;34:422-8.
17. Loutradis D, Theofanakis CH, Anagnostou E, et al. Genetic Profile of SNP(s) and Ovulation Induction. Curr Pharm Biotechnol. 2012;13:417-25.
18. Maheshwari A, McLernon D, Bhattacharya S. Cumulative live birth rate: time for a consensus? Hum Reprod. 2015;30: 2703-7.
19. Magnusson A, Källen K, Thurin-Kjelbberg A, et al. The number of oocytes retrieved during IVF: a balance between efficacy and safety. Hum Reprod. 2018;33:58-64.
20. Munné S, Magli C, Adler A, et al. Treatment-related chromosome abnormalities in human embryos. Hum Reprod. 1997;12:780-4.
21. Nargund G, Frydman R. Towards a more physiological approach to IVF. Reprod Biomed Online. 2007;14:550-2.
22. Orvieto R, Vanni VS, Gleicher N. The myths surrounding mild in vitro fertilization (IVF). Reprod Biol Endocrinol. 2017;15:48.
23. Pellicer A, Polan ML, De Cherney AH. Improved oocyte quality through improved ovarian induction regimen. Ann N Y Acad Sci. 1988;541:46-59.
24. Pinborg A, Hougaard CO, Nyboe Andersen A, et al. Prospective longitudinal cohort study on cumulative 5-year delivery and adoption rates among 1338 couples initiating infertility treatment. Hum Reprod. 2009;24:991-9.
25. Ruiz-Alonso M, Blesa D, Díaz-Gimeno P, et al. The endometrial receptivity array for diagnosis and personalized embryo transfer as a treatment for patients with repeated implantation failure. Fertil Steril. 2013;100:818-24.
26. Santos MA, Kuijk EW, Macklon NS. The impact of ovarian stimulation for IVF on the developing embryo. Reproduction. 2010;139:23-34.
27. Sato A, Otsu E, Negishi H, et al. Aberrant DNA methylation of imprinted loci in superovulated oocytes. Hum Reprod. 2007;22:26-35.
28. Sekhon L, Shaia K, Santistevan A, et al. The cumulative dose of gonadotropins used for controlled ovarian stimulation does not influence the odds of embryonic aneuploidy in patients with normal ovarian response. J Assist Reprod Genet. 2017;34:749-58.
29. Shapiro BS, Daneshmand ST, Desai Jm Garner FC, et al. The risk of embryo-endometrium asynchrony increases with maternal age after ovarian stimulation and IVF. Reprod Biomed Online. 2016;33:50-5.
30. Siristatidis C, Sergentanis TN, Kanavidis P, et al. Controlled ovarian hyperstimulation for IVF: impact on ovarian, endometrial and cervical cancer—a systematic review and meta-analysis. Hum Reprod Update. 2013;19:105-23.
31. Sunkara SK, Rittenberg V, Raine-Fenning N, et al. Association between the number of eggs and live birth in IVF treatment: an analysis of 400135 treatment cycles. Hum Reprod. 2011;26:1768-74.
32. Testart J, Belaisch-Allart J, Frydman R. Relationships between embryo transfer results and ovarian response and in vitro fertilization rates: analysis of 186 human pregnancies. Fertil Steril. 1986;45:237-43.
33. The Practice Committee of the American Society for Reproductive Medicine. Diagnostic evaluation of the infertile female: a committee opinion. Fertil Steril. 2012;98:302-7.

34. Ubaldi F, Bourgain C, Tournaye H, et al. Endometrial evaluation by aspiration biopsy on the day of oocyte retrieval in the embryo transfer cycles in patients with serum progesterone rise during the follicular phase. Fertil Steril. 1997;67:521-6.
35. Vaughan DA, Leung A, Resetkova N, et al. How many oocytes are optimal to achieve multiple live births with one stimulation cycle? The one-and-done approach. Fertil Steril. 2017;107:397-404.
36. Verberg MF, Macklon NS, Nargund G, et al. Mild ovarian stimulation for IVF. Hum Reprod Update. 2009;15:13-29.
37. Verpoest W, Fauser BC, Papanikoilaou E, et al. Chromosomal aneuploidy in embryos conceived with unstimulated cycle IVF. Hum Reprod. 2008;23:2369-71.
38. Wennerholm UB, Hamberger L, Nilsson L, et al. Obstetric and perinatal outcome of children conceived from cryopreserved embryos. Hum Reprod. 1997;12:1819-1925.
39. Wong KM, Mastenbroek S, Repping S. Cryopreservation of human embryos and its contribution to in vitro fertilization success rates. Fertil Steril. 2014;102:19-26.
40. Wood JR, Dumesic DA, Abbott DH, et al. Molecular abnormalities in oocytes from women with polycystic ovary syndrome revealed by microarray analysis. J Clin Endocrinol Metab. 2007;92:705-13.
41. Zhu L, Li Y, Xu A. Influence of controlled ovarian hyperstimulation on uterine peristalsis in infertile women. Hum Reprod. 2012;27:2684-9.

34

CHAPTER

Optimizing Sperm Selection Methods

Alpesh Doshi

INTRODUCTION

Sperm obtained immediately after ejaculation are unable to fertilize eggs. Under *in vivo* conditions, after deposition in the female tract, spermatozoa undergo through a set of functional changes to acquire fertilization capacity. This process, known as *capacitation*, involves nuclear alterations as well as modifications to the flagellar movement pattern (hyperactivation) and endows sperm with the ability to carry out the acrosomal reaction. In conjunction with the physiological changes, there is *in vivo* an active migration from the cervical tract, which only allows motile spermatozoa to follow their path. This physic feature of displacement toward the oviduct implies a reduction of available sperm cells from an initial concentration of 10^7–10^8 spermatozoa to 10^3 arriving to the uterotubal junction, decreasing to a hundredth arriving to the cumulus oophorus complex, and reducing even more to a tenth, which will be close to the zona pellucida but only one will be penetrating into the oocyte. Sperm preparation methods for assisted reproduction technology (ART) seek to mimic *in vitro* this natural selection process before performing any further insemination technique. This chapter will discuss the different preparation and enhancing techniques currently used to optimize sperm selection.

CONSIDERATIONS FOR TREATMENT SELECTION

The quality of a sperm sample is one of the key factors when it comes to determine the most adequate ART treatment. In standard *in vitro* fertilization (IVF) integrity of sperm function, it is essential for sperm cells to be able to bind to the oocyte's zona pellucida, undergo the acrosome reaction, and fusing with the oolemma for fertilization to take place. Opposite to this, most of spermatozoa functions are not essential when intracytoplasmic sperm injection (ICSI) is the method chosen. Consequently, clinical decision on treatment is dependent on results of previous semen analysis (Flowchart 1).

Semen analysis is the most used diagnostic test by ART centers to assess male fertility. Based on a qualitative and quantitative analysis at a macroscopic and microscopic level, andrologists assess the appearance, liquefaction, viscosity, pH, volume, sperm cell concentration, motility, progression, morphology, and presence or absence of agglutination and other non-spermatic cells according to the most recent World Health Organization (WHO) standards for the evaluation of human semen. *Semen culture* is a complimentary test performed to evaluate whether a chronic infection is the cause of subfertility. Samples that show resistance to determinate antibiotics should be considered for ICSI only to prevent colonization of the culture dishes and potentially impairing embryo development.

In some cases, the body recognizes the sperm as foreign agents and creates antisperm antibodies that bind to them in order to be intercepted by the immune system lowering their fertilizing potential. This examination is specially recommended to patients whose testicles have been injured or have been exposed to certain surgeries (i.e. vasectomy, vasectomy reversal, or biopsy) or if there is a suspicion of a prostate gland infection. To evaluate this phenomenon, *mixed agglutination reaction (MAR) test* can be performed

Flowchart 1: Male factor algorithm for treatment selection. Semen analysis is the basic test that gives clinician an idea on testicular functions by assessing parameters such as sperm count, motility, and morphology. Other complimentary examinations can be done in order to have a complete male profile when the sample to study is considered to be within the normal parameters or close to them following the WHO criteria. These include semen culture, MAR Test and sperm DNA fragmentation.

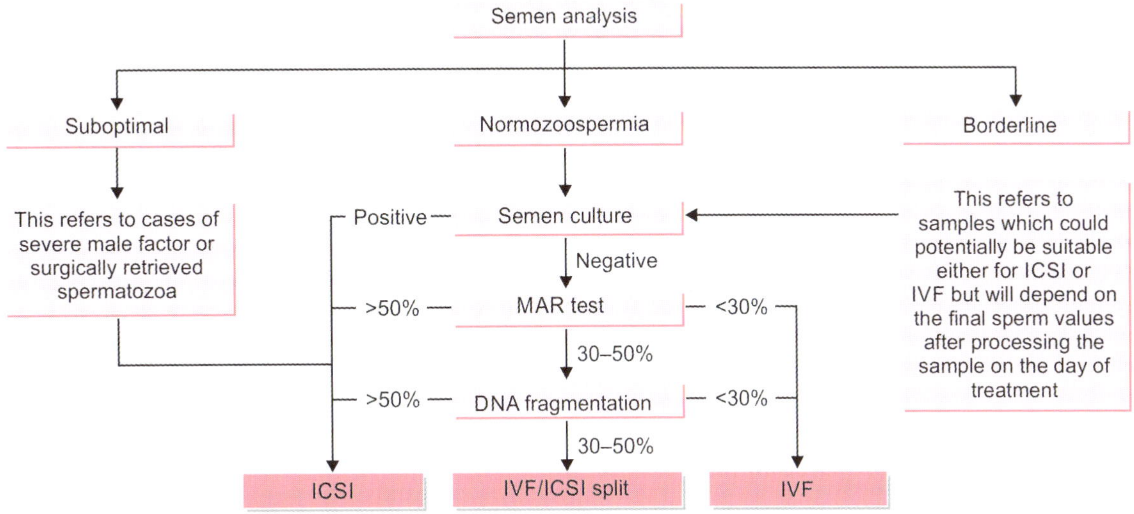

(DNA: deoxyribonucleic acid; ICSI: intracytoplasmic sperm injection; IVF: *in vitro* fertilization; MAR: mixed agglutination reaction)

as a complement to the semen analysis. According to the WHO criteria for the examination and processing of human semen, when more than 50% of sperm is covered with antibodies [immunoglobulin A or immunoglobulin G (IgA or IgG)], the rest result is considered to be positive and an immunologic infertility becomes evident. In those cases, ICSI is highly recommended as the insemination method. It has been described that physiological sperm functions, such as penetration into the cervical mucus or *in vivo* fertilization, are impaired when ≥50% of the motile sperm cells have antibodies antisperm attached. When the percentage of attached sperm to antibodies is less than 30%, sperm function is not compromised and the test result is considered to be normal (Fig. 1). For all those cases, where 30–50% of sperm are covered with antibodies an IVF-ICSI split is recommended as an insemination strategy, since these patients will be considered to have a slightly positive test.

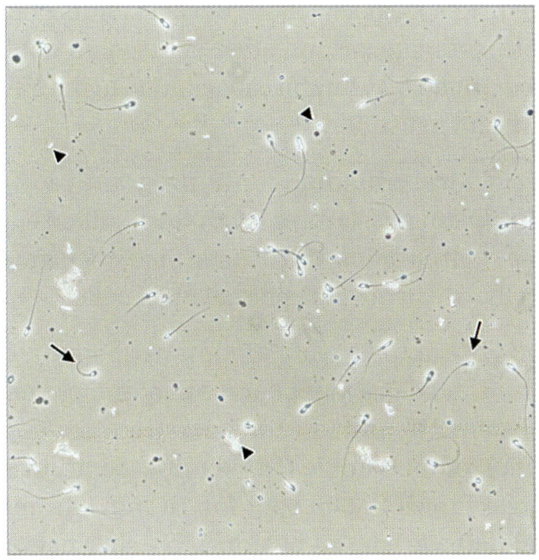

Fig. 1: Mixed agglutination reaction test (negative) semen is mixed with latex beads treated with specific antibodies that detect potential antibodies antisperm attached to sperm cells (arrows). When the interaction of the beads (arrowheads) with the antibodies antisperm occurs, it becomes visually evident by observing an agglutination phenomena of sperm cells under the microscope. The test is considered to be positive when >50% of the motile spermatozoa have beads attached.

Complimentary to the previous examinations, there is a further test in order to complete a male profile and that is the analysis of *sperm DNA fragmentation*. One of the causes of suboptimal results during ART can be related to the use of sperm cells with high DNA fragmentation, which are associated with low fertilization rates. Different tests are available on the market and their results help clinicians to advice on the insemination method to minimize the effect of sperm DNA fragmentation. Different tests agree that samples displaying a fragmentation level of <30% are at low risk, therefore male infertility could not be explained only by sperm fragmentation. Any fragmentation level between 30%

and 50% puts the individual at risk of male infertility and IVF will be suggested. Only samples where fragmentation levels are over a 50% are at risk of IVF failure, and ICSI should be advised to couples coming for ART treatment.

SPERM SELECTION METHODS

The ultimate method should not only be fast and cost-effective for isolation motile spermatozoa but also ought not to cause physiological damage to the gametes while eliminating nonviable spermatozoa and other agents [including other cells, decapacitation factors, or reactive oxygen species (ROS)]. The methods described below can be differentiated in (1) those provided by the separation techniques (Figs. 2A to D), (2) improvement methods after preparing the sample, or (3) selection techniques during insemination.

Selection Provided by Sperm Separation Techniques

Simple Wash Method

This method, although being quick and less complex, is not advised for normozoospermic samples, if our aim is to enhance sperm selection. Because of its simplicity, nonviable spermatozoa and other cells would not be fully separated, which may inhibit capacitation in the fraction of sperm we aim to use.

Concept: Culture media, containing antibiotics and protein supplements, is mixed with the liquified ejaculate. Following centrifugation, the seminal fluid is separated from sperm cells, which are concentrated in a pellet.

Protocol: For samples with suboptimal parameters (i.e. low volume and density or poor motility and progression), culture media is added in a 1:1 ratio after complete liquefaction of the sample (15–30 min). Centrifuge at low centrifugal forces (1,000 rpm for 10 min) to minimize potential damage caused by nonviable spermatozoa and leukocytes. Following centrifugation, remove supernatant down to the sperm pellet and resuspend in approximately 100 μL of culture media in a round bottom tube. Place the prepared sample with the loosen cap to allow gas exchange into the incubator for equilibration until insemination.

This technique implies that sperm cells are pelleted before final resuspension. This will be one of the major concerns of all techniques that display similar features due to the increased levels of ROS generated from cell to cell contact between sperm, debris, and plasma leukocytes (Box 1).

Swim-up

Initially described by Mahadevan and Baker, the swim-up method can be performed using a semen sample following complete liquefaction or as an enhancing selection method on a spermatozoa pellet. Despite being one of the oldest methods, it is still in use in a wide number of laboratories worldwide.

Concept: Sperm wash medium is layered on top of a liquefied semen sample. Motile sperm will move out, if the sample into the washing media.

Protocol: Restricted to ejaculates with high sperm count and motility, the basis of its methodology relies on the self-propelled movement of spermatozoa. For its preparation, several aliquots of liquefied semen (or a preprepared pellet) are taken and placed at the bottom of round-bottom tubes under a layer of culture media. The tubes are incubated for 60 minutes at 37° at an angle of 45°. Viable and motile sperm should be found in the supernatant, which will be removed with a Pasteur pipet. Alternatively, for viscous samples, semen sample can be diluted and centrifuged and pellet overlaid with culture media.

Similarly to simple wash methods, swim-up techniques are usually not complex and relatively inexpensive, although less than 10% of the spermatozoa exposed to this technique are recovered. Although the fraction of recovered sperm is lower than the one obtains from other techniques, it is very clean and contains high concentrations of motile sperm. Therefore, the quality of the initial sample must contain high concentrations of sperm to guarantee the success. Centrifugation of the sample can led to peroxidative damage with nonviable sperm and white cells. This phenomenon becomes evident when the sperm concentration is lower than 10^6/mL after swim-up methods in a good quality sample.

Density Gradient

Density gradient centrifugation (DGC) allows greater recovery of motile sperm but the percentage of progressive motile sperm is usually lower than with swim-up techniques. This technique protects sperm cells from trauma of centrifugation.

Concept: This method separates cells based on their density so progressive motile spermatozoa are selected at the same time that leukocytes, debris, and immature or nonviable sperm cells are discarded. Highly motile sperm cells actively move in the direction of the gradient and can go through the phases faster than poorly motile or immotile spermatozoa.

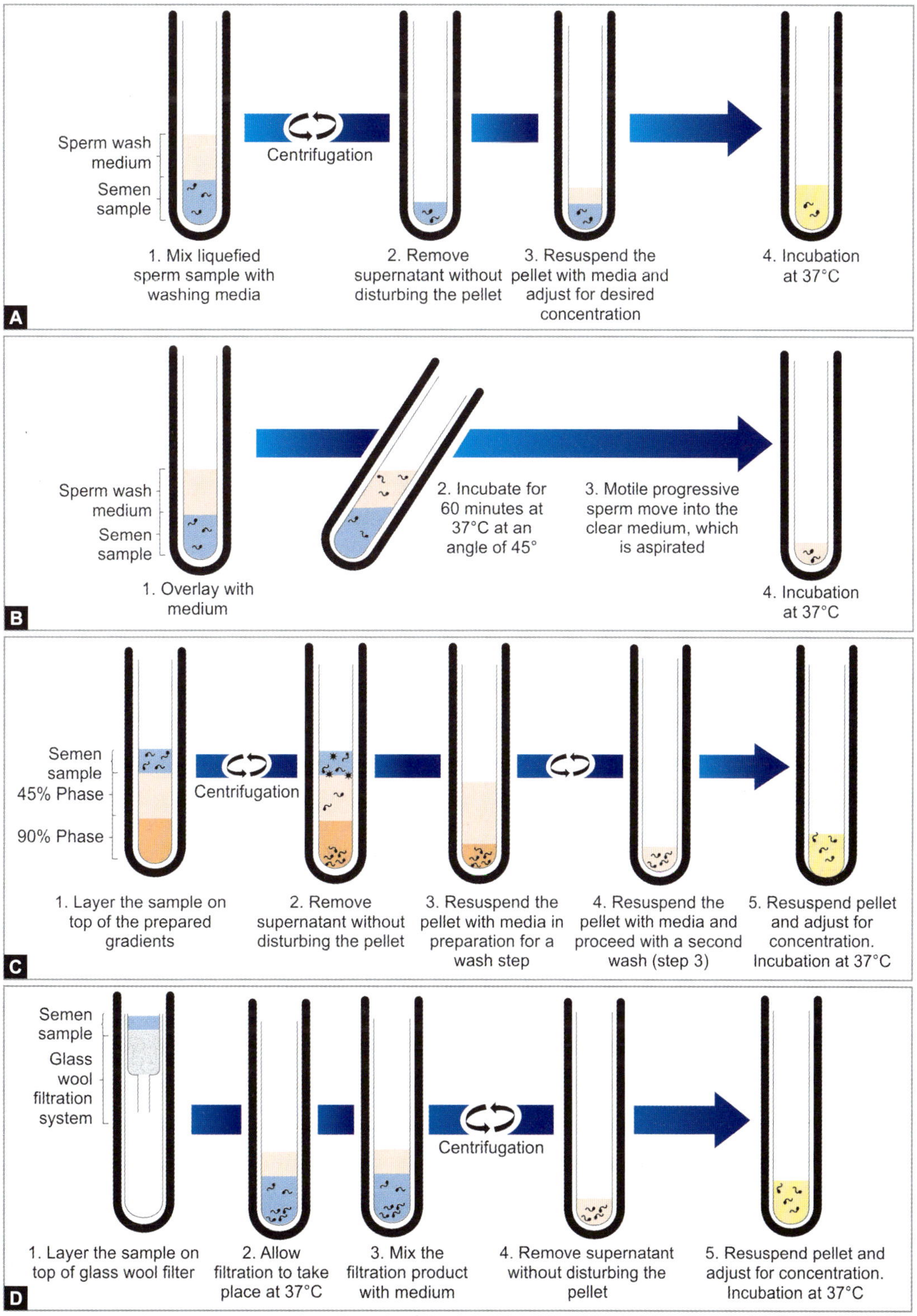

Figs. 2A to D: Sperm preparation techniques. (A) Simple wash method allows to concentrate sperm cells by mixing the semen sample with culture media. Mechanical centrifugation generates a rich pellet of spermatozoa but other cells present in the plasma would not be fully separated; (B) Swim-up method can be performed on a whole sample or on a prepared sample to maximize selection. Progressive motile sperm cells are selected by their ability to move out of the seminal plasma into the fresh culture media; (C) Using density gradient techniques provides an optimum selection given that other cell types and debris are separated in this process. This method uses centrifugal forces to separate cells by their different density; (D) Glass wool filtration techniques use a commercial filter that separates sperm cells similarly to density gradient techniques but with a less clear fraction as a result.

BOX 1 Reactive oxygen species induced damage.

Free radicals or reactive oxygen species (ROS) are chemically reactive molecules containing oxygen, which are generated during mitochondrial oxidative metabolism as well as in other cellular responses. *In vitro*, morphologically abnormal sperm cells and leukocytes present in the ejaculate generate free radicals that can irreversible damage viable sperm, impairing their fertilizing potential. Interestingly, leukocytes produce 100-times more ROS than sperm cells. Sperm plasma membranes are rich in polyunsaturated fatty acids, which are peroxidated in presence of ROS decreasing sperm functions. Moreover, free radicals induce strand breaks in the sperm DNA. Sperm cells prepared following simple washing methods most certainly will be at a higher risk of providing an altered genome to the embryo.

Protocol: Colloidal suspension of silica particles stabilized with covalently-bonded hydrophilic silane supplied in HEPES is the component included in the density gradient. Commonly used protocol for ART comprises two different phases: (1) an upper phase (45%) and (2) a lower phase (90%). Following complete liquefaction, layer the sperm sample over prepared gradients (1 mL for each phase) in conical tubes and allow the sample to centrifuge at 1,000 rpm for 20 minutes. A maximum of 3 mL of semen should be layered on the top of each gradient to guarantee a good recovery. Sperm pellet will be resuspended and washed twice in 3 mL of equilibrated culture media at 1,000 rpm for 10 more minutes. Transfer final pellet into a 5 mL round-bottom tube and resuspend unequilibrated culture media ensuring a final density of <30 million spermatozoa. The tube must be kept in the incubator for equilibration until insemination. Asthenozoospermic samples can be distributed over gradients but reducing its volume to less than 1 mL per phase.

As a result of using DGC methods, the final sample is a substantial and clean fraction, rich in motile spermatozoa. Low quality samples can be processed with this method with good results. The different phases ensure the elimination of debris and leukocytes, which implies that ROS effect is significantly minimized. Although additional centrifugation steps are required in this method, some studies point that levels of DNA fragmented sperm are equal or even reduced when compared with swim-up techniques.

Glass Wool Filtration

First described by Paulson and Polakoski in 1997, the basis for the separation of viable sperm from debris and other cells is the self-propelled movement of the sperm cells and a filtration effect of glass wool fibers.

Concept: Glass wool filtration aims to separate motile progressive spermatozoa from other contents of semen by a mechanical effect provided by glass fibers.

Protocol: Previous to use, loos glass particles must be eliminated by flushing the column with 2–3 mL of sterile medium. Column must be then placed on a new sterile tube and filled with no more than 3 mL of liquefied semen. Allow filtration to take place in an incubator at 37°C and immediately after the whole sample has gone through, wash with fresh medium. Filtrated sample must be diluted with fresh medium in the ratio 1:5 with fresh medium and centrifuge 10 minutes at 1,000 rpm. The pellet will be then resuspended in fresh medium and adjusted for concentration before insemination.

Using glass wool fiber columns, the leukocyte concentration is reduced in a 90% therefore reducing the ROS effect significantly. Because all the ejaculate can be used, this technique is suitable for samples with lower concentrations. Similar to density gradient techniques, the glass-wool filtration results in a higher percentage of normal chromatin condensed sperm cells. As a disadvantage, the fraction obtained in the end of the process is not as clean as the one obtained with swim-up methods.

Enhancing Methods

Magnetic-activated Cell Sorting

This technique is a new efficient and noninvasive method that represents a new evolution in sperm selection in assisted reproduction, which results in samples of highly purified spermatozoa with low fragmentation of their DNA. The application of this technique is indicated to patients with increased percentage of sperm with fragmented DNA, low fertilization or embryo quality, and severe male factor among others.

Concept: Magnetic-activated cell sorting (MACS) separates apoptotic sperm cells from nonapoptotic spermatozoa. Phosphatidylserine residues from the inner membrane of the spermatozoa are translocated to the outside membrane in those experiencing apoptosis. Annexin V, conjugated with magnetic beads, has a strong affinity for phosphatidylserine residues. Therefore, annexin V will bind those sperm exhibiting compromised membrane integrity.

Protocol: 100 μL of MACS solution is mixed with an aliquot of 100 μL of a prepared sperm sample allowing an incubator period of around 15 minutes. Before time finishes, place the provided column in the MACS separator magnetic field and prepare it by hydrating it with the buffer provided. Apply the suspension on the column and collect the filtered result in a bottom round tube.

Semen samples prepared using density gradients followed by MACS show higher viability and a lower population of apoptotic sperm cells. It has been reported that annexin V-negative spermatozoa (non-apoptotic) were associated with an increase in cleavage and pregnancy rates in severe male factor cases. This will be probably related to the fact annexin V-negative sperm cells have lower amounts of DNA damage, decreased caspase activation, higher motility, and increased oocyte interaction when compared to annexin V-positive (apoptotic) spermatozoa. This technique cannot be used by its own since it needs other techniques to remove other substances in the semen that may compromise fertilization potential of sperm cells.

Microsort

As a result of research and improvement in the ART field, recent technologies have emerged to perform a further sperm selection based on the amount of genetic material these cells contain. Developed by the Genetics and IVF Institute in Fairfax (Virginia), Microsort uses flow cytometry sorting to separate sperm cells with different sex chromosome content. Despite the controversial debates about the ethics of sex selection for nonmedical reasons, this technology is available in different countries.

This technique is complementary to processing techniques previously discussed and will be performed on a prepared sample. Following resuspension, different aliquots are stained with a special fluorescent compound (Hoechst 33342) that binds to the sperm's DNA. Ready prepared and stained sperm is then sorted by a flow cytometer, where sperm cells go individually through a laser and the system will select those desired from the rest of the sample. X-sperm will shine brighter since they carry 2.8% more DNA material compared with sperm containing the Y chromosome. Sorting process of each sample takes around 7 hours, so it is advised to plan ahead the process if the unit is planning to offer it, since sample will probably need cryopreservation.

Compounds to Stimulate Sperm Motility

In cases where no motility is detected to a sperm sample, either before or after preparation, viability of sperm can be assessed by the use of products whose composition have theophylline. Sperm motility can be assessed after mixing 1:1 a sperm aliquot with theophylline solution directly on a slide. Theophylline's action is based on increasing the intracellular levels of cyclic adenosine monophosphate (cAMP), phenomenon that only viable sperm will reveal. The use of this compound is highly recommended in cases of surgically retrieved sperm at the insemination time to easily spot the suitable sperm.

Selection Methods during Insemination

Classically, there are two main insemination techniques through which fertilization can be achieved—(1) conventional insemination or IVF, where oocytes and sperm are cultured together and (2) ICSI, where a sperm is inserted directly into the oocyte. For IVF techniques, there is no further selection we can achieve from the laboratory since natural selection will take place thanks to the cumulus cells and will be determined by sperm parameters and ability to undergo the acrosomal reaction. On the other hand, during insemination performing ICSI, embryologists can select sperm based on its motility and progression.

Intracytoplasmic Morphologically Selected Sperm Injection

Sperm cells morphology can be easily assessed during semen analysis and has been consistently associated with fertilization success or failure. Intracytoplasmic morphologically selected sperm injection (IMSI) technique is a variation of ICSI and uses a higher power magnification to visualize different structures (acrosome, nucleus, mitochondria, tail, postacrosoma lamina, and neck) of the sperm morphology in order provide a further selection step before injecting the oocytes. In ICSI cases, the micromanipulator is set to an optical magnification of 200×–400× whereas in IMSI cases, magnification is 6,000× and contrast must be adjusted so that the adequate illumination is achieved (Figs. 3A and B).

Initial studies have shown that IMSI, using spermatozoa selected under high magnification, is associated with higher pregnancy rates in couples with repeated implantation failure. This ultraselection of sperm is potentially interesting in cases of repeated IVF failure and/or in cases of high sperm DNA fragmentation. To date, no evidence of an effect on live birth or miscarriage has been described yet and the improvement in clinical pregnancy rate must be further analyzed with big and robust studies. Furthermore, an inconsistency across different randomized controlled trials (RCTs) is evident and calls for further research in the field since current evidence would not support the clinical use of IMSI.

Physiological Intracytoplasmic Sperm Injection

Through physiological intracytoplasmic sperm injection (PICSI), it is intended to find a less subjective system of choosing sperm for ICSI, and is performed using a molecule similar to it, which envelops the oocyte naturally, hyaluronan (Box 2). Hyaluronan is the main constituent of the cumulus matrix and is known to play a role in the

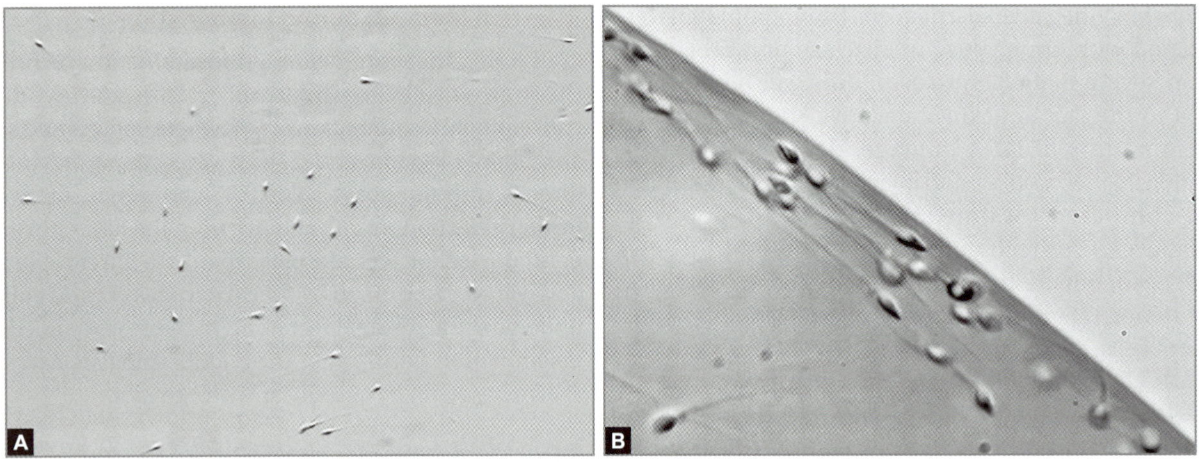

Figs. 3A and B: Microscope magnification for sperm selection. (A) Conventional intracytoplasmic sperm injection (ICSI) is performed setting up the micromanipulator to an optical magnification of 200×–400×. At this magnification, sperm cells are selected based predominantly on motility and progression; (B) Intracytoplasmic morphologically selected sperm injection (IMSI) magnification (6000×) allows embryologists to select spermatozoa based on its morphology as well as by its motility and progression.

BOX 2 Hyaluronic acid binding.

During the spermatogenesis process, the sperm experiences different stages of maturation before acquiring the ability to fertilize. Within these, we found the capacitation process, a series of molecular phenomena that occurs in the sperm after maturation in the epididymis and which gives the sperm the ability to undergo the acrosomal reaction. Only in those spermatozoa that can undergo this process, the plasma membrane of the equatorial and postequatorial segment acquires fusogenic capacity. The acrosome is a small deposit located at the apical end of the sperm head that contains enzymes such as proteins, glycosides, lipases, phosphatases, among others. Hyaluronic acid binding sites on the sperm plasma membrane are an indicator of maturity and its binding to hyaluronic acid in the cumulus matrix causes the release of enzymes that will digest this matrix in order to move toward the oocyte.

selection of competent sperm during IVF. In contrast with traditional ICSI, after sperm preparation with the desired method, and previous to insemination, spermatozoa are cultured in a special dish containing a few drops of a synthetic material similar to hyaluronan. Sperm cells with affinity to this compound will be found in these drops and embryologists will be able to load those to the ICSI dish to perform the insemination (Table 1).

This novel technique is usually indicated in patients with high levels of sperm DNA fragmentation, previous failed ICSI treatment or repeated miscarriages after embryo replacement. Similarly to IMSI, evidence to date is still insufficient to show any differences in pregnancy rates between PICSI and standard ICSI. Robust RCTs urge to evaluate the effect of this technique for it to be considered suitable for the clinical use.

KEY POINTS

- Capacitation is an essential process sperm cells must undergo in order to acquire fertilization capacity.
- Semen analysis is a diagnostic test to assess male fertility, which evaluates key sperm parameters such as sperm cell concentration, motility, and morphology.
- Immune infertility can be caused by the presence of antisperm antibodies.
- The mixed antiglobulin reaction test may be included in some semen analyses to detect the presence of antisperm antibodies.
- Analysis of sperm DNA fragmentation can be useful for treatment selection in couples with previous low fertilization rates.
- The ideal sperm selection method should be fast, easily reproducible and should minimize physiological damage to sperm cells.
- Simple wash method is the one elected for samples with suboptimal parameters (i.e. cryptozoospermia) or surgically retrieved sperm. The main disadvantage is the lack of elimination of other cells that may impair capacitation and affect fertilization potential.
- Reactive oxygen species are compounds generated due to mitochondrial oxidative metabolism and can cause irreversible damage to sperm function.
- Reactive oxygen species are produced by sperm cells and leukocytes predominantly in cell-to-cell interaction scenarios.

TABLE 1 Comparison between the different methods for sperm preparation.

	Low sperm samples	*Normal sperm count*	*Sperm yield*	*Reactive oxygen species ROS damage*	*Leukocyte elimination*	*Time*	*Other comments*
Simple wash	√	√	+++	↑↑	×	20′	• Quick and easy • Not advised for samples with contamination
Swim-up	×	√	+	↑	×	60′	• Quick and easy • Fraction with highly progressive motile sperm • Reduced of percentage of normally chromatin-condensed spermatozoa
Density gradient	√	√	++	↓	√	50′	• Best removal of debris and other cell types • Potential risk of endotoxins
Glass wool	√	√		↓	√	30′	• Remnants of debris present • Increased number of spermatozoa with intact acrosome
Density gradient + MACS	√	√	+++	↓↓	√	70′	Only method to separate apoptotic spermatozoa

(ROS: reactive oxygen species; MACS: magnetic-activated cell sorting)

- Good sperm motility is needed for selecting sperm using swim-up techniques.
- Density gradients separate cells based on their density allowing motile progressive sperm to be separated from leukocytes, debris, and nonviable spermatozoa.
- Reactive oxygen species effect is significantly minimized using density gradients and glass wool filtration techniques.
- Glass wool filters can separate sperm cells from others, reducing up to a 90% leukocyte concentration at the final fraction.
- Magnetic activated cell sorting is a complimentary technique useful to separate sperm cells undergoing an apoptotic process (programmed cell death).
- Microsort is a flow cytometry-based technique that allows separation of sperm cells given their sexual chromosome content.
- Intracytoplasmic sperm injection is an insemination technique where spermatozoa are selected under low magnifications and introducing it inside of a mature oocyte.
- Intracytoplasmic morphology sperm injection is a modified version of conventional ICSI, where spermatozoa are selected based on its morphology using higher magnifications (6,000×).
- Physiological ICSI requires a prior incubation period to identify sperm cells with affinity to hyaluronic acid.

EDITORS' COMMENTS

A number of semen processing techniques have been developed to select the optimal sperm fraction for use with IVF and ICSI. DGC and swim-up procedures have been used as standard semen preparation techniques for ICSI for more than 2 decades.[1] These methods are based on the principle of removing contaminants (cellular debris, microorganisms, red blood cells, and exfoliating cells). Overall, these traditional sperm selection techniques are unable to select sperm fractions with optimal DNA integrity and functional characteristics.[1] Advanced sperm selection techniques have now been introduced to optimize the selection of high quality sperm for ICSI. These selection methods are based on sperm surface charge (electrophoresis and zeta potential), apoptosis (MACS and glass wool), membrane maturity (hyaluronic acid binding), or ultramorphological sperm assessment.[1] A Cochrane review evaluated the effect of sperm selection using hyaluronic acid binding on ICSI outcomes and no differences were observed in clinical pregnancy rates, live birth rates, and miscarriage rates. These results were corroborated by a larger meta-analysis of seven studies and 1,437 ICSI cycles. The authors did not find improvements in fertilization rate or pregnancy rate with sperm selection using hyaluronic acid compared with conventional sperm selection for ICSI. Lastly, the studies comparing IMSI with conventional ICSI have yielded conflicting results, and a 2013 Cochrane review concluded that the results from the existing RCTs do not support the use of IMSI in routine practice. In summary, existing evidence is insufficient to recommend advanced sperm selection techniques for use in ICSI in clinical practice. Further studies are required to determine whether any of these advanced sperm selection techniques could be recommended in specific subgroups of men with low semen quality undergoing ICSI.[1]

Recently, use of testicular sperm for ICSI from non-azoospermic men with high sperm DNA fragmentation in the ejaculated semen has gained increased attention.[2] The biological plausibility relies on the use of sperm collected from the seminiferous tubules that have not undergone oxidative stress attack during the passage through the male genital track.[3] Preliminary results have indicated that the use of testicular in preference over ejaculated sperm for ICSI might increase live birth rates and decrease miscarriage rates in men with confirmed seminal DNA damage.[4]

REFERENCES

1. Esteves SC, Roque M, Bedoschi G, et al. Intracytoplasmic sperm injection for male infertility and consequences for offspring. Nat Rev Urol. 2018;15:535-62.
2. Esteves SC. Testicular versus ejaculated sperm should be used for intracytoplasmic sperm injection (ICSI) in cases of infertility associated with sperm DNA fragmentation | Opinion: Yes. Int Braz J Urol. 2018;44:667-75.
3. Esteves SC. Should a couple with failed in vitro fertilization or intracytoplasmic sperm injection and elevated sperm DNA fragmentation use testicular sperm for the next cycle? Eur Urol Focus. 2018;4:299-300.
4. Esteves SC, Roque M, Bradley CK, et al. Reproductive outcomes of testicular versus ejaculated sperm for intracytoplasmic sperm injection among men with high levels of DNA fragmentation in semen: systematic review and meta-analysis. Fertil Steril. 2017;108:456-67.e1.

SUGGESTED READING

1. Abshagen K, Behre HM, Cooper TG, et al. Influence of sperm surface antibodies on spontaneous pregnancy rates. Fertil Steril. 1998;70:355-6.
2. Aitken RJ, Clarkson JS. Cellular basis of defective sperm function and its association with the genesis of reactive oxygen species by human spermatozoa. J Reprod Fertil. 1987;81:459-69.
3. Amiri I, Ghorbani M, Heshmati S. Comparison of the DNA fragmentation and the sperm parameters after processing by the density gradient and the swim up methods. J Clin Diagn Res. 2012;6:1451-3.
4. Berger T, Marrs RP, Moyer DL. Comparison of techniques for selection of motile spermatozoa. Fertil Steril. 1985;43:268-73.
5. Calogero AE, Fishel S, Hall J, et al. Correlation between intracellular cAMP content, kinematic parameters and hyperactivation of human spermatozoa after incubation with pentoxifylline. Hum Reprod. 1998;13:911-5.
6. Chi HJ, Kim SG, Kim YY, et al. ICSI significantly improved the pregnancy rate of patients with a high sperm DNA fragmentation index. Clin Exp Reprod Med. 2017;44:132-40.
7. Dirican EK, Ozgun OD, Akarsu S, et al. Clinical outcome of magnetic activated cell sorting of non-apoptotic spermatozoa before density gradient centrifugation for assisted reproduction. J Assist Reprod Genet. 2008;25:375-81.
8. Ford WCL. The role of oxygen free radicals in the pathology of human spermatozoa: implications of IVF. In: Matson PL, Lieberman BA (Eds). Clinical IVF Forum; Current Views in Assisted Reproduction. Manchester, UK: Manchester University Press; 1990. pp. 123-39.
9. Franken DR. How accurate is sperm morphology as an indicator of sperm function? Andrologia. 2015;47:720-3.
10. Henkel R, Ichikawa T, Sanchez R, et al. Differentiation of ejaculates showing reactive oxygen species production by spermatozoa or leukocytes. Andrologia. 1997;29:295-301.
11. Jayaraman V, Upadhya D, Narayan PK, et al. Sperm processing by swim-up and density gradient is effective in elimination of sperm with DNA damage. J Assist Reprod Genet. 2012;29:557-63.
12. Mahadevan M, Baker G. Assessment and preparation of semen for in vitro fertilization. In: Wood C, Trounson A (Eds). Clinical In Vitro Fertilization. Berlin: Springer; 1984. pp. 83-97.
13. McDowell S, Kroon B, Ford E, et al. Advanced sperm selection techniques for assisted reproduction. Cochrane Database Syst Rev. 2014;(10):CD010461.
14. Osman A, Alsomait H, Seshadri S, et al. The effect of sperm DNA fragmentation on live birth rate after IVF or ICSI: a systematic review and meta-analysis. Reprod Biomed Online. 2015;30:120-7.
15. Shoukir Y, Chardonnens D, Campana A, et al. Blastocyst development from supernumerary embryos after intracytoplasmic sperm injection: a paternal influence? Hum Reprod. 1998;13:1632-7.
16. Teixeira DM, Barbosa MA, Ferriani RA, et al. Regular (ICSI) versus ultra-high magnification (IMSI) sperm selection for assisted reproduction. Cochrane Database Syst Rev. 2013;(7):CD010167.
17. van der Ven HH, Jeyendran RS, Al-Hasani S, et al. Glass wool column filtration of human semen: relation to swim-up procedure and outcome of IVF. Hum Reprod. 1988;3:85-8.
18. World Health Organization. WHO laboratory manual for the examination and processing of human semen, 5th edition. Geneva: World Health Organization; 2010.

35

CHAPTER

Cryopreservation in ART

Rajvi H Mehta

INTRODUCTION

Cryopreservation is the process of cooling and storing cells, tissues or organs at very low temperatures with the word cryos originating from the Greek word kryos which means cold. One of the earliest observations in this field was when Spallanzani reported in 1776 that sperms cooled in snow for 20 minutes became motionless but later regained motility. One of the defining moments in the science of cryobiology is the pivotal discovery that the use of glycerol, a permeating solute, provided protection to the cells at low temperatures (Polge et al., 1949). Later, Bunge and Sherman (1954) and Bunge et al. (1954) reported on the first human pregnancies following the transfer of frozen-thawed human sperms. Since then our understanding of the principles and the techniques of freezing have refined leading to better outcome following the use of cryopreserved gametes and embryos. Cryopreservation is now an essential component of all assisted reproductive technology (ART) programs.

PRINCIPLES OF CRYOPRESERVATION

Water is major component of all living cells and is necessary for all its metabolic activity. Cellular metabolism diminishes when water from a cell is removed. Therefore, any technique intended to preserve cells aims to first remove all the water from the cells. Thus, the metabolic activity of a cell slows down and completely ceases when it is cooled to low temperatures and they remain suspended in this state when stored at very low temperature. Temperatures, which are as low as –196°C.

REMOVING WATER FROM CELLS

There are three distinct ways of removing water from cells. These are:

1. Converting intracellular water from the fluid state to the solid state of ice by lowering the temperature.
2. Formation of extracellular ice which creates an osmotic imbalance whereby water from the cells migrates out by what is termed as the "osmotic effect".
3. By cooling cells to such low temperatures very quickly wherein the water in the cells gets converted to a glass-like state termed as a vitrified state without the formation of intracellular ice.

The rate of cooling determines how the removal of water from the cells occurs, whether there is intracellular ice crystal formation or osmotic effect. If the cooling rate is high then there is increased ice formation whereas when the cooling rate is slow then there is less ice formation but a greater osmotic imbalance. Therefore, an ideal cooling rate has to be determined whereby damage by either of these effects is minimized (Figs. 1A and B).

The major limiting factor for cell survival following cryopreservation is the intracellular ice crystal formation. This weakness had been long recognized when Luyet stated in Biodynamica that "Crystallization is incompatible with living beings and should be avoided whenever possible." These ice crystals can have sharp edges which in turn damage the intracellular organelles be it endoplasmic reticulum, Golgi, RNA or mitochondria. Therefore, minimizing ice crystal formation ensures minimal damage to the cell and higher survival rate following thawing.

Slow cooling	*Rapid cooling*
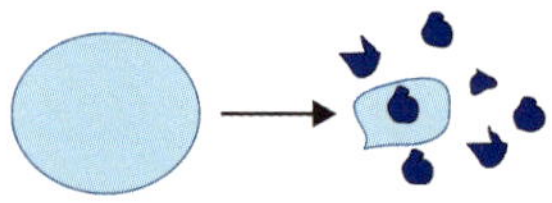	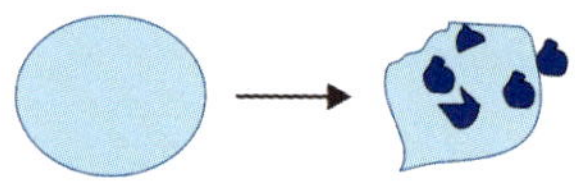
A	**B**
Gradual cooling of the cell suspension	Rapid cooling of the cell suspension
Less ice crystal formation	Greater formation of ice crystal
Less damage of intracellular organelles	Greater risk of intracellular organelle damage
More osmotic imbalance	Less osmotic imbalance
Can be used for larger cells with greater water content	Applicable for smaller cells with less intracellular water
Ideal for embryos	Ideal for sperms

Figs. 1A and B: Rate of (A) slow cooling and (B) rapid cooling.
Source: https://alcor.org/Library/html/vitrification.html

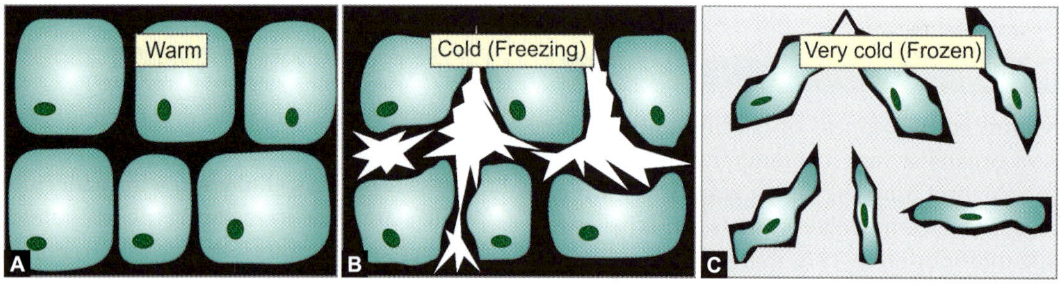

Figs. 2A to C: Changes that occur during slow freezing.
Source: https://alcor.org/Library/html/vitrification.html

MECHANISMS OF CELL DAMAGE DURING FREEZING

In a warm solution, there is water in as well as between the cells. As the temperature is lowered, the process of freezing starts. When the rate of cooling is slow then there is a formation of ice between the cells. This leads to the dehydration of the cells as there is increased extracellular ice formation as depicted in Figures 2A to C.

The white space indicates ice crystal formation in Figure 2B. Finally cells get squashed by the ice crystals leading to membrane damage.

IDEAL RATE OF COOLING

The survival rate of cells depends upon the rate of cooling and an ideal rate of cooling has been determined for many cell types and that the optimum cooling rate generally appears as inverted "U" (Fig. 3) (Mazur et al., 1972).

Mazur in this landmark paper on the fundamentals of cryobiology explained that the second half of the inverted "U" (i.e. at higher cooling rates), came from the supercooling (cooling of the solute below its freezing point) induced by cooling at a rate that prevented the cell from maintaining an equilibrium between the intracellular and extracellular milieu. As the cell and the surrounding media cool below freezing, pure water is precipitated out of the extracellular media as ice. This causes an increase in extracellular concentration, which, at slow enough cooling rates, causes the cell to lose water and increase intracellular concentration. When cooling rates are too rapid, water cannot leave the cell quickly enough to maintain equilibrium with the external medium and supercools. Since the probability of ice formation increases with the degree of supercooling, the faster the cooling rate the more likely ice will form inside the cell, a major factor of cell death in cryopreservation procedures.

MITIGATING THE DETRIMENTAL EFFECTS OF FREEZING

The detrimental effects of freezing are mitigated by the use of solutions termed as cryoprotectants. These are

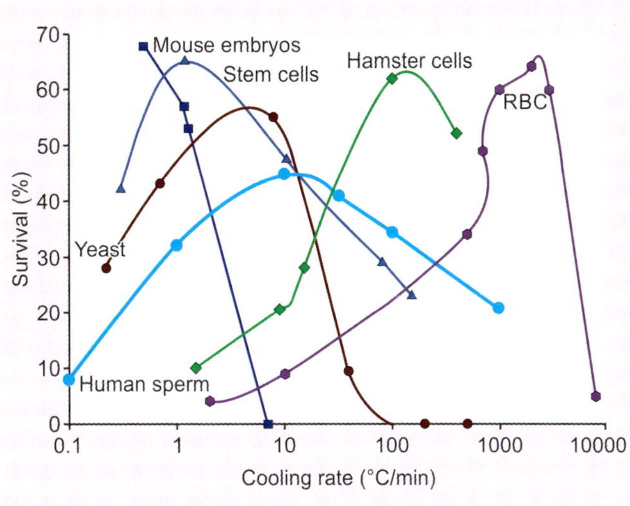

Fig. 3: The ideal rate of cooling.
Source: Adapted from Walters EM, Benson JD, Woods EJ, et al. History of sperm cryopreservation. In: Pacey AA, Tomlinson MJ (Eds). Sperm Banking: Theory and Practice. Cambridge: Cambridge University Press; 2009.

highly viscous solutions which can either permeate within the cell or could be impermeable. When they permeate, they increase the solute concentration within the cell and thereby reduce intracellular ice crystal formation. These croprotectants get into the extracellular space, slow down the movement of the water molecules and prevent them from gathering together to form ice.

Although these cryoprotectants mitigate all the detrimental effects of freezing, they themselves are toxic when cells are exposed to them at high concentrations or for longer periods of time. Therefore, an "optimal" concentration and time for which the cells should be exposed to the cryoprotectant has to be determined and an ideal protocol for its removal is equally crucial. The concentration and time of exposure to the cryoprotectant would be dependent on the type of the cells to be cryopreserved especially their dimension and the intracellular water content.

Some of the most commonly used cryoprotectants are the nonpermeating cryoprotectant such as sucrose and permeating cryoprotectants such as dimethyl sulfoxide, propanediol and glycerol.

FACTORS DETERMINING THE SUCCESS OF CRYOPRESERVATION

- The type and concentration of cryoprotectant.
- The duration of exposure to the cryoprotectant.
- The cell dimension and the amount of water content.
- The cooling rate.
- The optimal protocol for removal of the cryoprotectant.

This can be done by monitoring cells under a microscope while cooling and noting the percentage of cells which freeze intracellularly at a given temperature and degree of supercooling. After these parameters are established a theoretically optimized protocol can be developed which obeys the fundamental principles (Karlsson et al., 1993). Further research is needed in this area as rightly suggested by Walters et al. (2009). A large amount of work is involved in establishing such cryobiological parameters but the outcome would be quite significant as currently many cryopreservation protocols have been empirically derived.

VITRIFICATION

Vitrification is a process whereby the intracellular water gets converted to a state of "glass" without the intermediary solid phase of "ice" formation (Luyet and Hodapp, 1938). This technique therefore reduces the extent of cryoinjury that occurs either due to ice crystal formation or osmotic effect. To achieve this state, one needs very high concentration of cryoprotectants and an extremely high rate of cooling. A cell suspension on vitrification appears totally transparent as compared with one that has been cooled by either of the earlier described methods.

MECHANISMS OF COOLING DURING VITRIFICATION

When large concentrations of cryoprotectants are added to the cells, these substances prevent the movements of the water molecules and thereby freezing of the solution

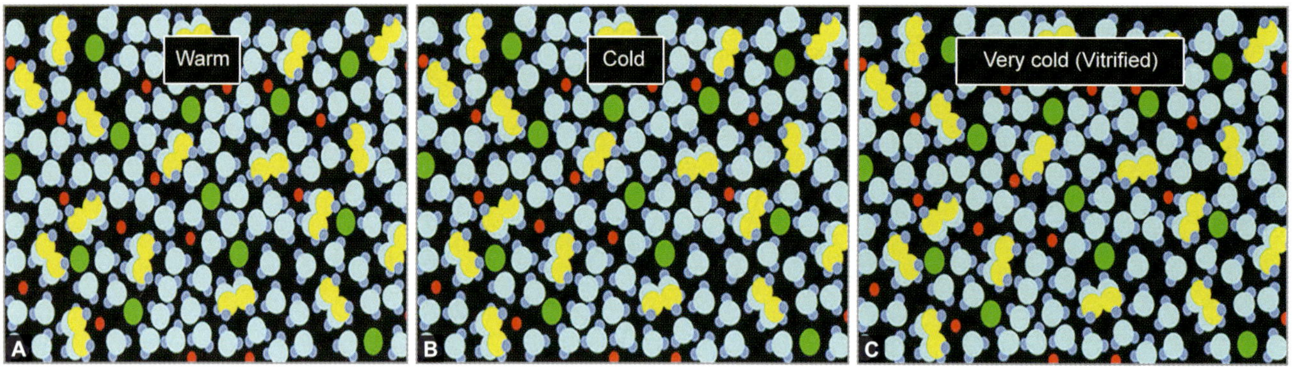

Figs. 4A to C: Changes that occur during the cooling process of vitrification.
Source: https://alcor.org/Library/html/vitrification.html

as the temperature is lowered. The molecules get locked at temperature –100°C and lower.

In Figures 4A to C, water molecules are depicted in blue, the cryoprotectant in yellow and the cells are green and red. In the presence of high concentration of cryoprotectants, the molecules just move slower and slower when they are cooled and finally get locked in a place and a solid is formed. Water thus becomes solid without freezing, i.e. vitrified. (http://www.alcor.org/Library/html/vitrification.html).

Three factors affect the probability of vitrification: the cooling rate, viscosity and volume.

The probability of vitrification is directly proportional to the cooling rate and inversely proportional to the volume. Increasing the viscosity or cooling rate, or decreasing the volume will each increase the probability of vitrification. In the past, vitrification was achieved simply by plunging the sample into liquid nitrogen (LN) at –196°C (Rall and Fahy, 1985). In this method, heat transfer from the sample into the LN leads to the evaporation of LN around the sample, resulting in the formation of a nitrogen gas layer, which acts as an insulator. This insulation reduces the heat transfer and makes it impossible to achieve uniform and rapid cooling rate.

The efficacy of vitrification therefore depends upon the kind of carrier system on which the cells can be placed to maximize heat transfer and the skills of the cryobiologist whereby he/she can mix the sample with the cyroprotectant, load it on the carrier and plunge into LN in the shortest possible time. For human embryos, this entire procedure has to be accomplished within a minute.

FACTORS DETERMINING THE SUCCESS OF CRYOPRESERVATION

The success of cryopreservation is the ability to retrieve viable and functionally active cells following thawing or cooling. The factors which determine the success of cryopreservation are nothing but a summarization based on the fundamental principles of cryobiology. These factors include:

1. *The size of the cells and the water content within the cells*. The post-thaw recovery is better in smaller cells. Therefore, cryopreservation of sperms is much easier than cryopreservation of eggs as the latter are one of the largest cells in the human body.
2. *The type of cryoprotectant used and the concentration and its permeability*. Higher the concentration better is the cryopreservation but all these solutions are toxic and therefore a balance has to be attained between the concentrations that can optimize cryodamage without toxicity.
3. *The rate of cooling***.** This in turn would depend upon the cell type especially the permeability of the cell membrane. It is also influenced by the container in which the samples are frozen for slow or rapid freezing or the carriers on which the samples are cooled for vitrification. Therefore, cooling in straws as the thickness of the walls is much thinner than cooling in vials is often better. Cooling in vials is used efficiently for cells like sperms.
4. *Storage temperature*. All metabolic activity of cells ceases when stored at –196°C in LN. Sherman (1963) had reported that storing human sperm at (LN) temperature (–196°C) was superior to storage at –75°C. In addition, no loss of motility was observed when the sperms were stored in LN for 1 year; however, there was a decline in motility after storage at –75°C.
5. The rate of warming/cooling.

CRYOPRESERVATION IN ASSISTED REPRODUCTIVE TECHNOLOGY

As mentioned earlier, semen cryopreservation and use of frozen-thawed sperms for insemination was first reported in the 1950s. With the concern about transmission of the human immunodeficiency virus (HIV) through infected semen, it became mandatory to cryopreserve and quarantine donor semen, retest the donor after 3 months and then release the semen sample for insemination. This made the use of cryopreservation of semen a routine procedure in ART clinics and semen banks.

CRYOPRESERVATION OF EMBRYOS

Trounson and Mohr (1983) were the first to report on the cryopreservation of human embryos and a live birth following the transfer of the thawed embryos. It is now routine to stimulate the ovaries for recovering multiple oocytes but to prevent the risk of multiple pregnancies and multiple births, a maximum of three embryos are transferred and the rest cryopreserved for use in the subsequent cycles. It was slow freezing that was being used as rapid freezing leads to the development of ice crystals which often damage blastomeres.

CRYOPRESERVATION OF OOCYTES

Although cryopreservation of embryos became routine, cryopreservation of oocytes still baffled cryobiologists. Oocytes being the largest cell in the body and a high content of cytoplasm made it difficult to cryopreserve them as the potential of ice crystal damage was very high. Chen (1986) did manage to achieve a pregnancy with the fertilization of a frozen-thawed oocyte. However, for the next 15 years, oocyte cryopreservation still remained an experimental procedure. It was only after the successful standardization of vitrification that oocyte cryopreservation became possible (Kuleshova et al., 1999).

INDIA'S CONTRIBUTION TO HUMAN EMBRYO CRYOPRESERVATION

It is pertinent to mention here that although it is Trounson and Mohr (1983) who are credited with the birth of the first baby following the transfer of frozen-thawed embryos; it was later discovered that Dr Subhas Mukherjee was the first to cryopreserve human embryos and transfer them to a natural cycle leading to the birth of Durga aka Kanupriya in 1978 (Anand Kumar, 1997).

CRYOPRESERVATION OF HUMAN REPRODUCTIVE TISSUES: THE PURPOSE

As of date, semen, sperms, oocytes, zygotes, 2–8 cell embryos, blastocysts and ovarian and testicular tissues have been successfully frozen and thawed. The reasons for which they are frozen and their efficacy is variable. Sperms/semen and embryos from various species, laboratory animals, domestic animals as well as endangered species have been frozen. The principles behind cryopreservation remain the same but the actual protocols may differ. This section is only focusing on the need and purpose of cryopreservation of reproductive cells and tissues in humans.

PURPOSE FOR CRYOPRESERVATION OF SEMEN/SPERMATOZOA

Patients with cancer: When young adults in their reproductive age group have been diagnosed with cancer then there is likelihood that there could be some damage to their testis following radiation or chemotherapy. This could either lead to infertility or potential genetic damage. Therefore, in such patients, it is advisable to store the semen sample prior to the onset of chemotherapy or radiation therapy.

Semen donors: With a potential high risk of transmission of HIV or hepatitis virus through semen, it is now mandatory to freeze and quarantine semen samples from donors for 3–6 months prior to thawing and releasing them to a recipient. Blood samples of all semen donors are tested for infectious diseases prior to enrolling them as donors. Even if they test negative by an HIV/hepatitis antibody test at that point of time, they could still have been infected in the very near past which may not yet be reflected in the blood sample tested. Therefore, the semen samples are frozen stored, donor retested for infectious viral diseases and then if he still tests negative then the samples are released for use.

For later use when male partner is not available during treatment: Male partners in certain professions like the military or working in the different countries stay away from their spouses for long periods of time. Semen samples of male partners of such couples can be stored so that the female partner can be inseminated even when the partner is not available.

As a "backup" in case of difficulty in getting samples during infertility treatment with ARTs: It is a well-established fact that many couples undergo a lot of anxiety during infertility treatment with ART. There are some instances when the male partner is unable to provide a semen sample on the day of the procedure of ART. Therefore, semen samples when collected and stored in the early stages of treatment serve as a backup in case of the male not able to provide the sample. Often, just knowing that there is a stored sample gives psychological relief to the male and reduces anxiety on the day of the procedure.

For pooling samples: In some individuals, the sperm concentration which may be low but not very low to go in for the more demanding ARTs like *in vitro* fertilization (IVF) and embryo transfer or intracytoplasmic sperm injection (ICSI). In such individuals, several samples can be stored, pooled and then can be inseminated in the female partner. Storing and pooling of semen samples may be a more cost-effective and less demanding method of treating infertility due to borderline oligozoospermia.

PURPOSE FOR CRYOPRESERVATION OF OOCYTES

Before cancer therapy: Like sperms and semen, oocytes are preserved for women, in the reproductive age group or those who have not yet completed their families, undergoing treatment for cancer. Oocyte preservation is yet not as efficacious as semen/sperm freezing. Also recovering oocytes is a complex procedure necessitating ovarian stimulation and follicular aspiration which can take about 2 weeks. In many instances, it may not be possible to delay cancer treatment till oocytes have been retrieved. In some cases, it may be deleterious to the woman, especially those with reproductive cancers, to undergo ovarian stimulation. In such cases, attempts can be made to retrieve oocytes from the ovaries without stimulation wherein it may not be possible to even recover the oocytes.

Delaying pregnancy: Childbearing is being delayed in many societies, especially urban societies and professionals and with the biological clock ticking, women may want to prefer to preserve their oocytes. Women take this decision if they are not psychologically or financially prepared for a pregnancy; they may not have found a suitable life partner or would not want a pregnancy as that could interfere with professional goals especially those working in the entertainment or fashion industry. Being aware that the quality of the oocytes deteriorates with age and the rapid decline after 35–37 years, many women do consider preserving their healthy oocytes for future use.

Oocyte donation: Donated oocytes can be cryopreserved for future use as and when the recipient is ready for the procedure. Although, unlike semen and sperms, it is not mandatory to quarantine the donated oocytes prior to use since the protocol for preserving oocytes is not as efficacious as that for sperms.

Partner unable to provide sample on day of ART: In some rare incidents, a male partner is unable to provide the semen sample for IVF or there are not adequate sperms for ICSI and there is no backup sample then on may need to cryopreserve the oocytes.

PURPOSE FOR CRYOPRESERVATION OF ZYGOTES

It is common practice in all ART clinics to hyperstimulate the ovaries to retrieve more than oocyte and therefore more than one embryo following IVF or ICSI. However, only two or maximum of three embryos are transferred while the rest are preserved. Some clinics prefer to preserve the fertilized eggs at the two pronuclei stage (zygotes) rather than embryos.

Advantages of zygote freezing: Zygotes have no meiotic spindles and the nuclear material is membrane bound, there is very low risk of any chromosomal damage as compared to that with dividing cells such as within an embryo or maturing oocyte.

Disadvantages: All eggs that fertilize do not develop into embryos. Therefore, one could be freezing zygotes which had no development potential which would have easily been "screened out" if these were allowed to develop further. As of now, the pregnancy rate following frozen-thawed zygote transfer is reported to be about 15% (Mocanu et al., 2008).

There are countries like Germany and Italy which did not permit embryo freezing and therefore they needed to freeze zygotes despite the limitations.

Cryopreservation of embryos: As mentioned earlier, women undergo ovarian stimulation for ART. The excess of embryos are stored for use in the subsequent cycles thereby reducing the risk of multiple pregnancy as well as need for ovarian stimulation and pick-up.

In patients who have been hyperstimulated and at a risk of ovarian hyperstimulation syndrome (OHSS), a pregnancy accompanied by an increase in beta-hCG levels can seriously aggravate OHSS. In such cases, a pregnancy is not desired and therefore it is advisable to store the embryos for use in the subsequent cycles.

Ovarian and testicular tissue preservation: This is recommended in cases of young adults wherein mature germ cells may not be retrievable. Furthermore, preservation of tissues is considered to be simpler as compared with cells. However, the outcome following ovarian tissue transplantation following thawing needs lot more standardization.

CRYOPRESERVATION PROTOCOLS

Slow freezing: There are several protocols available for the cryopreservation of oocytes and embryos. Basically, the

TABLE 1 Comparison of slow freezing versus vitrification.

	Slow freezing	*Vitrification*
Cryopreservation concentration	1.5 M	3–5 M
Volume	0.3–1 mL	<1 μL
Contact between LN and cells	No	Yes (open system)
Cooling rate	~0.5°C/min	~25–50,000°C/min
Freezing	Slow	Ultrarapid
Thawing/Warming	Slow	Rapid
Time taken	>180 min	1 sec

(LN: liquid nitrogen)

cells are gradually exposed to relatively low concentration of permeating cryoprotectants usually glycerol or dimethyl sulfoxide (DMSO) in the range of 1.0–1.5 M for oocytes or 1.35–1.5 M for embryos, which are added to the culture medium. Other protectants are also in widespread use, alone or in various combinations. These include permeating cryoprotectants such as ethylene glycol (EG) and propylene glycol (Chen et al., 2005; Luz et al., 2009) and nonpermeating ones such as sucrose, glucose, or fructose (Diez et al., 2001; Barcelo-Fimbres and Seidel 2007). The oocytes/embryos are then loaded in small volumes into straws and cooled to about –5°C to –7°C where they are kept for several minutes to equilibrate. After equilibration, the solution is seeded to initiate extracellular freezing, and then cooled slowly, at about 0.3–0.5°C/minute, to anywhere between –30°C and –65°C. Once at the desired temperature, the straws are plunged into LN for storage. When following this procedure, seeding of the extracellular solution and a very slow cooling rate ensure that freezing will take place only outside the cytoplasm, resulting in outward movement of osmotically active water from the cells and their gradual dehydration until they reach the temperature at which the intracellular matrix vitrifies (Saragusty and Arav, 2011).

*Vitrification***:** Vitrification needs to be carried out with very low volumes (<1 μL) for efficient heat transfer and solution with very high concentrations of cryoprotectants and high viscosity. This low volume and high viscosity makes handling a little difficult and this needs to be done at very high speed to minimize the exposure and toxicity of the cryoprotectants. The cooling rates are as high as –50,000°C/minute. It has been shown that increasing the cooling rates improves the survival rates by up to 37% (Arav and Zeron, 1997).

To attain these very high cooling rates, different devices and carriers are used for "carrying' the cells. These could be "open" systems wherein the cells are directly exposed to LN. These include an electron microscope grids or commercially available carriers such as cryoloops and cryoleafes with vitrifit. These give excellent cooling rate but there is a risk of potential contamination of LN or contamination with LN. To overcome this, equipment which sterilize LN are now available (Parmegiani et al., 2009).

A closed system is one where the samples are stored in carriers wherein they are not directly exposed to LN. Matsumoto et al. (2001) have provided a detailed list of the different carrier devices.

COMPARISON OF SLOW FREEZING VERSUS VITRIFICATION

Comparison of slow freezing versus vitrification has been shown in Table 1.

Although it takes about 3 hours for slow freezing, the time taken by the cryobiologist to process the cells for slow freezing or vitrification is nearly the same. Whatever time is taken for slow freezing is automated and does not require operator's time and several samples can be processed at the same time. The actual time taken for vitrification is just a few seconds but one needs to process one or two eggs or embryos at a time. Therefore, if there are many eggs or embryos to be frozen then the time taken for vitrification may be much higher than that for slow freezing.

EDITORS' COMMENTS

This chapter provides readers an overview of principles and practices of cryobiology applied to ART. In recent years, practitioners have witnessed a shift from "slow freezing" protocols to "vitrification" methods using different carriers and cryoprotectants. Nowadays, competent ART programs have mastered the fundamental principles of cryobiology and obtained over 85% and 70% cryosurvival rates for blastocysts and oocytes, respectively.[1] These achievements allowed the introduction of commercial egg banks and gave infertile couples the possibility of family planning with aid of gametes and embryos cryopreservation. Advances in embryo and oocyte cryopreservation techniques have also changed the metrics of ART. Clinicians now rely of cumulative live birth rates (LBRs) as the indicator to best reflect the effectiveness of an ART program.[2] Furthermore, sperm freezing has evolved and now allows cryopreservation of low sperm numbers in special carriers mimicking vitrification of embryos and oocytes.[3,4] Recovery of spermatozoa is high, and good-quality epididymal (or testicular) sperm will invariably be obtained in obstructive azoospermia, thus a single operation suffices for numerous subsequent IVF procedures, and the vast majority of samples can be successfully cryopreserved in straws using the established low-cost technique.[5] However, this is not the case for the vast majority of men with nonobstructive azoospermia undergoing sperm retrieval. In such cases, the number of spermatozoa harvested from the seminiferous tubules can be very small and repeat procedures are not always feasible.[6] Therefore, the possibility of freezing low sperm numbers in small carriers, and recovery of viable sperm for intracytoplasmic sperm injection is greatly advantageous.

REFERENCES

1. Alpha Scientists In Reproductive Medicine. The Alpha consensus meeting on cryopreservation key performance indicators and benchmarks: proceedings of an expert meeting. Reprod Biomed Online. 2012;25(2):146-67.
2. Esteves SC. Efficacy, efficiency and effectiveness of gonadotropin therapy for infertility treatment. Med Express. 2015;2(3):M150302.
3. Esteves SC. Novel concepts in male factor infertility: clinical and laboratory perspectives. J Assist Reprod Genet. 2016;33(10):1319-35.
4. Yovich JL, Esteves SC. Storage of sperm samples from males with azoospermia. Reprod Biomed Online. 2018;37(5):509-10.
5. Miyaoka R, Esteves SC. Predictive factors for sperm retrieval and sperm injection outcomes in obstructive azoospermia: do etiology, retrieval techniques and gamete source play a role? Clinics (Sao Paulo). 2013;68:111-9.
6. Esteves SC. Clinical management of infertile men with nonobstructive azoospermia. Asian J Androl. 2015;17:459-70.

SUGGESTED READING

1. Anand Kumar TC. Architect of India's first test tube baby: Dr Subhas Mukerji, 16 January 1931 to 19 July 1981. Curr Sci. 1997;72:526-31.
2. Arav A, Zeron Y. Vitrification of bovine oocytes using modified minimum drop size technique (MDS) is effected by the composition and the concentration of the vitrification solution and by the cooling conditions. Theriogenology. 1997;47:341.
3. Barcelo-Fimbres M, Seidel GE Jr. Effects of either glucose or fructose and metabolic regulators on bovine embryo development and lipid accumulation in vitro. Mol Reprod Dev. 2007;74:1406-18.
4. Bunge RG, Keettel WC, Sherman JK. Clinical use of frozen semen: report of four cases. Fertil Steril. 1954;5:520-9.
5. Bunge RG, Sherman JK. Frozen human semen. Fertil Steril. 1954;5:193-4.
6. Chen C. Pregnancy after human oocyte cryopreservation. Lancet. 1986;1:884-6.
7. Diez C, Heyman Y, Le Bourhis D, et al. Delipidating in vitro-produced bovine zygotes: effect on further development and consequences for freezability. Theriogenology. 2001;55:923-36.
8. Karlsson JO, Cravalho EG, Borel Rinkes IH, et al. Nucleation and growth of ice crystals inside cultured hepatocytes during freezing in the presence of dimethyl sulfoxide. Biophys J. 1993;65:2524-36.
9. Kuleshova L, Gianaroli L, Magli C, et al. Birth following vitrification of a small number of human oocytes: case report. Hum Reprod. 1999;14:3077-9.
10. Luyet BJ, Hodapp EL. Revival of frog's spermatozoa vitrified in liquid air. Proc Soc Exp Biol NY. 1938;39:433-4.
11. Luz MR, Holanda CC, Pereira JJ, et al. 99 Survival rate and in vitro development of in vivo-produced and cryopreserved dog embryos. Reprod Fertil Dev. 2009;22:208-9.
12. Matsumoto H, Jiang JY, Tanaka T, et al. Vitrification of large quantities of immature bovine oocytes using nylon mesh. Cryobiology. 2001;42:139-44.
13. Mazur P, Leibo SP, Chu EH. A two-factor hypothesis of freezing injury. Evidence from Chinese hamster tissue-culture cells. Exp Cell Res. 1972;71:345-55.
14. Mocanu EV, Cottell E, Waite K, et al. Frozen-thawed transfer cycles: are they comparable with fresh? Ir Med J. 2008; 101:181-4.
15. Parmegiani L, Cognigni GE, Filicori M. Ultra-violet sterilization of liquid nitrogen prior to vitrification. Hum Reprod. 2009;24:2969.
16. Polge C, Smith AV, Parkes AS. Revival of spermatozoa after vitrification and dehydration at low temperatures. Nature. 1949;164:666.
17. Rall WF, Fahy GM. Ice-free cryopreservation of mouse embryos at –196°C by vitrification. Nature. 1985;313:573-5.
18. Saragusty J, Arav A. Current progress in oocyte and embryo cryopreservation by slow freezing and vitrification. Reproduction. 2011;141:1-19.
19. Sherman JK. Improved methods of preservation of human spermatozoa by freezing and freeze-drying. Fertil Steril. 1963;14:49-64.
20. Trounson A, Mohr L. Human pregnancy following cryopreservation, thawing and transfer of an eight-cell embryo. Nature. 1983;305:707-9.
21. Walters EM, Benson JD, Woods EJ, et al. History of sperm cryopreservation. In: Pacey AA, Tomlinson MJ (Eds). Sperm Banking: Theory and Practice. Cambridge: Cambridge University Press; 2009.

36

CHAPTER

Morphokinetics in ART

Keshav Malhotra

INTRODUCTION

Ever since the inception of in vitro fertilization (IVF), selecting what goes back has always been based on the morphological evaluation, whether it is a 4 cell, 8 cell or a top quality blastocyst, grading embryo quality based on the morphology is still considered the best prognostic indicator for an assisted reproductive technology (ART) outcome (Pirkevi et al., 2016), but the fact is that conventional morphological selection is still poorly linked to implantation and live birth rates (LBRs). The past decade or so has worked on combining morphology and kinetics and we now have a new field known as morphokinetics which seems to be a very promising venture to select the best possible embryo thus hoping to improve the chances of conception (Pirkevi et al., 2016). Monitoring of the dynamic morphology with the various systems available in the market has given us the chance to evaluate the exact timings of cell division and the aberrations that come with it (Wong et al., 2010). In a conventional setup, the embryos would have to be moved from the incubator to the microscope for evaluation once or sometimes even twice a day, whereas a time-lapse system would take images every 5–10 minutes and allow for real-time continuous monitoring without the embryos being subjected to any stress of temperature and pH change, along with this one can also now pinpoint the exact timing of the various cell divisions also observe multinucleation and the formation and absorption of fragmentation. When you combine all of these parameters and compare it with conventional embryo selection, we now have an obvious extra set of parameters to consider before choosing an embryo for transfer (Meseguer et al., 2011; Wong et al., 2010).

TIME-LAPSE TECHNOLOGY: DIFFERENT SYSTEMS AVAILABLE RIGHT NOW

There are numerous time-lapse systems (Figs. 1A to E) in use as of now, the most common ones being Primo vision (Vitrolife) and Embryoscope (Vitrolife) which use bright-field imaging in their technology. EEVA or early embryonic viability assessment (Auxogyn) is based on the dark-field imaging, all of these systems use and inverted microscope which is programmed to take pictures at set intervals ranging from 5 minutes to 20 minutes. The images are then patched to each other using a software creating a time-lapse video of the embryonic growth, and these can be played at any speed and even rewound to certain time points making embryo assessment highly detailed (Kovacs, 2014). The Embryoscope is basically an incubator which has the time-lapse system incorporated within it, here the embryos are cultured in microdrop wells and the dish is brought into view sequentially where the images are then taken, in this system each dish can culture 12 embryos and the system can take 6 dishes in one go. The newer model (Embryoscope+) can incorporate 16 embryos and 12 dishes. The embryos can be evaluated in 7 focal planes and it utilizes red LED light which is of a low intensity 635 nm and the amount of exposure is also limited to 0.5 seconds per image, thus the total exposure to light which was earlier thought to be a compromising factor is actually lesser than the conventional monitoring systems. The system is incorporated with an annotation software which can also grade the embryos on D3 and D5 and now newer versions are incorporating technology which would make annotations automatic and less time-consuming.

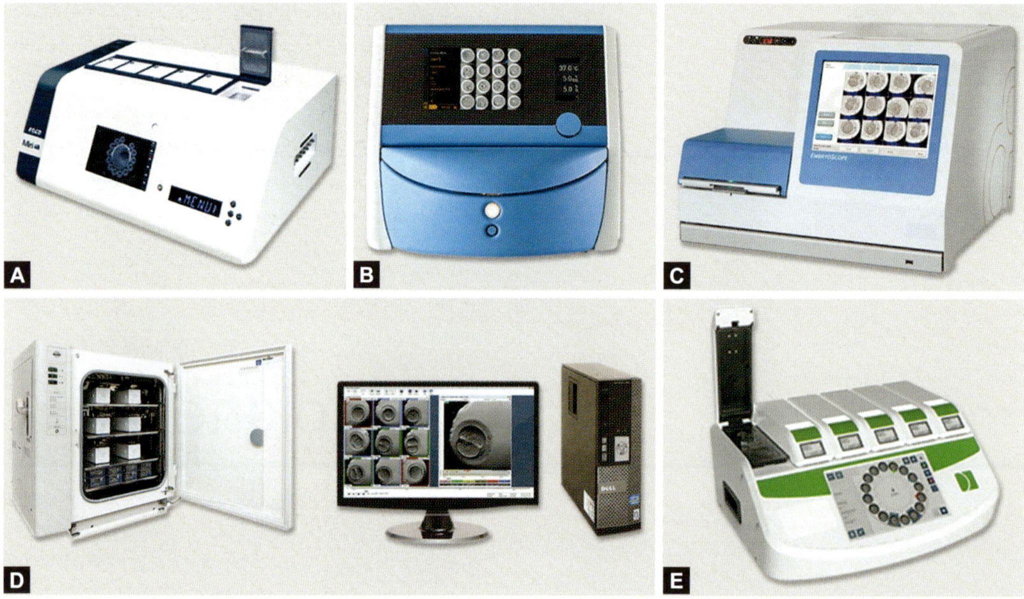

Figs. 1A to E: Various time-lapse incubators available. (A) Esco Miri; (B) Embryoscope plus; (C) Embryoscope; (D) Primo vision; (E) Gavi.

Primo vision is another form of a time-lapse imaging device which can be placed directly into a conventional incubator, thus making it more cost-effective. Here also the embryos are cultured in multiwell dishes and each device can only incorporate 1 dish which contains about 16 wells.

Early embryonic viability assessment like the Primo vision requires a device to be placed into a traditional incubator and utilizes dark-field observation to provide an improved assessment of the cell membranes of the blastomeres and record cleavage events. The software, based on its patented prediction system, selects which 4-cell embryo has the best chance to become a blastocyst.

Esco has also come up with a time-lapse system named as Miri. The Miri has six individual chambers and in this system the camera moves to the dish, opening the chambers does not interrupt the culture conditions of the other dishes. Each dish of the Miri can culture up to 14 embryos and the system has a software which can help in annotating the embryonic growth.

Another common time-lapse is the Geri by Genea Biomedx. Like the Miri this incubator also has six individual chambers. All chambers have their own camera, dedicated to capture images in 11 focal planes and the image of the embryo is taken every 5 minutes. Having a dedicated camera gets rid of the need to move the dishes, thus making things simpler.

Other companies are also foraying into this field and we can expect this technology to grow rapidly in the coming few years.

Safety of the Equipment

Any new technology when it enters into any stream needs to prove its safety and it was the same with time-lapse. Many thought that light exposure during the observations and the electromagnetic field or the heat generated due to the moving parts can all be potentially harmful for the embryos. It was found that overall light exposure was significantly lesser in these devices as compared to standard monitoring of embryos. No difference in fertilization rates, cleavage and blastulation rates and many have concluded that there are no safety issues with using these devices (Kovacs, 2014).

Observations by Time-lapse

It was actually in 1997 when Payne et al. described the first set of observations made using this technology. Of the 50 oocytes cultured, there were no differences in fertilization and embryo quality but they noted variations in polar body extrusion and pronuclear (PN) appearance, also noted some significant differences between good and bad embryos throughout development. Since then many have studied various parameters and many prediction models have been made. Embryonic morphokinetics were studied by Meseguer et al. and they analyzed 247 embryos which had data for implantation. Based on his work, it was found that direct cleavage division from a single cell to 3 cells or a reduced time as 2 cells (<5 hours), uneven blastomeres at the first division (>25% difference) and multinucleation of 4-cell embryos was directly linked with very low

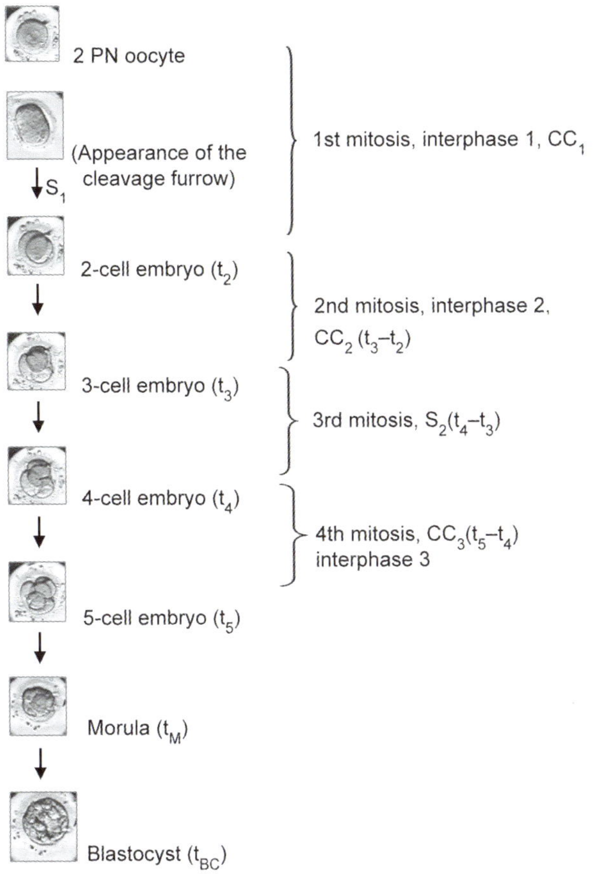

Fig. 2: Embryo development and various time points.
Source: Kovacs P Embryo selection: the role of time-lapse monitoring. Reprod Biol Endocrinol. 2014;12:124.

implantation potential. They also studied the various cell division time points which are shown in the Figure 2.

TIME-LAPSE IMAGING: A PREDICTIVE AS WELL AS A SELECTIVE TOOL

We know that culturing embryos to blastocyst and subsequently transferring the best blastocyst can result in achieving high implantation and LBRs (Gardner et al., 1998). Multiple studies have proposed that embryos should be graded at multiple points and a cumulative score should be considered before transfer but even these models can have certain limitations as far as prognosticating the embryonic potential to implant (Racowsky et al., 2009; ALPHA Scientists in Human Reproductive Medicine, 2011; Hossain et al., 2016). Embryo evaluation definitely becomes better with multiple observations at fixed time points but with the conventional way of scoring embryos, this would cause fluctuations in the environment and there can be potential stress on the embryo which can do more harm than good as far as implantation and LBRs are concerned. This creates a big dilemma and most clinics would not follow the multiple time point scoring system in their laboratories. Time-lapse monitoring brings forward a way to observe embryos without disturbing their culture environment and thus can potentially improve the scoring of embryos and potentially improve the implantation rate and reduce the multiple pregnancy rate (Wong et al., 2010).

How does It Help in Embryo Selection?

Time-lapse gives us so much information about the kinetics and the dynamic morphology (Fig. 3) of embryos. It can help in identifying abnormal cell division, multinucleation, direct cleavage, reverse cleavage, blastomere exclusions, early or late compaction, etc. (Fig. 4), there is just so much information that we can derive from this technology. And only now we are understanding the effects of all these parameters and their correlation with blastulation, implantation and even live birth (Castelló et al., 2016; Ebner et al., 2017). When time-lapse came into the clinical IVF scenario, it caused a lot of controversies regarding its implementation and whether its use would improve outcomes and whether it would be cost-effective. Though there were quite a few papers showing benefits of this, it is still unclear whether these results in improvement of outcomes and whether this improvement is because of uninterrupted culture or due to the scoring and selection based on morphokinetics. It is a known fact that embryos showing early cleavage but within the normal developmental limits have a better blastulation rate and prognosis.

And this parameter can be observed using the Embryoscope. Most clinics have now shifted to Day 5 culture and now have to do multiple embryo assessments each day which increases the workload and also reduces the accuracy of judgment especially on heavier days, another reason to incorporate time-lapse systems.

Fragmentation is another thing which can be tracked really well using time-lapse, there has been data which has shown the dynamic pattern of fragmentation (Fig. 5), where fragments were reabsorbed by the blastomeres, some suggest that this could be a way of auto repair of embryos, others have linked it to aneuploidy and poor implantation rates.

A lot of researchers have tried to correlate morphokinetics with aneuploidies. A study by Chavez et al. showed that euploid embryos followed a very tight morphokinetics pattern (S_1: 14.4 ± 4.2 minutes, CC_2: 11.8 ± 0.71 hours, S_2: 0.96 ± 0.84 hours), the prediction of aneuploidy was difficult

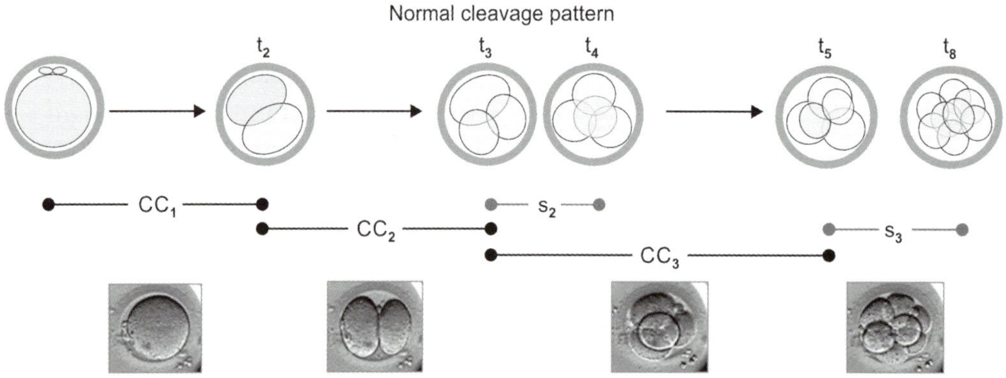

Fig. 3: Embryo development and important endpoints to assess implantation potential.

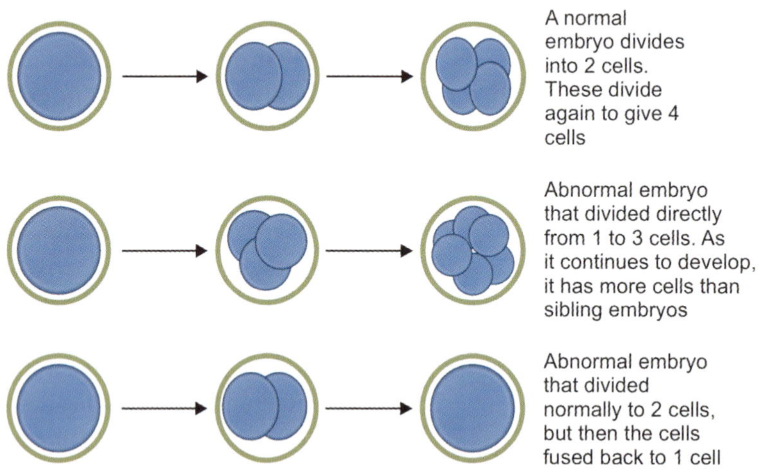

Fig. 4: Different patterns of embryo cleavage.

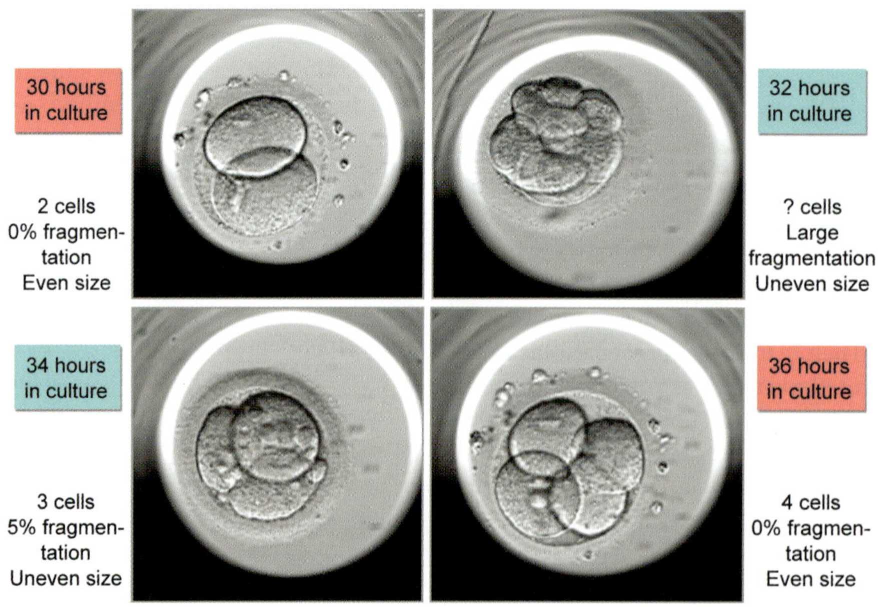

Fig. 5: Dynamic changes in fragmentation during embryo development.

but many of the studied embryos showed patterns outside the normal kinetics and also were more likely to have had a higher chance of embryonic fragmentation. Another study by Basile et al. showed that the embryos which were euploid had a higher chance to fall in the kinetic ranges of t_5 CC_3 and t_5-t_2 morphokinetics. Campbell et al., 2013 showed that euploid embryos tend to have a significantly short time to start of compaction, start of blastulation and time to blastocyst expansion. Sadly all of these studies have a very small cohort of embryos and patients thus we cannot really come to a conclusion whether time-lapse can actually predict aneuploidy but there is a lot of scope in this field. Researchers also studied the competence of frozen oocytes and tried using various morphokinetics time points to analyze their competence.

LIMITATIONS OF EXISTING MODELS

We have to take into consideration that the existing model of embryo scoring is a bit flawed. It is common practice for an embryologist to remove the culture dish once a day to assess the growing embryo. This assessment only gives us an idea about the morphology and the fragmentation in embryos. It is important to note that embryos do not react well to changes in the culture environment and a daily assessment, especially if it is prolonged, can result in altering the pH of the media and also cause temperature fluctuations. When using a time-lapse monitoring system, these flaws of conventional assessment are eliminated. This monitoring also collects massive data for advanced embryonic assessment from zygote to blastocyst (Cruz et al., 2013). Several groups have studied and correlated morphokinetics with the potential to implant and the potential to result in a live birth. They have also tried to correlate euploidy with morphokinetics. The logic behind prediction of euploidy and blastulation is based on the idea that the embryonic growth and live birth could be determined using developmental endpoints during early embryonic development. Using this prediction scoring, it is suggested that the time to pregnancy could be reduced and can also help in reduction of costs. Also certain time-lapse technologies allow selection of embryos based on certain criteria which are fed into the incubator and thus they predict which embryos to transfer/freeze (Fig. 6).

LIMITATION OF MORPHOKINETICS

The concept of monitoring of embryos without taking them out of the incubator seems great but taking a closer look at this, it has been found that though the device is safe and has not caused any harm on the embryo but the studies that have showed positive outcome does suffer from methodological flaws. Apart from being retrospective, which obviously has its limitations and studies like the one from Meseguer et al. show the same. Most of the reviewed studies already show promising results but suffer from methodological issues. First, essentially all of the cited studies have a retrospective design. Retrospective study design cannot account for differences in the patient populations or culturing conditions. It is well known that patients with similar characteristics could have a different treatment outcome in different clinics. It was shown that the results of using time-lapse varied quite a lot in a multicentric study (Dal Canto et al., 2012) and differentiating between the patient characteristic, culture conditions, etc. as probable reasons for the variation, could not be deciphered (Campbell et al., 2013). Genetics seems to have a more prominent role in the development of the embryo. It is one of the most important jobs of the ART practitioners to choose embryos which will implant from embryos which would not. Studies like the one from (Campbell et al., 2013) have shown that euploid embryos have a more synchronous division pattern

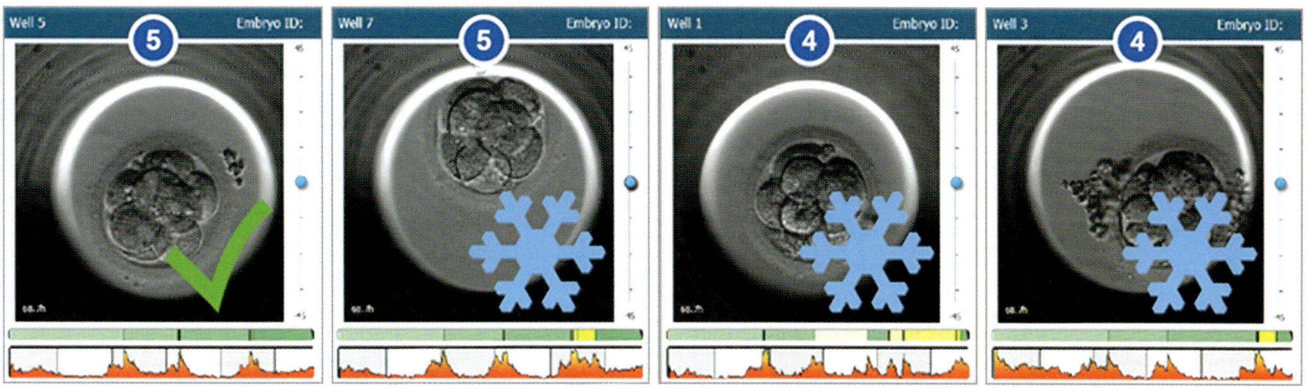

Fig. 6: Decision-making using Kids score on Embryoscope (Vitrolife).

following certain time frames which could be used as markers for ploidy, whereas the aneuploid ones usually fall out of range. But these morphokinetics patterns can differ from center to center and could also depend on the clinics transfer policy (Fleming et al., 2008; Hashimoto et al., 2012; Hlinka et al., 2012). The studies which have studied these parameters have had embryos being transferred at day 2 and also at day 5 so to conclude on the morphokinetics and the implantation potential based on these studies becomes a rather difficult task. Blastulation rates and implantation are prime prognostic indicators of the treatments being offered, but LBR still remains as one of the most important markers for cycles (Oxford University Press; 2000). Some of the important studies, especially the ones deciding on the morphokinetics do not have enough clinical data to support them. Though this pattern is changing now with the newer studies on time-lapse but it still is difficult at this point to propagate the use of time-lapse for all. In a noted commentary by Wells et al. in 2010, it was stated that data on the correlation between ongoing pregnancy rate (OPR) and LBR is not conclusive as of now. With most following a retrospective pattern and lacking proper tested time frames as markers for implantation, two randomized control trials (RCTs) published on the same and comparing conventional incubation to morphokinetics selection included only good prognosis patients or patients for oocyte donation. Rubio did a large study and did report an increased OPR for couples who utilized the time-lapse monitoring system, but again whether these could be attributed to the selection using the software or to the differences in the culture conditions are something that could not be inferred. The utilization rate was higher in the time-lapse thus suggesting that the conditions for culture are optimal or even better than the standard systems available. As this study also utilized a good prognosis pool of patients, it could be said that time-lapse could help this particular pool of patients in reducing the time to pregnancy, but for the other groups it could be expected that the number of embryos falling in the high potential group would be less and it needs to be determined whether the technology can actually be beneficial if the number of embryos to choose from is limited.

CONCLUSION

With the use of time-lapse in a clinical setup, the embryologist can now monitor the embryos in more detail and track the morphokinetics and evaluate them in much detail. This is definitely different from the conventional monitoring that we usually do in laboratories. We have learnt a lot from this technology in the last decade and we now have a better understanding of how embryos grow, how they divide, etc. we also know that the static monitoring can be flawed as reverse cleavage and direct cleavage do happen in some embryos and they are obviously not the best to transfer. This technology also helps in tracking fragmentation and also gives us a better selection when fragmentation is resorbed. And while we have uses which are quite fascinating, the full potential of this technology is yet to be achieved. More research is needed on morphological markers of aneuploidies and even selecting embryos when morphological parameters are evidently deranged as in certain cases of polycystic ovary syndrome (PCOS). It is a fantastic tool for quality control in the laboratory and can also be a great teaching tool for trainings as well. And even though we need more data on determining the effects on pregnancy and implantation rates, whether they improve because of uninterrupted culture or because of the advanced scoring, it is still a fantastic incubator to be put into laboratories but the cost-effectiveness and justification of its use has to be seen.

EDITORS' COMMENTS

1. In IVF technology, a morphokinetic "era" has started though not widely available to many embryologists due to cost factor, the Embryoscope is a boon, proposed a noninvasive, safe and reliable tool for detailed embryo study.
2. Reduced handling, detailed and undisturbed monitoring, better embryo selection, etc. are few more benefits of time-lapse evaluation of embryo using Embryoscope.
3. The continuous time-lapse monitoring of morphokinetic parameters like cleavage events, cell cycle intervals, initiation of blastulation, etc. can aid in assessing the embryo better and in turn help in the transfer of the best "embryo".
4. In spite of its initial high promise, various sections of ART clinicians and embryologist have questions its role in improving IVF outcomes.

SUGGESTED READING

1. ALPHA Scientists in Reproductive Medicine; ESHRE Special Interest Group Embryology. Istanbul consensus workshop on embryo assessment: proceedings of an expert meeting. Reprod Biomed Online. 2011;22(6):632-46.
2. Bland M. An Introduction to Medical Statistics, 3rd edition. Oxford: Oxford University Press; 2000.
3. Campbell A, Fishel S, Bowman N, et al. Modelling a risk classification of aneuploidy in human embryos using non-invasive morphokinetics. Reprod Biomed Online. 2013;26:477-85.

4. Castelló D, Motato Y, Basile N, et al. How much have we learned from time-lapse in clinical IVF? Mol Hum Reprod. 2016;22(10):719-27.
5. Cruz M, Garrido N, Gadea B, et al. Oocyte insemination techniques are related to alterations of embryo developmental timing in an oocyte donation model. Reprod Biomed Online. 2013;27:367-75.
6. Dal Canto M, Coticchio G, Mignini Renzini M, et al. Cleavage kinetics analysis of human embryos predicts development to blastocyst and implantation. Reprod Biomed Online. 2012; 25:474-80.
7. Ebner T, Oppelt P, Radler E, et al. Morphokinetics of vitrified and warmed blastocysts predicts implantation potential. J Assist Reprod Genet. 2017;34(2):239-44.
8. Fleming TR, Sharples K, McCall J, et al. Maintaining confidentiality of interim data to enhance trial integrity and credibility. Clin Trials. 2008;5:157-67.
9. Gardner DK, Vella P, Lane M, et al. Culture and transfer of human blastocysts increases implantation rates and reduces the need for multiple embryo transfers. Fertil Steril. 1998;69(1):84-8.
10. Hashimoto S, Kato N, Saeki K, et al. Selection of high-potential embryos by culture in poly (dimethylsiloxane) microwells and time-lapse imaging. Fertil Steril. 2012;97:332-7.
11. Hlinka D, Kalatova B, Uhrinova I, et al. Time-lapse cleavage rating predicts human embryo viability. Physiol Res. 2012; 61:513-25.
12. Kovacs P. Embryo selection: the role of time-lapse monitoring. Reprod Biol Endocrinol. 2014;12:124.
13. Meseguer M, Herrero J, Tejera A, et al. The use of morphokinetics as a predictor of embryo implantation. Hum Reprod. 2011;26(10):2658-71.
14. Payne D, Flaherty SP, Barry MF, et al. Preliminary observations on polar body extrusion and pronuclear formation in human oocytes using time-lapse video cinematography. Hum Reprod. 1997;12(3):532-41.
15. Pirkevi Çetinkaya C, Kahraman S. Morphokinetics of embryos—where are we now? J Reprod Biotechnol Fertil. 2016;5.
16. Racowsky C, Ohno-Machado L, Kim J, et al. Is there an advantage in scoring early embryos on more than one day? Hum Reprod. 2009;24(9):2104-13.
17. VerMilyea MD, Tan L, Anthony JT, et al. Computer-automated time-lapse analysis results correlate with embryo implantation and clinical pregnancy: a blinded, multi-centre study. Reprod Biomed Online. 2014;29:729-36.
18. Wells D. Embryo aneuploidy and the role of morphological and genetic screening. Reprod Biomed Online. 2010;21:274-7.
19. Wong CC, Loewke KE, Bossert NL, et al. Non-invasive imaging of human embryos before embryonic genome activation predicts development to the blastocyst stage. Nat Biotechnol. 2010;28(10):1115-21.

37

CHAPTER

Preimplantation Genetic Screening and Diagnosis

Yuvraj Jadeja, Niket Patel, Piyush Chudasama

INTRODUCTION

Screening and diagnosis of genetic condition by preimplantation genetic testing (PGT) for monogenic diseases and/or numerical and structural chromosomal abnormalities are the basis for embryo testing aimed at recognizing euploid embryo in a cohort produced during *in vitro* fertilization (IVF) cycle. The aim of PGT is to diagnose whether an embryo is affected by monogenic disease and/or chromosomal impairment thus preventing its implantation of an abnormal fetus limiting the risks underlying the transfer of a chromosomally abnormal embryo. In recent years, PGT has gained a lot of momentum, various studies supporting and equally good number opposing its role in IVF outcomes have been published. PGT in recent times has also come under a lot of criticism due to a lot of ethical as well as scientific reason but there is no doubt that PGT has been one of the most talked about important breakthrough in IVF. An important aspect of this technique is the possibility that the procedure itself can adversely affect the quality of embryo. Many approaches to biopsy have been put forward. Cleavage stage biopsy of the blastomere was most commonly accepted approach. Polar body (PB) biopsy, cleavage stage biopsy and trophectoderm biopsy all have been probed in detail for its advantages and disadvantages.

Preimplantation genetic testing has two subgroups under its banner, in the form of: (1) preimplantation genetic screening (PGS), and (2) preimplantation genetic diagnosis (PGD). Chromosomal abnormalities are one of the major causes of pre- and postimplantation embryo wastage reflected by decreased implantation and increased miscarriage. Hence chromosomal evaluation of the embryos in these patients and the selection of normal embryos could increase the rate of pregnancy and healthy offspring.

Recently the society has renamed PGD/PGS to:

- Preimplantation genetic testing
- Preimplantation genetic testing for aneuploidy (PGT-A)
- Preimplantation genetic testing for chromosomal structural rearrangements (PGT-SR) like translocation, inversions
- Preimplantation genetic testing for single or multiple gene disorders (PGT-M).

With development of prenatal diagnostic techniques like amniocentesis and chorionic villus sampling (CVS), noninvasive prenatal testing (NIPT), it has been possible for couples at risk of genetic diseases to give birth to healthy babies. However, the experience of prenatal diagnosis (PND) followed by termination of pregnancy in case an abnormality if detected can be an unwelcome memory. PGT is essentially an alternative to PND, which helps in negative selection of affected embryo prior to implantation, i.e. before the onset of pregnancy and thus obviates the stress and emotional trauma associated with termination of pregnancy.

Preimplantation genetic testing, a highly specialized field incorporating the latest techniques of assisted reproductive technology (ART) and genetics, is an early form of PND bringing the hope of healthy babies to couples at risk of transmitting genetic disorders to their offspring. The patient opting for this testing has to undergo IVF/intracytoplasmic sperm injection (ICSI). A cell is removed from the oocyte or the embryo followed by cytogenetic or molecular diagnosis for particular genetic disorders.

The aim of doing PGD on an embryo is to identify whether the embryo carries a genetic abnormality. The other alternative techniques available for diagnosis of an unfavorable pregnancy by unhealthy embryo are only available in the postconception period, which are procedures like amniocentesis or CVS. These are invasive procedures and also done during the pregnancy period. In these diagnostic procedures, termination of pregnancy will be the ultimate option if there are positive findings. The beauty of PGD is that it helps to transfer the good embryos without any genetic abnormalities to the uterus for implantation giving a healthy conceptus and healthy take home babies.

HISTORY OF PREIMPLANTATION GENETIC DIAGNOSIS

The first successful embryo biopsy was performed on rabbit embryo in 1968 by Edwards and Gardner. In mid-1980s, PGD on human embryo was developed in the United Kingdom as an alternative to current prenatal diagnoses. In the beginning, PGD was used to determine gender as an indirect means to avoid an X-linked disorder. In 1989 in London, the first unaffected child born was reported by performing PGD for an X-linked disorder by Handyside and colleagues.

Milestones in Preimplantation Genetic Diagnosis Technology

- 1990: First PGD for X-linked disorder by Handyside et al.
- 1995: PGD by fluorescence in situ hybridization (FISH) reported by Munne et al.
- 1996: PGD for chromosomal translocations.
- 2000: Preimplantation human leukocyte antigen (HLA) typing for Fanconi anemia.
- 2010: PGD for chromosomal disorders by microarray-based technology.
- 2010: Karyomapping for PGD for single gene disorders.
- 2013: Next-generation sequencing (NGS) for preimplantation aneuploidy testing.

INDICATIONS FOR PREIMPLANTATION GENETIC TESTING

Couples with a history of recurrent miscarriage produce chromosomally abnormal embryos with a significant higher percentage. In 22% of these couples, the chromosomal abnormality is present in all the embryos and the percentage of abnormal embryos is similar in subsequent attempts. Preimplantation testing can help identify chromosomally normal embryo, thus reducing the chances of abortion in this patients. It also helps to increase the pregnancy rate and reduce abortion rates in cases of older age women, women with previous unsuccessful IVF attempts, women who have undergone repeated termination because of an abnormality diagnosed prenatally and in known carriers of genetic defects like chromosomal translocations. Patients with balanced translocations usually present with subfertility and recurrent miscarriages. Couples morally and religiously opposed to termination of attested pregnancies diagnosed prenatally can also avail the advantages of this technique. Another indication is minimizing the psychological trauma incurred by couples who have had to undergo repeated terminations. The option of PGD offers them hope of normal child.

PREIMPLANTATION GENETIC TESTING

Preimplantation genetic testing is advised in the following conditions:

- Family history of X-linked disorders, have a 25% risk of having an affected embryo.
- Chromosome translocations, which can cause implantation failure, recurrent pregnancy loss, or mental or physical problems in offspring.
- Carriers of autosomal recessive diseases, the risk an embryo may be affected is 25%.
- Carriers of autosomal dominant diseases, the risk an embryo may be affected is 50%.
- Women of advanced maternal age.
- History of recurrent pregnancy loss.
- Repeated IVF failure.
- Male partner with severe male factor infertility.

SOURCES OF GENETIC MATERIAL FOR PREIMPLANTATION GENETIC TESTING

Preimplantation genetic testing utilizes three types of cell line for its analysis: (1) PBs from the oocyte/zygote stage, (2) blastomeres from cleavage stage embryos, and (3) trophectoderm cells of blastocysts. The most fundamental requirement is the experience and meticulousness of the embryologist for performing the biopsy without compromising the viability. The first step is to create a hole in the zona pellucida that surrounds the oocyte or embryo. Chemical drilling by acid Tyrode's solution was the initial method used, but the skepticism was for PB biopsy where acid Tyrode's would adversely affect subsequent oocyte development, and so mechanical means that tear the zona was introduced. The most recent development in PGT is the use of a laser for zona drilling, as it is the most precise and safest method.

Polar Body Biopsy

Polar body biopsy was initially considered advantageous since the technique involves disturbing the oocytes rather than embryos, precluding ethical and safety debates concerning human embryo biopsy, and the genetic material removed is not destined to become part of the developing embryo. For PGT-M of monogenic diseases, the technique predicts that the genotype of the oocyte is indirectly derived from the opposite diagnosis of the first PB (IPB). However, PB analysis may be complicated by recombination events, whereby if a crossover event occurs in a heterozygous primary oocyte which includes the region around the gene under analysis, the two daughter chromatids in IPB will have a "heterozygous" genotype. Due to this, analysis of the second PB (IIPB) is essential to define the status of the secondary oocyte. Thus, this determination may still be complicated. By the phenomenon of allelic dropout (ADO), which may occur during polymerase chain reaction (PCR) analysis of single cells, such that detection of a single allele in IPB cannot distinguish between a "true" genotype (when there has been no recombination event) or ADO (unless the gene maps closely to the centromere of a chromosome, where recombination is less likely to occur). The problem with the analysis of both IPB and IIPB needs manipulation twice of the samples for analysis, and furthermore out of those oocytes that are tested, a significant number will fail to fertilize or form embryos. Finally, the genotype of the paternal allele would remain unknown. PB analysis is definitely useful in detecting numerical chromosomal anomalies, since the highest numbers of aneuploidies are maternally derived. In clinical PGT cycles, PB biopsy has been used mainly for age-related aneuploidy or chromosomal analysis where the female carries a translocation, but is not preferred by most centers offering PGT.

Cleavage Stage Biopsy

On the 3rd day postinsemination, the fertilized embryos have reached 6–8 cells (cleavage stage embryos). At this stage, the cells are still totipotent and the embryos are usually not yet compacting. The quality of cleavage stage embryos in culture is variable but they can be evaluated morphologically as grade I (correct stage of development, regularly shaped, evenly sized blastomeres, and no fragmentation) to grade III (slow development, unequally sized blastomeres, at least one degenerate blastomere and/or a high level of fragmentation). Biopsy of blastomeres from cleavage stage embryos is preferred by most centers performing PGT. Hardy et al. describe the original protocol for this *cleavage stage biopsy*. Subsequent modifications to the protocol include the use of the same pipette for zona drilling and blastomere aspiration, the use of a laser for zona drilling, and in addition the use of calcium and magnesium-free media during the biopsy to reduce cell-cell adhesion, especially if the embryos have begun to compact. One of the main disadvantages of blastomere biopsy is the limited amount of material available for analysis and the entire debate of autocorrection. Many PGD centers recommend the biopsy and replicate analysis of two blastomeres from each cleavage stage embryo, although this approach is often limited by suboptimal embryo quality and/or development in culture.

Blastocyst Stage Biopsy

The blastocyst is a cavitated structure that develops about 5–6 days postinsemination. Biopsy of the blastocyst has a potential advantage over blastomere biopsy in that more cells may be extracted for analysis, and the biopsy procedure is technically less demanding than that of blastomeres or PBs. The trophectoderm cells do not contribute to the embryo proper, but eventually form the placenta and other extraembryonic tissue (comparable to an early CVS), partially reducing ethical considerations. The removal of up to about 10 cells from the trophectoderm does not appear to alter the early development of human embryos. Furthermore, although the use of sequential media for embryo culture supports the development of embryos to the blastocyst stage, only up to about 40–50% of preimplantation embryos develop to this stage *in vitro* with present protocols, limiting the application of this biopsy method for PGT.

PROTOCOLS FOR GENETIC ANALYSIS

Preimplantation genetic diagnosis for monogenic diseases and/or protocols for genotyping single cells for monogenic disorders are based on PCR. Since the first PCR-based PGD cases were performed, several inherent difficulties associated with single cell DNA amplification have become evident. These include potential sample contamination, total PCR failure, and ADO (when one of the alleles fails to amplify to detectable levels), all of which should be minimized for any PGD PCR protocol before clinical application. PCR failure and ADO are specific concerns that need to be minimized to optimize PCR results; single cell amplification rate of above 90% and an ADO rate of up to 10% is what most centers accept for maintaining quality assurance of the performing laboratory. PCR failure is undesirable, but ADO is more dangerous since it may lead to a misdiagnosis. Designing of protocols that monitor of ADO is imperative. The monogenic diseases for which PCR-based PGT protocols have been developed generally reflect those for which PND is already offered and includes a continuously growing list of autosomal recessive, dominant, and X-linked diseases. Here summarized are the disorders for which PGD has been most commonly applied. The molecular genetics associated with a disorder largely determines the type of protocol(s) selected for performing PGT.

Monogenic diseases for which PGD has been more commonly applied:

- *Autosomal recessive*: Cystic fibrosis, β-thalassemia (β-globin gene), sickle cell anemia (β-globin gene), spinal muscular atrophy (type I), Tay-Sachs disease, congenital adrenal hyperplasia.
- *Autosomal dominant*: Myotonic dystrophy, Huntington's disease, Charcot-Marie-Tooth disease type IA, Marfan syndrome, familial adenomatous polyposis coli.
- *X-linked*: Duchenne/Becker muscular dystrophy, hemophilia, fragile X syndrome, Wiskott-Aldrich syndrome, Lesch-Nyhan syndrome.

DIAGNOSTIC METHODS FOR PGD/PGS

Fluorescence in situ Hybridization

Fluorescence *in situ* hybridization was the initial method used in PGT technique. Schrurs et al. introduced it first time in 1993 to determine aneuploidy, Munne et al. further expanded its use in diagnosis of chromosomal translocation.

Molecular probes which are fluorescently labeled are used to identify chromosomes and their fragments via FISH technique.

The probes are specifically made for each run and are made up of complementary sequence to the fragmented DNA regions that are subjected to hybridization, the result of this technique is seen under the fluorescent microscope as a fluorescent signal.

Interphase nuclei are used for performing FISH after the biopsy taken for PGT, the cells extruded (blastomeres) are placed in a solution that is hypotonic solution, methanol and acetic acid for digestion and fixation.

Though the ideal situation would be able to diagnose the entire panel of 24 chromosomes in one go, but as it is only possible to use 5–9 probes most at once it requires 2-3 rounds in FISH.

And that is specifically the reason why PGT-FISH has limitations in diagnosis; it only targets most common abnormality in involving chromosomes 13, 15–18, 21, 22.

The reliability of the FISH technique in PGT has also been questioned many times on fallacies in performing the procedure and errors in steps such as fixation of cells, attaching of probes, multiple washing as well as artifacting which are all issues due to which, this procedure has been criticized and imprecise with high error rates.

There were also many studies that proved, i.e. in 2007, a study was conducted on 206 patients in PGT-FISH arm and 202 patients in the control arm whose age group were of 35–41 years, revealed a significantly lower rate of pregnancies in the first arm (25%) as against control arm (37%).

Apart from the few disadvantages of FISH, mentioned before, it is also a method that requires extraction of cells for D3 embryo which can also potentially disturb their blastocyst development ability and also because the number of chromosomes analyzed is limited, it is not the method of choice today. In this regard, one could say that PGT-FISH with normal reporting does not mean it is 100% "healthy" and normal embryos.

Diagnosis of translocation can also be done on FISH, other methods however successfully replaced FISH now.

Diagnosis of translocation is more reliable and precise with single-nucleotide polymorphism (SNP) and NGS and comparative genomic hybridization (CGH).

Comparative Genomic Hybridization

Molecular cytogenetics introduced CGH in the year 1992 and was first used by Kallioniemi et al. This technique could diagnose deletion/duplication of fragments in chromosomes without culturing of cells. Standard (normal) DNA which is fluorescent dye labeled and the DNA to be tested (from a patient) that is fluorochrome labeled are placed on a slide or metaphase plate. In this way, two genomes coded with different colors and cut enzymatically into small fragments reorganize on chromosomes using the rule of complementarity and competition for hybridization sites.

A predominance of one color over the other is the visible sign of quantitative difference. The main criticism in the role of the classic CGH run is the issue of low resolution, with an average of 10 Mbp, Array CGH is so an improved version introduced in PGT. It is more precise (2.9% no errors), highly specific (1.9% errors) and less time required for its run (analysis of up to 24 hours). Its drawback is that it cannot be used for a low-grade mosaicism diagnosis or single mutations, but research and observations throughout years have shown that such dysfunctions mostly have additional abnormalities, that can be detected with a CGH (such as aneuploidy), but nonetheless the hypothesis cannot be extrapolated into actual reporting.

Alfarawati et al. in 2011 were the first group report on delivery of the birth of healthy child subjected to CGH-based PGT. The indication was balanced translocation in parents, which diagnosis unbalanced translocation at embryonic stage.

Later Schoolcraft et al. reported significantly higher embryo implantation rate statistically from 46.6% to 72.2% ($p < 0.001$) in embryos tested biopsied at the blastocyst stage, frozen, verified and transferred after CGH-based PGT. As mentioned above, translocations are other common causes of application for PGT/CGH especially reciprocal translocations which can be balanced or unbalanced Robertsonian translocation.

Translocation in ART accelerates the failure rate, sometimes by as high as 85%, and these carriers will create abnormal embryos in ART unworthy of implantation. Therefore, it becomes mandatory that PGT simultaneously detects translocations along with numeric abnormalities.

Comparative genomic hybridization can be used in PGT for determination of translocations, translocating fragments which are not smaller than 6 Mbp can be easily picked up. Colls et al. in their study demonstrated the more precise use of CGH against FISH where the precision was based on detection of at least three chromosomal fragments that were translocated.

This study also demonstrated an important point, that is, it reiterated the necessity of PGT in selecting healthy embryo, as 26.4% of normal or balanced embryo when looked for aneuploidy were abnormal while having processed for diagnosis of translocations. The same inference of this thesis was also backed up in 2011 studies by Gutierrez-Mateo et al. in a group of 81 embryos diagnosed as normal or balanced with regard to translocations, 51 were simultaneously positive for aneuploidy. Fiorentino et al. and Pujol et al. also produced comparable results in their studies which were local published.

Single-Nucleotide Polymorphism (SNP) Analysis

These are placed in a genome where one nucleotide in a particular location is not the same as carried by the rest of its population and its diagnosis is called SNP analysis.

Methods using SNP markers utilize platforms/plates allowing determination of multiple SNPs. During a single analysis, there are large numbers of SNP methods based on hybridization, starter elongation, ligation or so-called invasive rupture, all of which favor the accessibility of this method.

Treff et al. designed a method where the entire set of 24 chromosomes was screened using SNP and was validated in 2010. Since then many ART clinics have used SNP technique and get good results.

Good outcomes were observed in diagnosis of balanced, unbalanced and Robertsonian translocation also using SNP platforms.

Next-generation Sequencing

Next-generation sequencing belongs to the group of massively parallel sequencing (MPS) methods that allow for parallel processing of an extremely large number of nucleic acid molecules. As a result of sequencing on a micro space scale, it has been possible to drastically increase the amount of information collected during one test, up to an entire human genome. The revolution NGS has brought to sequencing is much greater than what microarrays revolutionized CGH. Within subsequent years of its existence, the costs of equipment, disposables and chemicals have fallen, which has increased the accessibility and popularity of its use in research and medical fields.

Currently, more than ten NGS platforms are available. Post-light NGS, where semiconductor chips are used instead of laser-optic systems and color reactions allowing for translation of genetic information directly into binary signals, needs special mention. In preimplantation testing, NGS has become a better alternative than a CGH. NGS can be used in fresh and frozen cycles, and it is possible to analyze almost all types of genetic variability. It is the only method that allows for detection for aneuploidy as well as translocation of all chromosomes and mutations responsible for any single-gene disease, using one biopsy and one process.

At the same time using NGS, it is possible to study an entire genome with regard to different abnormalities such as aneuploidy, single-gene mutations or de novo mutations. It is quite costly to equip a laboratory with all of the equipment necessary to perform NGS procedures, but this technology allows for performance of analyses of many samples at the same time, thereby reducing the costs of a single analysis.

When NGS is used in PGD, it is necessary to isolate the DNA and amplify the whole genome (from a single cell or several cells). Then, the material is cut into small DNA fragments (of 100–200 base pairs) and placed on a 2 × 2 cm "chip". It seems incredible to place a hundred thousand DNA fragments from different patients on a single chip, but this is possible thanks to DNA barcoding. A sequence of each fragment is then compared to a reference sequence.

Currently, NGS is thought to be a future and target technology for PGD/PGS. As a gold standard for genetics sequencing, it allows for the almost 100% study of an entire gene/genome, and so it is possible to obtain a "perfect" analytical result.

Some technical considerations have to be made before planning of PGS:

- Biopsy should be taken by trained and experienced embryologist.
- While taking biopsy try to give minimal exposure of laser.
- Single cell biopsy is necessary to get actual aneuploidy result in case of 3rd day biopsy, while 5th day biopsy contains 4–8 cells.
- Cells of embryo biopsy should be taken in PBS and oil aspiration during biopsy should be avoided, otherwise library preparation would be compromised resulting in low library concentration.
- Biopsy storage and transportation should be done under cooling condition to prevent embryo cell damage.
- Library preparation reagents should be stored at appropriate temperature and frequent freeze-thaw cycle should be avoided to retain its self-life.
- All the reagents must be thawed properly and mix it well before adding to embryo biopsy tubes.
- Inserting micropipettes in the biopsy tubes must be avoided to eliminate chances of losing cell/s.
- Vigorous mixing by pipette and vortex should be avoided to prevent breakage of cells at initial stages.
- During library preparation, it should be incubated for optimum time with beads for proper binding. Ethanol removal from the beads is a crucial step in order to achieve higher purified library.
- Avoid over-drying of beads and improper ethanol concentration for optimum library yield.

MOSAICISM CHALLENGE

An imminent challenge of embryo selection by PGS has brought to light an entire new question of how to deal with mosaic embryos. Mosaic embryos are those embryos that have two or more cell lines with different karyotype. Malsegregation of chromosome at the time of early meiotic cleavage stage is its root cause. A mosaic embryo might have combination of diploid and aneuploidy cells or mixture of various aneuploidy cells. NGS as of now has confirmed that approximately 30% of cohort of D5 embryos are diploid aneuploidy mosaics.

The biggest challenge in PGS is that one cannot confirm that the biopsied cells are a complete and accurate representation of the entire embryo structure. A PGS euploid embryo could still have an aneuploidy cell line and vice versa.

Though there is a long-standing evidence that a mosaic embryo is not always lethal. In fact, mosaic aneuploidy embryos confined to placental tissues are seen in 1–2% of pregnancies and most of the cases have corresponding fetus that is chromosomally normal. Ambiguity still exists as some studies have found that discrepancies in rates of aneuploidy between inner cell mass (ICM) and trophectoderm of blastocyst.

The major concern is clinical implication of mosaic embryos arc not yet fully understood, there have been cases where a known mosaic embryo transferred have produced a chromosomally normal offspring, which has led to the entire concept of autocorrection in form of blastomere exclusion, multipolar divisions, endoreduplication of chromosome and fragment resorption. However, evidence points that mosaic embryos have less implantation potential.

RECOMMENDATIONS FOR THE LABORATORY

- For reliable detection of mosaicism, ideally 5 cells should be biopsied, with as little cell damage as possible.
- Validated to quantitatively measure copy number should be used. Ideally, a NGS methodology that can accurately and reproducibly measure 20% mosaicism in a known sample.
- For reporting embryo results, the suggested cutoff point for definition of mosaicism is >20%, so lower levels should be treated as euploid, >80% abnormal (aneuploid), and the remaining ones between 20% and 80% mosaic (euploid-aneuploid mosaic).

RECOMMENDATIONS FOR CLINICIANS

- Patients should be thoroughly counseled that any genetic test cannot be 100% accurate for a combination of technical and biological factors, including chromosome mosaicism.
- Transfer of blastocyst with euploid result should always be prioritized over those with mosaic aneuploid results.
- In the event of considering the transfer of a blastocyst with only mosaic aneuploidies, the following options should be discussed with the patients:
  - A possible another cycle of IVF with PGT testing to increase the chance of gaining a normal euploid blastocyst for transfer
  - Transfer of a blastocyst with mosaic aneuploidies for low risk chromosomes only, after appropriate genetic counseling if available
  - Appropriate monitoring and PND of any resulting pregnancy, preferably by early amniocentesis (<14 weeks gestation).

SUGGESTED GUIDELINES TO PRIORITIZE THE TRANSFER OF MOSAIC EMBRYOS

- Embryos showing mosaic euploid/monosomy are preferable to euploid/trisomies, given that monosomic embryos (excepting 45 X) are not viable
- If a decision is made to transfer mosaic embryos trisomic for a single chromosome, one can prioritize selection based on the level of mosaicism and the specific chromosome involved:
  - The preferable transfer category consists of mosaic embryos trisomic for chromosomes 1, 3, 4, 5, 6, 8, 9, 10, 11, 12, 17, 19, 20, 22, X, Y. None of these chromosomes involve the much adverse characteristics
  - Embryos mosaic for trisomies that are associated with potential for uniparental disomy (14 and 15) are of less priority
  - Embryos mosaic for trisomies that are associated with intrauterine growth retardation (chromosomes 2, 7, 16) are of lesser priority
  - Embryos mosaic for trisomies capable of live birth viability (chromosomes 13, 18, 21) are of the lowest priority for obvious reasons.

CONCLUSION

The initial concept of PGT appeared fairly simple, especially following the development of PCR-based DNA methodologies. However, a decade of practical application and advent of newer techniques such as FISH, CGH and now NGS has well proven that this is not the case, and although vast improvements have been made with the research, experience, and technological advances. PGT is still a challenging and multistep, labourious technique which mandates the close collaboration of an entire specialized team of experts. Efforts toward amelioration and simplification of protocols, mainly for genetic analysis and to develop more and more methods for disorders, but present technologies still limit its wider application. Other major drawback to the wider application of clinical PGT includes the necessity to involve IVF, (even if the couples are not infertile) the relatively low pregnancy and birth rate, and the high cost of a complete PGT cycle. With close ethical attention and the continuous trend of technological advancement, it can be foreseen that PGT could have an ever-widening role to play in averting serious inherited diseases, alongside PND.

EDITORS' COMMENTS

1. PGS/PGD is a screening test for monogenic diseases and/or numerical/structural chromosomal abnormalities in the cohort of embryos produced in IVF.
2. It is a molecular diagnostic test which utilizes techniques such as PCR, FISH, CGH array or NGS.
3. Indication includes advanced maternal age, recurrent pregnancy loss, repeated IVF failure and severe male factor and PGD especially for monogenic diseases.
4. Genetic material for PGS/PGD can be PBs, blastomere or trophectoderm from expanded blastocyst.
5. Despite of all the recent debates, PGS/PGD is still believed to increase the implantation potential to some extent, decrease the abortion rate, and reducing the time to conceive.

SUGGESTED READING

1. Alfarawati S, Fragouli E, Colls P, Wells D. First births after preimplantation genetic diagnosis of structural chromosome abnormalities using comparative genomic hybridization and microarray analysis. Hum Reprod. 2011;26:1560-74.
2. Carbone L, Chavez SL. Mammalian pre-implantation chromosomal instability: species comparison evolutionary considerations, and pathological correlations. Syst Biol Reprod Med. 2015;61(6):321-35.
3. Colls P, Escudero T, Fischer J, et al. Validation of array comparative genome hybridization for diagnosis of translocations in preimplantation human embryos. Reprod Biomed. 2012;24:621-9.
4. Eduardo CL, Marleen MJ, Carl BB. Preimplantation genetic testing: current status and future prospects. In: Shevach Friedler (Ed). In Vitro Fertilization: Innovative Clinical and Laboratory Aspects. InTech; 2012. pp. 137-56.
5. Fiorentino F, Spizzichino L, Bono S, et al. PGD for reciprocal and Robertsonian translocations using array comparative genomic hybridization. Hum Reprod. 2011;26(7):1925-35.
6. Greco E, Minasi MG, Fiorentimo F. Healthy babies after intrauterine transfer of mosaic aneuploid blastocysts. N Engl J Med. 2015;373(21):2089-90.
7. Grifo J, Colls P, Ribustello L, et al. Why do array-CGH (ACGH) euploid embryos miscarry? Reanalysis by NGS reveals undetected abnormalities which would have prevented 56% of the miscarriages. Fertil Steril. 2015;104(3):e14.
8. Gutiérrez-Mateo C, Colls P, Sánchez-García J, et al. Validation of microarray comparative genomic hybridization for comprehensive chromosome analysis of embryos. Fertil Steril. 2011;95(3):953-8.
9. Kallioniemi A, Kallioniemi OP, Sudar D, et al. Comparative genomic hybridization for molecular cytogenetic analysis of solid tumors. D Science. 1992;258:818-21.

10. Kalousek DK, Dill FJ. Chromosomal mosaicism confined to the placenta in human conceptions. Science. 1983;221(4611): 665-7.
11. Kalousek DK, Vekemans M. Confined placental mosaicism. J Med Genet. 1996;33(7):529-33.
12. Knapp M, Stiller M, Meyer M. Generating barcoded libraries for multiplex high-throughput sequencing. Methods Mol Biol. 2012; 840:155-70.
13. Liu J, Wang W, Sun X, et al. DNA microarray reveals that high proportion of human blastocysts from woman of advanced maternal age are aneuploid and mosaic. Biol Reprod. 2012;87(6):148.
14. Łukaszuk K, Pukszta S, Ochman K, et al. Narodziny zdrowego dziecka u pary z nosicielstwem translokacji Robertsonowskiej po zastosowaniu Genetycznej Diagnostyki Przedimplantacyjnej (PGD) z Sekwencjonowaniem Następnej. Generacji (NGS). ART Newsletter. 2014;2:31-3.
15. Mastenbroek S, Twisk M, van Echten-Arends J, et al. In vitro fertilization with preimplantation genetic screening. N Engl J Med. 2007;357:9-17.
16. Munné S, Scott R, Sable D, Cohen J. First pregnancies after preconcep- tion diagnosis of translocations of maternal origin. Fertil Steril. 1998;69(4):675-81.
17. Munné S. Preimplantation genetic diagnosis for aneuploidy and translocations using array comparative genomic hybridization. Current Genomics. 2012;13(6):463-70.
18. Pujol A, Benet J, Staessen C, et al. The importance of aneuploidy screening in reciprocal translocation carriers J Reproduction. 2006; 131:1025-35.
19. Schoolcraft WB, Fragouli E, Stevens J, et al. Clinical application of comprehensive chromosomal screening at the blastocyst stage. Fertil Steril. 2010;94:1700-6.
20. Schrurs BM, Winston RM, Handyside AH. Preimplantation diagnosis of aneuploidy using fluorescent in-situ hybridization: evaluation using a chromosome 18-specific probe. Hum Reprod. 1993;8(2):296-301.
21. Sobrino B, Brión M, Carracedo A. SNPs in forensic genetics: a review on SNP typing methodologies. Forensic Sci Int. 2005;154:181-94.
22. Tan YQ, Tan K, Zhang SP, et al. Single-nucleotide polymorphism microarray-based preimplantation genetic diagnosis is likely to improve the clinical outcome for translocation carriers. Hum Reprod. 2013;28:2581-92.
23. Treff NR, Su J, Tao X, et al. Accurate single cell 24 chromosome aneuploidy screening using whole genome ampli cation and single nucleotide polymorphism microarrays. Fertil Steril. 2010;94:2017-21.
24. Wu MY, Chao KH, Chen CD, et al. Current status of comprehensive chromosome screening for elective single-embryo transfer. Obstet Gynecol Int. 2014;2014:581783.

38

CHAPTER

In Vitro Maturation

Devika Gunasheela, Rajam Murali

INTRODUCTION

Maturation of immature eggs retrieved from small antral follicles in the laboratory is defined as *in vitro* maturation (IVM) of oocytes.

The principle of IVM is the maturation *in vitro* of the immature germinal vesicle (GV) stage oocytes collected from unstimulated ovaries to mature metaphase II (MII) stage oocytes (Figs. 1 and 2).

In vitro maturation was initially recommended in polycystic ovarian syndrome (PCOS) women to prevent adverse effects of controlled ovarian hyperstimulation (COH) using gonadotropins, to avoid ovarian hyperstimulation syndrome (OHSS), to reduce drug expenditure, and to lighten patient's stress.

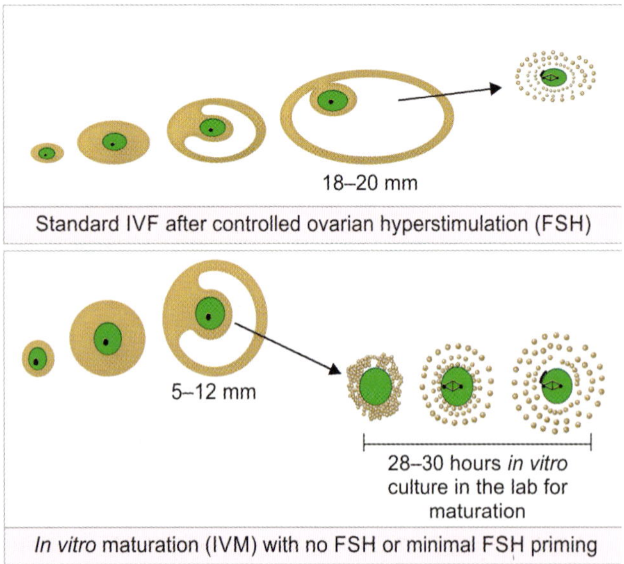

Fig. 1: Process of *in vitro* maturation.

In vitro maturation is a cost-effective substitute for conventional intracytoplasmic sperm injection (ICSI). IVM has been termed as a convenient and beneficial treatment for PCOS women because of less/no gonadotropin use.

In 1965, Robert Edwards established the spontaneous resumption of meiosis in GV oocytes and he encouraged and popularized the clinical and research work in IVM. He demonstrated that 50% of retrieved human immature oocytes gain maturity spontaneously *in vitro*.

The main obstacle to a favorable outcome in an IVM cycle is the lesser maturation rates of immature oocytes *in vitro*, approximately around 50%.

HISTORY

Pincus and Enzmann (1935) observed that immature oocytes in rabbits are able to mature naturally *in vitro*. In 1965, Robert Edwards showed that human GV oocytes collected in standard *in vitro* fertilization (IVF) cycles are capable of maturing in the laboratory to MII oocytes in 36 hours. In 1983, Veeck reported about the initial live birth by the transfer of embryos made from immature eggs retrieved in a standard IVF program.

In 1991, Cha published about the earliest triplet live birth from immature eggs retrieved from a donor with no gonadotropin stimulation. In 1994, Trounson documented that immature eggs collected from PCOS women with no gonadotropin stimulation has resulted in a live birth.

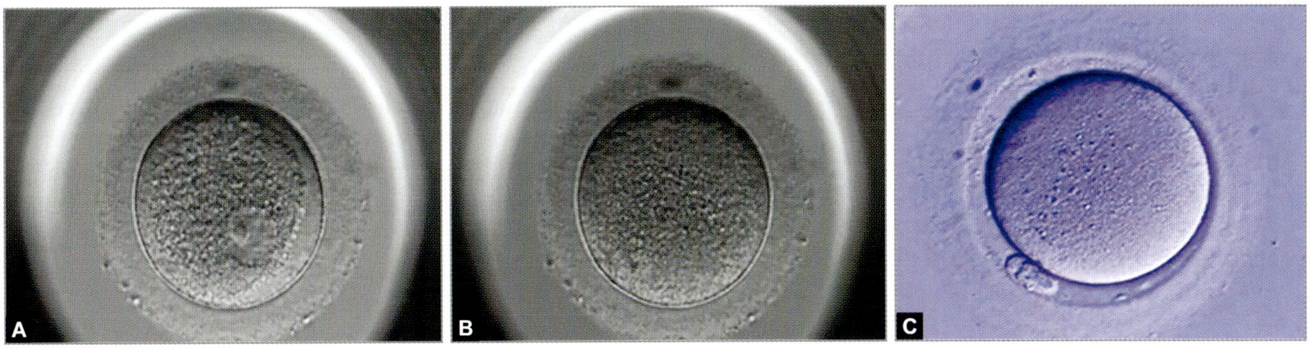

Figs. 2A to C: (A) GV oocyte; (B) MI oocyte; and (C) MII oocyte.
(GV: germinal vesicle; MI: metaphase I stage; MII: metaphase II stage)
Courtesy: Gunasheela Fertility Centre.

Mikkelson reported the earliest live birth from GV oocytes retrieved from a normo-ovulatory patient in 1999.

DEFINITION OF IVM AND ITS CONTROVERSIES

In early 90's, IVM was initiated in clinical practice as a simple, cheap, and patient friendly assisted reproduction technology (ART) procedure. The immature GV stage oocytes from small antral follicles can form mature MII stage oocytes in the IVF laboratory with less/no-hormonal stimulation. The fact that, immature oocytes in IVM cycles are less efficient than mature oocytes from conventional ICSI cycle has prompted the use of small priming doses of recombinant follicle-stimulating hormone (rFSH) and/or human chorionic gonadotropin (hCG) for final follicular triggering in IVM programs. As hCG trigger can cause oocytes in small antral follicles of size 10–13 mm to mature *in vivo*, there is scepticism about the interpretation of IVM among ART consultants worldwide.

In a latest article, few infertility specialists have suggested that IVM encompasses eggs retrieved from small and medium sized antral follicles after minimal FSH priming and hCG or gonadotropin-releasing hormone (GnRH) agonist triggering. Some ART specialists prefer to do IVM with no FSH priming or hCG triggering. As various ART clinics around the world, use different protocols for IVM like no gonadotropin stimulation or minimal FSH priming for 5–7 days with or without ovulation triggering, the reported laboratory and clinical outcomes are not similar.

In order to have a consistency in the reporting of IVM cycles from various parts of the world, IVM includes eggs collected from small- and medium-sized follicles when the size of the biggest follicle is less than 13 mm after FSH priming and/or hCG triggering. In IVM cycles using FSH/hCG, there is a possibility of collecting *in vivo* mature oocytes. Few researchers do not consider this as IVM as they state follicular diameter should not be the ground to establish the definition for IVM.

Some clinicians have retitled IVM cycles using gonadotropin priming and ovulation triggering as IVM combined with IVF in a modified natural cycle with early triggering. However, there is an on going dispute among IVF specialists about the best way to manage an IVM program in the ART clinic as well as in the laboratory.

PHYSIOLOGY OF OOCYTE MATURATION

The maturation of oocytes starts in utero prenatally and progresses throughout life by the process of folliculogenesis to attain developmental competence for fertilization. It takes almost 220 days for the small primordial follicles to grow into large preovulatory follicle. Human eggs gain nuclear and cytoplasmic maturity in antral follicles of size 2–5 mm. The human oocyte attains a size of about 100–120 μm at the antral follicle stage and it can complete meiosis in antral follicles of diameter 5 mm.

The last step in the maturation of human oocytes is the completion of meiosis before ovulation. In human oocytes, meiosis stops in the prophase I. Several external and intracellular signals promote or inhibit the meiotic arrest. Human oocytes when removed from follicular environment or denuded resume meiosis spontaneously within hours. This proves that the factors promoting meiotic arrest in human oocytes are in the neighboring follicular tissues. Nevertheless, the inhibitory signals for meiosis resumption in fish or frog oocytes appear to be internal within the oocyte itself.

In human oocytes, the most important factor inhibiting meiosis completion is the cyclic adenosine monophosphate (cAMP). cAMP is regulated by two enzyme groups, adenylcyclases (AC) which produces cAMP and phosphodiesterases (PDE) which degrades cAMP.

ACs are either stimulated (Gs) or inhibited (Gi) by G proteins and PDE are regulated by protein kinase A (PKA) phosphorylation.

Cyclic AMP in the oocyte prevents oocyte maturation. Hypoxanthine (PDE inhibitor) inhibits degradation of cAMP thus increasing cAMP levels to maintain meiotic arrest.

Theca cells surround the human oocyte in the outer most layer, which helps in steroidogenesis. The next layer is outer mural granulosa cells, which in turn surround the inner cumulus granulosa cells. The inner cumulus cells (CC) are the inner most layer closest to the human oocyte and they communicate with the oocytes via gap junctions.

Connexion 43 proteins form gap junctions and they are essential for oocyte growth, follicular development, and cumulus expansion. Gap junctions are also responsible for sustaining the meiotic arrest. The disruption of gap junctions during granulosa cell expansion corresponds with the resumption of meiosis and maturation of the oocyte.

Luteinizing hormone (LH) surge causes restoration of meiosis and ovulation. LH receptors are present in the outer theca cell layer and mural granulosa cell layers and are absent in inner cumulus granulosa cell layer covering the oocyte. LH surge causes paracrine factors like epiregulin and amphiregulin [members of epidermal growth factor (EGF) family] to be released from the outer theca and mural granulosa cell layers. These paracrine factors cause expansion of inner CC and disruption of gap junctions to restart meiosis. These paracrine growth factors activate CC to make testosterones, estrogen, progesterone, and follicular fluid-derived meiosis activating sterol (FF-MAS), which aids in the maturation of oocyte (Fig. 3).

WHY IVM AND IN WHOM?

Despite its lower efficiency than conventional IVF, IVM is used for a number of reasons to prevent OHSS and to reduce costs of COH. Even though the concept of segmented IVF by giving GnRH agonists for final follicular maturation and elective freezing of all embryos, has almost nullified OHSS risk, the curiosity in IVM as a patient friendly ART option has not disappeared. A number of benefits prompting the use of IVM are:

- No OHSS
- Low cost
- Increased convenience as less monitoring
- Comparable pregnancy rates
- Less duration and dose of gonadotropins.

The cumulative live birth rate in IVM cycles (per egg retrieval) is around 41% and is comparable to standard IVF cycles. The important factors contributing to the success of IVM include minimal gonadotropin priming, hCG triggering, good endometrial preparation in fresh cycles, reducing the incubation time of immature eggs to 30 hours from 48 hours, extending culture of embryos till blastocyst stage, and doing frozen thawed embryo transfers if endometrium is inadequate in fresh cycles.

The number of blastocysts formed are less in an IVM cycle compared to standard IVF cycle but the implantation rates of IVM embryos are equal and on par with the standard IVF embryos. Thus, IVM is more economical than standard IVF regarding blastocyst formation (Figs. 4A and B).

At present, GV oocytes have decreased maturation rates *in vitro* and *in vitro* mature eggs have reduced developmental competence. So, IVM is not recommended for all patients requiring ART.

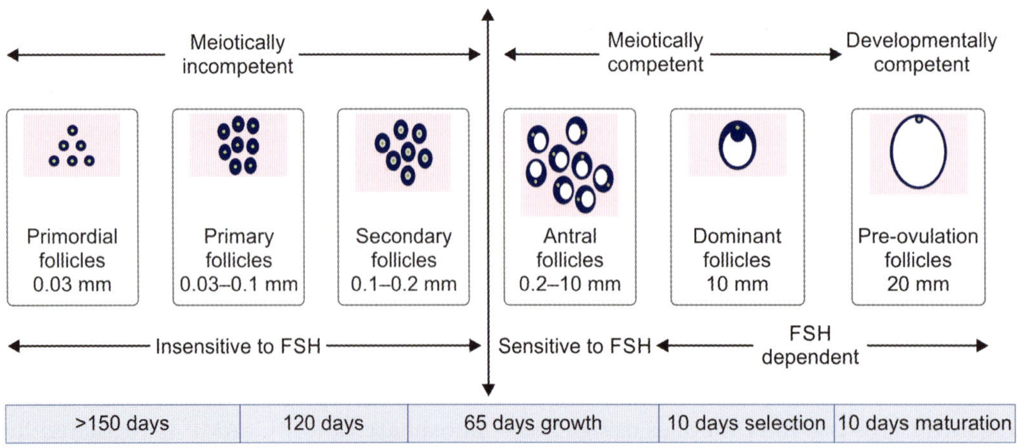

Fig. 3: Steps of oocyte maturation.
(FSH: follicle-stimulating hormone)

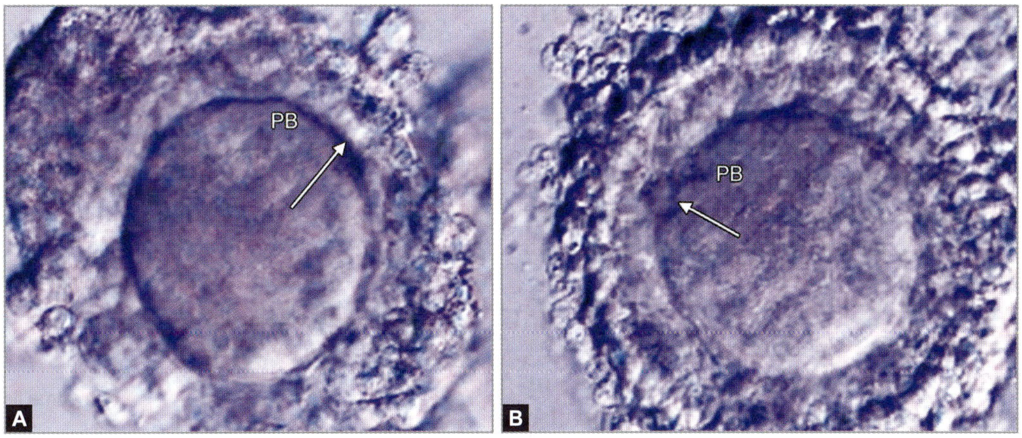

Figs. 4A and B: MII oocytes (*in vivo* matured) obtained in an IVM cycle.
(PB: polar body)
Courtesy: Gunasheela Fertility Centre.

Thus, the key factor of a successful and effective IVM program is choosing the correct patient and it seems that women with polycystic ovaries are the best possible choices for IVM. The quality of an *in vitro* mature oocyte in an IVM cycle is lesser when compared to an *in* vivo mature oocyte in a standard IVF cycle. The larger quantity or huge number of immature eggs collected in PCOS women compensates for the lesser quality of immature eggs. Serum anti-Müllerian hormone (AMH) is associated with the severity of PCOS and decides the number (quantity) of eggs collected in an ART cycle. Serum AMH, a surrogate of the number of immature eggs retrieved in an IVM cycle predicts success rates of an IVM program.

Women should be selected for IVM cycles based on:

- Previous history or risk of OHSS
- High antral follicle count (AFC) and high AMH in PCOS women
- Patients whose antral follicles are unresponsive to FSH
- Women with a history of cancer or other medical condition that will not endure elevated levels of estradiol
- Repeated poor responders or repeated poor embryo quality in previous ICSI cycles
- Fertility preservation in cancer patients before chemotherapy
- Limited time period for ART
- Salvage of immature oocytes obtained in a conventional IVF cycle.

Polycystic ovarian syndrome women having serum AMH more than 8.5 ng/mL and formation of more than five embryos in an IVM cycle were autonomous markers of live birth rate in IVM cycles with unstandardized coefficients of 0.078 and 0.113, respectively.

In vitro maturation can give ultimate hope in women with normal ovarian reserve and FSH/LH polymorphisms.

Protocols used in IVM

In vitro maturation involves collecting immature oocytes from small antral follicles and the largest follicle should not exceed a diameter of 12 mm to avoid adverse influences on the smaller follicles.

The IVM rates of immature oocytes in an IVM cycle are lower. This suggests that the immature oocytes are required to be in the follicular milieu a little longer to attain developmental competence.

The maturation of an immature oocyte can be augmented by giving 10,000 units of hCG 36–38 hours prior to egg collection. In hCG triggered IVM cycles, few *in vivo* matured oocytes are collected along with immature oocytes. In IVM cycles without hCG trigger, all collected oocytes are at GV stage at the time of egg retrieval. Incubation of collected immature oocytes is done in the IVF laboratory for 24–30 hours in culture media supplemented with EGF and 1:10 ratio of rFSH: rLH. Currently, IVF laboratories have started using IVM culture media available in the market such as SAGE (Coopersurgical) IVM medium and Medi-Cult IVM medium, which are IVF quality control certified. The matured eggs are fertilized by ICSI and the laser assisted hatching performed on the resulting blastocysts before transferring them into the women's uterus.

Minimal gonadotropin priming and use of hCG trigger in IVM cycles increase the clinical and laboratory outcome of IVM cycles when compared to no gonadotropin or hCG use.

Gonadotropin priming and hCG triggering improve the developmental competence of immature oocytes. The various protocols used in IVM cycles are:

- No gonadotropins and no hCG trigger (pure IVM)
- Short (<6 days) and low dose (75 IU) FSH stimulation with no hCG trigger
- Only hCG trigger and no gonadotropins
- Short and low dose FSH stimulation and hCG trigger
- Estrogens suppression IVM cycles (oral estrogens are given from Day 3 of menstrual cycle to suppress the formation of dominant follicle. No ultrasound monitoring is required).

IVM Oocyte Retrieval

In an IVM cycle, hCG trigger is planned when the biggest follicle reaches a size of 10–12 mm and when the endometrial thickness is more than 7 mm. This is to avoid the harmful paracrine signals released from the dominant follicle to affect the smaller immature follicles.

When the follicles do not grow beyond 10 mm as in anovulatory PCOS patients, egg retrieval is planned when the biggest follicle size is equal to or less than 10 mm and the reported clinical pregnancy rates and the implantation rates were comparable (27.0 and 13.6%, respectively). Collection of GV oocytes from the ovary is possible in all phases of the menstrual cycle (early follicular phase or late follicular phase or luteal phase of menstrual cycle).

The needles used for aspiration of immature follicle are slightly shorter with a short bevel so that there is no leakage of fluid. For oocyte retrieval (OR) in IVM cycles, use of double lumen needle is preferred over single lumen needle to decrease the number of pricks on the vaginal and ovarian tissues. The 17 gauge outer needle has a file structure on the apex and used to pierce the vagina and penetrate the capsule of ovary for support during follicular aspiration. The inner needle is 19 gauged and is introduced into the outer needle for follicular aspiration using reduced pressures (40–70 mm Hg) when compared to OR in conventional IVF cycles (80–100 mm Hg) (Fig. 5).

Rotating the inner aspiration needle inside the follicle and moving it in a forward and backward direction multiple times with continuous negative pressures scrapes the inner surface of the follicle completely without leaving an immature oocyte. By changing the orientation and depth of outer needle, the inner needle aspirates all small follicles in the ovary without multiple extra vaginal pricks.

In IVF OR, the follicles are larger with expanded CC, but in IVM OR, most of the follicles are small and have compacted CC. The smaller inner aspiration needle is blocked with blood clots and tissues during IVM OR. The inner needle is flushed with heparinized media to remove the clogging whenever there is inadequate suction pressure.

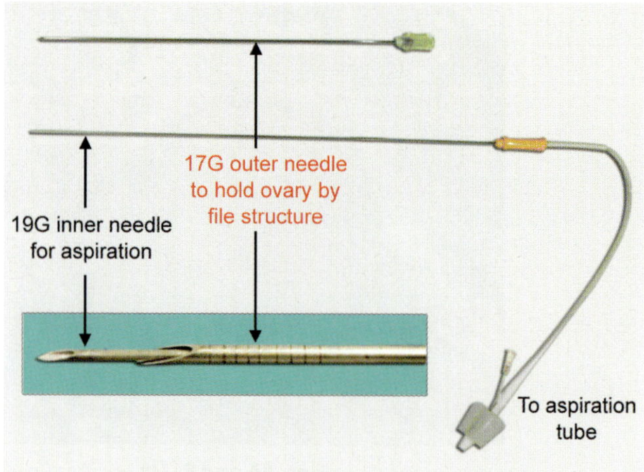

Fig. 5: Double needle system used for IVM.

On the other hand, 17 gauge 25-mm long Swemed needles which are normally used for standard IVF can also be used for aspirating immature follicles.

In our center, we have had experience using both the 16G beveled IVM needle (COOK) and the 17G needle (COOK). We have had equally good results with both the needles.

LABORATORY AND EMBRYOLOGICAL ASPECTS OF IVM

In IVM cycles using hCG and/or gonadotropins, the distention, scattering, and spreading of granulosa or CC surrounding the eggs helps to dissociate and separate the oocyte from the follicle and thus makes follicular aspiration and oocyte identification a simpler procedure.

During OR, the aspirated fluid is received in collection tubes filled with media and two units of heparin to prevent coagulation of the bloody aspirates. The two methods to recognize immature oocytes are the strainer and the direct method. First, directly under the stereomicroscope, the oocytes with expanded cumulus complex are recognized. Next, a cell strainer (nylon mesh with 70-mm holes) filters the rest of the follicular fluid to aid the detection of immature oocytes with compact CC. The structure of the collected oocytes in an IVM cycle is categorized into three groups as:

1. Expanded CC
2. Condensed or compacted CC
3. Scanty CC.

Immature oocytes with expanded CC are collected in IVM cycles only when hCG is used for triggering. The expanded cumulus complexes help to increase the

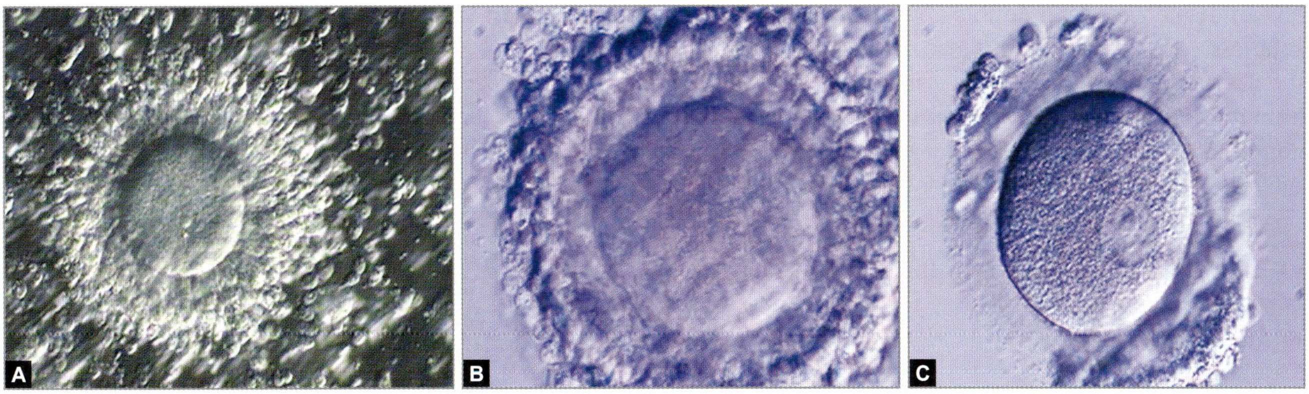

Figs. 6A to C: (A) Germinal vesicle (GV) stage oocyte with dispersed CC; (B) GV stage oocyte with compacted CC; (C) GV stage oocyte with sparse CC.
Courtesy: Gunasheela Fertility Centre.

maturation rate and developmental competence of the immature eggs. The mature oocytes retrieved from smaller follicles produce good quality blastocysts comparable to the blastocysts formed from a MII oocyte from a larger follicle. Collecting *in vivo* matured oocytes along with immature oocytes in an IVM cycle improves the clinical pregnancy rates. The optimal time interval between egg retrieval and hCG trigger in an IVM cycle is 38 hours rather than 36 hours as it aids maturation *in vivo* and helps to increase the maturation rates of immature oocytes. In IVM cycles, ICSI rather than IVF is opted to fertilize the mature eggs.

After 1–4 hours of first polar body extrusion, ICSI is performed on the *in vitro* matured oocytes and the exact time of ICSI performance can be assisted by a live spindle imaging system. In our study on the ideal time to perform ICSI of oocytes matured *in vitro* (Gunasheela D et al., unpublished data), we observed that the fertilization rate was higher about 83.1% when ICSI was performed between 3–6 hours after first polar body extrusion. This is in contrast to the fertilization rates of 40% and 64% when ICSI done at less than 3 hours and more than 6 hours, respectively. The total number of good quality blastocysts formed in an IVM cycle will decide the day of embryo transfer and the number of blastocysts to be transferred.

Recognition of *in vivo* mature or MII oocytes after IVM OR is an essential step in the IVF laboratory. Under stereomicroscope using the spreading method, it is easy to detect the oocytes having GV in their cytoplasm. Differentiating MII oocytes from MI oocytes is really difficult before stripping the CC. In hCG triggered IVM cycles, about 6% of the retrieved eggs are at MI (GVBD) stage. Approximately, one-third of those MI oocytes can mature on the same day of egg collection (Day 0) to MII stage oocytes and ICSI is done on the same day evening on those MII oocytes.

Oocytes are assessed early in the morning on Day 1 of egg collection for maturity and if there are MII oocytes, they are inseminated with male partner sperms.

It is not required to check again for the maturity of GV oocytes on the evening of egg collection (Day 0). In a study on the size of immature oocytes and its relation with nuclear maturation (Gunasheela D et al., unpublished data), we found that GV stage oocytes with average diameter less than 102 µm did not mature *in vitro* even after 28 hours of culture.

Our analysis showed that GV stage oocytes that matured *in vitro* had larger diameters (>110 µm), than those GV stage oocytes that did not mature. The diameter did not change from GV to MI stage, but decreased after first polar body extrusion (MII oocytes). The average diameter of the *in vitro* matured oocyte is equal to the *in vivo* matured oocytes in IVM cycles and *in vivo* mature oocytes from standard IVF cycles (Figs. 6 A to C).

ENDOMETRIAL PREPARATION IN IVM CYCLES

Patients receive estradiol valerate (progynova 2 mg) beginning one day prior to OR, increased in a stepwise fashion up to 12 mg per day till pregnancy check date.

Luteal support is provided by vaginal progesterone tablets 400 mg twice daily starting from the OR day till pregnancy check date. If endometrial thickness is less than 7 mm, patients are counseled for vitrification of embryos for frozen thawed embryo transfer in the next cycle. Pregnancy check by serum beta hCG is done 2 weeks after embryo transfer and luteal support with estrogens and progesterone is extended until the first trimester of pregnancy.

SAFETY OF IVM

The blastocysts formed from *in vitro* matured oocytes do not have extra chromosomal and epigenetic defects. However, few studies have raised doubts about the efficiency and safeness of IVM cycles, but these studies were done on the *in vitro* mature oocytes from a standard IVF cycle. The immature oocytes in a conventional IVF cycle are inherently abnormal and have high DNA damage as they do not restart meiosis after hCG trigger for final follicular maturation.

The pregnancy rates are low in an IVM program due to:

- The cytoplasm and nuclear maturation of the oocyte are not simultaneous.
- In the endometrium, the window of implantation has not yet opened.
- Suboptimal culture conditions.

The rates of chromosomal aneuploidies by FISH are comparable in the blastocysts from IVM and conventional IVF cycles (58.7% vs 57.4%, respectively). Blastocysts from oocytes matured *in vitro* 48 hours after OR showed greater aneuploidy rate compared with blastocysts from *in vivo* mature oocytes and *in vitro* mature oocytes 24 hours after OR. Fertilization and cleavage rates are lower in the oocytes matured 48–52 hours after OR (Day 2) and they had higher DNA damage compared with oocytes matured on Day 0 or Day 1.

Approximately, more than 5,000 PCOS women worldwide have given birth to babies after IVM treatment, (Chian et al., 2013, Sonigo et al., 2016, and Fadini et al., 2012). Babies born after IVM procedures show normal growth and development. The pregnancy after IVM has a favorable obstetric outcome and the congenital deformity rate is similar compared with pregnancies after standard IVF and ICSI (Buckett WM et al., 2007 and Soderstorm-Anttila et al., 2006). The epigenetic changes caused by IVM in the newborns are negligible and rare. *In vitro* mature oocytes or babies born after IVM have not showed significant epigenetic changes causing ill health. It is important to track the progress of health of children born after an IVM program.

THE GUNASHEELA EXPERIENCE

We started our IVM program in 2002 and till date over 600 cycles of IVM have been performed at our center.

We would like to present our small study (from June 2013 to June 2017), where we compared the ART outcomes in 222 PCOS women with AMH >10 ng/mL who opted for either IVM (FSH/hCG priming) or standard ICSI (antagonist protocol) (Flowchart 1).

Flowchart 1: Algorithm showing study of Gunasheela.

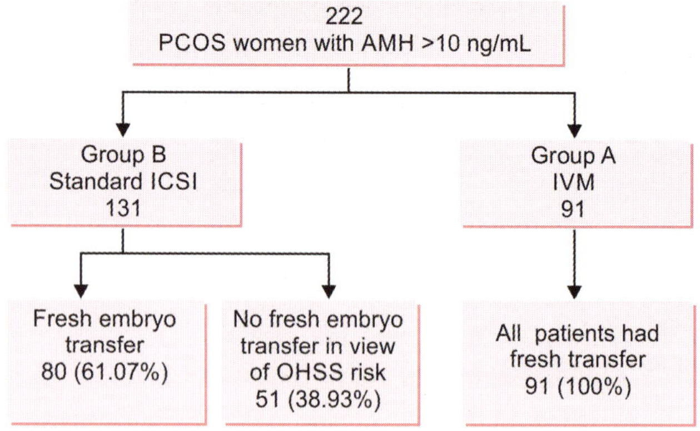

(AMH: anti-Müllerian hormone; ICSI: intracytoplasmic sperm injection; IVM: *in vitro* maturation; PCOS: polycystic ovarian syndrome; OHSS: ovarian hyperstimulation syndrome)

From Day 3 or 5 of the menstrual cycle, minimal gonadotropin priming with 75 units of rFSH is given for duration of 5–7 days. When the largest follicle attains a diameter of 10–12 mm and endometrial thickness is above 7 mm, rhCG trigger is given. Oocytes are retrieved 38 hours after trigger. A 17-gauge single lumen needle is used for aspiration using a suction pressure 80 mm Hg.

The immature eggs are isolated in follicle flushing culture media. The CCs are stripped from the oocytes 3 hours after retrieval to evaluate oocyte maturity. *In vivo* mature oocytes found on the day of collection are injected with partner sperm the same day. The rest of the immature eggs are incubated in Quinns IVM medium (supplemented with rFSH, rLH, and EGF) for 28 hours to finish the maturation process. *In vitro* mature oocytes are inseminated with the husband's sperm after 3–6 hours of extrusion of first polar body (the optimal ICSI timing of GV oocytes in IVM cycle Gunasheela et al. ESHRE 2017). The embryos were incubated using global single step culture media, in Tri-gas benchtop incubators.

In IVM cycles, the duration and the amount of gonadotropin used and the mean expenditure of drugs in Indian Rupees (INR) were considerably lesser when compared to conventional IVF cycles ($p \leq 0.0001$). There was no OHSS in IVM cycles compared to conventional ICSI cycles (17.56%). The clinical pregnancy rate per fresh embryo transfer (48.35% vs 63.75%) was comparable between the IVM and the standard ICSI groups, respectively.

Minimally stimulated IVM is a simple, safe, and inexpensive option because it avoids the risk of OHSS entirely (Dahan et al., 2016; Seyhan et al., 2014). Even in segmented IVF cycles (triggering the final follicular maturation with GnRH agonist and elective vitrification all blastocysts), cases of severe OHSS have been reported (Fatemi et al., 2014 and Devroey et al., 2011). The cost of frozen embryo transfer cycle is an additional expense.

RESULTS (TABLES 1 TO 3 AND FIG. 7)

Results are given in Tables 1 to 3 and Figure 7.

IVM IN FERTILITY PRESERVATION

As most cancer patients cannot delay their life-saving cancer treatment, they do not have sufficient time to do COH to retrieve mature eggs for fertility preservation before radiotherapy and chemotherapy. High estrogen levels and COH are contraindicated in few cancer patients. In such patients, immature eggs can be collected from small antral follicles in all phases of menstrual cycle, be it follicular or luteal phase.

In the IVF laboratory, immature oocytes can be collected from excised ovarian tissue intended for cryopreservation in cancer patients (*ex vivo*). The collected immature oocytes are matured *in vitro* and injected with husband sperms and the embryos formed are vitrified for later use. These integrated methods of preserving fertility in young cancer patients may fulfill their dreams of parenthood later in life. Immature oocytes are collected for fertility preservation.

- *In vivo* oocyte collection by transvaginal aspiration in the follicular phase or luteal phase
- Intraoperative aspiration from the ovaries
- *Ex vivo* oocyte collection is from resected ovarian cortex in laboratory.

Ex vivo OR avoids the spread of tumor within the abdominal cavity and prevents upstaging of the cancer. The maturation rate in fertility preservation is 30–60%. Young age and absence of gonadotropin priming are the reasons

TABLE 1 Baseline characteristics of PCOS women with AMH levels > 10 ng in Group A and Group B.

Baseline Characteristics	*Group A IVM cycles (n = 91)*	*Group B ICSI cycles (n = 131)*	*p-value*
Mean age (years)	29.60 ± 3.83	29.91 ± 3.59	0.682
BMI (kg/m^2)	26.64 ± 2.10	25.61 ± 3.47	0.076
Duration of infertility (Years)	6.73 ± 3.57	6.014 ± 2.99	0.295
AFC (n)	35.58 ± 9.33	32.73 ± 2.66	0.053
AMH (ng/mL)	17.33 ± 5.70	16.62 ± 2.70	0.450
FSH (IU/L)	5.21 ± 1.30	4.88 ± 1.35	0.225
LH (IU/L)	9.193 ± 4.46	7.89 ± 2.85	0.101
Days of stimulation (days)	5.98 ± 1.13	9.81 ± 1.19	0.0001
Dose of gonadotropins (IU)	532.09 ± 171.26	1,496.12 ± 438.38	0.0001
Average cost of gonadotropins per cycle (INR)	14,223.06 ± 4,577.81	39,991.50 ± 11,718.06	0.0001

(AMH: anti-Müllerian hormone; AFC: antral follicle count; FSH: follicle-stimulating hormone; ICSI: intracytoplasmic sperm injection; IVM: *in vitro* maturation; LH: luteinizing hormone)

TABLE 2 Laboratory outcomes in IVM (Group A) and ICSI cycle (Group B).

Parameters	*Group A IVM cycles (n = 91)*	*Group B ICSI cycles (n = 131)*	*p-value*
Total no. of oocytes	23.67 ± 13.28	13.78 ± 6.14	0.0001
No. of *in vivo* matured oocytes	4.37 ± 7.74 18.44%		
No. of immature oocytes	19.31 ± 10.35 81.55%		
Maturation rate	10.65 ± 5.96 55.17%		
Fertilization rate (%)	10.31 ± 5.86 68.71%	8.74 ± 3.95 76.12%	0.100
Cleavage rate (%)	9.81 ± 5.94 95.14%	8.59 ± 3.83 98.22%	0.198

(AMH: anti-Müllerian hormone; ICSI: intracytoplasmic sperm injection)

TABLE 3 Pregnancy outcome between IVM cycles (Group A) and ICSI cycles with fresh embryo transfer (Group B).

Parameters	*Group A IVM cycles (n = 91)*	*Group B ICSI cycles with Fresh ET (n = 80)*	*p-value*
Clinical pregnancy rate/cycle	48.35%	38.93%	0.3942
Clinical pregnancy rate/ET	48.35%	63.75%	0.3942
Implantation rate	21.26%	40.06%	0.0180
Multiple pregnancy rate	11.36%	17.64%	0.449
Biochemical pregnancy rate	4.31%	2.5%	0.2279
Abortion rate	18.18%	15.6%	0.6988
OHSS in patients with fresh ET	0%	10% (8/80)	–
mild OHSS in segmented IVF/ICSI	–	29.41% (15/51)	–
No. of frozen embryos	2.38	3.98	0.9190
No. of transferred embryos on Day 5	2.19 ± 0.57	1.77 ± 0.32	0.0001

(ICSI: intracytoplasmic sperm injection; IVF: *in vitro* fertilization; IVM: *in vitro* maturation; PCOS: polycystic ovarian syndrome; OHSS: ovarian hyperstimulation syndrome ; ET: embryo transfer)

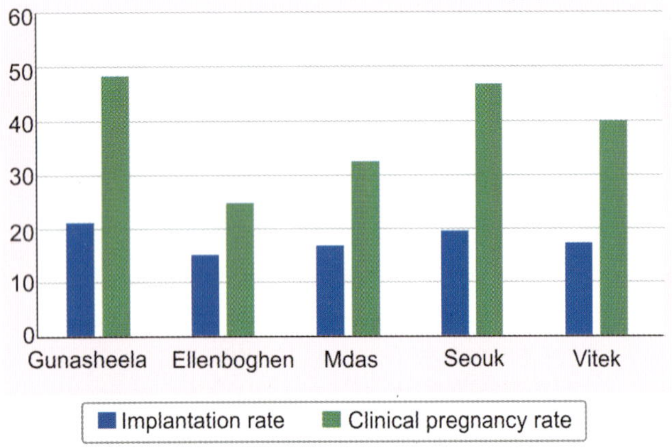

Fig. 7: IVM cycle outcome in various studies.

for the comparatively lesser maturation rates. Vitrification is used for freezing the *in vitro* mature oocytes and embryos.

In Brussels, a young nulliparous woman required therapeutic embolization of the left uterine and the right ovarian artery for pelvic arteriovenous (AV) malformation following ovarian injury, which usually results in premature ovarian failure. 13 GV oocytes are retrieved *ex vivo* in the laboratory before vitrification of ovarian cortex for fertility preservation. IVM of *ex vivo* collected oocytes and the resultant embryos are cryopreserved. Transfer of the thawed embryos resulted in the birth of a term healthy baby in July 2015.

In a 21-year-old nulliparous, women with FIGO stage IIIC grade 1 serous cancer of the ovary, fertility is preserved by conserving the uterus and GV oocytes were collected *ex vivo* from left oophorectomy specimen in the laboratory. IVM of the GV oocytes and the embryos formed were frozen. The cryopreserved embryos are warmed and replaced later which produced a healthy live birth (Prasath EB et al.).

Retrieving immature oocytes as a procedure is technically more difficult when compared to retrieving mature oocytes. The reasons for this are that:

- The largest follicle size during retrieval of immature oocytes is only 1.2 cm. Hence, the ovaries are still small and very mobile. So during OR, the ovaries tend to slip away from the needle. This can be managed by applying manual pressure on the lower abdomen to fix the ovary or by using double-lumen needle where the outer needle fixes the ovary and the inner aspirates the small follicles.
- Quite often, it is difficult to assess the presence of the needle within the follicle, as the follicle size is very small. The needle can often get clotted with blood—may have to be flushed which results with multiple punctures in the vaginal fornix which can lead to bleeding.
- The embryologists should be trained to identify these very small oocytes using a cell strainer, which will maximize the number of oocytes retrieved. Identifying immature oocytes is a laborious and time-consuming procedure, which has a learning curve.
- There is still a higher miscarriage rates in pregnancy produced by *in vitro* matured oocytes and this can be attributed to culture media whose formula still has to be perfected.

CONCLUSION

Minimal FSH priming in IVM cycles gives comparable live birth rates in PCOS women at a low cost with no OHSS. Improvement in IVM culture mediums and novel strategies for endometrial preparations may enhance success rates. IVM can be used safely in fertility preservation of hormone sensitive cancer patients. It could be the method of choice when cancer therapy should be started as soon as possible. IVM does not appear to pose any increased risk of poor obstetric outcomes or congenital abnormality compared to IVF or other ART. Research on using cAMP culture systems or including paracrine factors, like GDF9 (growth differentiation factor 9) and BMP15 (bone morphogenetic protein 15) to refine the maturation process *in vitro* can result in promisingly good clinical outcomes.

SUMMARY

- *In vitro* maturation is gaining popularity worldwide and is becoming an alternative to IVF in select populations.
- There are controversies in the definition depending on the usage of gonadotrophin or hCG.
- Oocytes maturation is dependent on several factors like intracellular signaling pathways, gap junctions in the cumulus cells, steroids, growth factors, etc.
- Advantages of IVM would be no OHSS and low costs.
- Protocols differ from clinic to clinic worldwide with IVM.
- Germinal vesicle oocytes <102 µm do not resume meiosis *in vitro*.
- Comparable pregnancy rates in PCOS patients with IVM or IVF
- No major congenital or epigenetic abnormalities noted in children born after IVM.

EDITORS' COMMENTS

1. Despite the current limitations, IVM continues to attract growing interest in consideration of potential novel applications in human ART.
2. *In vitro* maturation in connection with ovarian tissue cryopreservation (OTC) provides a unique platform for fertility preservation as well as to compare multiple culture media compositions and improves basal maturation conditions for IVM.
3. Implantation and pregnancy rate are much higher in replacement cycles using frozen embryos obtained after IVM compared to fresh transfer due to inadequate endometrial receptivity in fresh cycle.
4. Scope of IVM is now widening from PCO to oncofertility and now even becoming tried in poor responders in endometriosis.

SUGGESTED READING

1. Albertini DF, Carabatsos MJ. Comparative aspects of meiotic cell cycle control in mammals. J Mol Med. 1998;76:795-9.
2. Albertini DF, Combelles CM, Benecchi E, et al. Cellular basis for paracrine regulation of ovarian follicle development. Reproduction. 2001;121:647-53.
3. Anderiesz C, Ferraretti A, Magli C, et al. Effect of recombinant human gonadotrophins on human, bovine and murine oocyte meiosis, fertilization and embryonic development in vitro. Hum Reprod. 2000;15(5):1140-8.
4. Atkinson P, Koch J, Ledger WL. GnRH agonist trigger and a freeze-all strategy to prevent ovarian hyperstimulation syndrome: a retrospective study of OHSS risk and pregnancy rates. Aust N Z J Obstet Gynaecol. 2014;54(6):581-5.
5. Ben-Ami I, Komsky A, Bern O, et al. In vitro maturation of human germinal vesicle-stage oocytes: role of epidermal growth factor-like growth factors in the culture medium. Hum Reprod. 2011;26(1):76-81.
6. Buckett WM, Chian RC, Holzer H, et al. Obstetric outcomes and congenital abnormalities after in vitro maturation, in vitro fertilization, and intracytoplasmic sperm injection. Obstet Gynecol. 2007;110(4):885-91.
7. Cha KY, Koo JJ, Ko JJ, (1991). Pregnancy after in vitro fertilization of human follicular oocytes collected from nonstimulated cycles, their culture. Fertil Steril. 1991;55: 109-13.
8. Chang EM, Song HS, Lee DR, et al. In vitro maturation of human oocytes: Its role in infertility treatment and new possibilities. Clin Exp Reprod Med. 2014;41(2):41-6.
9. Conti M, Andersen CB, Richard F, et al. Role of cyclic nucleotide signaling in oocyte maturation. Mol Cell Endocrinol. 2002;187:153-9.
10. Coticchio G. IVM in need of clear definitions. Hum Reprod. 2016;31(7):1387-9.
11. Dahan MH, Tan SL, Chung J, et al. Clinical definition paper on in vitro maturation of human oocytes. Hum Reprod. 2016;31(7):1383-6.
12. Das M, Son WY, Buckett W, et al. In-vitro maturation versus IVF with GnRH antagonist for women with polycystic ovary syndrome: treatment outcome and rates of ovarian hyperstimulation syndrome. Reprod Biomed Online. 2014;29:545-51.
13. De Vos M, Smitz J, Thompson JG, et al. The definition of IVM is clear-variations need defining. Hum Reprod. 2016;31(11):2411-5.
14. Edwards RG. Maturation in vitro of human ovarian oocytes. Lancet. 1965;2:926-9.
15. Eftekhar M, Khalili MA, Aflatoonian A, et al. Successful pregnancy following a novel endometrial preparation in a PCOS patient undergoing IVM: a case report. J Assist Reprod Genet. 2012;29(4):335-6.

16. Fadini R1, Dal Canto MB, Mignini Renzini M, et al. Effect of different gonadotrophin priming on IVM of oocytes from women with normal ovaries: a prospective randomized study. Reprod Biomed Online. 2009;19(3):343-51.
17. Farsi MM, Kamali N, Pourghasem M. Embryological Aspects of oocyte in vitro maturation. Int J Mol Cell Med. 2013;2(3): 99-109.
18. Fatemi HM, Popovic-Todorovic B, Humaidan P, et al. Severe ovarian hyperstimulation syndrome after gonadotropin-releasing hormone (GnRH) agonist trigger and "freeze-all" approach in GnRH antagonist protocol. Fertil Steril. 2014;101(4):1008-11.
19. Grynberg M, Poulain M, le Parco S, et al. Similar in vitro maturation rates of oocytes retrieved during the follicular or luteal phase offer flexible options for urgent fertility preservation in breast cancer patients. Hum Reprod. 2016;31(3):623-9.
20. Gunasheela D, Murali R, Menon JG, et al. In-vitro maturation in women with polycystic ovaries and high anti-Müllerian hormone levels. Minerva Ginecol. 2018;70(1):120-1.
21. Guzman L, Ortega-Hrepich C, Polyzos NP, et al. A prediction model to select PCOS patients suitable for IVM treatment based on anti-Mullerian hormone and antral follicle count. Hum Reprod. 2013;28(5):1261-6.
22. Jamnongjit M, Hammes SR. Oocyte maturation: The coming of age of a germ cell. Semin Reprod Med. 2005;23(3):234-41.
23. Junk SM, Yeap D. Improved implantation and ongoing pregnancy rates after single-embryo transfer with an optimized protocol for in vitro oocyte maturation in women with polycystic ovaries and polycystic ovary syndrome. Fertil Steril. 2012;98(4):888-92.
24. Mahajan N, Gupta S, Sharma S, et al. Early onset ovarian hyperstimulation syndrome despite use of segmentation approach and ovarian hyperstimulation syndrome prophylaxis. J Hum Reprod Sci. 2015;8(4):234-8.
25. Martins Wde P, dos Reis RM, Ferriani RA, et al. Endometrial preparation for in vitro oocyte maturation: Early use of estrogen increases endometrial tissue and requires lower daily dosage: A cross over trial in 'mock' cycles. J Assist Reprod Genet. 2006;23(5):241-6.
26. Mikkelsen AL, Lindenberg S. Benefit of FSH priming of women with PCOS to the in vitro maturation procedure and the outcome: A randomized prospective study. Reproduction. 2001;122(4):587-92.
27. Park CW, Lee SH, Yang KM, et al. Cryopreservation of in vitro matured oocytes after ex vivo oocyte retrieval from gynecologic cancer patients undergoing radical surgery. Clin Exp Reprod Med. 2016;43(2):119-25.
28. Park JY, Su YQ, Ariga M, et al. EGF-like growth factors as mediators of LH action in the ovulatory follicle. Science. 2004;303:682-4.
29. Peng XR, Hsueh AJ, LaPolt PS, et al. Localization of luteinizing hormone receptor messenger ribonucleic acid expression in ovarian cell types during follicle development and ovulation. Endocrinology. 1991;129:3200-7.
30. Pliushch G, Schneider E, Schneider T, et al. In vitro maturation of oocytes is not associated with altered deoxyribonucleic acid methylation patterns in children from in vitro fertilization or intracytoplasmic sperm injection. Fertil Steril. 2015;103(3):720-7.
31. Prasath EB, Chan ML, Wong WH, et al. First pregnancy and live birth resulting from cryopreserved embryos obtained from in vitro matured oocytes after oophorectomy in an ovarian cancer patient. Hum Reprod. 2014;29(2):276-8.
32. Rose BI, Laky D. A comparison of the Cook single lumen immature ovum IVM needle to the Steiner-Tan pseudo double lumen flushing needle for oocyte retrieval for IVM. J Assist Reprod Genet. 2013;30(6):855-60.
33. Rose BI. The case for more active management of endometrial development in ivm: decreasing the miscarriage rate and increasing the clinical pregnancy rate. J Reprod Endocrinol Infert. 2015;1:4.
34. Segers I, Mateizel I, Van Moer E, et al. In vitro maturation (IVM) of oocytes recovered from ovariectomy specimens in the laboratory: a promising "ex vivo" method of oocyte cryopreservation resulting in the first report of an ongoing pregnancy in Europe. J Assist Reprod Genet. 2015;32(8): 1221-31.
35. Seok HH, Song H, Lyu HW, et al. Application of serum anti-Müllerian hormone levels in selecting patients with polycystic ovary syndrome for in vitro maturation treatment. Clin Exp Reprod Med. 2016;43(2):126-32.
36. Shalom-Paz E1, Almog B, Wiser A, et al. Priming in vitro maturation cycles with gonadotropins: salvage treatment for nonresponding patients. Fertil Steril. 2011;96(2):340-3.
37. Shavit T, Ellenbogen A, Michaeli M, et al. In-vitro maturation of oocytes vs in-vitro fertilization with a gonadotropin-releasing hormone antagonist for women with polycystic ovarian syndrome: can superiority be defined? Eur J Obstet Gynecol Reprod Biol. 2014;179:46-50.
38. Shirasawa H, Terada Y. In vitro maturation of human immature oocytes for fertility preservation and research material. Reprod Med Biol. 2017;16(3):258-67.
39. Son WY, Chung JT, Chian RC, et al. A 38-h interval between hCG priming and oocyte retrieval increases in vivo and in vitro oocyte maturation rate in programmed IVM cycles. Hum Reprod. 2008; 23(9):2010-6.
40. Son WY, Chung JT, Demirtas E, et al. Comparison of in-vitro maturation cycles with and without in-vivo matured oocytes retrieved. Reprod Biomed Online. 2008;17(1):59-67.
41. Son WY, Chung JT, Herrero B, et al. Selection of the optimal day for oocyte retrieval based on the diameter of the dominant follicle in hCG-primed in vitro maturation cycles. Hum Reprod. 2008;23(12):2680-5.
42. Son WY, Tan SL. Laboratory and embryological aspects of hCG-primed in vitro maturation cycles for patients with polycystic ovaries. Hum Reprod Update. 2010;16(6):675-89.
43. Son WY, Yoon SH, Lim JH. Effect of gonadotrophin priming on in-vitro maturation of oocytes collected from women at risk of OHSS. Reprod Biomed Online. 2006;13(3):340-8.

44. Thompson JG, Gilchrist RB. Pioneering contributions by Robert Edwards to oocyte in vitro maturation (IVM). Mol Hum Reprod. 2013;19(12):794-8.
45. Trounson A, Wood C, Kausche A. (1994). In vitro maturation and the fertilization and developmental competence of oocytes recovered from untreated polycystic ovarian patients. Fertil Steril. 1994;62(2): 353-62.
46. Vitek W, Robins JC. In vitro maturation. Obstet Gynaecol. 2013;15:215-9.
47. Walls ML, Hunter T, Ryan JP, et al. In vitro maturation as an alternative to standard in vitro fertilization for patients diagnosed with polycystic ovaries: a comparative analysis of fresh, frozen and cumulative cycle outcomes. Hum Reprod. 2015;30(1):88-96.
48. Yang SH, Son WY, Yoon SH, et al. Correlation between in vitro maturation and expression of LH receptor in cumulus cells of the oocytes collected from PCOS patients in HCG-primed IVM cycles. Hum Reprod. 2005;20(8):2097-103.
49. Zhang XY, Ata B, Son WY, et al. Chromosome abnormality rates in human embryos obtained from in-vitro maturation and IVF treatment cycles. Reprod Biomed Online. 2010;21: 552-9.

39

CHAPTER

Microfluidics in ART

Manish Pandya

WHAT IS OUR GOAL IN ASSISTED REPRODUCTIVE TECHNOLOGY?

We have to optimize production of preimplantation embryos for use in assisted reproductive technology (ART) and get maximum implantation and very good carry home baby rate with least possible chance of abortion.

Our embryologist is trained in a way to handle gametes in very delicate manner with all possible do no harm of Hippocratic oath to mimic as natural as possible to get maximum result.

Now we have very good culture media available for growth of embryo and sequential maturation in CO_2 incubators either bench top or conventional.

Still we are fighting with negative effects done by manipulation, denudations, chemical application such as hyaluronidase and media incubation, osmotic imbalance, pH changes, shifts in temperature, mechanical stress, etc.

So to minimize negative effects on gametes *in vitro*, what we can do is modification of the platforms on which gametes and embryos are handled, and we can also modify and improve culture condition.

At present, we are using all polystyrene test tube, petri dishes, organ culture wells like center well or four well plates for culture of varying number of cells and variable amount of media, and different amount of sperm concentration.

To overcome all above negatives and laboratory hazards, an idea came into action is "back to nature "and we can give gametes an environment same as nature and formulation of culture again same as nature, pathways to meet ovum and sperm same as nature and final maturation process near to same as nature

What is ideology behind these are:

- We have to make culture media same as composition of fluid in female genital tract to get best of its ability.
- Make same biometric approach to culture platforms attempting to recapitulate the conditions experienced by embryo *in vitro*.
- Gametes and embryos are exposed to the constricted "moist environment" of female genital tract and surrounded by variously oriented glycoproteins and are gently moved via ciliated epithelium.
- Give embryo the same path from fallopian tube to uterine cavity so that ovum and sperm can travel the same path as from posterior fornix to garden of ampulla in fallopian tube.
- So, we can change largely static environment of gametes and embryo to novel *in vivo* environment *in vitro*.

So, a novel idea occurred to make inert synthetic polymers, bathed in a relative ocean of media making *in vitro* same as *in vivo*.

Microfluidic technology and other novel culture platforms offer a means to further manipulate culture conditions *in vitro* in the hopes of creating an environment that is more suitable for gametes and embryo development and function.

So basic idea is to offer the potential to revolutionize the fundamental approach what we are utilizing within *in vitro* fertilization (IVF) laboratories and allow the replacement of manual manipulation within automation of specific steps.

Nowadays, we have some platforms utilizing fluid movements on the macro level for dynamic cultures employing microfluidics.

We may develop vibrational embryo culture and tilting culture both in same device to phenol mimic the female genital tract.

So, what we mean by microfluidic is the technology by which the utilization of fluid movements in a micro- or nanoenvironment like fluid density, viscosity, and size or geometry.

At macro level, the flow of fluid within the system leading to turbulence so in microfluidics we can make flow streamlined and predictable just like laminar flow on fluids through microchannels with no mixing, except by diffusion across the fluid–fluid interface.

These all are done at very small microscales so fluid viscosity and surface tension become a main feature of fluid flow pattern.

So, now we are moving from macrodroplet to microdroplet to microfluidics for gamete and embryo culture and eliminating larger dynamic fluid movements (Figs. 1A to C).

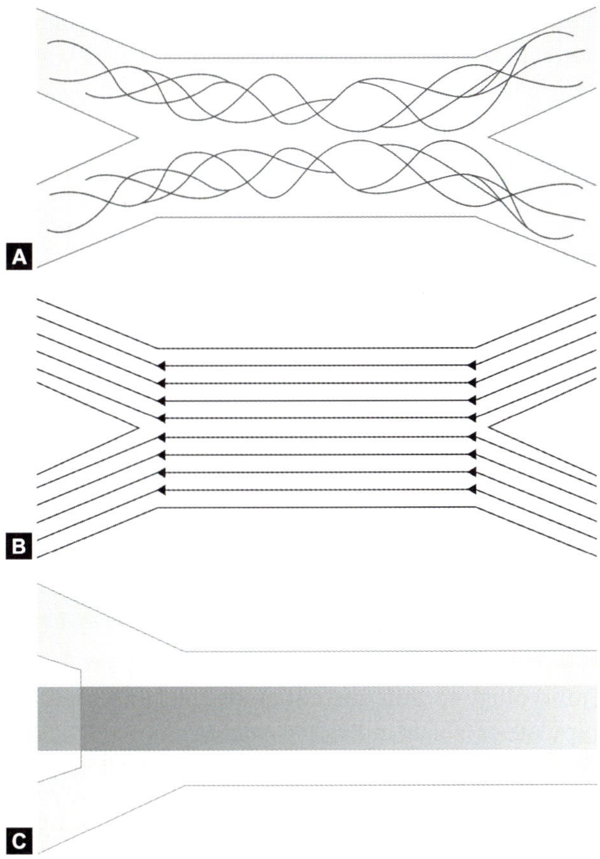

Figs. 1A to C: (A) Turbulent flow; (B) Laminar flow; (C) Media flow.

Microlaminar Flow

So now great challenges in fabrication of microfluidic device for use in ART to make more biocompatible material and approach to improve techniques in IVF.

So, we have to make perfusion-based microfluidic platforms for adherent cell culture.

At present material tested for devices composed of:

- Polydimethylsiloxane (PDMS)
- Silicone
- Borosilicate glass
- Pyrex
- Quarts
- Combinations of above materials.

There may be different material for microchannel and actual surface on which cell lies which is main critical consideration for cell attachments and cell culture; so manufacturing this device requires great technology that involves photolithography, moulding, and chemical or mechanical etching channel.

At present material available is PDMS as it has certain advantages like flexibility, ease of soft lithography patterning, and ease of use under microscopy as it has low auto fluorescence and we can make rapid, repeatable, precise, and less expensive production with ensure sterility for clinical use in ART.

One of benefit of microfluidics is the ability to achieve dynamic media flow platforms.

Although we have tried prior attempts on macroscale proven in efficient and subsequently not used on large scale or ground.

So we have unique nature of microfluidics media perfusion and movement that are more amenable for wide spread use whether perfusion systems are recirculating or nonrecirculating.

Main principle of new platform systems, is perfusion devices, has to operate successfully for over a week.

First few microfluidics devices are based on gravity driven passive flow with hydrostatic pressure in media reservoirs as an integral part for media driven flow down microchannels.

The simplicity of above device is advantageous but it is very difficult to regulate flow speed or volume changes over time frame particularly when height of media columns diminishes an alternative to that is made by externally attached syringes for input and output ports.

Alternative to syringe driven flow another approach is use of Hamilton syringes attached to a programmable infusion pump but very difficult for use in close incubator, as it requires external tubing and machinery.

Tilting device gives an improved method for gentle movement of media and embryo and gives associated benefits and same we have seen in large volume macro-droplets culture.

Vibrating devices developed using dynamic fluid movements and flow may be helpful as gentle agitation on human embryo is found to be beneficial.

Recently, Braille pumping system using piezoelectric actuators has been used successfully to peristaltically move media along microchannels during embryo culture and embryo remain undisturbed and these devices are very compact and can fit in single incubators easily in multiples.

Nowadays, most intriguing concept for regulating media flow within a microfluidic device entails use of the expansive characteristics of a 3D matrix—a hydrogel to regulate flow through channels and this technology gives full control over media channels through mechanical responses in hydrogel to external stimuli such as light, pH, and biological clues.

Factors for consideration for best microfluidic device:

- Which material and design should be used?
- How to operate and what is success?
- Ease of manipulation embryo within device and how to remove it?
- What is level of compatibility with embryologist and IVF laboratory?

Best Design

It should be nontoxic and must pass all quality test control assay. They are biocompatible with ability to sterilize with ultraviolet (UV) light, ethanol, or ethylene oxide, or can be autoclavable. PDMS is now-a-days more compatible with above criteria and can be used traditionally in gamma radiation also.

In best design, microfluidics platforms, we are using very small amount of media so properties like medium viscosity, pH, and density of cells are most important criteria for consideration.

Operation of Device

During operation, there must be good coordination between dynamic culture and media flow with perfusion regulatory in device with ability to avoid bubble formation within channels to control bubble trap and in case of failure or media halts easy correction should be available.

Ease of Manipulation and Removal of Embryos

Most difficult and challenging problem is construction of device much friendly to use in IVF laboratory by embryologist with great ease and no disturbance to embryo without stress.

As we are using very small amount of media, we must think of pH, evaporation, osmolality, and temperature rapid shift and design must incorporate an embryologist friendly system to assess cells within funnels.

EMBRYOLOGIST COMPATIBILITY

Microfluidics device needs to be friendly enough to fit into all conventional incubators without any problem of tubing and apparatuses and should be of low cost.

ANDROLOGY AND MICROFLUIDICS

Different devices made of silicone were used for sperm evaluation since 1993, like interception via cervical mucus, hyaluronic acid, spermicide, antisperm antibody bed, etc.

Polydimethylsiloxane is a passive gravity-driven device, where the hydrostatic pressure of two separate inlet reservoirs droving the media flow down to a converging microfluidics channel which are available in market and used by embryologist for poor sperm sample to isolate good quality sperm for ICSI.

Basic idea behind this device is that only motile sperm can travel the border that separates the parallel streams of diluted semen and fresh medium, and microchannels allow motile sperm to swim away from debris and nonmotile sperm (Figs. 2 and 3).

Modification of PDMS microfluidics sperm sorter device is to increase hydrophilicity with a coasting such as polyethylene glycol methacrylate (PEG-MA) is of great help.

Recently, we have a device with idea of developing a system which can do sorting of X and Y bearing sperm and ability to laser cut tail of sperm so we can use them directly for ICSI with ease.

In conventional sperm preparation with any method, we require centrifugation, which leads to damage of sperm DNA, and formation of ROS but initial results with use of microfluidics for andrology show significantly lower damage to DNA and higher motility.

EMBRYOLOGY AND MICROFLUIDICS

Like andrology, it is very challenging to use microfluidics in embryology to utilizing adherent cells and ability to manipulate or isolate individual cells.

So, devices are made to use in *in vitro* maturation (IVM), IVF, and embryo culture:

- Device for IVM
- Device for IVF
- Device for embryo culture.

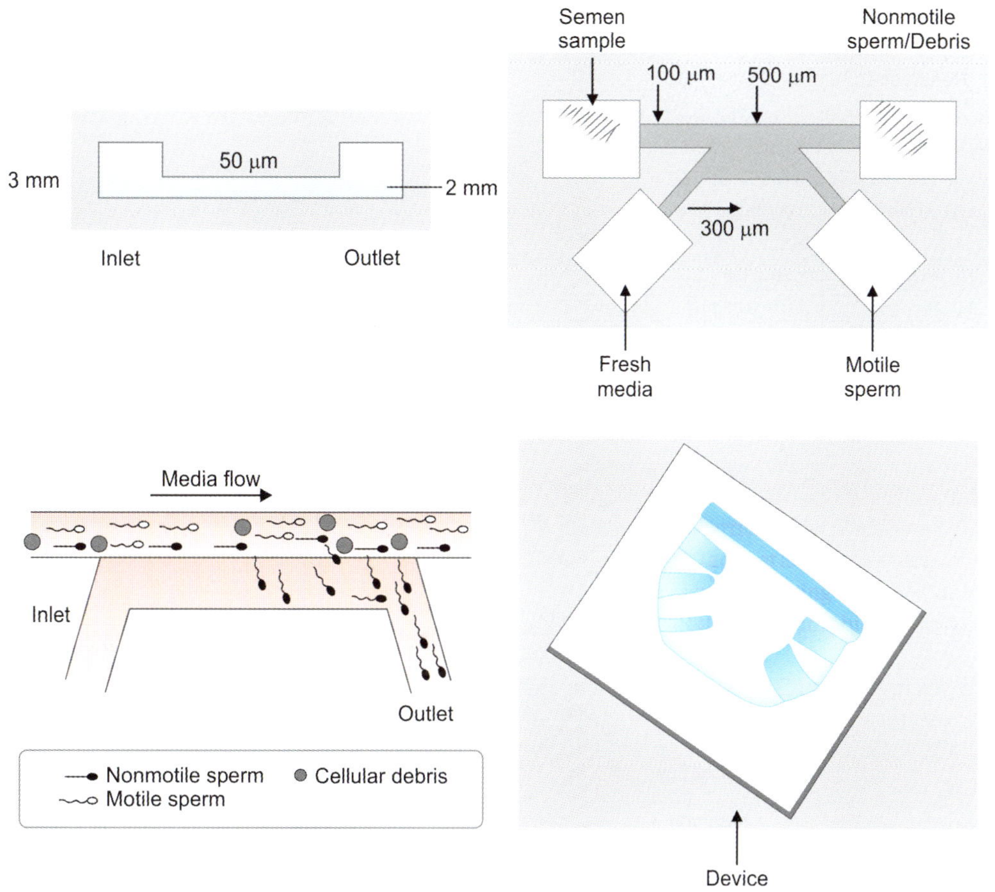

Fig. 2: Microfluidic sperm sorter.

In vitro maturation is need of hour to reduce OHSS, cost and health risk at reduced cost; with help of microfluidics, we may improve success rate.

Initial experiment with PDMS microchannels success rate is 71% in development of MII.

Oocyte matured on 200 micro M wide microchannels containing approximately 8 or 500 micro M drops, oocyte maturation consists of two components: (1) nuclear and (2) cytoplasmic maturations. In 8 μL droplet, cumulus cell expansion will be diminished, may be due to size and volume limitation. In experiments done by Walter et al., static microchannels show enhancement in oocyte cytoplasmic maturation.

It has been shown in bovine oocyte that they will mature in dynamic microfluidics device with braille pin regulated media flow.

In vitro fertilization and microfluidics are based on to mimic same *in vivo* environment by gravity driven sperm flow to prevent poly spermia and limit the time for sperm near to ovum. Sperm motion path is dependent on flow rate and it will make sperm no longer capable of independent movement and also influenced by contours of device because of all these quality microfluidics devices have immense implication in successful IVF.

Use of low concentration of sperm in microfluidic devices had given higher pregnancy rate compare to control where high concentration of sperms was used because of increased concentration of sperm near vicinity of ovum.

In vitro fertilization not only entails mixing of sperm and eggs, but also requires manipulation of presumptive zygote to remove cumulus cells in order to visualize pronuclei. Microfluidics device does not exist that can remove cumulus and even zona pellucidae (Figs. 4 and 5).

EMBRYO CULTURE

Exhaustive studies have been conducted for embryo culture *in vitro* in microfluidic platform and we have seen even two cells, four cells, and hatching blastocyst formation at 72 and 96 hours.

However, there is no observable beneficial effect on embryo development to culture organ well dishes.

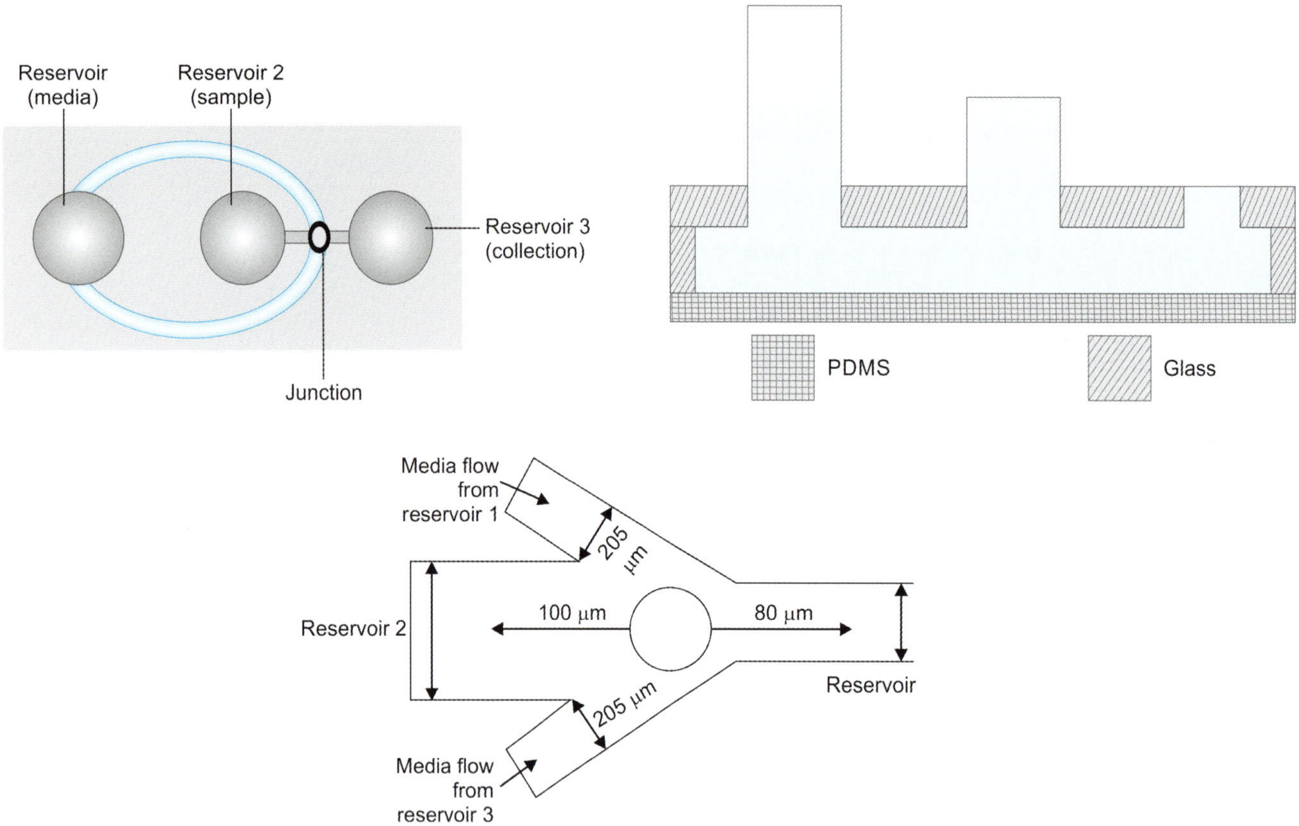

Fig. 3: Sperm separation device.
(PDMS: polydimethylsiloxane)

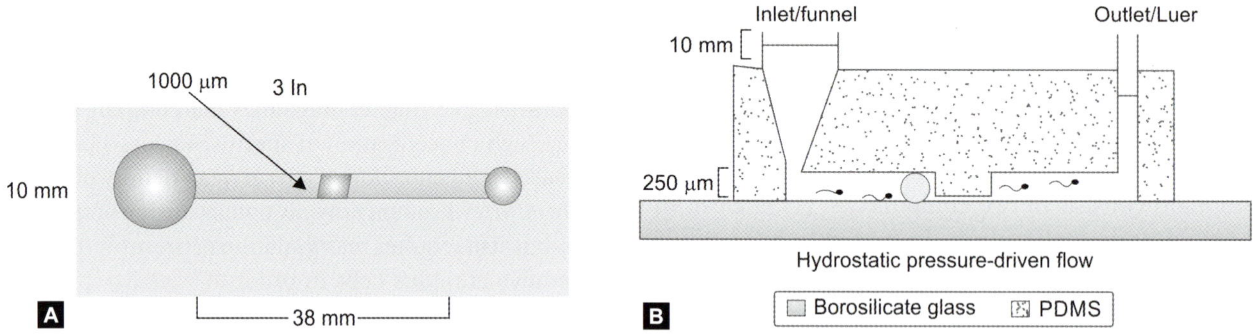

Figs. 4A and B
(PDMS: polydimethylsiloxane)

It has been seen in mouse embryo model that they were loaded into funnel reservoir, and medium was added to the bottom of funnel via the action of Braille actuator, and it was seen regardless of media flow pattern back and front versus flow through or fast versus slow growth in dynamic device showed greater hatching of blastocysts and significantly higher cell number than static control (Figs. 6A to E).

Bormann and colleagues had presented data on beneficial effect of Braille-driven media flow and have found that good number of embryos has reached morula stage in

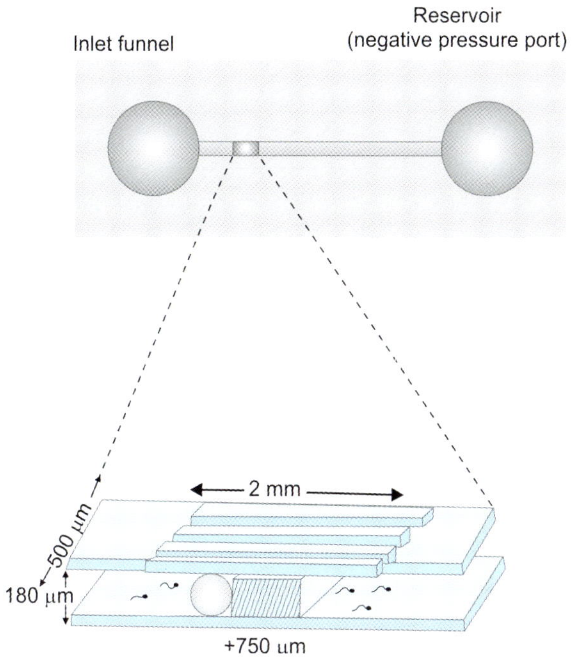

Fig. 5: Microfluidic device composed of polydimethylsiloxane to perform IVF "on chip".

48 hours, blastocyst stage in 72 hours and hatching around in 96 hours and gives less fragmentation.

Womb-on-a-chip design in which endometrial cells are grown in a lower chamber and embryo is cultured in upper chamber separated by thin membrane, so allows embryo to interact with secreted factors from endometrial cells shows development of two cells and blastocyst rate similar to 50 μL droplet. Cell numbers are higher and implantation rate and live offspring rate is good (Figs. 7A to C).

On same principle, Opticell^{TM} by Mizuno gives chromosomally normal embryos that give live offspring. They have cultured two cell frozen human embryos in microfluidic device and got good blastocyst development compare to static device.

We can have same microfluidic device in which oocyte has been fertilized using microwell media and sperm via gravity-driven hydrostatic pressure after fertilization media replaced by culture media and flow through the channel same device, where we get higher number of blastocyst formation compare to control.

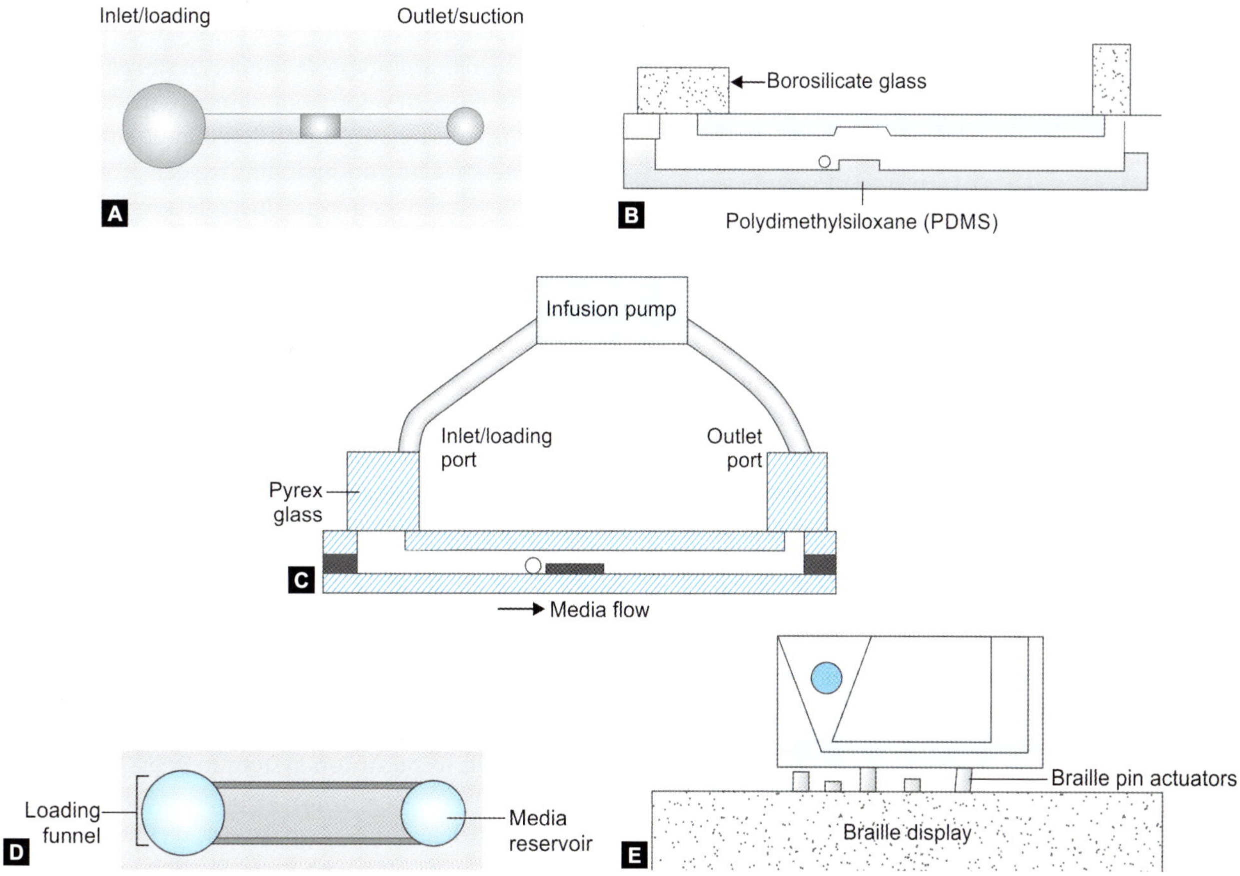

Figs. 6A to E: Microfluidic device of polydimethylsiloxane (PDMS) using Braille actuators to drive media.

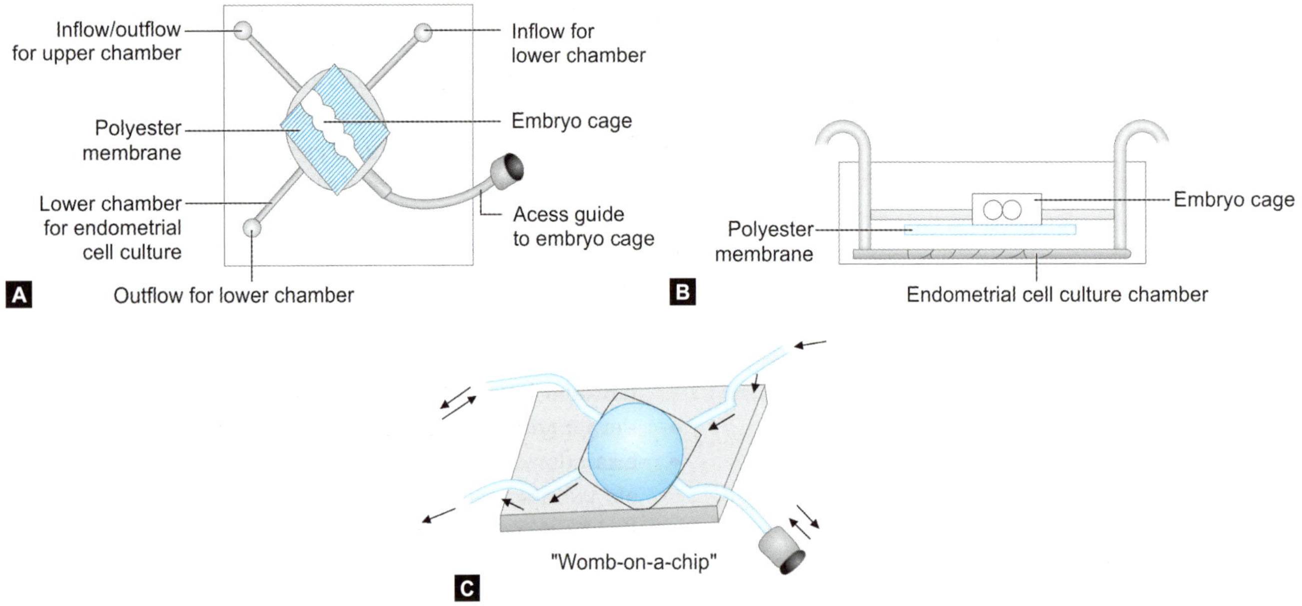

Figs. 7A to C: Microfluidic perfusion system.

Big question is how microfluidics helps in improvement of result, hypothesized that autocrine and paracrine factors secreted by gametes or embryo are localized due to confining nature of microfluidics.

Research is going on various secretion form oocyte and embryo as secretome as noninvasive markers as embryo developmental competence.

As secretion form cultured cell gives beneficial effect as well as quantity of embryo, volume of media and surface area are also additional factors for better outcome.

We have seen beneficial effect of group culture with good quality embryo and volume of media on static culture.

We have observed that harmful metabolic products like ammonia can be easily removed by dynamic device same we can do with small microdroplet and replacement with fresh culture media shows no benefit on embryo development.

A common factor between static and microfluidics device is constrictive nature of micro device and all embryos are staying in very small area and give cell proximity and spacing same as group culture.

There is difference of a well and small nanowell, with extremely small amount of media with reduced spacing for direct contact to make physical contact.

It is postulated that doing culture in extremely small volume droplets and microfluidic device results in reduction in localized oxygen tension because of confined spaces.

In static culture, we have reduced oxygen level from atmospheric level of around 20% to 5–7% , which is very good for embryo development same in microfluidics.

We have used 5% CO_2 in air so there will be reduction in oxygen content, 5% oxygen in dynamic device shows improved results.

It has seen that embryo developed in stirred in dynamic device has more development compare to static culture because of media renewal due to flow may be either building up or depletion of factors including oxygen proves that this advance development may be due to less oxygen.

When flow is used in both micro and macro devices, it can stimulate embryos and give them sense of sheer stress, which will activate different intracellular signaling pathways that lead to apoptosis mild stimulation to embryo, may mimic action of ciliated epithelium of fallopian tube—active embryo hypothesis.

At present we have all kind of culturing devices in form of channel, funnel, in flow and out flow, co-culturing, and so many, so it is very difficult to understand that which is better.

Still research will throw light on divergence of gene expression patterns, molecular signaling pathways, and some biochemical endpoints.

There is some practice consideration like bioavailability means material should be nontoxic, operator friendly, disposable, and user friendly design.

Operation in perfusion system may be recirculating, ability to be used over 5–6 days, air bubbles can cause failure so can able to detect and can make easy rectification, it must have easy visualization with rapid loading and unloading with ability to isolate and monitor individual cells.

Device must be fit in conventional incubators, user friendly, and take less time for setup.

Till date, we are not able to find device, which can do all integral function involved in field of embryology because it is about involving multiple steps.

It is sure that microfluidic can offer revolution in field of IVF made easy.

KEY POINTS

- For the optimization of preimplantation embryos, we must do least harm.
- Embryologist must handle the gamete very delicately to get maximum result.
- Back to nature is main motto off microfluidics device.
- In anthology to get good motile sperm, we have very good microfluidics device in market.
- For embryo culture, Braille-driven microchip device is available.
- Womb-on-a-chip designed mimic more of a natural cycle IVF.
- Microfluidics can offer revolution in IVF made easy.

EDITOR'S COMMENTS

1. Microfluidics is interdisciplinary work, which involves biologists as well as bioengineers, which is growing fast nowadays.
2. Still data from clinical trials are required for making future evidenced-based decisions regarding the application of microfluidics in human ART.
3. Microfluidics from sperm selection in IUI and IVF has now come into regular time and use but requires more data to prove its efficacy.
4. Microfluidics for sperm preparation can be an easy and cost-effective option low resource settings where advanced embryology laboratory equipment and skilled technicians are not available.

SUGGESTED READING

1. Manish R Pandya, Vijaykumar Chelur N. The Techniques of IVF Made Easy. Jaypee Brothers Medical Publishers; 2015.

40

CHAPTER

Co-culture Techniques in ART

Harsha Bhadarka, Kruti Patel

INTRODUCTION

The past few decades have seen remarkable advancement in culture media for assisted reproduction technology (ART) and treatment for infertile couple to improve culture condition *in vitro*. Fundamental research on the metabolic activity of mammalian embryos demonstrated very peculiar requirements in the embryogenesis *in vitro*. Bernard in the late 1800s introduced the idea that the surrounding environment of living tissues has crucial role. Therefore to facilitate such studies organs and tissues should be studied *in vitro* in a suitable formulated medium.

Actually, most of ART culture media presently in use are not optimum for the *in vitro* development of human embryo. Moreover, advance research is required to bring down stress to embryo culture system and find out specific embryos from cohort, which are more likely to give result. The first success of human *in vitro* fertilization (IVF) by Robert Edwards was achieved in a basic medium, prepared with chemicals. This medium was a modified Ham's F10 or T6 supplemented with maternal serum and a modified Earle's balanced salt solution. Another specifically designed media for human IVF was human tubal fluid (HTF). HTF contains serum albumin or whole serum, which was proved to be beneficial for day 2 or day 3 human embryo cultures, and has continued in utilization for long time. Use of maternal serum, HTF, is supposed to provide natural nourishment like *in vivo* to embryo. The design of media is complex, consisting of specific components, and its concentrations in order to reduce the stress on a developing embryo. Particularly, the culture media is an essential part in successful *in vitro* interactions between gametes and later embryonic development. Thus to reduce this stress during embryo development and to provide natural culture conditions an idea of culturing embryo with another type of growing cells arose. Two different schools of thought led to two different systems for human embryo culture: one is the "back-to-nature" means culturing in sequential media, and "let-the-embryo-decide" means culturing in single-step media. These media are available commercially and the research is still continued by different groups of scientists.

Co-culture technique means growing of embryos in a culture media on top of a mono layer of feeder cells, it appeared as an effective strategy to mimic *in vivo* culture environment. In animal and human culture systems, feeder cells tend to secrete several growth factors and cytokines. This method aims to improve the culture medium for embryos *in vitro* and leads to better embryo morphology, with higher possibilities of reaching up to the blastocysts stage, and thus leading to a possible implantation and healthy pregnancy. However, one hypothesis is that, the presence of unwanted growth factors that are secreted during co-culture system may lead to uncontrollable *in vitro* conditions resulting in developmental alterations during early embryogenesis.

A various types of cells, either commercially obtained cell lines or cultured cells established from surgical specimens or abattoir, have been claimed to support human embryo growth *in vitro*. Till date feeder layer of different cells like Vero cell, bovine uterine fibroblast, bovine oviductal epithelial cell, human granulosa cell, cumulus cell, ampullary cell, human oviductal cell, and human endometrial cell co-culture, and sequential co-culture with human ampullary cells and endometrial cells have been used and demonstrated improvement in human embryo development.

Vero cell (cell line derived from green monkey kidney) is the commercially available cell line, which has been utilized extensively for the study of human embryo co-culture. These cells are easy to handle, highly controlled, and manipulate and also it can be easily incorporated into an IVF laboratory set up. Favorable results on embryo co-cultured with Vero cells, as a feeder layer, have been reported by several investigators (Menezo et al., 1990; Zetova et al., 1993; and Magli et al., 1995), except by Sakkas et al., 1994. Wiemer et al., (1993) reported a beneficial effect of co-culturing of bovine oviduct cells and achieving improved embryonic development and pregnancy rate for only patients with normal male factor.

As compare to embryos cultured in only culture medium, co-cultured embryos have better morphology in terms of lesser fragmentation and blastomere swelling and increased in-embryo variation in zona pellucida thickness. Increased blastocyst rate in co-cultured embryo and natural hatching has also been observed. It is not commonly used, as it requires extra techniques and high-skilled practices.

MECHANISMS

There are different mechanisms involves, which include the release of embryotrophic factors and the detoxification of the culture medium by removal of heavy metal cations, free radicals, or metabolic inhibitors. The aim of the co-culture technique is to supply factors that will permit the embryo to cross the critical stage of MZT (maternal to zygotic transition), allowing for full development. Such cytokines and growth factors must be active during the first 3 days of culture to increase the metabolism of the embryo, thereby increasing its potential to develop and implant.

Initially, co-culture system by Biggers et al. (1962) developed in the mouse, supported a paracrine effect. Paracrine effect defines cell-to-cell communication in which a cell releases a signal to stimulate changes in nearby cells, which leads to improvement in the growth of these cells. These signaling molecules or paracrine factors distributed over a very short distance, and help in improvement of embryonic growth. These embryos were cultured on feeder layer of hormonally primed oviducts. In 1984, Camous et al. had studied bovine embryos co-culture with bovine trophoblastic tissue which was depend on autocrine function. It is a form of cell signaling where a cell releases chemical messenger that binds to autocrine receptors on that cell, leading to alterations in the cell. Live calves were produced after more than 5 days of co-culture.

There are many different factors, which may have impact on result of co-culture, which includes indication for IVF treatment, type of feeder layer, period of time of co-culture technique, and criteria for the patient selection (Plachot, 1996). Due to risk factors concerning disease transmission from nonhuman or homologous feeder cell lines and also 2002 FDA warning of categorizing the use of non-human feeder cell lines as xenotransplantation, co-culture is now restricted to the use of autologous cumulus cells and endometrial cells.

Role of different growth factors in commercial culture media is known, to evaluate their competency on embryo culture, implantation and pregnancy rate, as alternate approach respective growth factors in certain proportions have been supplemented precisely to culture medium (Table 1).

Co-culture cell lines have also been involved in reduction of harmful elements like hypoxanthine and oxygen metabolites, which are known to interfere in embryo culture.

Most commonly, cumulus cells, endometrium cells, the walls of the ovarian follicles, and the fallopian tube cells are in use as feeder cells in assisted reproduction.

AUTOLOGOUS ENDOMETRIAL CO-CULTURE

Studies have been done using prepubertal oviduct cells as feeder layers and tubal or uterine cells in co-culture which confirmed the role of the endometrium during the window of implantation and the use of endometrial cells in co-culture as a method to get better implantation rate makes sense. Several studies indicate evidence of a

TABLE 1 Role of different growth factors in commercial culture media.

Growth factors	*Beneficial effects*
IGF-I (insulin-like growth factor)	Reduction of cellular apoptosis and increased the number of morphologically normal embryos
GM-CSF (granulocyte-macrophage colony-stimulating factor)	Produced more blastocyst embryo and improved IVF outcome
PAF (platelet activating factor)	Positive effect on live birth rates in assisted reproduction
HB-EGF (heparin-binding epidermal growth factor)	Improvement of growth and hatching capacity of blastocysts embryo
LIF (leukemia-inhibiting factor)	Better pregnancy rates

cross-talk between the embryo and the endometrium. Beside promoting embryo development, it also activates specific paracrine factors that increase the probability of implantation. De los Santos, in 1996, proved that a co-culture system with human endometrial epithelial cells tends to increased embryonic paracrine markers production and embryos cultured in endometrial epithelial cells control definite fundamental adhesion molecules and improve uterine receptivity. Spandorfer et al. in 2001, marked the presence of leukemia inhibitory factor (LIF) in co-culture media and showed a positive correlation of embryo growth and clinical pregnancy rates with LIF levels.

Desai et al. demonstrated embryotrophic properties of endometrium cell line and compared with both Vero cells and human oviductal cells as a co-culture system. In 2003, they reported a new noninteracted human endometrial co-culture system using this endometrial cell line and Transwell plates. With this technology, embryos are benefited from secreted embryotrophic components while preventing connection with endometrial cells, thus reduce the hypothetical risk of disease transmission. The role of co-culture procedures about perinatal safety is unknown. The result of embryo transferred on cleavage-stage and blastocysts stage, after co-culture, has same perinatal outcomes as compare to IVF without co-culture.

An autologous endometrial co-culture cycle involves following steps:

- After counseling, when a patient is ready for the procedure, she has to undergo an endometrial biopsy in previous cycle of treatment, where small piece of her endometrium is removed in sterile condition.
- This sample is then enzymatically treated with trypsin/ethylenediaminetetraacetic acid (EDTA) solution and washed for two to three times before freezing.
- The patient then undergoes a regular IVF stimulation as per clinic's protocol.
- On the day of human chorionic gonadotropin (hCG) injection, biopsy of endometrial cells is thawed and plated in single culture media contained 100 μL droplets.
- On the day of retrieval, intracytoplasmic sperm injection (ICSI) is performed and injected oocytes were placed on cultured endometrial cell.
- The embryo development is closely monitored.
- The patient's embryos are transferred either on day 3 or blastocyst stage, into her uterus with ultrasonography guidance (Figs. 1 and 2).

Advantages and Disadvantages

- Endometrial cells can be easily obtained through biopsy in a previous cycle.
- Though, specific protocols for autologous endometrial cell co-culture differ from center to center but the basic principles are the same.
- It is invasive but comparatively pain free.
- The procedure can also provide better embryo quality and embryo development.
- However, till date there is no harmful effects on embryo growth with co-culture are reported. The use of autologous endometrial cells prevents chance for transmission of disease.
- The risks of endometrial co-culture are minimal.
- Complications related to uterine infection or damage caused by endometrial biopsy are very rare.

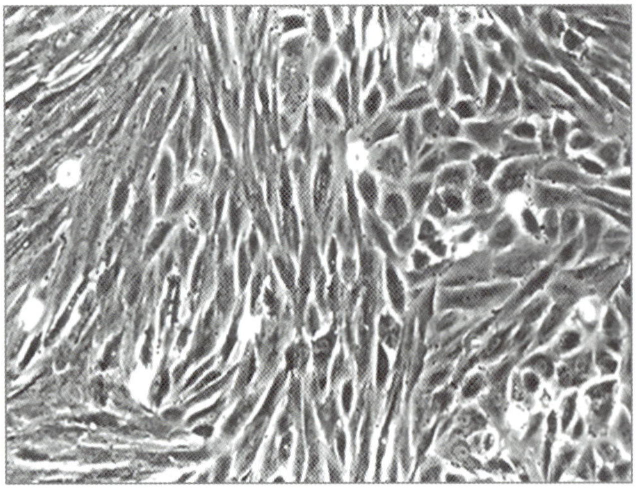

Fig. 1: Endometrial co-culture.

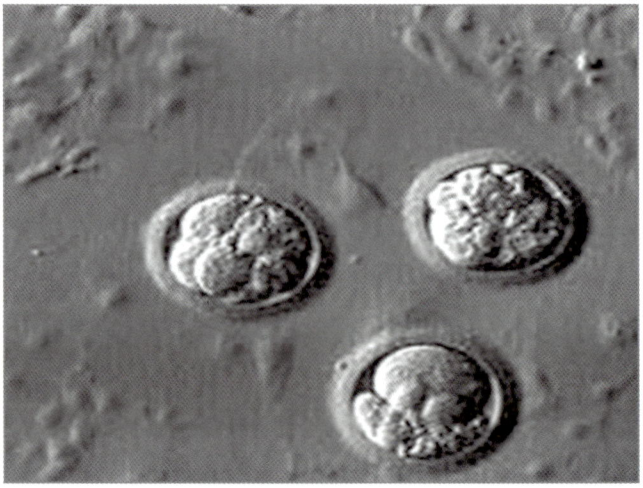

Fig. 2: Embryos grown with endometrial co-culture.

- Over all advantages, it is not routinely used as it requires more time than routine IVF cycle.
- Moreover, it also requires prior freezing in previous cycle of treatment and later it requires thawing at the time of patient's IVF cycle.

AUTOLOGOUS CUMULUS CELL CO-CULTURE

During the past two decades, scientific studies have been published on improvement of *in vitro* cultured embryos in assisted reproduction. Particularly, cumulus cells that impact the oocyte development, physiologically connected to oocyte maturation and also instantly available, easily harvested after follicular aspiration for IVF and successfully used to assist in embryo culture. It is proven that different growth factors released by cumulus cells can enhance oocyte maturation and support embryo developments during *in vitro* culture. Similarly, as they take part in cross-cellular processes under *in vivo* conditions. During such co-culture these cells seem to be responsible for better embryo quality, increased numbers of embryos, also provide an advantageous effect on pregnancy rates in IVF.

During preimplantation, the detection of different receptors responsible for various growth factors on the surface of embryos represents the importance of exchange and impact of stage specific morphogenetic products between developing embryo and surrounding cells. Such molecular cross communication can inadequately take place in commercial culture media that deprive embryos of crucial growth factors. This may simply potential risks related to standardized IVF technique since early embryos through their receptors cannot respond and interact with the particular growth factors. Hence, it is anticipated that cumulus cells with their particular released growth factors more closely resemble the physiologic surroundings in favor of improvement of embryo culture in *in vitro* conditions. Supplementation of autologous cumulus cell into the culture medium and presence of several growth factors during co-culture have contributed to this qualitative and quantitative betterment of embryogenesis and ultimately final ART outcome.

Another benefit of cumulus cells in conventional IVF method is—they are one of the sources of sperm chemoattractants that surrounds the oocyte. Progesterone, proved to be secreted from cumulus cells. As per Oren-Benaroya et al. (2008), there are other different components, which were confirmed as sperm chemoattractant.

Sperm chemotaxis has been identified toward various female origins as follicular fluid, oviduct fluid, and conditioned medium from the cumulus cells and the oocyte. Also human sperm seems to be guided by chemotaxis toward the oocyte in the female genital tract, similarly, which may also attract sperm during incubation of COC with washed sperm and increases fertilization.

Parikh et al. 2004 presented a novel method for embryo transfer with the use of cumulus cells where during embryo transfer, some amount of cumulus cells were loaded with the cleaved or expanded embryo in the catheter, which may increases the uterine receptivity and enhances the implantation rate. Denudation of cumulus oocyte complex with hyaluronidase is done in routine ICSI protocol.

Some embryologists keep some cumulus cells during this procedure, which surround the oocyte and take advantage of cumulus cell in embryo culture.

CUMULUS CO-CULTURE METHOD

Cumulus co-culture technique involves the following steps:

- Once a patient is ready for the procedure after counseling, she undergoes egg retrieval procedure after stimulation as per clinic protocol.
- After 2–3 hours incubation from the retrieved eggs, cumulus cells were mechanically removed with help of 26G needle and washed it with culture medium, keep it in 50 μL (another method for harvesting cumulus cells is, during denudation with hyaluronidase for ICSI, recovered cumulus cells are repeatedly washed with culture medium and use for co culture.
- Then oocytes were denuded by exposure to hyaluronidase for ICSI.
- ICSI done by standard protocol of embryology laboratory.
- Injected oocytes were plated and incubated on monolayers of cumulus cells, single oocyte was kept per droplet at 37°C in triple gas incubator.
- The embryos, which are cultured on monolayer of cumulus cells, are supervised for its development (Figs. 3 and 4).
- The patient's embryos transferred into her uterus.

Advantages

- After oocyte retrieval, the cumulus cells are usually discarded.
- No extra invasive procedure, extra time, and expense require for the procedure.
- No need to freeze and thaw the cells.

Limitations

Obviously, it requires skilled embryologist. Because improper handling may cause infection or may damage oocyte.

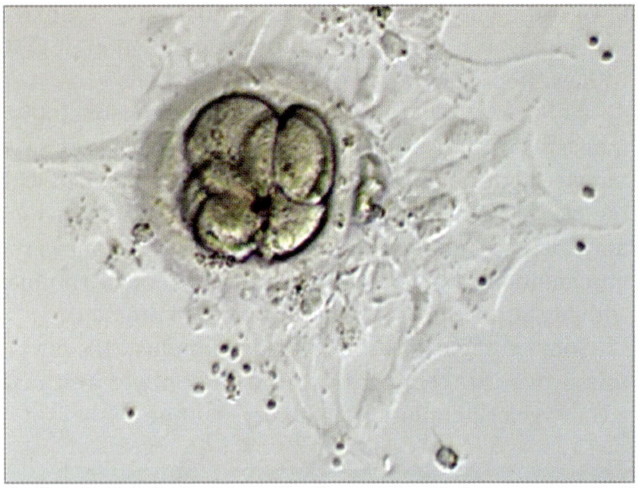

Fig. 3: Embryos cultured on monolayer of cumulus cells.

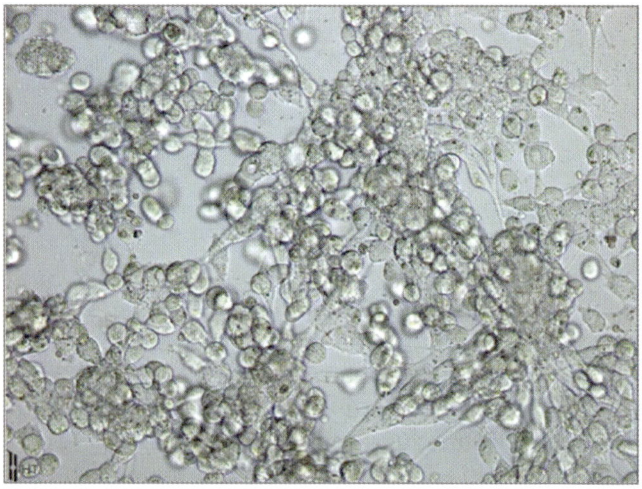

Fig. 4: Cumulus cells.

CO-CULTURE WITH FALLOPIAN TUBE EPITHELIAL CELLS

Fallopian tube cells were obtained according to Yeung et al. (6, from female who underwent tubal ligation during previous cycle of treatment) (Fig. 5).

- Samples were enzymatically treated with trypsin/EDTA solution and the cells were collected after centrifugation.
- Oviductal cells were cultured in culture media for 48 hours and frozen after confirming viability and infection.
- The patient then undergoes a regular IVF cycle in next month as per clinic protocol.
- On the day of hCG injection, frozen fallopian epithelial cells were thawed and cultured in single culture media contained 100 μL droplets.
- On the day of retrieval, ICSI done as per embryology laboratory protocol and injected oocytes were placed in droplets on cultured cell, which already growing.
- The embryos are closely supervised for development.
- The patient's embryos are transferred into her uterus under ultrasonography guidance for implantation and pregnancy.

Limitations

As autologous Fallopian tube cells are extremely difficult to obtain in humans and there are less data available for its beneficial effects, so these methods are no more in use for human assisted reproduction.

Co-culture of Donor human fallopian cells has been done in past and resulted in improvement of fertilization as well as implantation rate but risk of disease transmission will also be there.

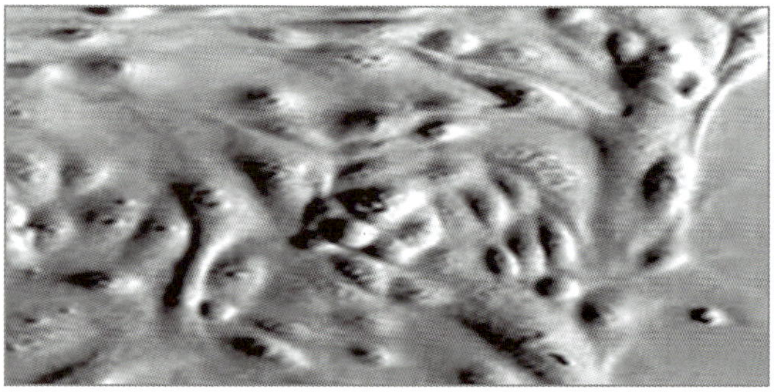

Fig. 5: Fallopian tube epithelial cells.

CONCLUSION

The co-culture of embryos should not be considered a first choice of fertility treatment as the method is still comparatively new with less data, so its potential long-term effects are not known.

Co-culture can be an effective treatment for indicated patients, who have poor embryo morphology in past cycle, failed previous IVF cycles, and male factor infertility.

Bongso et al. (1992) were able to demonstrate a positive effect using human oviduct cells for a group of patients with tubal, idiopathic, or male factor infertility who had failed at least two previous IVF attempts.

Instead of adding individual growth factors to improve standard culture condition, if we supplement standard culture medium with autologous cumulus cells then it mimics a physiological environment of uterus and fulfills the biological requirements of the developing embryo.

EDITORS' COMMENTS

1. Multiple co-culture techniques have been around in ART for a long time; various cell lines such as tubal, endometrial, etc. have been tried.
2. Autologous cumulus cells co-culture is technically easy and gives better results without any harm to embryos. It mimics the natural environment to the embryo.
3. Cumulus cells are discarded during the ICSI procedure and also it does not require any other extra surgical procedure to harvest it, as compared to other cells like endometrial and fallopian tubal cells.
4. It seems a good alternative instead of adding individual growth factors to the commercial media.

SUGGESTED READING

1. Anderson RA, Sciorio R, Kinnell H, et al. Cumulus gene expression as a predictor of human oocyte fertilisation, embryo development and competence to establish a pregnancy. Reproduction. 2009;138:629-37.
2. Barmat LI, Worrilow KC, Paynton BV. Growth factor expression by human oviduct and buffalo rat liver coculture cells. Fertil Steril. 1997;67(4):775-9.
3. Barnet DK, Bavister BD. What is the relationship between the metabolism of preimplantation embryos and their developmental competence? Molecular Reproduction and Development. 1996;43:378-83.
4. Benkhalifa M, Demirol A, Sari T, et al. Autologous embryo-cumulus cell co-culture and blastocyst transfer in repeated implantation failures: a collaborative prospective randomized study. Zygote. 2012;20(2):173-80.
5. Biggers JD. Thoughts on embryo culture conditions. Reprod Biomed Online. 2001;4:30-8.
6. Biggers JD, Gwatkin RBL, Brinster RL. Development of mouse embryos in organ culture of fallopian tubes on a chemically defined medium. Nature. 1962;194:747-9.
7. Bongso A, Fong CY, Ng SC, et al. Human embryonic behavior in a sequential human oviduct-endometrial coculture system. Fertil Steril. 1994;61:976-8.
8. Bongso A, Ng S, Fong C, et al. Improved pregnancy rate after transfer of embryos grown in human Fallopian tubal cell coculture. Fertil. Steril. 1992;58:569-74.
9. Bongso A, Ng SC, Sathananthan H, et al. Improved quality of human embryos when co-cultured with human ampullary cells. Hum Reprod. 1989;4:706-13.
10. Camous S, Heyman Y, Meziou W, et al. Cleavage beyond the block stage and survival after transfer of early bovine embryos cultured with trophoblastic vesicles. J Reprod Fertil. 1984;72:479-85.
11. Carrel D, Peterson C, Jones K, et al. A simplified coculture system using homologous, attached cumulus tissue results in improved human embryo morphology and pregnancy rates during in vitro fertilization, J Assist Reprod Genet. 1999;16:344-9.
12. Cross JC, Werb Z, Fisher SJ. Implantation and the placenta: key pieces of the development puzzle. Science. 1994;266(5190):1508-18.
13. De los Santos MJ, Mercader A, Frances A, et al. Role of endometrial factors in regulating secretion of components of the immunoreactive human embryonic interleukin-1 system during embryonic development. Biol Reprod. 1996;54(3): 563-74.
14. Desai N, Abdelhafez F, Bedaiwy MA, et al. Live births in poor prognosis IVF patients using a novel non-contact human endometrial co-culture system. Reprod Biomed Online. 2008;16(6):869-74.
15. Desai N, Goldfarb J. Co-cultured human embryos may be subjected to widely different microenvironments: pattern of growth factor/cytokine release by Vero cells during the co-culture interval. Hum Reprod. 1998;13:1600-5.
16. Desai NN, Goldfarb JM. Growth factor/cytokine secretion by a permanent human endometrial cell line with embryotrophic properties. J Assisted Reprod Genet. 1996;13(7):546-50.
17. Desai NN, Kennard EA, Kniss DA, et al. Novel human endometrial cell line promotes blastocyst development. Fertil Steril. 1994;61:760-6.
18. Drakakis P, Vlismas A, Partsinevelos G, et al. Gene expression of hormones and hormone receptors and growth factors and receptors in 8-cell human embryos and their role in early embryonic development. Hum Reprod. 2010;25(S1):i013-6.
19. Dunglison GF, Barlow DH, Sargent IL. Leukaemia inhibitory factor significantly enhances the blastocyst formation rates of human embryos cultured in serum-free medium. Hum Reprod. 1996;11(1):191-6.
20. Edwards RG, Purdy JM, Steptoe PC, et al. The growth of human preimplantation embryos in vitro. Am J Obstet Gynecol. 1981;141:408-16.
21. Edwards RG. Test-tube babies. Nature. 1981;293:25-6.
22. Freeman MR, Whitworth CM, Hill AH. Granulosa cell coculture enhances human embryo development and pregnancy rate following in vitro fertilization. Hum Reprod. 1995;10:408-14.
23. Freshney RI. Culture of animal cells. 4th edition. New York: Wiley-Liss; 2000.
24. Fukui Y, Mcgowan LT, James RW, et al. Factors affecting the in vitro development to blastocysts of bovine oocytes matured and fertilized in vitro. J Reprod Fertil. 1991;92(1):125-31.
25. Gardner DK, Lane M. Culture and selection of viable blastocysts: a feasible proposition for human IVF? Hum Repod Update. 1997;3:367-82.
26. Gardner DK, Lane M. Embryo culture systems. In: Trouson AO, Gardner DK (Eds). Handbook of in Vitro Fertilization, Second Edition. Boca Raton: CRC Press; 1999. pp. 205-64.
27. Gil PI, Guidobaldi HA, Teves ME, et al. Chemotactic response of frozen-thawed bovine spermatozoa towards follicular fluid. Anim Reprod Sci. 2008;108(1-2):236-46.
28. Kawamura K, Chen Y, Shu Y, et al. Promotion of human early embryonic development and blastocyst outgrowth in vitro using autocrine/paracrine growth factors. PloS One. 2012;7(11):e49328.

29. Kim D, Kim M, Kang H, et al. The supplementation of granulocyte-macrophage colony stimulating factor (GM-CSF) in culture medium improves the pregnancy rate in human ART programs. Fertil Steril. 2001;76(3:S1):S6.
30. Lighten AD, Moore GE, Winston RM, et al. Routine addition of human insulin-like growth factor-I ligand could benefit clinical in-vitro fertilization culture. Hum Reprod. 1998;13(11):3144-50.
31. Lin Y, Hwang J, Seow K, et al. Effects of growth factors and granulosa cell co-culture on in vitro maturation of oocytes. Reprod Biomed Online. 2009;19:165-70.
32. Loutradis D, John D, Kiessling AA. Hypoxanthine causes a 2- cell block in random-bred mouse embryos. Biol Reprod. 1987;37(2):311-6.
33. Magli MC, Gianaroli L, Ferraretti AP, et al. Human embryo coculture: results of randomized prospective study. Int J Fertil. 1995;40;254-9.
34. Mansour RT, Aboulghar MA, Serour GI, et al. Co-culture of human pronucleate oocytes with their cumulus cells. Hum Reprod. 1994;9:1727-9.
35. Markmann JF, Desai NM, Bassiri H, et al. Prolonged survival of class I deficient mouse islet allografts but not xenografts. Transplant Proc. 1994;26(2):748.
36. Martin KL, Barlow DH, Sargent IL. Heparin-binding epidermal growth factor significantly improves human blastocyst development and hatching in serum free medium. Hum Reprod. 1998;13(6):1645-52.
37. Menezo Y, Elder K. The enhancers of oocyte competence. In: Tosti E, Boni R (Eds). Oocyte maturation and fertilization: a long history for a short event. Sharjah: Bentham Science Publishers Ltd; 2011. pp. 64-70.
38. Menezo YJR, Guerin JF, Czyba JC. Improvement of human early embryo development in vitro by co-culture on monolayer of Vero cells. Biol Reprod. 1990;42:301-6.
39. O'Neill C. The role of PAF in embryo physiology. Hum Reprod Update. 2005;11(3):215-8.
40. Oren-Benaroya R, Orvieto R, Gakamsky A, et al. The sperm chemoattractant secreted from human cumulus cells is progesterone. Hum Reprod. 2008;23:2339-45.
41. Paria BC, Dey SK. Preimplantation embryo development in-vitro: cooperative interactions among embryos and role of growth factors. Proc Nat Acad Sci U S A. 1990;87(12):4756-60.
42. Parikh FR, Nadkarni SG, Naik NJ, et al. A novel way of enhancing pregnancy rates in ART cycles-cumulus co-culture and cumulus aided embryo transfer. Obstet Gynecol India. 2004;54:571-4.
43. Plachot M. Co-culture of embryos and feeder cells. Hum Reprod. 1996;11:35-42.
44. Quinn P, Kerin JF, Warnes GM. Improved pregnancy rate in human in vitro fertilization with the use of a medium based on the composition of human tubal fluid. Fertil Steril. 1985;44:493-8.
45. Richter KS, The importance of growth factors for preimplantation embryo development and in-vitro culture, Curr Opin Obstet Gynecol. 2008;20(3):292-304.
46. Roudebush WE, Massey JB, Kort HL, et al. Exposure of preimplantation embryos to platelet-activating factor increases birth rate. J Assist Reprod Genet. 2004;21:297-300.
47. Sakkas D, Jaquenoud N, Leppens G, et al. Comparison of results after in vitro fertilized human embryos are cultured in routine medium and in coculture on Vero cells: a randomized study. Fertil Steril. 1994;61:521-5.
48. Simon C, Gimeno MJ, Mercader A, et al. Embryonic regulation of integrins beta 3, alpha 4, and alpha 1 in human endometrial epithelial cells in-vitro. J Clin Endocrinol Metabol. 1997;82(8):2607-16.
49. Spandorfer SD, Navarro J, Levy D, et al. Autologous endometrial coculture in patients with in-vitro-fertilization (IVF) failure: correlations of outcome with leukemia inhibiting factor (LIF) production. Am J Reprod Immunol. 2001;46(6):375-80.
50. Spanos S, Becker DL, Winston RM, et al. Antiapoptotic action of insulin-like growth factor-I during human preimplantation embryo development. Biol Reprod. 2000;63:1413-20.
51. Tazuke SI, Giudice LC. Growth factors and cytokines in endometrium, embryonic development, and maternal: embryonic interactions. Semin Reprod Endocrinol. 1996;14(3):231-45.
52. Thibodeaux JK, Menezo Y, Roussel JD, et al. Coculture of in-vitro fertilized bovine embryos with oviductal epithelial cells originating from different stages of the estrous cycle. J Dairy Sci. 1992;75(6):1448-55.
53. Thouas GA, Dominiquez F, Green MP, et al. Review: soluble ligands and their receptors in human embryo development and implantation. Endocr Rev. 2015;36(1);92-130.
54. Vithoulkas A, Goudas VT, Levanduski M, et al. Embryo co-culture with autologous granulosa cell clusters in comparison to regular embryo culture in ART. Fertil Steril. 2011;96(S3):S59.
55. Vithoulkas A, Goudas VT, Levanduski M, et al. Growth factors associated with embryo co-culture and autologous granulosa cell clusters compared to regular embryo culture in IVF. Fertil. Steril. 2014;102(S3):e218.
56. Vithoulkas A, Goudas VT, Levanduski M, et al. Growth factors IGF-I and IGF-II in human embryo co-culture with autologous granulosa cell clusters compared to regular embryo culture in IVF. Fertil Steril. 2016;106(S3):e362.
57. Wiemer KE, Cohen J, Amborski GF, et al: In-vitro development and implantation of human embryos following culture on fetal uterine fibroblast cells. Hum Reprod. 1989;4:595-600.
58. Wiemer KE, Cohen J, Wiker SR, et al. Co-culture of human zygotes on fetal bovine uterine fibroblasts: Embryonic morphology and implantation. Fertil Steril 1989;52:503-8.
59. Wiemer KE, Hoffman DI, Maxson WS, et al. Embryonic morphology and rate of implantation of human embryos following co-culture on bovine oviductal epithelial cells. Hum Reprod. 1993;8:97-101.
60. Yeung WSB, Ho PC, Lau EYL, et al. Improved development of human embryos in vitro by a human oviductal cell coculture system. Hum Reprod. 1992;7:1144-9.
61. Zetova L, Mardesic T, Mikova M, et al. Improved development of human embryos cultured on a Vero cell monolayer. J Assist Reprod Genet. 1993;10:234-6.
62. Ziebe S, Loft A, Povlsen BB, et al. A randomized clinical trial to evaluate the effect of granulocyte-macrophage colony-stimulating factor (GM-CSF) in embryo culture medium for in vitro fertilization. Fertil Steril. 2013;99(6):1600-9.

41

CHAPTER

Oocyte Activation

Takashi Yamaguchi, Keiji Kuroda, Masahiko Ito, Atsushi Tanaka

INTRODUCTION

After ovulation, meiosis is arrested at the second meiotic metaphase in mammalian mature oocytes that are surrounded by zona pellucida and cumulus cells. Sperms approach the egg, bind, and penetrate the zona pellucida. The membrane of the sperm and the ovum are fused, leading to the integration of the sperm nucleus in the egg cytoplasm. The sperm entry stimulates calcium ions (Ca^{2+}) increase resulting in cortical reaction and meiosis reinitiation. In mature oocytes, the contents in cortical granules laid right under the plasma membrane are secreted to the perivitelline space upon the cortical reaction of the granule-oocyte membrane fusion. Zona pellucida glycoprotein is modified by the proteinases and ovoperoxidase, which presents in the released contents, resulting in the protein denaturation. This is why the sperm binding and penetration of the zona pellucida are disturbed. In addition, sperm receptors on the cell membrane of the egg are also altered. Collectively, other sperms are not allowed to fuse with the egg, resulting in prevention of multisperm fertilization.

Fertilization is not successful when the fertilization ability of the oocytes or sperms is impaired. Intracytoplasmic sperm injection (ICSI) method has contributed remarkably to the improvement of fertilization rates; however, many couples cannot obtain fertilized eggs even with the use of ICSI. In some infertile couples, the fertilization rate is 25% or less in eggs that appear to be morphologically normal. For the treatment of such cases, the artificial activation of the eggs is one of the possible solutions. We present here the efficacy of various oocyte activation procedures from the cytological (embryogenesis) and biochemical (intracellular Ca^{2+} responses) perspectives.

FERTILIZATION AND OOCYTE ACTIVATION

Sperm penetration triggers a rise of Ca^{2+} concentration in the egg at the point of sperm fusion, leading to the spreading of a Ca^{2+} wave across the entire egg. Transient Ca^{2+} rises (Ca^{2+} spikes) are repeated and continue until pronuclei formation (Ca^{2+} oscillations). As shown in Figure 1C, during the ICSI procedure, a series of Ca^{2+} oscillations is also induced, however, the Ca^{2+} wave starts at the site of sperm injection and propagates radially in the egg. Ca^{2+} oscillations are required for the resumption and completion of the meiosis, known as oocyte activation, including the dyad chromosome separation process (the second meiotic anaphase), extrusion of the second polar body, and the male and female pronuclei formation, leading to cleavage of the embryo. Ca^{2+} ions are released from the endoplasmic reticulum through inositol 1,4,5-trisphosphate (IP3) receptors into nucleoplasm. The initiator of Ca^{2+} oscillations is a cytosolic sperm factor, secreted at the site of sperm-egg fusion. A strong candidate sperm factor is a sperm-specific IP3-producing enzyme, phospholipase C zeta (PLCζ). The reasons that support this theory are as follows:

- Sperm extract immune-precipitated with anti-PLCζ antibody treatment suppressed the Ca^{2+} release completely in the eggs.
- Injection of PLCζ RNA induced Ca^{2+} oscillations that closely resemble those at fertilization, leading to the development into blastocysts parthenogenetically.

- Injection of recombinant PLCζ protein could also elicit Ca^{2+} oscillations in the oocytes.
- Transgenic PLCζ knockdown mice demonstrated decreased ability of oocyte activation with impaired Ca^{2+} oscillation and inability to conceive.

FERTILIZATION FAILURE

Oocyte penetration by human sperm requires motility, capacitation, and acrosome reaction during *in vivo* fertilization, but not ICSI. The success of the fertilization can be recognized with the extrusion of the second polar body and formation of male and female pronuclei, even if the azoospermia cases of round spermatid cell and immature spermatogenic cell injection can be performed. The risk factors of the fertility impairment can be classified into cases derived from the gametes themselves and the circumstance surrounding the gametes *in vivo*. The former concerns the quality and quantity of gametes, and the latter is related to problems in the internal circumstance of the female reproductive tract. Common problems that affect sperm fertility are spermatogenesis, spermiogenesis, conditions of the female reproductive tract, chemical composition in the tubal fluid surrounding oocyte-cumulus complex, the interaction with the zona pellucida, membrane fusion, and egg activation. On the other side, egg fertility is influenced by egg reserve, oogenesis, egg nuclear and cytoplasmic maturation, the nature of the zona pellucida, and membrane fusion. The ability of the egg to activate itself (to resume the second meiosis and cooperate with the penetrating sperm) as well as the process leading to nuclear fusion also affects egg fertility.

We performed an analysis of the potential causes why the oocytes fail to form pronuclei after ICSI. As for the sperm, the lack of the sperm factor, which initiates the egg activation, appears to be responsible for this phenomenon. On the egg side, the lack of egg activation by the Ca^{2+} signaling, which is induced by the sperm factor, is the main cause.

TREATMENT OF FERTILIZATION FAILURE

Intracytoplasmic Sperm Injection

Intracytoplasmic sperm injection is the most useful treatment to overcome severe male factors infertility (asthenozoospermia or oligozoospermia) and fertilization failure with conventional *in vitro* fertilization. The exact causes of fertilization failure after ICSI are debatable.

Nowadays, fertilization rates after ICSI are high, roughly 70–80%. Yet, fertilized eggs are not recognized in 1–5% of ICSI cycles, as in oocyte fertilization failure.

Assisted Oocyte Activation

In most cases of fertilization failure after conventional *in vitro* fertilization, ICSI can solve it, yet fertilization failure is recognized in 1–5% of ICSI oocytes. Our previous report showed that the main reason of fertilization failure after ICSI was impaired oocyte activation. Assisted oocyte activation (AOA) can induce cellular Ca^{2+} increase in the eggs. AOA is a beneficial treatment for couples with a history of fertilization failure following ICSI. AOA includes mechanical, electrical and chemical stimulations (Table 1). The popular AOA agents, which are clinically used for human eggs, are calcium ionophores and electrical pulses; however, a standard AOA has not been established yet. Abnormal form or dysfunction of PLCζ is involved in egg activation failure, therefore PLCζ is a key enzyme for treatment of severe fertilization deficiency. The efficiency of each AOA procedure for human oocyte activation including human PLCζ (hPLCZ1) RNA injection is reviewed.

Mechanical Activation

In 2002, mechanical egg activation was reported by Tesarik et al. as modified ICSI. This modified ICSI consists of the aspiration of ooplasm from the oocyte periphery and reinjection into the center of the oocyte two or three times.

TABLE 1 Assisted oocyte activation.

Assisted oocyte activation	*Procedure*
Mechanical activation (cytosolic aspiration and injection)	Tesarik J et al. 1994
Electrical stimulation	Yanagida K et al. 1997
Chemical activation:	
• Strontium chloride	Kishikawa H et al. 1999
• 6-Dimethylaminopurine	Szöllösi MS et al. 1993
• Phorbol esters	Cuthbertson Cobbold KS and PH, 1985
• Thimerosal	Fissore RA et al. 1995
• Calcium ionophore (A23187)	Steinhardt RA et al. 1974, Tesarik J et al. 1994, Eldar-Geva T et al. 2003
• Calcium ionophore and puromycin	Murase Y et al. 2004
• Calcium ionophore and ionomycin	Vanden Meerschaut et al. 2014
PLCζ[1]	K Swann et al. 2013, Nomikos M and Kashir J et al. 2017 Yamaguchi T et al. 2017

[1] No report of human birth

Yet, these findings have not been reproduced, thus it has not spread around the world as an AOA procedure. We demonstrated that modified ICSI induced only a small single Ca^{2+} rise (Fig. 1A).

Chemical Activation

Many chemical agents are applicable for AOA including strontium chloride, puromycin, 6-DMAP, phorbol esters, thimerosal, and calcium ionophore. Ionomycin and calcimycin (A23187) in calcium ionophores have been widely used as AOA agents in clinical practice. Calcium ionophores can convey Ca^{2+} from outside to inside oocytes to induce an influx of Ca^{2+} when they go through the plasma membrane. Although, the mechanism of egg activation by calcium ionophores is still unclear, several reviews have concluded that calcium ionophores raise the fertilization and cleavage rates in couples with reported fertilization deficiency in ICSI procedure. Montag et al. analyzed the benefit of calcium ionophore in couples with a history of fertilization failure. They found an increase of fertilization rate after continuous ICSI and AOA with calcium ionophore compared with the rate after ICSI in the patients with low (<30%) fertilization rate after ICSI treatment (0–41.6% in patients with reported fertilization failure and 19.3–44.4% in patients with low (1–29%) fertilization rates). In our previous experiments, AOA using calcium ionophore brought one long-lasting Ca^{2+} rise in the eggs (Fig. 1B). Calcium ionophores are easy to use, however, the pattern of cellular Ca^{2+} increase was different from physiological Ca^{2+} oscillations.

Electrical Activation

Electrical oocyte activation was reported as piezoelectric ICSI by Yanagida et al. in 1999. Electrical pulses can make micropores in the surface of eggs, and induce Ca^{2+} influx, leading to oocyte activation. Baltaci et al. reported the effectiveness of electric activation for the cases with a history of fertilization deficiency using a BTX Electro-cell manipulator with single pulse of 1.5 kV/cm DC for 100 µs for 20 min after ICSI procedure. Fertilization rate after ICSI with electrical pulses was 62% and significantly higher compared with that following ICSI only in fertilization failure cases (62% and 12%, respectively, p <0.001). In our previous research, human eggs were stimulated with a single electrical pulse of 1.2 kV/cm DC for 99 µs. Figure 1D demonstrated cellular Ca^{2+} responses in human eggs following an electrical pulse. Some oocytes Ca^{2+} spikes were triggered; however, they differed from Ca^{2+} oscillations after ICSI in terms of duration and frequency of spikes of Ca^{2+} oscillations.

PLCZ1 mRNA Injection

The hPLCZ1 RNA injection has a potential for clinical application as an egg-activating agent. We injected hPLCZ1 RNA (100 ng/µL) into eggs and measured fluorescent intensity using fluorescence microscopy (Fig. 1E). First Ca^{2+} spike was observed 23.6 min after hPLCZ1 RNA injection, followed by repetitive transient spikes. The Ca^{2+} oscillations pattern caused by hPLCZ1 RNA was very similar to the one found in the eggs after sperm injection. We found that Ca^{2+} oscillations by hPLCZ1 are similar to natural oscillations, but not exactly the same. We also found the appropriate concentration of hPLCZ1 RNA for induction of optimal Ca^{2+} oscillations pattern in human eggs. In patients who experienced fertilization failure after ICSI, ICSI-AOA may restore the fertilization rate especially in the case of displaying abnormal Ca^{2+} oscillation pattern in ICSI. hPLCZ1 RNA injection has a possibility as a more effective treatment to induce natural Ca^{2+} oscillations and oocyte activation in the patients with a history of low or failed fertilization.

CONCLUSION

The main cause of fertilization failure after ICSI is egg activation failure. Conventional AOA procedures and agents are possible solutions for severe fertilization failure; however, they cannot induce the pattern of physiological Ca^{2+} increases observed at normal fertilization and may have potential cytotoxicity or mutagenicity on eggs and embryos. In contrast, use of hPLCZ1 RNA can render the optimal and physiological Ca^{2+} oscillations, resulting in the parthenogenetic blastocyst formation. Although hPLCZ1 RNA seems to be ideal for parthenogenetic egg activation, safety of RNA injection into human eggs is still unknown. So far, hPLCZ1 RNA has a potential for clinical application as an AOA. Further studies of the genomic and epigenetic effect of PLCZ1 RNA injection on human eggs and babies are required.

EDITORS' COMMENTS

1. Though the concept of oocyte activation seems promising, it has not lived up to its expectations. Its major indications are severe male factor, POR, higher age patients, and prior fertilization failure.
2. Calcium tonophore seems the most feasible applicable technique for oocyte activation these days.
3. Electrical activation has shown most promising results. Puromycin, ionomycin, and various other activation have been tried till date, with postphospholipase zeta is becoming the new technique on the block.

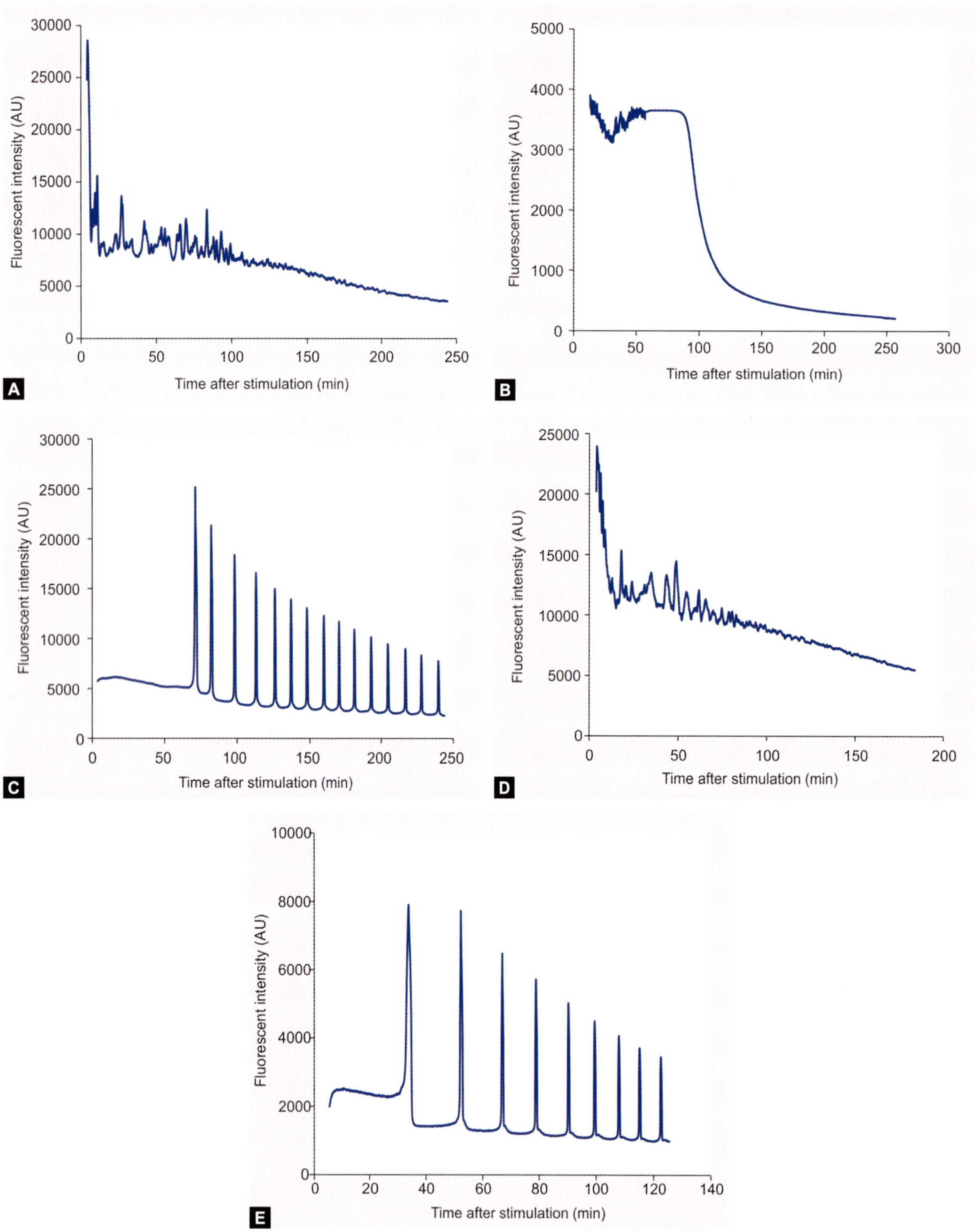

Figs. 1A to E: Induction of Ca^{2+} responses in human eggs by various artificial oocyte activation agents and procedures. (A) Ca^{2+} responses in human eggs induced by mechanical activation with a procedure of cytosolic aspiration and reinjection; (B) ionomycin treatment; (C) ICSI; (D) electrical stimulation; (E) and human PLCZ1 (hPLCZ1) RNA injection (100 ng/µL). The time of stimulation was set as the zero time.

SUGGESTED READING

1. Baltaci V, Ayvaz OU, Unsal E, et al. The effectiveness of intracytoplasmic sperm injection combined with piezo-electric stimulation in infertile couples with total fertilization failure. Fertil Steril. 2010;94(3):900-4.
2. Cox LJ, Larman MG, Saunders CM, et al. Sperm phospholipase Czeta from humans and cynomolgus monkeys triggers Ca^{2+} oscillations, activation and development of mouse oocytes. Reproduction. 2002;124(5):611-23.
3. Cuthbertson KS, Cobbold PH. Phorbol ester and sperm activate mouse oocytes by inducing sustained oscillations in cell $Ca2^{+}$. Nature. 1985;316(6028):541-2.
4. Ferrer-Buitrago, M Dhaenens L, Lu Y, et al. Human oocyte calcium analysis predicts the response to assisted oocyte activation in patients experiencing fertilization failure after ICSI. Hum Reprod, 2018;33(3):416-25.
5. Fissore RA, Pinto-Correia C, Robl JM. Inositol trisphosphate-induced calcium release in the generation of calcium oscillations in bovine eggs. Biol Reprod. 1995;53(4):766-74.
6. Heytens E, Parrington J, Coward K, et al. Reduced amounts and abnormal forms of phospholipase C zeta (PLCzeta) in spermatozoa from infertile men. Hum Reprod. 2009; 24(10):2417-28.
7. Kashir J, Jones C, Lee HC, et al. Loss of activity mutations in phospholipase C zeta (PLCzeta) abolishes calcium oscillatory ability of human recombinant protein in mouse oocytes. Hum Reprod. 2011;26(12):3372-87.
8. Kimura Y, Yanagimachi R. Intracytoplasmic sperm injection in the mouse. Biol Reprod. 1995;52(4):709-20.
9. Kishikawa H, Wakayama T, Yanagimachi R. Comparison of oocyte-activating agents for mouse cloning. Cloning. 1999;1(3):153-9.
10. Knott JG, Kurokawa M, Fissore RA, et al. Transgenic RNA interference reveals role for mouse sperm phospholipase Czeta in triggering Ca^{2+} oscillations during fertilization. Biol Reprod. 2005;72(4):992-6.
11. Kouchi Z, Fukami K, Shikano T, et al. Recombinant phospholipase Czeta has high Ca^{2+} sensitivity and induces Ca^{2+} oscillations in mouse eggs. J Biol Chem. 2004;279(11): 10408-12.
12. Kuroda K, Ito M, Shikano T, et al. The role of X/Y linker region and N-terminal EF-hand domain in nuclear translocation and Ca^{2+} oscillation-inducing activities of phospholipase Czeta, a mammalian egg-activating factor. J Biol Chemi. 2006;281(38):27794-805.
13. Li LJ, Zhang FB, Liu SY, et al. Human sperm devoid of germinal angiotensin-converting enzyme is responsible for total fertilization failure and lower fertilization rates by conventional in vitro fertilization. Biol Reprod. 2014;90(6):125.
14. Mangoli V, Dandekar S, Desai S, et al. The outcome of ART in males with impaired spermatogenesis. J Hum Reprod Sci. 2008;1(2):73-6.
15. Masui Y. From oocyte maturation to the in vitro cell cycle: the history of discoveries of Maturation-Promoting Factor (MPF) and Cytostatic Factor (CSF). Differentiation. 2001;69(1):1-17.
16. Miyazaki S, Ito M. Calcium signals for egg activation in mammals. J Pharmacol Sci. 2006;100(5):545-52.
17. Miyazaki S, Shirakawa H, Nakada K, et al. Essential role of the inositol 1,4,5-trisphosphate receptor/Ca^{2+} release channel in Ca^{2+} waves and Ca^{2+} oscillations at fertilization of mammalian eggs. Dev Biol. 1993;158(1):62-78.
18. Montag M, Koster M, van der Ven K, et al. The benefit of artificial oocyte activation is dependent on the fertilization rate in a previous treatment cycle. Reprod Biomed Online. 2012;24(5):521-6.
19. Murase Y, Araki Y, Mizuno S, et al. Pregnancy following chemical activation of oocytes in a couple with repeated failure of fertilization using ICSI: case report. Hum Reprod. 2004;19(7):1604-7.
20. Nakano Y, Shirakawa H, Mitsuhashi N, et al. Spatiotemporal dynamics of intracellular calcium in the mouse egg injected with a spermatozoon. Mol Hum Reprod. 1997;3(12):1087-93.
21. Nasr-Esfahani MH, Deemeh MR, Tavalaee M. Artificial oocyte activation and intracytoplasmic sperm injection. Fertil Steril. 2010;94(2):520-6.
22. Nomikos M, Kashir J, Swann K, et al. Sperm PLCzeta: from structure to Ca^{2+} oscillations, egg activation and therapeutic potential. FEBS Lett. 2013;587(22):3609-16.
23. Rankin TL, Coleman JS, Epifano O, et al. Fertility and taxon-specific sperm binding persist after replacement of mouse sperm receptors with human homologs. Dev Cell. 2003;5(1):33-43.
24. Rogers NT, Hobson E, Pickering S, et al. Phospholipase Czeta causes Ca^{2+} oscillations and parthenogenetic activation of human oocytes. Reproduction. 2004;128(6):697-702.
25. Ross PJ, Beyhan Z, Iager AE, et al. Parthenogenetic activation of bovine oocytes using bovine and murine phospholipase C zeta. BMC Dev Biol. 2008;8:16.
26. Sanusi R, Yu Y, Nomikos M, et al. Rescue of failed oocyte activation after ICSI in a mouse model of male factor infertility by recombinant phospholipase Czeta. Mol Hum Reprod. 2015;21(10):783-91.
27. Sasagawa I, Kuretake S, Eppig JJ, et al. Mouse primary spermatocytes can complete two meiotic divisions within the oocyte cytoplasm. Biol Reprod. 1998;58(1):248-54.
28. Saunders CM, Larman MG, Parrington J, et al. PLC zeta: a sperm-specific trigger of $Ca^{(2+)}$ oscillations in eggs and embryo development. Development. 2002;129(15):3533-44.
29. Sfontouris IA, Nastri CO, Lima ML, et al. Artificial oocyte activation to improve reproductive outcomes in women with previous fertilization failure: a systematic review and meta-analysis of RCTs. Hum Reprod. 2015;30(8):1831-41.
30. Shirakawa H, Kikuchi T, Ito M. Calcium Signaling in Mammalian Eggs at Fertilization. Curr Top Med Chem. 2016;16(24):2664-76.

31. Steinhardt RA, Epel D. Activation of sea-urchin eggs by a calcium ionophore. Proc Natl Acad Sci U S A. 1974;71(5): 1915-9.
32. Stricker SA. Comparative biology of calcium signaling during fertilization and egg activation in animals. Dev Biol. 1999;211(2):157-76.
33. Swann K, Ozil JP. Dynamics of the calcium signal that triggers mammalian egg activation. Int Rev Cytol. 1994;152:183-222.
34. Swann K, Saunders CM, Rogers NT, et al. PLCzeta(zeta): a sperm protein that triggers Ca^{2+} oscillations and egg activation in mammals. Semin Cell Dev Biol. 2006;17(2):264-73.
35. Szollosi MS, Kubiak JZ, Debey P, et al. Inhibition of protein kinases by 6-dimethylaminopurine accelerates the transition to interphase in activated mouse oocytes. J Cell Sci. 1993;104(Pt 3):861-72.
36. Tanaka A, Nagayoshi M, Takemoto Y, et al. Fourteen babies born after round spermatid injection into human oocytes. Proc Natl Acad Sci U S A. 2015;112(47):14629-34.
37. Tesarik J, Mendoza C. Spermatid injection into human oocytes. I. Laboratory techniques and special features of zygote development. Hum Reprod. 1996;11(4):772-9.
38. Van der Westerlaken L, Helmerhorst F, Dieben S, et al. Intracytoplasmic sperm injection as a treatment for unexplained total fertilization failure or low fertilization after conventional in vitro fertilization. Fertil Steril. 2005;83(3): 612-7.
39. Yamaguchi T, Ito M, Kuroda K, et al. The establishment of appropriate methods for egg-activation by human PLCZ1 RNA injection into human oocyte. Cell Calcium. 2017;65: 22-30.
40. Yamaguchi T, Kuroda K, Tanaka A, Watanabe S. Fertilization Failure. In: Kuroda K, Brosens JJ, Quenby S, Takeda S (Eds). Treatment Strategy for Unexplained Infertility and Recurrent Miscarriage. Singapore: Springer Singapore; 2018. pp. 7-17.
41. Yanagida K, Katayose H, Yazawa H, et al. The usefulness of a piezo-micromanipulator in intracytoplasmic sperm injection in humans. Hum Reprod. 1999;14(2):448-53.
42. Yanagida K, Morozumi K, Katayose H, et al. Successful pregnancy after ICSI with strontium oocyte activation in low rates of fertilization. Reprod Biomed Online. 2006;13(6): 801-6.
43. Yoon SY, Jellerette T, Salicioni AM, et al. Human sperm devoid of PLC, zeta 1 fail to induce $Ca^{(2+)}$ release and are unable to initiate the first step of embryo development. J Clin Invest. 2008;118(11):3671-81.

42

CHAPTER

Triple Parenting

Harsha Bhadarka, Arpita Patel

INTRODUCTION

Louise Joy Brown was the first baby born through *in vitro* fertilization (IVF) treatment on July 25th 1978 in England. According to the International Committee for Monitoring of Assisted Reproductive Technology (ICMART) 2017, after this major outbreak in the world of reproductive biology, approximately 5 million babies have been born with the use of same technique. Also many advancements have taken place in assisted reproductive technology (ART) such as improvement in fertility drugs, techniques of egg retrieval, intracytoplasmic sperm injection (ICSI), laser assisted hatching (LAH), and methods of embryo transfers have changed, time-lapse imaging has been introduced for better selection of embryo, preimplantation genetic diagnosis (PGD) and preimplantation genetic screening (PGS) techniques give safer and accurate prediction of the genetic makeup of an embryo, cryopreservation of egg and embryo has improved but still the fertilization and implantation rates are not satisfactory.

Newer technologies along with advanced treatment will ultimately enhance the success rates for IVF cycle. One of such techniques involves mitochondrial transfer or triple parenting.

Triple Parenting: Triple parenting is a procedure in which unhealthy mitochondrial DNA (mtDNA) from mother's egg is manipulated or replaced with a healthy mtDNA from a donor woman. A child resulted from such technique has almost all DNA from his mother and father, only small amount of mtDNA comes from donor. Majority of our genes (20,000) are present in nucleus whereas only 37 genes are present in mitochondria. Thus, the embryo resulted will contain nuclear DNA from parents and majority of mtDNA from donor. So, it is termed as *triple parenting.*

By the use of such technique, we are able to reduce transmission of mutant or unhealthy mtDNA into next progeny.

Mitochondria are present in the cytoplasm of a cell, which are known as powerhouses of a cell because they are responsible for production of the majority of adenosine triphosphate (ATP). During embryonic development, ATP imparts an important role. Proteins that are involved in production of ATP are encoded by genes which are present in nucleus as well as in mitochondria that requires coordination between nuclear and mitochondrial genomes, which is important for survival of the cell. If ATP production is affected, organs such as heart, brain, liver, central nervous system, which require high energy, are also affected. In tissues, if cells have identical mtDNA, it is known as homoplasmy. But if cells have mixed types of mtDNA, which is rare, it is known as heteroplasmy. During natural fertilization, different mechanisms result into heteroplasmy.

Mitochondrial inheritance is strictly maternal which means if a woman has disease caused by mutations in mtDNA then she will inherit these mutations to her future children. In order to treat this, mitochondrial transfer techniques are good option.

INDICATIONS

Mitochondrial DNA Disease

Assisted reproduction technology offers an opportunity to females having increased chances of inheriting mtDNA disease in next generation. These opportunities include PGD or to opt for donor oocytes. However, both options have their pros and cons.

Preimplantation genetic diagnosis is comparatively unsuccessful in reporting mtDNA mutations. PGD does not offer any remedial solutions, as it only gives diagnostic result of mutations. On an average out of 200, every single child is victim of mitochondrial diseases. Most of them show only mild signs. In some cases, it leads severe medical conditions which are around one in 6,500. Mitochondrial disorders are noncurable.

Advanced Maternal Age or Age-related Infertility

Nowadays, the most common thing in infertility is, women are delaying childbirth beyond 35 years which ultimately leads to high reactive oxygen species (ROS) at cellular levels in body. High ROS levels reduce metabolic function and energy production. The relation between age, high ROS levels and metabolic decline was evidenced many years ago.

Age-related ROS leads to unceasing buildup of mutations which impacts the potentiality of the mtDNA disease, DNA genome to replicate. Therefore, patients with higher age show dysfunction which initiates with molecular level to cell, tissue and lastly it affects organ.

Female reproductive physiology is not as per cultural and social inclinations which result in infertility related to age; ultimately it leads to fetal abnormality and aneuploidy.

Diabetic Patients

Patients with history of diabetes generally have elevated level of oxidative stress that affects mitochondrial ultrastructure, rises mtDNA copy number and decreases ATP levels and metabolism of tricarboxylic acid (TCA) cycle.

The increase in number of mtDNA copy is astounding which shows that diabetic mother may play a role in stimulation of mitochondrial biogenesis or she may obstruct the oocyte degradation.

Studies in mice with diabetes have shown that oocytes which are ovulated give high frequency of aneuploidies, which are supposed to be result of meiotic spindle defects and misalignment of chromosome in the process of meiotic cell division. It is reported by many researchers that abnormal development of oocytes is result of toxic environment due to diabetic conditions as it is supposed to activate mitochondrial defects. The association between dysfunction in mitochondria and resistance in insulin shows that offsprings developed from oocytes with defective mitochondria are prone to preaccumulated obesity and insulin resistance.

So, in this manner, it is shown that abnormal mitochondrial metabolism is responsible for transmission of intergenerational metabolic disorders.

PREVENTION IN NEXT GENERATION

There are many ways for such women to have child. Some of the ways are either they can go for adoption or else have treatment like IVF cycle with donated eggs given by healthy egg donor. By this way, the resulting child does not have DNA from mother. Those women with desire to have their own genetical child, options like IVF with PGD in embryos, by which mitochondrial mutations can be known or if during pregnancy parents want to know about their fetus whether it is normal or affected then they have chorionic villus sampling (CVS) test at 10–12 weeks of pregnancy, or amniocentesis test during 14–20 weeks of pregnancy. Mitochondrial diseases can be known in both test, but disadvantage of this technique is that they may lead to lower risk of miscarriage. If substantial mutations are there in mitochondria of all eggs then these test are not useful at all.

Mitochondrial transfer offers patients one of the best advanced options to stop mtDNA disease to be transmitted into their next generation through ART.

The practice of mitochondrial transfer as ART procedure is near to realism. In this chapter, we have furnished summary of mitochondrial transfer techniques.

Procedures which prevent mitochondrial diseases:
There are mainly four kind of mitochondrial transfer techniques:
1. Ooplasmic transfer (cytoplasmic transfer)
2. Pronuclear transfer
3. Spindle transfer
4. Blastomere transfer.

Ooplasmic Transfer (Cytoplasmic Transfer) (Fig. 1)

The main reason for failure in assisted reproduction with higher aged female is ooplasmic deficiencies due to increase in chromosomal abnormalities as women grows older. It is common to see autosomal trisomy in pregnant women older than 40 years and that is mainly due to predivision of chromosomes.

Basically, in cytoplasmic transfer, fertile egg donor donates cytoplasm which is used by women having faulty eggs. It is very good option for the ones who are having advanced maternal age due to less functionality of their eggs. It is also useful for patients with history of unexplained infertility at young age and repeated implantation failure. Patients who are suffering from mitochondrial disease can be beneficial with this technique.

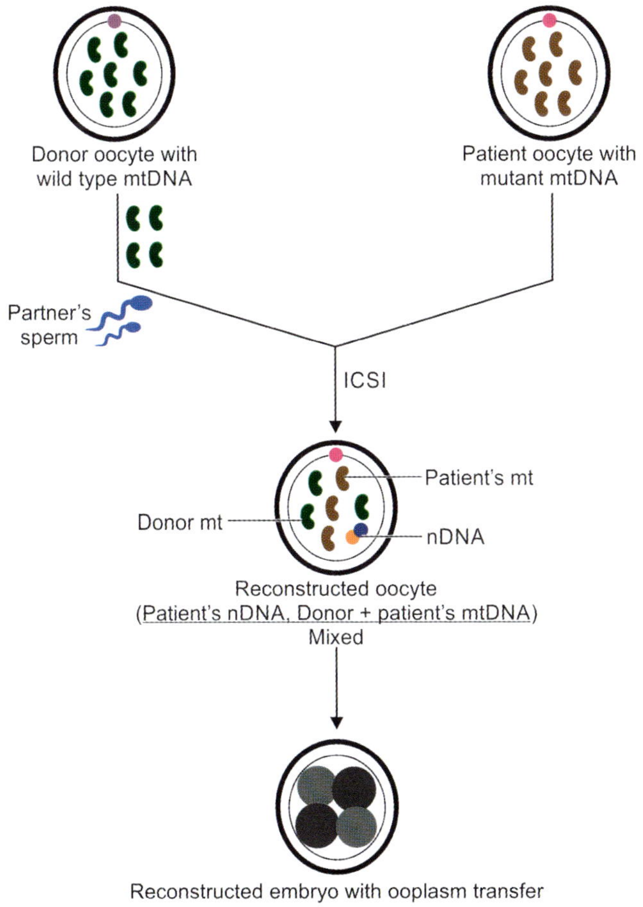

Fig. 1: Ooplasmic transfer or cytoplasmic transfer. (mt: mitochondria; mtDNA: mitochondrial DNA; ICSI: intracytoplasmic sperm injection)

Ooplasm plays important role in oocyte activation and maturation from germinal vesicle to MII phase. Ooplasmic regulators regulate the activity of ooplasmic events. Cohen et al. announced human pregnancy in 1997 using donor ooplasm transfer into patient's oocyte. Till date about 30 healthy babies are born worldwide.

Procedure

- In ooplasm transfer, stimulation is done in such a way that both, donor and patient's egg are retrieved on same day or frozen eggs of donor can be used.
- After eggs are retrieved, denudation with hyaluronidase is done followed by ICSI as per protocol of IVF laboratory.
- During ICSI procedure, a sperm is immobilized and it is aspirated with some amount (approximately 15–17%) of ooplasm from donor oocytes in injecting needle by avoiding suction of spindle.
- The affected oocyte is injected with the healthy ooplasm and spermatozoa by mixing properly, with gentle suction in injecting needle, of donor and recipient cytoplasm.
- Care should be taken to avoid leakage of cytoplasm and damage from the injection area of the oocyte.

Advantage

For patients having history of recurrent IVF failure, fertilization failure or bad quality embryo, this procedure improves quality of embryo.

Limitations

- Ooplasmic transfer requires compulsory oocyte denudation followed by ICSI.
- It is believed that in this technique small quantity (approximately 15%) of ooplasm transferred may not overcome mutant mtDNA of recipient's oocyte.
- Moreover, it is still a question to transfer more volume of ooplasm in recipient oocyte as it may have its side effects.
- It is shown in various studies that after ooplasm transfer chances of chromosomal anomalies and birth defects increase which creates doubt for its clinical application.
- In this technique, mtDNA heteroplasmy in the new born may result into ethical issues.
- For all these reasons, this technique has not been the primary focus of research for the prevention of mtDNA disease.
- It is also evident that no major impact of mtDNA on the child from donor has been reported yet.

Pronuclear Transfer (Fig. 2)

The first child born using this technique is a baby boy of a Jordanian couple in which mother was carrier of Leigh syndrome, which is found in her mitochondria. Due to this condition, they have lost two children. As mitochondrial inheritance is maternal, mother passes genes for this disease to her child. So, to reduce chances of passing those affected mtDNA, John Zhang along with his colleagues performed a new technique, which involves fertilizing both the mother's egg and a donor egg with the partner's sperm. At pronuclear stage, the nucleus from the donor's fertilized oocyte is discarded and replaced by nucleus from the mother's fertilized oocyte. Hence, now resultant embryo has healthy mtDNA from the donor and nuclear DNA from parents. This procedure is known as pronuclear transfer.

Procedure

- Pronuclear transfer includes the transferring pronucleus from one zygote to another.
- This technique involves fertilization of donor egg/s having healthy mitochondria with the intending male parent sperm.

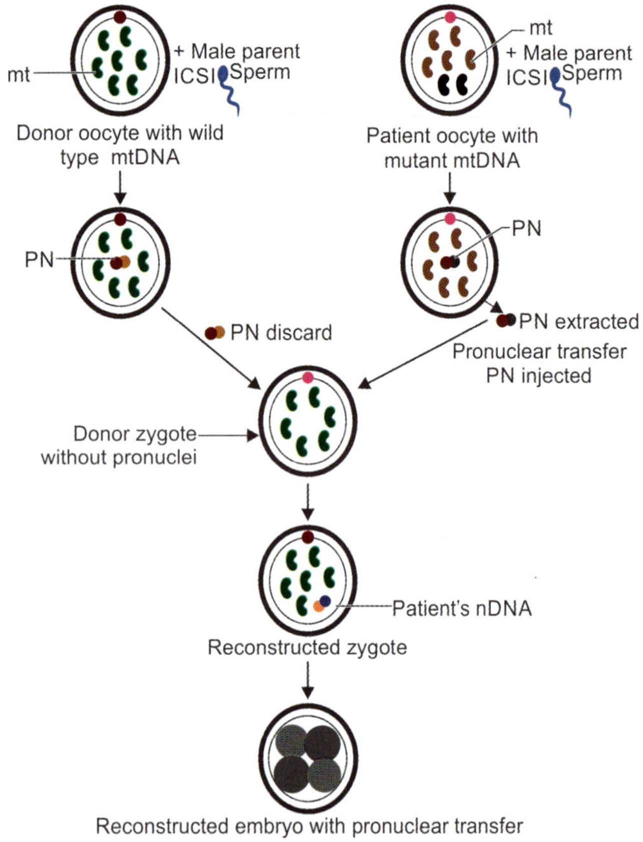

Fig. 2: Pronuclear transfer.

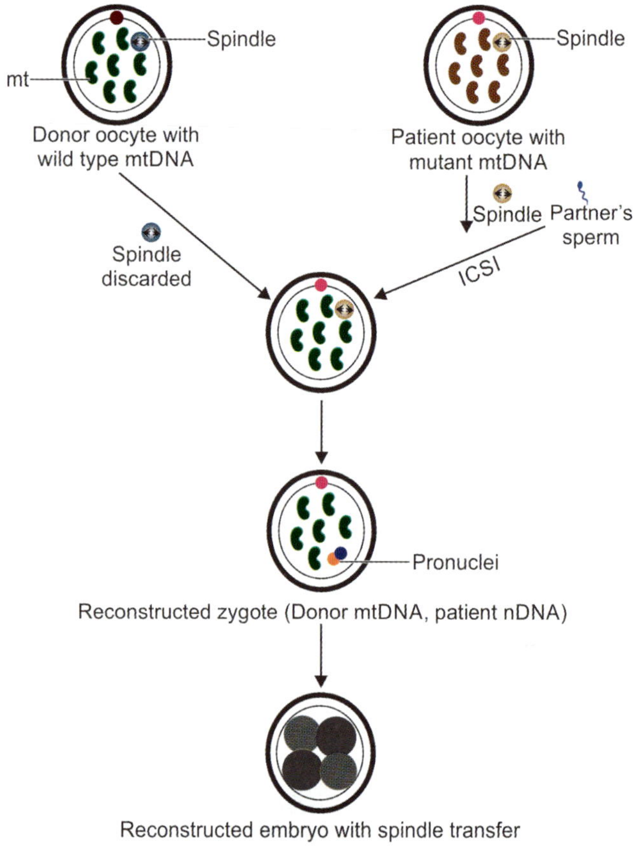

Fig. 3: Spindle transfer.

- At the same time, the intending female parent's affected oocytes are fertilized with the intending male parent sperm.
- Fertilized oocytes are allowed to develop to the pronuclear stage.
- With the help of micromanipulator, the pronucleus of zygotes resulted from donor oocytes is discarded and pronucleus from affected oocytes was extracted and carefully inserted into enucleated healthy oocyte with the help of inactivated viral vector.
- Now the zygotes contain nuclear DNA from parents and mtDNA from donor.

Advantages

- Advantage as compared to spindle transfer technique is that ICSI is not mandatory.
- By using an inverted microscope, pronucleus can be very easily visualized than spindles.

Limitations

- From an ethical point of view, main disadvantage of this technique is that half of the embryos formed with affected zygotes which will be enucleated are discarded.
- In nuclear transfer method, the use of inactivated viral vector (SeV—Sendai virus, also known as HVJ-E) by Craven and Tachibana raises a question about the future effects of it on embryonic development. However, Tachibana demonstrated that the lack of SeV genetic material in resulted embryos by reverse transcription polymerase chain reaction (RT-PCR) analysis shows that the viral vector does not have any possible harm in next generations.
- As this is a new procedure, it has been applied by Craven L and team on zygotes which are abnormally fertilized having either one or three pronuclei. In order to prove its efficacy and safety, this technique requires more assessment in an animal model, as that has been done with spindle transfer.

Spindle Transfer (Fig. 3)

It is also referred as maternal spindle transfer. This technique aims in preventing transmission of mitochondrial disease by inheritance of donor mtDNA and parental nuclear DNA in the offspring. Maternal spindle transfer is a same technique like pronuclear transfer to eliminate the inheritance of mitochondrial disease. The major difference between both the techniques is that maternal spindle transfer requires unfertilized eggs and pronuclear transfer requires early embryos at pronuclear stage.

Researchers of Oregon Science and Health University claimed in 2009 that they had successfully done maternal spindle transfer technique in rhesus macaques and they reported that the macaques' eggs were normally fertilized and had normal embryo development. Three healthy progenies were produced with the help of this technique. The presence of mtDNA from healthy donor oocytes and nuclear DNA from maternal spindle was analyzed through genetic tests.

It also proved that regular blood and body weight were comparable with experimental controls. The Newcastle group is still trying the maternal spindle transfer technique on human embryos. No results in human have been published yet.

Procedure

- Healthy oocyte from donor and oocyte of patient with faulty chromosome retrieved on same day.
- Denudation of all oocyte should be done with hyaluronidase as per ICSI protocol.
- With the help of polarized microscope and micromanipulators, spindle from the donor eggs is discarded.
- Same way, the spindle is aspirated from mother's egg and is introduced into the enucleated donor egg with the intended father's sperm by ICSI procedure.
- The chromosome-free egg, having the unhealthy mitochondria, is discarded.
- The resultant egg so formed contains healthy mitochondria from the donor and nuclear DNA from the mother.
- Hence, so formed embryo will be transferred into the intending mother's uterus.

Limitations

- It requires donor oocyte denudation as the oocyte can only be fertilized through ICSI.
- It is more costly because the spindle can only be visualized by using specialized instrument, along with an imaging system that uses polarized light birefringence.
- The chromosome-spindle complex is a delicate structure so needs to be handled with extreme care, as the DNA is not as stable as in pronucleus. Hence, it demands skilled embryologist.
- Ideally, the first polar body should be removed with the spindle from the donor oocyte as the polar body can be reabsorbed during later fusion of the karyoplast, and produce polyploidy.
- At metaphase II, chromosome scattering can happen, and this evidence of spindle alteration has been found to occur because of temperature changes and higher maternal age.
- Craven suggested that spindle transfer should be performed under highly regularized environment with negligible risk of damage, that otherwise could result in aneuploidy during manipulation of the spindle.

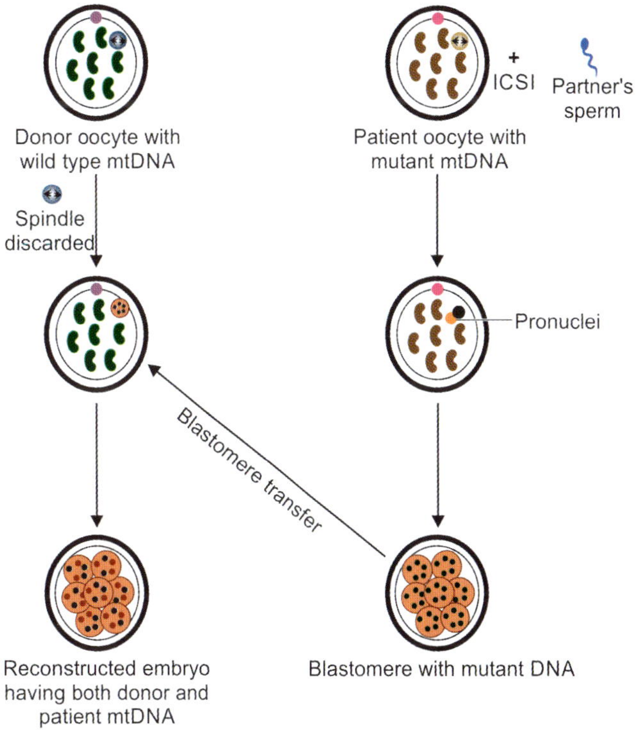

Fig. 4: Blastomere transfer.

Blastomere Transfer (Fig. 4)

This procedure has not been applied clinically and no studies have been published in humans, as it is similar to reproductive cloning and involves the same micromanipulation procedures, using postzygotic nuclear transplantation.

- Blastomere transfer involves transplantation of a blastomere from an unhealthy embryo into an enucleated healthy donor oocyte.
- However, the embryo will inherit mtDNA from the healthy donor oocyte, but it is still not clear if this technique can successfully prevent mtDNA disease in the resultant offspring.

- Apart from karyoplast which contains most of nuclear material along with very less mitochondria, an entire cell with blastomere is fused to the recipient oocyte.
- Moreover, bovine studies have discovered heteroplasmy in mtDNA in the consequent embryos.

CONCLUSION

- The role of cytoplasm in human biological process of oocyte development and activation is not clearly studied but efforts are ongoing to understand it, at both cellular as well as molecular level. Some actions like meiotic maturation, conception and genome activity in embryo relate both cytoplasmic and nuclear processes. The cytoplasmic events involve mRNA, maternal proteins, energy substrates, various energy-related components and many factors that are yet to be observed.
- Psychological counseling should be given properly about pros and cons of the specific technique, impact of techniques on fetus, etc.
- Ethical and clinical consent is mandatory for all the techniques prior treatment.
- However, with evolutions in mitochondrial transfer techniques, many ethical issues have been raised in the health sectors regarding these new treatment options.
- These techniques demand huge number of healthy oocyte donors to perform research and for its clinical application. It has been proposed that in order to manage this number, a regulation would have to be implemented that would assure the donor's well-being, through proper recruitment and deciding a limitation on the number of donations per donor, which protects them against the adverse effects of repeated ovarian hyperstimulation.
- *Germline modifications*: Germline refers to the genetic material which is inherited through generations of a family. If alteration to mtDNA is made, it will continue down the germline. Hence, children born through this technique would have a genetic linkage to three people: their parents and the donor.
- Safety-related involvements have also been raised that children born after mtDNA replacement may still show anomalies because of incompatibilities between "unmatched" nuclear and mitochondria genomes.
- Moreover, the question of compatibility between the mother's nuclear genes and donor's mitochondrial genes also arises. Though there is not much data on humans, experiments on mice have shown that such incompatibility may lead to obesity, metabolic disorders, accelerated aging and other problems.
- Carryover of abnormal mtDNA from the mother's egg during the procedure might be expected. However, evidence showed that this carryover was usually less than 2% of the total mtDNA in the final embryos.
- A person born with genetic material from three people might have a conflicted self.
- Studies must be conducted in animal models on mitochondria-nucleus connection, transmission of mtDNA to the offspring, especially with respect to the variable transmission of heteroplasmy due to the bottleneck effect symptoms of mitochondrial diseases, before we can successfully implement these techniques in routine.
- Since animal studies have limitations in predicting outcomes in humans, subsequent research in humans would be necessary.

EDITORS' COMMENTS

1. Triple parenting treatment is a modality for patient with mitochondrial disease and those who want to go for egg donation treatment.
2. The treatment should be done after proper counseling about pros and cons of the particular treatment.
3. Informed content should be mandatory for all the treatment.
4. Still, more data is required about children born through this option and the safety of this treatment is yet to be proven.
5. Triple parenting is yet legally not permitted in most of the countries around the world.

SUGGESTED READING

1. Almeida PA, Bolton VN. The effect of temperature fluctuations on the cytoskeletal organisation and chromosomal constitution of the human oocyte. Zygote. 1995;3:357-65.
2. Battaglia DE, Goodwin P, Klein NA, et al. Influence of maternal age on meiotic spindle assembly in oocytes from naturally cycling women. Hum Reprod. 1996;11:2217-22.
3. Brown DT, Herbert M, Lamb VK, et al. Transmission of mitochondrial DNA disorders: possibilities for the future. Lancet. 2006;368:87-9.
4. Calabrese V, Lodi R, Tonon C, et al. Oxidative stress, mitochondrial dysfunction and cellular stress response in Friedreich's ataxia. J Neurol Sci. 2005;233:145-62.
5. Cohen J, Scott R, Schimmel T, et al. Birth of infant after transfer of anucleate donor oocyte cytoplasm into recipient eggs. Lancet. 1997;350(9072):186-7.
6. Craven L, Elson JL, Irving L, et al. Mitochondrial DNA disease: new options for prevention. Hum Mol Genet. 2011;20:R168-74.

7. Craven L, Tuppen HA, Greggains GD, et al. Pronuclear transfer in human embryos to prevent transmission of mitochondrial DNA disease. Nature. 2010;465(7294):82-5.
8. Ferreira CR, Meirelles FV, Yamazaki W, et al. The kinetics of donor cell mtDNA in embryonic and somatic donor cell-derived bovine embryos. Cloning Stem Cells. 2007; 9:618-29.
9. Greggains GD, Lister LM, Tuppen HA, et al. Therapeutic potential of somatic cell nuclear transfer for degenerative disease caused by mitochondrial DNA mutations. Sci Rep. 2014;4:3844.
10. Harman D. Aging: a theory based on free radical and radiation chemistry. J Gerontol. 1956;11:298-300.
11. Hassold T, Chiu D. Maternal age-specific rates of numerical chromosome abnormalities with special reference to trisomy. Hum Genet. 1985;70(1):11-7.
12. Hook EB. Rates of chromosome abnormalities at different maternal ages. Obstet Gynecol. 1981;58:282-5.
13. Huang CC, Cheng TC, Chang HH, et al. Birth after the injection of sperm and the cytoplasm of tripronucleate zygotes into metaphase II oocytes in patients with repeated implantation failure after assisted fertilization procedures. Fertil Steril. 1999;72:702-6.
14. Jacobs LJ, deWert G, Geraedts JP, et al. The transmission of OXPHOS disease and methods to prevent this. Hum Reprod Update. 2006;12:119-36.
15. Kirkwood TB. A systematic look at an old problem. Nature. 2008;451:644-7.
16. Kirkwood TB. Understanding the odd science of aging. Cell. 2005;120:437-47.
17. Maritim AC, Sanders RA, Watkins JB 3rd. Diabetes, oxidative stress, and antioxidants: a review. J Biochem Mol Toxicol. 2003;17:24-38.
18. Steinborn R, Schinogl P, Zakhartchenko V, et al. Mitochondrial DNA heteroplasmy in cloned cattle produced by fetal and adult cell cloning. Nat Genet. 2000;25:255-7.
19. Tachibana M, Amato P, Sparman M, et al. Towards germline gene therapy of inherited mitochondrial diseases. Nature. 2013;493:627-31.
20. Tachibana M, Sparman M, Sritanaudomchai H, et al. Mitochondrial gene replacement in primate offspring and embryonic stem cells. Nature. 2009;461:367-72.
21. Taylor RW, Turnbull DM. Mitochondrial DNA mutations in human disease. Nat Rev Genet. 2005;6:389-402.
22. Thorburn DR, Dahl HH, Singh KK. The pros and cons of mitochondrial manipulation in the human germ line. Mitochondrion. 2001;1:123-7.
23. Turner N, Robker RL. Developmental programming of obesity and insulin resistance: does mitochondrial dysfunction in oocytes play a role? Mol Hum Reprod. 2015;21:23-30.
24. Wang Q, Ratchford AM, Chi MM, et al. Maternal diabetes causes mitochondrial dysfunction and meiotic defects in murine oocytes. Mol Endocrinol. 2009;23:1603-12.

Index

Page numbers followed by *b* refer to box, *f* refer to figure, *fc* refer to flowchart, and *t* refer to table.

F

G

H

Q

R

W

X

Y

Z